Cell therapy is a rapidly developing area, drawing on cell biology, molecular biology, virology, immunology, cell quantitation techniques, and biomedical engineering. It has potential in many clinical settings, in the treatment of cancer and other diseases.

This volume in the series *Cancer: Clinical Science in Practice* examines the current state and future prospects of cell therapy, which seems likely to have a profound impact on health care, as profound as the production of proteins by recombinant DNA technology. The coverage is broad, including the scientific principles of hemopoietic cell therapy, the technology of cell collection and preparation, current and likely future clinical applications of cell therapy, and the principles and practice of cellular immunotherapy.

Up-to-date and authoritative, volumes in this series are intended for a wide audience of clinicians and researchers with an interest in the applications of biomedical science to the understanding and management of cancer.

CELL THERAPY

■ CANCER: CLINICAL SCIENCE IN PRACTICE

General Editor

Professor Karol Sikora

Department of Clinical Oncology
Royal Postgraduate Medical School
Hammersmith Hospital, London

A series of authoritative review volumes intended for a wide audience of clinicians and researchers with an interest in the application of biomedical science to the understanding and management of cancer.

Also in this series
Molecular Endocrinology of Cancer
Edited by Jonathan Waxman

Tumor Immunology: Immunotherapy and cancer vaccines
Edited by A. G. Dalgleish and M. J. Browning

■ CELL THERAPY

Stem Cell Transplantation, Gene Therapy, and Cellular Immunotherapy

Edited by

George Morstyn

Amgen Inc
Thousand Oaks, California
and University of California,
Los Angeles School of Medicine
Los Angeles, California

William Sheridan

Amgen Inc
Thousand Oaks, California
and University of California,
Los Angeles School of Medicine
Los Angeles, California

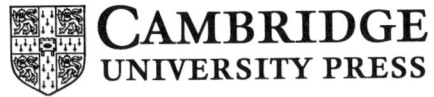

CAMBRIDGE
UNIVERSITY PRESS

PUBLISHED BY THE PRESS SYNDICATE OF THE UNIVERSITY OF CAMBRIDGE
The Pitt Building, Trumpington Street, Cambridge CB2 1RP, United Kingdom

CAMBRIDGE UNIVERSITY PRESS
The Edinburgh Building, Cambridge CB2 2RU, United Kingdom
40 West 20th Street, New York, NY 10011-4211, USA
10 Stamford Road, Oakleigh, Melbourne 3166, Australia

First published 1996
Reprinted 1996

Printed in the United States of America

Typeset in Stone Serif

A catalogue record for this book is available from the British Library

Library of Congess Cataloguing-in-Publication Data is available

ISBN 0-521-47315-2 hardback

Series Editor's Preface

The last decade has produced remarkable advances in our ability to dissect the various cell lineages that comprise one of the most fascinating human differentiation systems – the human bone marrow. Ultimately the transcriptional switches involved in controlling the expression of blocks of genes, that in turn encode for signals to replicate, differentiate and die will be identified. But already our knowledge can be applied successfully in the clinic.

The most obvious immediate potential benefit is our ability to escalate the dose of cancer chemotherapy. This would seem most likely to be of benefit in patients whose tumors are currently only partially responsive. The technology involved is developing rapidly and here the selection of stem cells, their characterization and expansion *in vitro* are vital processes. Ultimately high quality clinical trials are needed to ascertain the true role of such approaches in comparison to the best available conventional treatment.

Perhaps the most exciting potential of cell therapy is our ability to manipulate DNA so purposefully modifying the physiological properties of the cells to be returned to a patient. Gene therapy is one of the most rapidly advancing areas of medicine and of course the bone marrow is one of the most accessible and malleable organs in terms of genetic intervention.

The organization, regulation, and practicalities of cell therapy clearly pose major questions. These issues must be addressed whatever direction our healthcare system takes. This contribution provides a useful source book as well as a landmark at an extremely exciting time in the development of the whole field.

Karol Sikora

Preface

The biotechnology revolution started in the late 1970s following technological advances that allowed the production of large quantities of proteins by recombinant DNA technology. The 1990s are witnessing the beginning of another technological revolution due to our ability to produce large numbers of human cells outside the body and our ability to insert genes into these cells. Fundamental to this has been the discovery and industrial-scale production of cytokines controlling hemopoietic and lymphoid cell proliferation and development of increasingly sophisticated techniques for manipulation of DNA in mammalian cells.

The development of cellular therapy requires the coming together of cell biology, molecular biology, virology, cell quantitation techniques, and biomedical engineering. This book brings together reviews on applications of these research disciplines to cellular therapy in the hemopoietic and immune systems. We have organized the book into major sections covering basic biology, hemopoietic cell therapy, and cellular immunotherapy. Leaders in the field have covered the scientific principles, technology, clinical approaches, and future directions. We have not attempted to remove areas of overlap between chapters, so that a variety of perspectives could be presented on the different approaches to the many clinical and laboratory problems. We hope the book provides a snapshot of this evolving new area.

Cell therapy is a rapidly developing area with potential use in many clinical settings, such as cancer therapy and the correction of inborn errors of metabolism. Cell therapy includes the use of peripheral blood stem cells to support multiple cycles of intensive chemotherapy, gene therapy through the transfer of transfected cells, and T-cell vaccines.

The use of peripheral blood progenitor cells was begun in the early 1960s when Goodman and Hodgson published results of a study showing that hemopoiesis could be restored to mice receiving supralethal radiation if they were treated with infusions of allogeneic peripheral leukocytes (Goodman and Hodgson 1962). Northdurft et al. (1977) refined this work and showed that lethally irradiated dogs could be saved with cryopreserved peripheral blood mononuclear cells collected by apheresis and cryopreserved.

Cancer immunotherapy has a long history with many attempts at enhancing the immunologic response against established tumors. In the mid-1890s, Hericourt and Richert treated patients with an antitumor serum produced in dogs and donkeys (Currie 1972). Although cures were not obtained, there were some tumor regressions and benefits. Interest in immunotherapy has reawakened with the discovery of the interleukins and inflammatory cytokines and the increasing knowledge of the roles of lymphoid cell subsets. Understanding the mechanisms involved in the most successful form of anticancer cellular adoptive immunotherapy, the allogeneic graft-versus-leukemia effect, could prove important to new applications.

Gene therapy, another aspect of cell therapy, has the potential for treating inherited and acquired diseases by replacing genes within a patient's somatic cells. More than 4,000 genetic diseases have been identified, making gene therapy an extremely fertile area of research. Acquired immunodeficiency syndrome (AIDS) is caused by the retrovirus HIV-1, a virus able to transcribe its RNA to DNA and insert it into the DNA of a host cell, making AIDS an acquired genetic disease. Work is in the early stages, but results suggest an enormous potential for gene therapy in AIDS.

When it is clear what clinical benefits will flow from a particular form of cell therapy, we will need to decide whether the cells are produced in hospitals or blood banks of whether dedicated cell-therapy centers, much like cell factories, will be required. This type of decision will be made based on the complexity of the cellular manipulations and cultures, reimbursement issues, and the regulatory requirements, particularly if the product is considered to be the cells.

There are major scientific, clinical, and regulatory hurdles that still need to be overcome to bring the full potential clinical benefits of cell therapy to patients. Nevertheless, it seems clear that the problems can be solved and perhaps cellular therapy will have an even more profound impact on health care than did the production of proteins by recombinant DNA technology. The mid-1990s should be a very exciting period in the development of this field.

We would like to acknowledge those who assisted in the preparation of the book: Lawrence Transue, technical typist; and Jennifer Keysor and Danette Barron, graphic artists. This book was turned into reality by MaryAnn Foote, Ph.D. Without her sustained enthusiasm and persistence it would not have been possible.

George Morstyn, M.D., Ph.D.
William Sheridan, M.D.

REFERENCES

Currie, G.A. (1972) Eighty years of immunotherapy: a review of immunological methods used for treatment of human cancer. *British Journal of Cancer*, **26**, 141–53.

Goodman, J.W., and Hodgson, G.S. (1962) Evidence for stem cells in the peripheral blood of mice. *Blood*, **19**, 702–14.

Northdurft, W., Bruch, C., Fliedner, T.M., and Ruber, E. (1977) Studies on the regeneration of the CFU-C population in blood and bone marrow of lethally irradiated dogs after autologous transfusion of cryopreserved mononuclear blood cells. *Scandinavian Journal of Haematology*, **19**, 470–81.

Contents

Contributors

Aliza Ackerstein, R.N.
*Department of Bone Marrow Transplantation
Hadassah University Hospital
Jerusalem, Israel*

Joseph H. Antin, M.D.
*Hematology-Oncology Division
Brigham and Women's Hospital
Boston, Massachusetts*

Frederick R. Appelbaum, M.D.
*Professor of Medicine
Fred Hutchinson Cancer Research Center
University of Washington
Seattle, Washington*

James O. Armitage, M.D.
*Professor and Chair
Department of Internal Medicine
University of Nebraska Medical Center
Omaha, Nebraska*

Karen Auditore-Hargreaves, Ph.D.
*CellPro, Inc
Bothell, Washington*

Russell Basser, F.R.C.P.
*Ludwig Cancer Institute
The Royal Melbourne Hospital
Victoria, Australia*

Scott I. Bearman, M.D.
*University of Colorado Health Sciences Center
Denver, Colorado*

C. Glenn Begley, M.D., Ph.D.
*The Walter and Eliza Hall Institute of Medical Research
The Royal Melbourne Hospital
Victoria, Australia*

Ronald Berenson, M.D.
Mercer Island, Washington

Philip J. Bierman, M.D.
University of Nebraska Medical
  Center
Omaha, Nebraska

Michael Bishop, M.D.
University of Nebraska Medical
  Center
Omaha, Nebraska

David Bodine, Ph.D.
Laboratory of Gene Transfer
National Institutes of Health
Bethesda, Maryland

Wolfram Brugger, M.D.
Department of Medicine II
Eberhard-Karls-Universitat
  Tübingen
Tübingen, Germany

Randal A. Byrn, Ph.D.
Harvard Medical School
Boston, Massachusetts

Pablo T. Cagnoni, M.D.
University of Colorado Health
  Sciences Center
Denver, Colorado

Michael A. Caligiuri, M.D.
Departments of Hematologic
  Oncology and Bone Marrow
  Transplantation
Roswell Park Cancer Institute
Buffalo, New York

William E. Carson, M.D.
Department of Surgery
Roswell Park Cancer Institute
Buffalo, New York

Benjamin P. Chen, Ph.D.
Systemix, Inc
Palo Alto, California

John P.A. Crown, M.D.
St. Vincent's Hospital
Elm Park, Ireland

David C. Dale, M.D.
Professor of Medicine
Department of Medicine
University of Washington
Seattle, Washington

Cynthia E. Dunbar, M.D.
Hematology Branch
National Institutes of Health
Bethesda, Maryland

Pamela G. Dyson, B.Sc.
Hanson Center for Cancer Research
Adelaide, Australia

David Fennelly, M.D.
Memorial Sloan-Kettering Cancer
  Center
New York, New York

Richard Fox, F.R.A.C.P.
Professor of Medicine
Department of Clinical
  Haematology and Medical
  Oncology
The Royal Melbourne Hospital
Victoria, Australia

Judith C. Gasson, Ph.D.
Professor of Medicine and
  Biological Chemistry
University of California, Los
  Angeles School of Medicine
Los Angeles, California

Ursula Gehling, M.D.
University of Colorado Health
  Sciences Center
Denver, Colorado

John Goldman, M.D.
Department of Haematology
Royal Postgraduate Medical School
London, UK

John Gribben, M.D., Ph.D.
Harvard Medical School
Dana-Farber Cancer Institute
Boston, Massachusetts

David Haylock, B.App.Sc.
Hanson Center for Cancer Research
Adelaide, Australia

Shelly Heimfeld, Ph.D.
CellPro, Inc
Bothell, Washington

Ronald Hoffman, M.D.
University of Illinois
College of Medicine
Chicago, Illinois

Christopher J. Hogan, Ph.D.
University of Colorado Health
  Sciences Center
Denver, Colorado

Roy B. Jones, M.D.
University of Colorado Health
  Sciences Center
Denver, Colorado

Christopher Juttner, M.D.
Systemix, Inc.
Palo Alto, California

Lother Kanz, M.D.
Professor of Medicine
Department of Hematology/
  Oncology/Immunology
Universitätsklinik
Tübingen, Germany

Stefan Karlsson, M.D., Ph.D.
National Institutes of Health
Bethesda, Maryland

William Kidwell, Ph.D.
Cellco, Inc
Germantown, Maryland

Monica Krieger, Ph.D.
CellPro, Inc
Bothell, Washington

W. Conrad Liles, M.D., Ph.D.
University of Washington School of
  Medicine
Seattle, Washington

Michael Lill, M.D.
Department of Medicine
University of California, Los
  Angeles School of Medicine
Los Angeles, California

Kirsten Maakestad, B.S.
University of Washington
School of Medicine
Seattle, Washington

Vera Malkovska, M.D.
The Washington Cancer Institute
  at Washington Hospital Center
Washington, D.C.

Rosemary Mazanet, M.D., Ph.D.

*Amgen Inc
Thousand Oaks, California
and University of California,
Los Angeles School of Medicine
Los Angeles, California*

Jeffrey A. Medin, M.D.

*National Institutes of Health
Bethesda, Maryland*

Makoto Migita, M.D.

*National Institutes of Health
Bethesda, Maryland*

Stefan Miltenyi

*Miltenyi Biotec
Bergisch Giadbach, Germany*

Lori Minasian, M.D.

*Department of Medicine
Medical College of Georgia
Augusta, Georgia*

Malcolm A. Moore, Ph.D.

*James Ewing Laboratory of
    Developmental Hematopoiesis
Memorial Sloan-Kettering Cancer
    Center
New York, New York*

Shoshana Morecki, Ph.D.

*Department of Bone Marrow
    Transplantation
Hadassah University Hospital
Jerusalem, Israel*

George Morstyn, F.R.C.P., Ph.D.

*Amgen Inc
Thousand Oaks, California
and University of California,
Los Angeles School of Medicine
Los Angeles, California*

Lee M. Nadler, M.D.

*Professor of Medicine
Harvard Medical School
Boston, Massachusetts*

Arnon Nagler, M.D.

*Department of Bone Marrow
    Transplantation
Hadassah University Hospital
Jerusalem, Israel*

Elizabeth Naparstek, M.D.

*Department of Bone Marrow
    Transplantation
Hadassah University Hospital
Jerusalem, Israel*

Larry Norton, M.D.

*Professor of Medicine
Cornell University Medical College
    and Memorial Sloan-Kettering
    Cancer Center
New York, New York*

Reuven Or, M.D.

*Department of Bone Marrow
    Transplantation
Hadassah University Hospital
Jerusalem, Israel*

Susanne Osanto, M.D., Ph.D.

*Department of Clinical Oncology
University Hospital Leiden
Leiden, The Netherlands*

David Porter, M.D.
Division of Hematology-Oncology
University of Pennsylvania Medical
  Center
Philadelphia, Pennsylvania

George Raptis, M.D.
Memorial Sloan-Kettering Cancer
  Center
New York, New York

Diether Recktenwald, Ph.D.
AmCell Corporation
Sunnyvale, California

Margo R. Roberts, Ph.D.
Cell GeneSys
Foster City, California

Dennis Sasaki, M.A.
Systemix, Inc
Palo Alto, Calfornia

Peter Schrier, Ph.D.
Department of Clinical Oncology
University Hospital
Leiden, The Netherlands

William Sheridan, M.D.
Amgen Inc
Thousand Oaks, California
and University of California, Los
  Angeles School of Medicine
Los Angeles, California

Elizabeth J. Shpall, M.D.
University of Colorado Health
  Sciences Center
Denver, Colorado

Paul Simmons, Ph.D.
Hanson Center for Cancer Research
Adelaide, Australia

Shimon Slavin, M.D.
Professor of Medicine
Department of Bone Marrow
  Transplantation
Hadassah University Hospital
Jerusalem, Israel

Paul Sondel, Ph.D.
Professor of Pediatrics, Human
  Oncology, and Genetics
Comprehensive Cancer Center
University of Wisconsin, Madison
Madison, Wisconsin

Marion Subklewe, M.D.
Department of Hematology/
  Oncology/Immunology
Universitatsklinik
Tubingen, Germany

Luen Bik To, M.D.
Hanson Center for Cancer Research
Adelaide, Australia

Ann Tsukamoto, Ph.D.
Systemix, Inc
Palo Alto, California

Frits van Rhee, M.R.C.P.
Department of Haematology
Royal Postgraduate Medical School
London, UK

**Edmund K. Waller, M.D.,
  Ph.D.**
Department of Medicine
Emory School of Medicine
Atlanta, Georgia

Glossary of Terms

aa	amino acid
AAV	adeno-associated virus
Ab	antibody
ABMT	autologous bone-marrow transplant
AD	advanced disease
ADA	adenosine deaminase
ADCC	antibody-dependent cellular cytotoxicity
Ag	antigen
AIDS	acquired immunodeficiency syndrome
A-LAK	adherent lymphokine-activated cells
ALL	acute lymphocytic leukemia
allo-CCI	allogeneic cell-mediated cytokine-activated immunotherapy
allo-CMI	allogeneic cell-mediated immunotherapy
AML	acute myeloid (acute nonlymphocytic) leukemia
ANC	absolute neutrophil count
AP	accelerated phase
APC	antigen-presenting cell
ASA	arylsulphatase A
ASCT	autologous skin cell transplant
ASM	acid sphingomyelinase
ATC	doxorubicin, paclitaxel, and cyclophosphamide
AZT	zidovudine (azidothymidine)
baso-CFC	basophil colony-forming cell

BACOP	bleomycin, Adriamycin, cyclophospha-mide, vincristine, and prednisone
BC	blast crisis
BCG	bacille Calmette-Guérin
BCNU	carmustine
BCS	bovine calf serum
BCT	blood cell transplantation
BFU-E	blastoforming unit–erythroid
Bl-CFC	blast colony-forming cell
BLPD	B-cell lymphoproliferative disease
BM	bone marrow
BMT	bone-marrow transplantation
BU/CY	busulfan and cyclophosphamide
BU/THIO/CY	busulfan, thiotepa, and cyclophosphamide
CAF	cyclophosphamide, doxorubicin, and fluorouracil
CAFC	cobblestone area–forming cell
CALGB	cancer and leukemia group B
CB	cord blood
CDE	cyclophosphamide, doxorubicin, and etoposide
CFC	colony-forming cell
CGD	chronic granulomatous disease
CHOP	cyclophosphamide, doxorubicin, vincristine, and prednisone
CI	continuous infusion
CLL	chronic lymphocytic leukemia
CMI	cell-mediated immunity
CML	chronic myeloid leukemia
CMV	cytomegalovirus
CMV chemo	cisplatin, methotrexate, and vinblastine
CNS	central nervous system
CODE	cisplatin, vincristine, doxorubicin, and etoposide
COP-BLAM	cyclophosphamide, vincristine, prednisone, bleomycin, doxorubicin, and procarbazine
CP	chronic phase
CPB	cyclophosphamide, cisplatin, and carmustine
CR	complete remission/response
CSF	colony-stimulating factor

CTL	cytotoxic T lymphocyte
dGTP	deoxyguanosine triphosphate
DHAP	dexamethasone, cytarabine, and cisplatin
DHFR	dihydrofolate reductase
DICEP	dose-intensive cyclophosphamide, etoposide, and cisplatin
DMEM	Dulbecco's modified eagles medium
DMSO	dimethyl sulfoxide
DTH	delayed-type hypersensitivity
E. coli	*Escherichia coli*
E-BFC	erythroid burst-forming cell
EBV	Epstein-Barr virus
E-CFC	erythroid colony-forming cell
EDTA	ethylenediamine tetraacetic acid
Eo	eosinophil(s)
Eo-CFC	eosinophil colony-forming cell
Eo-CSF	eosinophil colony-stimulating factor, IL-5
EPO	erythropoietin
FA	Fanconi's anemia
FACS	fluorescence-activated cell sorting
FAGC	Fanconi's anemia group C gene
FDA	U.S. Food and Drug Administration
FITC	fluorescein
FL	*flt2/flk3* ligand
4-HPC	4-hydroperoxycyclophosphamide
5-FU	5-fluorouracil
GALV	gibbon ape leukemia virus
G-CSF	granulocyte colony-stimulating factor
GC	glucocerebroside
GD	Gaucher's disease
GEMM-CFC	granulocyte-erythroid-macrophage-monocyte colony-forming cells
GM-CFC	granulocyte-macrophage colony-forming cell
GM-CSF	granulocyte-macrophage colony-stimulating factor
GVHD	graft-versus-host disease
GVL	graft-versus-leukemia
Gy	Gray
HAMA	human anti–mouse antibody
HBV	hepatitis B virus
HC	histocompatibility complex
HCm	histocompatibility molecule

HD	Hodgkin's disease
HDCE	high-dose cyclophosphamide and etoposide
HDS	high-dose sequential (chemotherapy)
HDT	high-dose therapy
HES	hydroxyethyl starch
HGF	hemopoietic growth factor
HIV	human immunodeficiency virus
HLA	human leukocyte antigen
HPLC	high-performance liquid chromatography
HPPC	high-proliferative-potential cells
HPP-CFC	high-proliferative-potential colony-forming cell
HPV	human papilloma virus
HSA	heat-stable antigen
HSC	hemopoietic stem cell
HSCS	high-speed cell sorter
Hu	human
ICE	ifosfamide, cyclophosphamide, and etoposide
IFN	interferon
IL	interleukin
IM	intramuscular, intramuscularly
IMDM	Iscove's modification of Dulbecco's medium
IP	intraperitoneal/intraperitoneally
ITR	inverted terminal repeat
IU	international unit
IV	intravenous, intravenously
kb	kilobase
KS	Kaposi's sarcoma
LAD	leukocyte adhesion deficiency
LAK cell	lymphocyte-activated killer cell
LANAK	lymphokine-activated natural killer cells
LDH	lactic dehydrogenase
LGL	large granular lymphocytes
LIF	leukemia-inhibiting factor
LMI	lymphokine-mediated immunotherapy
LPS	lipopolysaccharide
LTBMC	long-term bone-marrow culture
LTC-IC	long-term culture-initiating cell
LTR	long terminal repeat
MAA	melanoma-associated antigen

mAB	monoclonal antibody
MACOP-B	methotrexate, doxorubicin, cyclophosphamide, vincristine, prednisone, bleomycin, and cotrimoxazole
MBP	methotrexate, bleomycin, and predisone
M-CFC	macrophage/monocyte colony-forming cell
MDS	myelodysplastic syndromes
Mast-CFC	mast-cell colony-forming cell
mCi	millicurie
M-CSF	macrophage colony-stimulating factor
MDR	multidrug resistance
MGDF	megakaryocyte growth and differentiation factor (c-*mpl* ligand)
MIX-CFC	mixed colony-forming cell
MK	megakaryocyte
MK-BFC	megakaryocyte blast-forming cell
MK-CFC	megakaryocyte colony-forming cell
MLD	metachromatic leukodystrophy
MM	multiple myeloma
MNC	mononuclear cell
MoMuLV	Moloney murine leukemia virus
MRD	minimal residual disease
MRP	multidrug resistance–associated protein
MSC	mouse stem cell
MTD	maximum tolerated dose
Multi-CSF	multi–colony-stimulating factor, IL-3
MVAC	methotrexate, vinblastine, doxorubicin, and cisplatin
NCI	National Cancer Institute
NHL	non-Hodgkin's lymphoma
NIH	National Institutes of Health
NK cell	natural killer cell
NR	not reported
PB	peripheral blood
PBL	peripheral blood lymphocyte
PBMC	peripheral blood mononuclear cell
PBPC	peripheral blood progenitor cell
PBSC	peripheral blood stem cell
PCR	polymerase chain reaction
PE	phycoerythrin
PGK	phosphoglycerate kinase
PHA	phytohemaglutinin antigen

Ph chromosome	Philadelphia chromosome
PIV	peripheral intravenous
PMA	phorbol myrisate acetate
PMN	polymorphonuclear neutrophil
PMVEC	porcine brain microvascular endothelial cells
PNP	purine nucleoside phosphorylase
PO	orally
PR	partial remission/response
PSCT	peripheral stem-cell transplant
PTFE	polytetrafluoroethylene
q	every
r	recombinant
RAC	U.S. Recombinant DNA Advisory Committee
RBC	red blood cell
RCCA	renal cell carcinoma
RFLP	restriction fragment length polymorphism (patterns)
rHu	recombinant human
RRE	rev-responsive element
RT-PCR	reverse transcriptase polymerase chain reaction
SA	splice acceptor
SAB	single-chain antibody
S-CFC	spleen colony-forming cell
SC	subcutaneous, subcutaneously
SCCHN	squamous cell carcinoma of head and neck
SCF	stem-cell factor
SCID	severe combined immunodeficiency (syndrome)
SCLC	small-cell lung cancer
SD	splice donor
SLE	systemic lupus erythematosus
SWOG	Southwest Oncology Group
TAA	tumor-associated antigen
TAR	*trans*-activating region
TATA	tumor-associated transplantation antigen
TBI	total-body irradiation
TIL	tumor-infiltrating lymphocyte
TNF	tumor necrosis factor

UR	universal receptors
UV	ultraviolet
VAPEC-B	vincristine, Adriamycin, prednisolone, etoposide, cyclophosphamide, and bleomycin
VATH	vinblastine, doxorubicin, thiotepa, and fluoxymesterone
VIC-E	VP16, ifosfamide, carboplatin, and epirubicin
VIP	etoposide
WBC	white blood cell
WCC	white cell count

Note of Terminology of Progenitor Cells: We have adopted a standard terminology for hemopoietic progenitor cells of the following style: granulocyte-macrophage colony-forming cell = GM-CFC (= CFU-GM or colony-forming unit, granulocyte-macrophage).

Aspects of Hemopoiesis and the Immune System Important for Cell Therapy

Overview of Hemopoiesis and Hemopoietic Reconstruction

MALCOLM A. S. MOORE

The hemopoietic system generates every day approximately 200×10^9 red blood cells (RBC) with a mean life span of 120 days, 125×10^9 platelets with a life span of 8 days, and 50×10^9 white blood cells (WBC) with life spans of 6 to 8 hours for neutrophils, or months or years for certain lymphocyte subpopulations. This steady-state production is sustained by a marrow population of 5 to 10×10^{11} cells containing approximately 1% progenitor cells and approximately 0.01% candidate stem cells. Selective increases in cell production of five- to tenfold can readily be obtained, for example, in RBC, when excessive red cell loss or destruction is occurring (as in sickle cell anemia), or in granulocytes as a response to infectious episodes. This can be achieved by the entry of quiescent cells into cycling, by increasing the number of amplification divisions during neutrophil development, and by reducing cell population doubling times and/or prolongation of the life span of mature cells. Granulocyte colony-stimulating factor (G-CSF) increases circulating neutrophils by the former mechanisms (Lord et al. 1989), while granulocyte-macrophage colony stimulating factor (GM-CSF) produces an increase by shortening the cell-cycle time of progenitors (Aglietta et al. 1989) and prolonging the neutrophil life span (Colotta et al. 1992). The regenerative capacity of the system is likewise remarkable, as seen most dramatically by the relatively rapid recovery of normal mature blood cell production following allogeneic or autologous transplantation of the equivalent of only about 1% of the total marrow (1 to 5×10^{10} cells) into myeloablated individuals.

Our understanding of the physiology of progenitor cells has been obtained over the last 27 years by analysis of in vitro clonogenic assay systems supported by an ever-increasing family of hemopoietic growth factors. Lineage-restricted progenitors for all differentiation pathways can be identified, as can oligopotential and multipotential progenitors. The absence of self-renewal capacity serves to distinguish progenitors from true stem cells that possess extensive self-renewal as well as multilineage differentiation potential. Conventional models show hemopoiesis as a series of sequential compartments of cells, beginning with a "black box" containing the stem cell. Actually, the system is a continuum of cell types with a progressive restriction in differentiation and proliferation potential, but with a strong stochastic component at the single-cell level (Ogawa 1993) (Fig. 1.1). The action of hemopoietic growth factors should be considered as permissive, facilitating the expression of a differentiation program rather than instructive, imparting commitment to an otherwise uncommitted cell. The concept of self-renewal of stem cells must also be questioned, since hemopoietic stem cells, like all somatic cells, have a finite doubling potential before exhibiting "decline" or proliferative senescence; for example, in serial bone-marrow transplantation (BMT) studies (Mauch and Hellman 1989). The mechanism of this decline has been attributed to progressive loss of chromosomal telomere base pairs with cell division (Vaziri et al. 1993, 1994). Thus, the progeny of each stem-cell division differs from the parent by a small but measurable and irreversible loss in proliferative potential. This difference

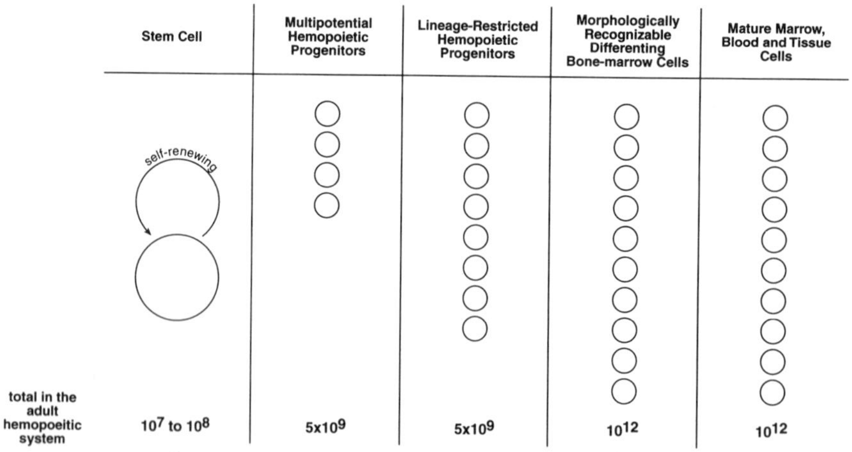

Stem Cell	Multipotential Hemopoietic Progenitors	Lineage-Restricted Hemopoietic Progenitors	Morphologically Recognizable Differenting Bone-marrow Cells	Mature Marrow, Blood and Tissue Cells
self-renewing	○○○○	○○○○○○○	○○○○○○○○○○	○○○○○○○○○○

total in the adult hemopoeitic system	10^7 to 10^8	5×10^9	5×10^9	10^{12}	10^{12}

Figure 1.1 The clonal hierarchy of hemopoietic populations. Multipotential stem cells generate committed progenitor cells. The progenitor cells generate morphologically identifiable cells that form the mature cells of the peripheral circulatory system.

can be revealed in long-term, competitive repopulation assays in mice (Harrison et al. 1993), where proliferative differences in stem-cell populations can be attributed to age differences or hemopoietic insults such as chemotherapy or radiation that deplete the stem-cell pool (Moore 1992).

Measurement of the quantity and quality of stem cells in humans is currently achieved by a number of surrogate in vitro assays that, in animal models, have been shown to correlate with long-term repopulating cells. The long-term culture-initiating cell (LTC-IC) assay measures the numbers of secondary granulocyte-macrophage colony-forming cells (GM-CFC) generated after 5 to 8 weeks of co-culture of hemopoietic cell populations with BM stroma (Sutherland et al. 1990) or stromal cell lines (Goldstein et al. 1993). A variation of this assay is the cobblestone area–forming cell (CAFC) assay with stromal co-culture and scoring of foci of hemopoietic cells that appear darker under phase-control microscopy with a characteristic cobblestone arrangement developing at 5 to 8 weeks (Breems et al. 1994). A stromal cell–independent assay is provided by the delta assay. This involves serial suspension cultures with secondary recloning for up to 5 weeks, initiated with populations enriched for stem cells such as CD34$^+$ cells or subsets, or 4-hydroperoxycyclophosphamide (4-HC)– or 5-fluorouracil (5-FU)–treated cells, in the presence of a combination of hemopoietic growth factors (Moore 1991; Muench, Firpo, and Moore 1993; Shapiro et al. 1994). Cumulative expansion of progenitors and total cells provides an index of the proliferative potential of the input population; however, with adult cell populations, the delta assay underestimates the stem cell population, since many of the cells are quiescent and not readily activated into cell cycle with currently available cytokine combinations (Lansdorp and Dragowska 1993). Xenograft assays have been developed to provide a measure of long-term repopulating capacity (and secondary transfer potential) of human hemopoietic cells engrafted in severe combined immunodeficiency (SCID) mice with human cytokine support (Lapidot et al. 1992) or within human fetal bone grafts (Kyoizumi et al. 1992) or following injection into fetal sheep (Srour et al. 1993). While cumbersome and, at best, semiquantitative, in vivo assays provide confirmation of the stem-cell quality of cell populations defined by certain phenotypic characteristics.

Both stem cells and committed progenitors express the CD34 antigen, but the former lack or have very low levels of antigens associated with lineage-specific differentiation and expressed on progenitors (Watt and Visser 1992). CD34$^+$ cell populations lacking CD38 or expressing low levels of CD45RA and CD71 contain the stem cells (and other cells including certain stromal precursors) (Lansdorp and

Dragowska 1993; Lansdorp, Dragowska, and Mayani 1993). HLA-DR is absent or expressed at low levels on adult stem cells (Moore et al. 1980), but is variably present on fetal and neonatal stem cells (Apperley 1994). The Thy-1 antigen, as in the mouse, is present on all stem cells, but is also expressed on a proportion of adult committed progenitors (Craig et al. 1993). The tyrosine kinase receptors c-kit and flk-2 are expressed on both stem cells and progenitors, but some c-kit–positive cells with stem-cell function can be flk-2–negative (Zeigler et al. 1994). Stem cells can be selected by their ability to exclude the mitochondrial-binding dye rhodamine[123]. This exclusion is due to the activity of the multidrug resistance gene (MDR1), whose p-glycoprotein is strongly expressed in stem cells (Chaudhary and Roninson 1991).

In adult marrow, 1% to 2% of nucleated cells are CD34+, and of these, approximately 1% lack CD38. By functional assay, about 0.5% of CD34+ cells are LTC-IC (Sutherland et al. 1990; Goldstein et al. 1993), and based on an adult marrow cellularity of 10^{12} cells, the steady-state stem cell pool at maximum is in the range of 5 to 10 × 10^7 cells. Transplantation of mice with highly purified stem cells has shown that as few as 10 to 30 cells will provide long-term hematopoietic reconstitution and, if only 10% to 20% seed to the marrow or spleen, extremely few clones are needed to repopulate the animals for their life span. This observation has been proven by studies with genetically and/or retrovirally marked stem-cell transplants (Van Zant, Chen, and Scot-Micus 1991). By extrapolation based upon the relative size of the hemopoietic systems, 3.5 to 10 × 10^3 stem cells would be required for successful long-term engraftment in humans. In practice, successful long-term allotransplantation is undertaken with 1 to 3 × 10^{10} nucleated marrow cells or 1% to 3% of the total marrow population, containing 5 to 10 × 10^5 LTC-IC.

Peripheral blood (PB) hemopoietic transplantation has certain advantages over bone-marrow transplantation (BMT). The donor harvest is performed without a need for general anesthesia and avoids the usually minor, but not negligible, morbidity associated with bone-marrow (BM) stem-cell harvests. In donors with extensive marrow metastasis of tumor cells, PB transplants would reintroduce fewer malignant cells. More rapid platelet and neutrophil recovery (5 to 8 days faster) is seen with PB, when compared with BMT (Sheridan et al. 1992; Kritz et al. 1993; Shpall et al. 1994). This can be explained only partially by higher numbers of progenitors in the former source when harvesting is optimized by either hemopoietic growth factors alone or cytotoxic chemotherapy combined with hemopoietic growth factors. Circulating progenitors may be primed and may initiate proliferation more rapidly upon transplantation than their BM counterparts; however, their proliferative status in the circulation is, paradoxically, much lower than BM, with only 1% to 8% of PB CD34$^+$ cells in DNA synthesis, in contrast to 20% to 35% in BM (Flasshove et al. 1995). Current debate centers on the issue of whether PB can be qualitatively as well as quantitatively equivalent or superior to BM, particularly in terms of stem-cell content. Steady-state PB contains 100 to 200 progenitor cells/mL and approximately 3 LTC-IC/mL (Pettengell et al. 1993a, b), and successful allogeneic transplantation has been reported using pooled cells from nine leukaphereses (Russell and Hunter 1994). With this number of harvests, it is possible to collect 2.5 to 5 $\times$ 10^5 LTC-IC and 1 to 3 $\times$ 10^6 progenitors, sufficient to fulfill transplant requirements for both short-term and long-term reconstitution. Reduction in apheresis requirements for PB harvests is achieved by using various elicitation procedures that mobilize CD34$^+$ cells and progenitors from the marrow into the circulation (see Chapters 8 and 9). Increase in the numbers of circulating progenitors of up to many hundredfold can occur in the recovery phase after a chemotherapy-induced nadir (Juttner et al. 1989), and synergistic increases are seen when rHuG-CSF or rHuGM-CSF are also administered (Siena et al. 1989; Sheridan et al. 1992; To et al. 1994). Maximum progenitor harvests are obtained when the WBC counts recover to approximately 4,000/μL following cyclophosphamide, etoposide, or 5-FU. Either rHuG-CSF or rHuGM-CSF alone are also effective in increasing circulating progenitor numbers in the absence of chemotherapy rebound, when administered daily for 5 to 10 days (Sheridan et al. 1992; Chatta et al. 1994; Schneider et al. 1994; To et al. 1994). In primate studies, the combination of rHuG-CSF and the c-kit ligand/stem cell factor synergistically increased circulating progenitors, and megakaryocyte progenitors were particularly elevated (Andrews et al. 1994). In primate studies, the administration of a single dose of recombinant human interleukin (rHuIL)-1β (1 μg/kg) produced an approximate 30-fold increase in circulating progenitors, peaking at 4 days, and a 15- to 20-fold increase by 2 to 7 days in more primitive pre–colony-forming unit (CFU) populations, detected by secondary recloning (Gasparetto et al. 1994). Single doses of rHuG-CSF or PIXY (rHuGM-CSF/rHuIL-3 fusion protein) did not produce significant increase in progenitors in this model. Monoclonal antibody to the cytoadhesion receptor VLA$_4$ has been shown, in vivo, to mobilize progenitors into the circulation (up to 200-fold) in primates, suggesting that blocking of cytoadhesion receptors on primitive marrow cells may be a useful and safe strategy for increasing mobilization (Papayannopoulou and Nakamato 1993).

Comparison of CD34[+] cells mobilized by rHuG-CSF alone or by chemotherapy with or without rHuG-CSF or rHuGM-CSF showed that all protocols elicited cells with lower c-kit and CD71 expression and retention of less rhodamine123 when compared with marrow (To et al. 1994). All peripheralization procedures yielded CD34 cells with comparable cell expansion potential in vitro with multiple cytokine stimulation, although steady-state PB and chemotherapy-mobilized CD34[+] cells generated fewer GM-CFC at day 21 than rHuG-CSF mobilized or steady-state BM CD34[+] cells. An age-related difference in mobilizing capacity of rHuG-CSF has been reported in normal individuals, with 300 μg/day rHuG-CSF producing comparable neutrophil increases (15-fold) in young and elderly, but with twice as many progenitors mobilized in the young (mean age 23 years) as in the elderly (mean age 74 years) (Chatta et al. 1994).

There is a close correlation between circulating CD34[+] cells and progenitors in the circulation. When more primitive populations are quantitated by the delta or LTC-IC assay, a lack of correlation can be observed in some patients, particularly those previously treated, between primitive cell assays and CD34[+] cells or progenitors. In some studies of pretreated patients, no correlation was found between numbers of LTC-IC in the PB and the numbers of progenitors, CD34[+] cells, or time to engraftment (Sutherland et al. 1994). The proliferative potential of LTC-IC mobilized in extensively pretreated patients has been reported to be significantly lower than that of marrow LTC-IC (Sutherland et al. 1990; Schneider et al. 1994; Shapiro et al. 1994). In contrast, progenitor-cell production in long-term stromal co-culture of elicited PB mononuclear cells (MNC) of noncompromised donors was sustained longer (13 to 14 weeks) than when marrow cells were used (8 to 9 weeks) (Pettengell et al. 1993a, b). A significant correlation has been reported between LTC-IC content of PB and platelet recovery in a pediatric allotransplant study (Hirao et al. 1994). GM-CFC content correlated with early granulocyte recovery, but not with platelet recovery.

In hematologically noncompromised patients, a single apheresis at an optimum time after chemotherapy and rHuG-CSF treatment can provide sufficient progenitors and CD34[+] cells for a single transplant and preprogenitor populations measured by delta or LTC-IC assay are at least equivalent to a marrow harvest (Pettengell et al. 1993a, b; Schneider et al. 1994). LTC-IC frequencies are in the range of about $1/10^4$ WBC, and maximum LTC-IC recoveries of 1 to 2×10^6 are generally obtained in apheresis performed when the WBC count reaches 4 to $5 \times 10^3/\mu$L. Upon repeated cycles of apheresis, particularly with intervening cycles of chemotherapy, the recovery of LTC-IC declines with (in some cases, but not all) a decline in progenitors, even when $CD34^+$ cell recovery remains undiminished.

Umbilical cord blood (CB) is increasingly being considered for allogeneic or autologous transplantation. The establishment of cryopreserved banks of CB, currently underway in a variety of centers, provides a potentially greatly expanded pool of donors for unrelated transplants. While over 50 CB transplants have been undertaken, the procedure has, in general, been limited to a pediatric population, due to concern that insufficient cells would be present for effective adult reconstitution. Cell recoveries from 50 to 100 mL CB are in the range of 1 to 2 $\times$ 10^9 nucleated cells, with 1 to 2 $\times$ 10^6 $CD34^+$ cells, 2.5 to 5 $\times$ 10^5 progenitors, and 5 to 20 $\times$ 10^3 LTC-IC recoverable after cell separation (Moore and Hoskins 1994). Significant loss of $CD34^+$ cells and progenitors is observed when physical cell separation procedures are used to isolate CB populations, thus most transplants are done with unseparated blood.

Hemopoietic reconstitution is increasingly undertaken using cell populations subjected to cell separation to enrich for progenitors and deplete contaminating tumor cells (Shpall et al. 1994) or alloreactive T cells. Additional manipulative steps may be done in vitro, in attempts to purge malignant cells or to facilitate retroviral-based gene transduction. A central question in such procedures is the status of the stem-cell population, both numerically and functionally, particularly if in vitro hemopoiesis is sustained for a number of days prior to transplantation. Human marrow stroma (Moore et al. 1980; Sutherland et al. 1990; Pettengell et al. 1993a, b) or murine or human stromal-cell lines (Goldstein et al. 1993; Issaad et al. 1993) support human hemopoiesis in culture for 8 to 12 weeks, with maintenance or modest expansion of LTC-IC numbers to an extent greater than sustained by cytokine combinations alone. LTC-IC may be maintained for up to 2 months in culture of $CD34^+$ cells separated from stromal cells by a cell-impermeable membrane or with stromal-conditioned medium in the presence of various cytokine supplements (IL-3, macrophage inflammatory protein-1, leukemia-inhibiting factor [LIF], c-kit ligand, G-CSF) (Verfaillie, Catanzarro, and Wen-na 1994; Verfaillie and Miller 1994).

Leukemic cell purging has been achieved using ex vivo culture, and successful reconstitution of normal hemopoiesis has been reported following autologous transplantation of marrow taken during relapse of acute myeloid leukemia (AML) and maintained under long-term culture conditions for 10 days (Dexter and Chang 1994). The selective ability of such culture systems to support normal stem cells and restrict survival of leukemic cells may reflect differential cytoadhesion to marrow stromal elements, as demonstrated in chronic myeloid leukemia (CML) (Udomsakdi et al. 1992). In long-term culture of CML marrow, Philadelphia chromosome-negative (Ph⁻) LTC-IC can be maintained at input levels for 10 days, while Ph⁺ LTC-IC declined markedly and autologous transplantation of such cultured marrow resulted in a substantial proportion of patients showing Ph⁻ hemopoietic reconstitution (Barnett et al. 1994).

The use of stromal co-culture for ex vivo expansion of hemopoietic cells on a clinical scale has been achieved in a perfusion bioreactor system (Koller et al. 1993). A 6- to 10-fold expansion of cells, a 15- to 21-fold expansion of progenitors, and a 3- to 10-fold expansion of LTC-IC has been reported over 2 weeks in such a system, starting with unseparated BM. CB MNC have also been expanded in such a system in the presence of irradiated allogeneic marrow stroma and IL-3, IL-6, and c-kit ligand (Koller et al. 1992). The advantage of this system is that small volumes of unseparated cells can be used (e.g., 10 to 15 mL of marrow) that in a bioreactor of 350 to 700 mL volume can attain cell densities of 10^7/mL and provide sufficient cells for a transplant. In addition, lymphoid cells rapidly disappear under the culture conditions optimal for myeloid expansion, providing a purging procedure for T-cell depletion in the case of cells required for allogeneic transplantation, or for elimination of malignant lymphoid cells in patients with acute leukemia or lymphoma (Rummel and Van Zant 1994). In the case of solid tumors with a predisposition to home to the marrow environment, such as breast or prostatic cancer, and neuroblastoma, there is as yet no evidence of significant tumor cell loss in marrow-stromal co-culture, and reinfusion of viable tumor cells with the expanded hemopoietic cells is a possibility.

The feasibility of ex vivo expansion has been shown in marrow reconstitution of lethally irradiated mice. Following in vitro culture of 5-FU–resistant marrow (Muench et al. 1993) or of purified primitive precursors (Rebel et al. 1994) in the presence of c-kit and IL-1, and either IL-6 or recombinant human erythropoietin (rHuEPO), long-term repopulating ability remained intact over 1 to 2 weeks. In addition, transplantation of the greatly expanded population of GM-CFC, CFU, and high-proliferative potential progenitors was associated with a greatly accelerated recovery of neutrophils, platelets, and RBC, when compared with that in mice receiving nonexpanded stem-cell populations. In stroma-free cultures of CD34⁺ cells, stem-cell–enriched subsets thereof, or 4-HPC–treated CD34⁺ cells, progenitor-cell expansion of 40- to 250-fold can be obtained in 7 to 14 days using combinations of c-kit, IL-3, IL-6, and G-CSF, and in some cases, with further addition of IL-1, EPO, or GM-CSF (Haylock et al. 1992; Brugger et al. 1993; Henschler et al. 1994; Moore et al. 1994b; Schneider et al. 1994; Shapiro et al. 1994) (see also Chapter 13). Mobilized PB progenitors expand to an extent equal to or greater than marrow progenitors. The expansion potential of CB progenitors is important, since a single CB collection may yield insufficient progenitors for rapid engraftment of an adult. An average of 225-fold expansion of progenitors can be obtained at 2 weeks, with some umbilical CB harvests generating up to a 600-fold expansion by 14 days and 2,300-fold by 21 days (Moore and Hoskins 1994).

Preservation of stem cells in stromal-independent, cytokine-driven expansion systems has been measured using the LTC-IC assay. The consensus is that in 7- to 14-day cultures of adult marrow or PB, stem cells are maintained or, at the most, expanded two- to threefold (Lansdorp and Dragowska 1993; Lansdorp et al. 1993; Henschler et al. 1994; Moore et al. 1994). In contrast, LTC-IC expansion of 15- to 20-fold can be obtained over 1 to 2 weeks with fetal liver or CB as the starting source (Moore and Hoskins 1994). The use of a fluorescence tracking dye to label purified primitive hemopoietic cells from adult, neonatal, or fetal sources has shown that the majority of such adult cells are not induced to proliferate using a cytokine cocktail including c-kit, although the cells survive (Lansdorp et al. 1993). Phenotypically similar cells from fetal or neonatal sources do proliferate under comparable conditions.

The use of specific combinations of growth factors offers the potential of selective generation or expansion of particular hemopoietic populations that could be matched to the requirement of the transplant recipient. To date, this has mainly focused on myeloid and, specifically, neutrophil reconstitution. Extensive megakaryocyte lineage expansion, as measured by generation of CD61 or GPIIb/IIIa[+] cells, can be achieved using cytokine combinations that include c-kit, IL-3, and IL-6 or IL-11. The recent discovery of c-mpl ligand thrombopoietin, and the demonstration of its selective ability to stimulate megakaryocyte and platelet production, provides a growth factor for further selective ex vivo amplification of this lineage (Bartley et al. 1994; Kaushansky et al. 1994). Dendritic cells and their progenitors can readily be generated in large numbers in cultures of CD34[+] cells in the presence of c-kit, GM-CSF, and tumor necrosis factor (TNF) (Young, Szabolcs, and Moore 1994). Selective expansion systems also exist for natural killer (NK) cells (Miller et al. 1994) and B- and T-lymphocyte subpopulations. The ability to selectively expand stem cells without differentiation has proved an elusive goal. Some strategies incorporate inhibitors of cells immediately post–stem cell (e.g., macrophage inflammatory protein 1), in an attempt to build up stem-cell numbers and block accumulation of differentiated cells. It is possible, however, that the stem-cell self-renewal versus differentiation probability is not influenced by external signals of the type provided by the known family of hemopoietic growth factors. In the final analysis, the replicative potential of stem cells is of greater significance than their absolute number in a hemopoietic transplant, provided the recipient receives adequate short-term hemopoietic rescue. Insight into the replicative potential of stem cells has been provided by analysis of telomere length. DNA polymerase incompletely replicates the 3' termini of chromosomes which, in eukaryocytes, end in specialized nucleoprotein structures termed "telomeres." Measurements of telomere length in BM and PB and in in vitro–expansion cultures of fetal, neonatal, and adult hemopoietic progenitors have shown that 40 to 50 telomeric base pairs are lost per hemopoietic cell division, and approximately nine base pairs per year in peripheral leukocytes (Vaziri et al. 1993, 1994). Thus, under steady-state conditions, the stem-cell pool undergoes, on average, one division every 4 to 5 years and relatively few stem-cell divisions are needed to sustain hemopoiesis throughout life. In cytokine-driven expansion cultures of $CD34^+$, $CD45RA^{low}$, $CD71^{low}$ cells, telomere length was dependent on the age of the cells (fetal, neonatal, adult) and the number of cell doublings sustained in vitro (Vaziri et al. 1994). Under exponential expansion conditions, proliferative senescence is responsible for eventual termination of cultures of normal somatic cells as telomeres truncate to a point incompatible with normal mitotic activity. This "Hayflick" limit has been reported in all nontransformed somatic cells (Hayflick and Moorehead 1961). In the adult, a stem-cell pool of 5 to 10×10^7 cells divides every 4 to 5 years, based on telomere base-pair loss, generating in the process 5 to 6×10^{14} mature blood cells (i.e., one stem cell generates, on average, 5 to 10×10^6 mature cells). In a standard adult hemopoietic graft, 5 to 10×10^5 LTC-IC are transplanted, and if 10% home to the marrow environment, 10 to 11 divisions would restore the LTC-IC population, and with CB, with fewer LTC-IC, some 15 to 16 divisions would be required. In both instances, the doubling potential of the reconstituted stem-cell compartment would be more than sufficient for a lifetime of hemopoiesis. Furthermore, short-term, ex vivo–expanded hemopoietic cell populations in which stem cell numbers are maintained or modestly expanded would still be capable of long-term reconstitution, since their proliferative potential would remain considerable.

REFERENCES

Aglietta, M., Piacibello, W., Sanavio, F., et al. (1989) Kinetics of human hematopoietic cells after in vivo administration of granulocyte-macrophage colony-stimulating factor. *Journal of Clinical Investigation*, **83**, 551–5.

Andrews, R.G., Briddell, R.A., Knitter, G.H., et al. (1994) In vivo synergy between recombinant human stem cell factor and recombinant human granulocyte colony-stimulating factor in baboons: enhanced circulation of progenitor cells. *Blood*, **84**, 800–10.

Apperley, J.F. (1994) Meeting report: Umbilical cord blood progenitor cell transplantation. *Bone Marrow Transplantation*, **14**, 187–96.

Barnett, M.J., Eaves, C.J., Phillips, G.L., et al. (1994) Autografting with cultured marrow in chronic myeloid leukemia: results of a pilot study. *Blood*, **84**, 724–32.

Bartley, T.D., Bogenberger, J., Hunt, P., et al. (1994) Identification and cloning of a megakaryocyte growth and development factor that is a ligand for the cytokine receptor Mpl. *Cell*, **77**, 1117–24.

Breems, D.A., Blokland, E.A., Neben, S., and Ploemacher, R.E. (1994) Frequency analysis of human primitive hematopoietic stem cell subsets using a cobblestone area forming cell assay. *Leukemia*, **8**, 1095–104.

Brugger, W., Möcklin, W., Heimfeld, S., Berenson, R.J., Mertelsmann, R., and Kanz, L. (1993) Ex vivo expansion of enriched peripheral blood CD34$^+$ progenitor cells by stem cell factor, interleukin-1 (IL-1) IL-6, IL-3, interferon-γ, and erythropoietin. *Blood*, **81**, 2579–84.

Chatta, G.S., Price, T.H., Allen, R.C., and Dale, D.C. (1994) Effects of in vivo recombinant methionyl human granulocyte colony-stimulating factor on the neutrophil response and peripheral blood colony-forming cells in healthy young and elderly adult volunteers. *Blood*, **84**, 2923–9.

Chaudhary, P.M. and Roninson, I.B. (1991) Expression and activity of P-glycoprotein, a multidrug efflux pump, in human hematopoietic stem cells. *Cell*, **66**, 85–91.

Colotta, F., Re, F., Polentarutti, N., et al. (1992) Modulation of granulocyte survival and programmed cell death by cytokines and bacterial products. *Blood*, **80**, 2012–20.

Craig, W., Kay, R., Cutler, R.L., and Lansdorp, P.M. (1993) Expression of Thy-1 on human hematopoietic progenitor cells. *Journal of Experimental Medicine*, **177**, 1331–42.

Dexter, T.M. and Chang, J. (1994) New strategies for the treatment of chronic myeloid leukemia. *Blood*, **84**, 673–5.

Flasshove, M., Banerjee, D., Mineishi, S., Li, M.-X., Bertino, J.R., and Moore, M.A. (1995) Ex vivo expansion and selection of human CD34$^+$ peripheral blood progenitor cells after introduction of a mutated dihydrofolate reductase cDNA via retroviral gene transfer. *Blood*, **85**, 566–74.

Gasparetto, C., Smith, C., Gillio, A., Stoppa, A.M., Moore, M.A., and O'Reilly, R.J. (1994) Enrichment of peripheral blood stem cells in a primate model following administration of a single dose of rh-IL-β. *Bone Marrow Transplantation*, **14**, 717–723.

Goldstein, N.I., Moore, M.A., Allen, C., and Tackney, C. (1993) A human fetal spleen cell line, immortalized with SV40 T-antigen, will support the growth of CD34$^+$ long-term culture-initiating cells. *Molecular and Cellular Differentiation*, **1**, 301–21.

Harrison, D.E., Jordan, C.T., Zhong, R.K., and Astle, C.M. (1993) Primitive hematopoietic stem cells: direct assay of most productive populations by competitive repopulation with simple binomial, correlation and covariance calculations. *Experimental Hematology*, **21**, 206–19.

Hayflick, L. and Moorehead, P.S. (1961) The serial cultivation of human diploid cell strains. *Experimental Cell Research*, **25**, 585–621.

Haylock, D.N., To, L.B., Dowse, T.L., Juttner, C.A., and Simmons, P.J. (1992) Ex vivo expansion and maturation of peripheral blood CD34$^+$ cells into the myeloid lineage. *Blood*, **80**, 1405–12.

Henschler, R., Brugger, W., Luft, T., Frey, T., Mertelsmann, R., and Kanz, L. (1994) Maintenance of transplantation potential in ex vivo expanded CD34$^+$ selected human peripheral blood progenitor cells. *Blood*, **84**, 2898–903.

Hirao, A., Kawano, Y., Takaue, Y., et al. (1994) Engraftment potential of peripheral and cord blood stem cells evaluated by a long-term culture system. *Experimental Hematology*, **22**, 521–6.

Issaad, C., Croisille L., Katz, A., Vainchenker, W., and Coulombel, L. (1993) A murine stromal cell line allows the proliferation of very primitive human CD34^{++}/CD38- progenitor cells in long-term cultures and semisolid assays. *Blood*, **81**, 2916–24.

Juttner, C.A., To, L.B., Haylock, D.N., et al. (1989) Autologous blood stem cell transplantation. *Transplantation Proceedings*, **21**, 2929–31.

Kaushansky, K., Lok, S., Holly, R.D., et al. (1994) Promotion of megakaryocyte progenitor expansion and differentiation by the c-Mpl ligand thrombopoietin. *Nature*, **369**, 568–70.

Koller, M.R., Bender, J.G., Miller, W.M., and Papoutsakis, E.T. (1993) Expansion of primitive human hematopoietic progenitors in a perfusion bioreactor system with IL-3, IL-6, and stem cell factor. *Biotechnology*, **11**, 358–63.

Koller, M.R., Bender, J.G., Papoutsakis, E.T., and Miller, W.M. (1992) Effects of synergistic cytokine combinations, low oxygen, and irradiated stroma on the expansion of human cord blood progenitors. *Blood*, **80**, 403–11.

Kritz, A., Crown, J.P., Motzer, R.J., et al. (1993) Beneficial impact of peripheral blood progenitor cells in patients with metastatic breast cancer treated with high-dose chemotherapy plus granulocyte-macrophage colony-stimulating factor. *Cancer*, **71**, 2515–21.

Kyoizumi, S., Baum, C.M., Kaneshima, H., McCune, J.M., Yee, E.J., and Namikawa, R. (1992) Implantation and maintenance of functional human bone marrow in SCID-hu mice. *Blood*, **79**, 1704–11.

Lansdorp, P.M. and Dragowska, W. (1993a) Maintenance of hematopoiesis in serum-free bone marrow cultures involves sequential recruitment of quiescent progenitors. *Experimental Hematology*, **21**, 1321–7.

Lansdorp, P.M., Dragowska, W., and Mayani, H. (1993) Ontogeny-related changes in proliferative potential of human hematopoietic cells. *Journal of Experimental Medicine*, **178**, 787–91.

Lapidot, T., Pflumio, F., Doedens, M., et al. (1992) Cytokine stimulation of multilineage hematopoiesis from immature human cells engrafted in SCID mice. *Science*, **255**, 1137–41.

Lord, B.I., Bronchud, M.H., Owens, S., et al. (1989) The kinetics of human granulopoiesis following treatment with granulocyte colony-stimulating factor in vivo. *Proceedings of the National Academy of Sciences of the United States of America*, **86**, 9499–503.

Mauch, P. and Hellman, S. (1989) Loss of hematopoietic stem cell self-renewal after bone marrow transplantation. *Blood*, **74**, 872–6.

Miller, J.S., Klingsporn, S., Lund, J., Perry, E.H., Verfaillie, C., and McGlave, P. (1994) Large scale ex vivo expansion and activation of human natural killer cells for autologous therapy. *Bone Marrow Transplantation*, **14**, 555–62.

Moore, M.A. (1991) Clinical implications of positive and negative hematopoietic stem cell regulators. Review Stratton Lecture. *Blood*, **78**, 1–19.

Moore, M.A. (1992) Does stem cell exhaustion result from combining hematopoietic growth factors with chemotherapy? If so, how do we prevent it? Editorial. *Blood*, **80**, 3–7.

Moore, M.A., Broxmeyer, H.E., Sheridan, A.P., Meyers, P.A., Jacobsen, N., and Winchester, R.J. (1980) Continuous human bone marrow culture: Ia antigen characterization of probable human pluripotential stem cells. *Blood*, **55**, 682–90.

Moore, M.A. and Hoskins, I. (1994a) Ex vivo expansion of cord blood derived stem cells and progenitors. *Blood Cells*, **20**, 468–81.

Moore, M.A., Schneider, J.G., Shapiro, F., and Bengala, C. (1994) Ex vivo expansion of CD34$^+$ hematopoietic progenitors. In S. Gross (Ed.) *Advances in bone marrow purging and processing: Fourth International Symposium*. Proc 4th Int. Symp. on Bone Marrow Purging and Processing; 1993 September 16–17, Orlando, FL, pp. 217–28. New York, Wiley-Liss, Inc.

Muench, M.O., Firpo, M.T., and Moore, M.A. (1993) Bone marrow transplantation with interleukin-1 plus kit-ligand ex vivo expanded bone marrow accelerates hematopoietic reconstitution in mice without the loss of stem cell lineage and proliferative potential. *Blood*, **81**, 3463–73.

Ogawa, M. (1993) Differentiation and proliferation of hematopoietic stem cells. *Blood*, **81**, 2844–53.

Papayannopoulou, T. and Nakamoto, B. (1993) Peripheralization of hemopoietic progenitors in primates treated with anti-VLA$_4$ integrin. *Proceedings of the National Academy of Sciences of the United States of America*, **90**, 9374–8.

Pettengell, R., Morgenstern, G.R., Woll, P.J., et al. (1993a) Peripheral blood progenitor cell transplantation in lymphoma and leukemia using a single apheresis. *Blood*, **82**, 3770–77.

Pettengell, R., Testa, N.G., Swindell, R., Crowther, D., and Dexter, T.M. (1993b) Transplantation potential of hematopoietic cells released into the circulation during routine chemotherapy for non-Hodgkin's lymphoma. *Blood*, **82**, 2239–48.

Rebel, V.I., Dragawska, W., Eaves, C.J., et al. (1994) Amplification of Sca-1+Lin-WGA+ cells in serum-free cultures containing Steel factor, interleukin-6, and erythropoietin with maintenance of cells with long-term in vivo reconstituting potential. *Blood*, **83**, 128–36.

Rummel, S.A. and Van Zant, G. (1994) Future paradigm for autologous bone marrow transplantation: tumor purging and ex vivo production of normal stem and progenitor cells. *Journal of Hematotherapy*, **3**, 213–8.

Russell, N.H. and Hunter, A.E. (1994) Editorial: Peripheral blood cells for allogeneic transplantation. *Bone Marrow Transplantation*, **13**, 353–5.

Schneider, J.G., Crown, J.P., Wasserheit, C., et al. (1994) Factors affecting the mobilization of primitive and committed hematopoietic progenitors into the peripheral blood of cancer patients. *Bone Marrow Transplantation*, **14**, 877–84.

Shapiro, F., Yao, T.-J., Raptis, G., Reich, L., Norton, L., and Moore, M.A. (1994) Optimization of conditions for ex vivo expansion of CD34[+] cells from patients with stage IV breast cancer. *Blood*, **84**, 3567–74.

Sheridan, W.P., Begley, C.G., Juttner, C.A., et al. (1992) Effect of peripheral blood progenitor cells mobilized by filgrastim (G-CSF) on platelet recovery after high-dose chemotherapy. *Lancet*, **339**, 640–6.

Shpall, E.J., Jones, R.B., Bearman, S.I., et al. (1994) Transplantation of enriched CD34[+] autologous marrow into breast cancer patients folowing high-dose chemotherapy: influence of CD34[+] peripheral blood progenitors and growth factors on engraftment. *Journal of Clinical Oncology*, **12**, 28–33.

Siena, S., Bregni, M., Brando, B., Ravagnani, F., Bonadonna, G., and Gianni, A.M. (1989) Circulation of CD34[+] hematopoietic stem cells in the peripheral blood of high-dose cyclophosphamide-treated patients: enhancement by intravenous recombinant human granulocyte-macrophage colony-stimulating factor. *Blood*, **74**, 1905–2000.

Srour, E.F., Zanjani, E.D., Cornetta, K., et al. (1993) Persistence of human multilineage, self-renewing lymphohematopoietic stem cells in chimeric sheep. *Blood*, **82**, 3333–42.

Sutherland, H.J., Eaves, C.J., Lansdorp, P.M., Phillips, G.L., and Hogge, D.E. (1994) Kinetics of committed and primitive blood progenitor mobilization after chemotherapy and growth factor treatment and their use in autotransplants. *Blood*, **83**, 3808–14.

Sutherland, H.J., Lansdorp, P.M., Henkelman, D.H., Eaves, A.C., and Eaves, C.J. (1990) Functional characterization of individual human hematopoietic stem cells cultured at limiting dilution on supportive marrow stromal layers. *Proceedings of the National Academy of Sciences of the United States of America*, **87**, 3584–8.

To, L.B., Haylock, D.N., Dowse, T., et al. (1994) A comparative study of the phenotype and proliferative capacity of peripheral blood (PB) CD34[+] cells mobilized by four different protocols and those of steady-phase PB and bone marrow CD34[+] cells. *Blood*, **84**, 2930–9.

Udomsakdi, C., Eaves, C.J., Swolin, B., Reid, D.S., Barnett, M.J., and Eaves, A.C. (1992) Rapid decline of chronic myeloid leukemic cells in long-term culture due to a defect at the leukemic stem cell level. *Proceedings of the National Academy of Sciences of the United States of America*, **89**, 6192–6.

Van Zant, G., Chen, J.-J., and Scot-Micus, K. (1991) Developmental potential of hematopoietic stem cells determined using retrovirally marked allophenic marrow. *Blood*, **77**, 756.

Vaziri, H., Dragowska, W., Allsopp, R.C., Thomas, T.E., Harley, C.B., and Lansdorp, P.M. (1994) Evidence for a mitotic clock in human hematopoietic stem cells: loss of telomeric DNA with age. *Proceedings of the National Academy of Sciences of the United States of America*, **91**, 9857–60.

Vaziri, H., Schachter, F., Uchida, I., et al. (1993) Loss of telomeric DNA during aging of normal and trisomy 21 human lymphocytes. *American Journal of Human Genetics*, **52**, 661–7.

Verfaillie, C.M., Catanzarro, P.M., and Wen-na, L. (1994) Macrophage inflammatory protein 1, interleukin 3 and diffusible marrow stromal factors maintain human hematopoietic stem cells for at least eight weeks in vitro. *Journal of Experimental Medicine*, **179**, 643–9.

Verfaillie, C.M. and Miller, J.S. (1994) CD34[+]/CD33- cells reselected from macrophage inflammatory protein 1 + interleukin-3-supplemented "stroma-noncontact" cultures are highly enriched for long-term bone marrow culture initiating cells. *Blood,* **84**, 1442–9.

Watt, S.M. and Visser, W.M. (1992) Recent advances in the growth and isolation of primitive human haemopoietic progenitor cells. *Cell Proliferation*, **25**, 263–97.

Young, J.W., Szabolcs, P., and Moore, M.A.S. (1995) Identification of CFU-DCs among normal human CD34$^+$ bone marrow progenitors that are expanded by c-kit-ligand and yield pure dendritic cell colonies in the presence of GM-CSF and TNFα. *Journal of Experimental Medicine*, (in press).

Zeigler, F.C., Bennett, B.D., Jordan, C.T., et al. (1994) Cellular and molecular characterization of the role of the Flk-2/Flt-3 receptor tyrosine kinase in hematopoietic stem cells. *Blood*, **84**, 2422–30.

2

Effector Cells of Experimental and Clinical Cellular Adoptive Immunobiology

SHIMON SLAVIN

Major progress in recent years in both understanding the pathophysiology of various malignancies and development of new chemotherapeutic agents and new combinational chemotherapy protocols with documented efficacy based in prospective randomized clinical trials has led to substantial progress in treating patients with a variety of malignant hematological diseases and solid tumors. Development of better supportive care for pancytopenic, immunocompromised patients following high-dose myeloablative chemoradiotherapy supported by bone-marrow transplantation (BMT) has led to further progress in exploiting the dose-response effect of more intensive anticancer modalities; however, considering the experimental and clinical data suggesting a logarithmic dose-response relationship for most chemoradiosensitive tumors, and taking into consideration the potential multiorgan toxicity of available anticancer modalities at dose ranges sufficient to eradicate all tumor cells, it became obvious that for patients with advanced and bulky disease at the time of diagnosis, especially those relapsing following conventional chemotherapy and certainly high-dose chemoradiotherapy supported by autologous or allogeneic BMT, the probability of elimination of the last tumor cell by currently available chemoradiotherapy seems infinitesimal. Considering that in the past few years no major progress has been made in curing patients with malignant hematological diseases, lymphomas, and disseminated solid tumors by conventional modalities, the need for more innovative anticancer modalities seemed highly desirable. It became obvious that eradication of chemoresistant tumor cells should be approached with alternative strategies such as immunotherapy, which seems more promising than in the past.

Insights into the potential role of the immune system in eradicating cancer were obtained with development of suitable experimental models in parallel with development of inbred mice strains by transferring various tumor cells into mice (Outzen 1975; Moller 1976; Rygaardc and Povlsen 1976). These experiments showed that tumor cells could not be successfully transferred into animals with a different genetic background (Bashford 1904; Loeb 1906; Tyzzer 1909; Rous 1910; Little and Tyzzer 1915; Tyzzer 1916; Woglom 1929; Bittner 1932; Klein 1975; reviewed in Scott 1991). Subsequently, several investigators have demonstrated the feasibility of raising an autochthonous immune response against chemically induced tumors (Baldwin 1955, 1976; Prehn and Main 1957; Klein et al. 1960). Experimental immunotherapy with tumor-antigen (Ag) extracts or irradiated tumor cells that by themselves could not induce tumor regression was the next important development (Revesz 1960; Wolf 1969; Parr 1972). Unfortunately, such approaches seemed ineffective against nonimmunogenic tumors. It was subsequently suggested, and recently confirmed, that operational cure may be accomplished against nonimmunogenic or weakly immunogenic tumors despite continuous presence of few residual tumor cells, once a state of dormancy has been established by activation of the host's anticancer effector mechanisms or by induction of down-regulatory signals in the primary tumor or in the host (Wheelock 1979). It was recently shown, however, that following induction of successful tumor dormancy, complete eradication of clonogenic tumor cells may be required to achieve complete cure, suggesting that prevention of clonal proliferation of tumor cells may eventually result in complete eradication of the last tumor cell, most likely through apoptosis (Slavin, Ackerstein, and Weiss 1988a; Slavin et al. 1992). Until recently, none of the available methods using immunotherapy for the treatment of naturally occurring malignancies (which are largely nonimmunogenic) proved effective in clinical practice.

Documentation of tumor-specific or tumor-associated Ag by modern molecular biology technology (Boon 1983), and documentation of cytotoxic tumor-infiltrating lymphocytes (TIL) that can be expanded and activated in vitro and used for immunotherapy (Rosenberg et al. 1988), generated new hopes that tumor-specific immunotherapy may be inducible either by potentiating immune responses against well-defined tumor Ag or by passive (adoptive) transfer of in vitro–activated, autologous T lymphocytes (and possibly other cell subsets). It remains to be seen whether raising an immune response against tumor-specific antigens (TAA) will be a practical, realistic, and cost-effective mode of therapy for a large number of patients. Nonetheless, these recent studies suggested that it might be possible to augment immune responses against weak tumor-specific Ag or to induce tumor cells to express more immunogenic cell-surface determinants. Recent emphasis in immunotherapy is based on amplifying immune responses against autologous tumor cells by rendering tumor cells more immunogenic either through enhancing expression of cell-surface tumor-associated Ag using cytokines (Geiner et al. 1984; Leon et al. 1989; Jorge et al. 1992), or by introducing foreign peptides to be recognized by host cytotoxic T cells through xenogenization by viruses (Freedman et al. 1983; Okada et al. 1987; Shimizu et al. 1988; Furukawa et al. 1989; Iwaki et al. 1989; Schirrmacher 1989; Shoham et al. 1990; Archer, Bretscher, and Ziola 1990; Wallack and Sivanandham 1993), viral lysates, or well-defined peptides (Giorgio and Guido 1974).

Alternatively, attempts at induction of antitumor responses by amplification of host immune responses against weak autologous tumor Ag has been made by using nonspecific adjuvants; by exogenous supply of cytokines, such as interleukin-2α (IL-2α) and interferon-γ (IFN-γ), given with autologous tumor material plus antibody (Ab) against the tumor, or directly into the host (McCune et al. 1990; Hoover et al. 1993; Slavin, Ackerstein, and Weiss 1988; Rosenberg 1991; Pomer et al. 1992; Nagler et al. 1994). The latter approach may be most effective in the state of minimal residual disease (MRD) accomplished by autologous or allogeneic BMT (Slavin and Kedar 1988; Slavin et al. 1990a; Ackerstein, Kedar, and Slavin 1991; Slavin and Nagler 1991; Slavin et al. 1992c; Nagler et al. 1994). One of the most innovative approaches for inducing antitumor host immune responses involves in vitro genetic engineering of tumor cells by transduction of cytokine genes, which forces tumor cells to secrete cytokines that attract and amplify host immune responses against tentative tumor-associated or tumor-specific Ag (Eglitis et al. 1985; Miller 1992; Jaffee et al. 1992, 1993; Pardoll 1993; Foa et al. 1994; Tepper and Mule 1994). An alternative, yet similar, approach involves transduction of strong co-stimulatory signals to transform an inert tumor cell to an Ag-presenting cell (e.g., by insertion of B7, which serves as a ligand for CD28 present on CD4$^+$ T cells) (Townsend and Allison 1993). Insertion of "naked" DNA genes, by direct in vitro or in vivo injection of tumor cells, or following systemic administration of DNA material using DNA/liposome complexes in contrast to vector-mediated gene transduction into tumor cells, does not require elaborate genetic engineering technology in vitro (Plautz et al. 1993; Zhu et al. 1993), and represents a promising future approach for cancer immunotherapy by host effector cells. Whereas many of the above studies have suggested that various in vitro and in vivo manipulations may successfully induce host responses against tumor cells under favorable experimental conditions, there are no conclusive clinical data available to unequivocally confirm that such approaches are beneficial in humans. Clearly, treatment of MRD and/or prevention of disease in experimental animals is much easier to accomplish compared with treatment of established diseases in both experimental animals and in clinical practice, where tumor Ag may not only be too weak to generate effective antitumor effect but may also tolerize host T cells (Weiss et al. 1994). Tolerance may develop either through induction of an anergic state peripherally or through activation of negative signals by active suppressor cells (Naor 1979) that may down-regulate beneficial antitumor responses. In summary, although attempts to induce successful autologous antitumor responses in clinical trials remain speculative at best, recent data using innovative immunotherapy based on a better understanding of immune interactions between allogeneic donors' immunocompetent T cells and host tumor cells are encouraging.

In contrast to the limited capacity of autologous antitumor responses against nonimmunogenic or weakly immunogenic tumors, passive adoptive transfer of allogeneic lymphocytes can result in marked and beneficial clinical effect in eradication of otherwise chemoradioresistant tumor cells. This beneficial effect is probably due to recognition of tumor cell surface alloantigens (i.e., major or minor histocompatibility complex [HC] Ag), rather than tumor-specific Ag that may not exist. This chapter reviews the cell subsets involved in Ag-specific and Ag-nonspecific cell-therapy procedures. These include passive adoptive transfer of autologous immune effector cells such as T cells sensitized in vitro against autologous tumor-specific Ag, TIL, or in vitro–activated natural killer (NK) cells ("LAK" cells), as well as an alternative approach based on passive adoptive transfer of fresh immunocompetent allogeneic blood lymphocytes or in vitro–activated allogeneic blood lymphocytes, with or without further in vivo activation of effector cells with recombinant interleukin-2 (rIL-2). Allogeneic immune-mediated responses against tumor cells are much more effective than autologous responses and have been shown to induce complete and durable remissions in a substantial number of patients in the setting of allogeneic BMT. Cell therapy might become a most important tool for cancer therapy, especially in patients with malignant hematological diseases either as an adjuvant treatment of MRD or as the only effective modality for patients who fail to respond to initial chemotherapy.

■ EFFECTOR CELLS OF NATURAL RESISTANCE/ IMMUNOSURVEILLANCE AGAINST CANCER

Although the primary role of the immune system is protection against pathogenic infections, substantial evidence exists to suggest that the immune system can also protect its host from potentially cancerous mutations that may occur spontaneously as a result of viral or other pathogenic infections or in response to physicochemical events (Burnet 1970). Certain cancers, especially those of the hemopoietic compartment, are more common in recipients of chemotherapy or radiation and after long-term immunosuppression either for autoimmunity or as maintenance treatment for prevention of rejection of organ allografts (Klein 1978; Purtilo 1984; I. Penn, personal communication). Likewise, certain cancers, especially of the lymphoreticular system, are more common in animals with lack of T-cell immunity (Outzen et al. 1975; Rygaardc and Povlsen 1976; Moller 1976) as well as in patients with immunodeficiencies (Groopman 1987). On the other hand, T-cell–deficient athymic mice with no circulating T cells do not show increased incidence or shorter latency of cancers induced by carcinogens (Klein 1978; Purtilo 1984; I. Penn, personal communication), whereas they do feature increased incidence of virus infections normally controlled by T cells or secondary malignancies induced by viral particles.

NK cells are also believed to play some role against cancer based on a number of observations including increased incidence of tumors in NK-deficient mice, suggesting that NK cells may be able alone to prevent generation of certain cancers (Herberman, Nunn, and Lavrin 1975; Sendo et al. 1975; Hanna and Fidler 1980). Likewise, NK cells were shown to inhibit primary and metastatic tumors in experimental animals (Talmadge et al. 1980; Hanna and Burton 1981). NK cells driven by IL-2 in vitro and in vivo can be further potentiated to generate antitumor effects, suggesting that NK cells and activated LAK cells may play a role in vivo in both providing resistance against development of primary cancer as well as prevention of propagation of existing cancer. This suggests that such cells may be applied clinically for Ag-nonspecific, major or minor HC–independent treatment of cancer (Rosenberg 1991).

■ IMMUNE RESPONSES AGAINST TUMORS BY VARIOUS COMPONENTS OF THE IMMUNE SYSTEM

Theoretically, all the rules of the immune system apply to cancer immunotherapy as long as the tumor cell is immunogenic. Hence, tumors induced by viral agents that follow the rules of antiviral immunity (Melief and Kast 1992), chemically and UV light–induced tumors (Foley 1953; Prehn and Main 1957), as well as tumors induced by mutagenic changes induced either spontaneously or intentionally (Boon et al. 1989; Boon, van Pel, and de Plaen 1989) are frequently characterized by unique tumor-specific Ag. Immune response against tumor Ag, like other Ag, involves a sequence of events in which various components of the immune system participate, starting with recognition of nonself Ag. This leads through a secondary inflammatory reaction to activation and mobilization of macrophages and antigen-presenting cells (APC) that increase the available doses of tumor-Ag peptides and present them in the context of enhanced expression of class II histocompatibility molecules (HCM) to CD4$^+$ T cells. Once activated through engagement of T-cell receptor with the proper co-stimulatory signal generation by positive feedback, T-cell activation results in the production of cytokines, predominantly IL-2, and subsequent generation of CD8$^+$ cytotoxic cells that mediate cytolytic effects through recognition of tumor-associated peptides in the context of cell-surface class I HCM. Local immune responses may be further activated nonspecifically by recruitment of inflammatory cells that can participate in tumor cell destruction by phagocytosis or secretion of a variety of active mediators that can lead to active disintegration of tumor cells.

In addition to cell-mediated antitumor responses, generation of antibody (Ab) by CD4-dependent B-cell responses may lead to either an Ag-dependent cell-mediated cytotoxic effect or complement-mediated cytolysis of tumor cells.

As previously indicated, most spontaneously arising tumors in both experimental animals and humans are operationally nonimmunogenic and, therefore, induce no spontaneous cell-mediated or humoral antitumor responses (Hewitt, Blake, and Walder 1976). The artifical induction of antitumor effector cells targeted against modified tumor cells using a variety of innovative immune approaches is extremely attractive; however, the efficacy of such methods may be limited, due to the need to eradicate the unmanipulated tumor cells, which may not be recognized by immune cells sensitized against in vitro modified tumor cells, unless cross-reactive determinants or cryptic ligands cross-reactive with the original tumor cell-surface Ag become the target of immunotherapy. Whether or not amplification of immune responses against weak Ag by a variety of immunological maneuvers will also generate effective specific responses against cryptic cell-surface antigenic determinants cross-reacting against the original tumor remains to be seen. This chapter will focus on antitumor effector cells induced in experimental tumor-bearing hosts against immunogenic tumors. The possible immunotherapy of spontaneous nonimmunogenic tumors in experimental animals and humans by adoptive transfer of effector cells obtained from genetically matched donors in the context of BMT will be described. Cell therapy using immune lymphocytes specific against tumor-specific Ag may be theoretically attempted against immunogenic tumors, whereas adoptive transfer of effector cells recognizing tumor minor HC or major HC as targets may be attempted in treating nonimmunogenic tumors. Activation of blood lymphocytes from HLA-matched siblings that recognize minor HC determinants rather than tumor-specific Ag, or effector cells operating with no major HC restriction such as activated NK cells or macrophages, may be used clinically to induce direct antitumor effects in vivo. Under normal circumstances, certainly when dealing with immunogenic tumors, the main antitumor responses are T-cell dependent. NK cells do not appear to provide longlasting and self-perpetuating responses against tumor cells in vivo, except, perhaps, under conditions where class I–deficient tumor variants or metastases may be present, since the antitumor response of professional T cells is dependent on major HC, whereas NK-dependent antitumor responses may be predominant in class I–deficient tumor cells (Karre et al. 1986).

Generation of Tumor-Specific Helper T Cells with Specific Immunity Against a Given Tumor

Sensitization of the immune system against an existing tumor requires either direct recognition by CD4[+] T cells of tumor-specific or TAA in the context of self class II, or indirectly, tumor-specific or associated peptide processed by professional APC and presented to CD4[+] T cells in association with class II of APC. Proper sensitization of CD4[+] T cells leads to clonal expansion of specific immune cells with generation of memory T cells (CD4[+] CD45RO[+]) and requires cytokine production, predominantly IL-2. Generation of CD8[+] cytotoxic T cells for optimal in vivo cytolysis may also require IL-2 production by immune-specific CD4[+] T cells. Activation of immune-specific cells may generate a cascade of secondary inflammatory reactions that may contribute to disintegration and elimination of tumor cells through mechanisms involving macrophages and neutrophils, with further possible sensitization of bystanding immune cells against a variety of relevant and irrelevant immunogenic peptides. This leads to antigen-nonspecific responses in addition to specific immune response against the primary sensitizing tumor cell. This scheme requires presence of class II Ag on the tumor cell to be directly recognized by host CD4[+] T cells. Furthermore, sensitization of host CD4[+] T cells requires additional co-stimulatory signals, the principal one being interaction between CD28 on the CD4[+] T cell and B7-1, B7-2, or possibly B7-3 on the target cell (June et al. 1994). Even class II positive tumor cells cannot serve as proper immunogens without the proper co-stimulatory signals. It was recently shown that transduction of a gene coding for B7 into tumor cells may render them immunogenic (Townsend and Allison 1993). Likewise, our model proposes that class II negative tumor cells cannot be recognized directly by host CD4[+] T cells, but instead are recognized indirectly through class II cell-surface determinants of professional APC after proper processing of tumor-specific or tumor-associated peptides and their presentation in association with class II HCM of host APC.

Generation of Cytolytic Cells Against Tumor-Specific or Tumor-Associated Antigens

Antitumor effects are mediated predominantly by CD8[+] cytotoxic T lymphocytes, recognizing tumor-specific or tumor-associated peptides in association with tumor cell-surface class I (Mills and North 1985; Matis et al. 1986; Greenberg 1991). In some tumor model systems, CD4[+] T cells were shown to mediate effective antitumor responses mostly against virally induced (immunogenic) tumors (Fujiwara et al. 1984; Tomita et al. 1986; Greenberg 1991). Whereas CD4[+] effector cells provide the necessary help and IL-2 needed for activation and replication of effector cells, CD8[+] effector T cells are dependent on IL-2 provided either by CD4[+] T cells, or alternatively, by exogenous supply of IL-2. Most of the available data relate to the potential contribution of T cells bearing α/β as compared with the γ/δ T-cell receptor. Likewise, the exact function of major HC nonrestricted T lymphocytes is not well understood. Other cell subsets may also play minor or major roles in eradicating tumors in an Ag-nonspecific fashion depending on the experimental system used, including macrophages (Fidler and Schroit 1988), NK cells, and IL-2–activated NK cells (Rosenberg and Lotze 1986). CD4[+] T cells may mediate antitumor effects in vivo indirectly by recruiting and activating host macrophages and APC through active delayed-type hypersensitivity reactions, resulting in activated macrophage-mediated antitumor responses. Specific immune CD4[+] T cells may mediate antitumor response, indirectly, by effector cells reacting locally against the tumor in an Ag-nonspecific major HC nonrestricted fashion (Greenberg 1986). NK cells may play an important role especially in the absence of major HC class I cell-surface molecules (Karre et al. 1986). Hosts may defend themselves against evolving immunogenic cancers induced by tumorogenic viruses, mutagens, or chemical carcinogens by effector mechanisms operating in harmony against nonimmunogenic or weakly immunogenic tumor cells. Hosts with tumor cells that render the host immune cells tolerant against tentative tumor-specific Ag or TAA may be completely helpless and may benefit from exogenous supply of cytokines, or preferably adoptively transferred anticancer effector cells. These effectors may recognize tumor cells as minor alloantigens rather than by virtue of tumor-specific Ag, which may be absent, weak, concealed, or nonimmunogenic.

■ ADOPTIVE CELL THERAPY OF TUMORS BY AUTOLOGOUS IMMUNE CELLS

The Role of Specific Immune T Cells

The use of cell therapy through passive transfer of in vitro–expanded immune cells requires development of immunity against the tumor by in vivo or in vitro presensitization of host cells. Such an approach, utilizing immune cells specific for a given tumor, cannot be used in treating nonimmunogenic tumors. An example of one of the most extensively studied tumor models is FBL-3 (Friend retrovirus-induced erythroleukemia) in C57BL/6 (B6) mice (Cheever, Greenberg, and Fefer 1980, 1981; Cheever et al. 1982; extensively reviewed in Greenberg 1991). Injection of FBL (5×10^6 cells/recipient) into B6 mice results in lethal disease within 1 to 2 weeks. Neither chemotherapy alone (cytoxan 180 mg/kg) nor injection of immune cells alone (on day +5) are able to cure any of the mice inoculated with FBL, even at a cell dose as great as 5×10^8 cells per recipient. In contrast, mice cytoreduced with cytoxan and infused with immune T cells can be cured, provided that an adequate number ($\geq 5 \times 10^6$) of immune cells are passively transferred. Antitumor effects of adoptively transferred immune cells could be abolished by treatment with monoclonal anti–T-cell Ab. Likewise, immune cells irradiated before cell therapy failed to provide any in vivo antitumor effect, suggesting that cell division and expansion of specific immune T cells is a necessary prerequisite for active specific immunotherapy in vivo (Greenberg 1991). Depletion of specific immune T cells generated in the immune donor resulted in complete loss of therapeutic effects of cell therapy; similarly, in vivo elimination of host T lymphocytes (Thy1.2^+) had no significant effect on the activity of adoptively transferred immune T cells, suggesting that recruitment of host T lymphocytes played no major role in tumor eradication (Greenberg 1991). Similar in vivo antitumor effects could be obtained by in vitro–generated FBL-specific T-cell lines (Klarnet et al. 1987) and T-cell clones (Cheever et al. 1982). Elimination of tumor cells in hosts inoculated with FBL appears to be a slow process, since in vivo depletion of T cells in B6 mice treated with specific immune cells by injection of specific monoclonal antibody (mAB) against adoptively transferred donor immune cells within the first 50 days following cell therapy resulted in mortality due to escape of residual tumor cells in the host. Elimination of specific donor-immune T cells after day 50 had no similar effect because by that time complete elimination of all tumor cells was successfully accomplished by cell therapy.

The Role of Antigen-Specific CD4⁺ and CD8⁺ T-Cell Subsets in Autochthonous Tumor Cell Therapy

As previously shown by the well-studied FBL tumor model in B6 mice, both $CD4^+$ and $CD8^+$ T cells can mediate their effect in the absence of host $CD8^+$ and $CD4^+$ cells, respectively, in lethally irradiated thymectomized recipients reconstituted with T-cell–depleted B6 BM allografts. This model avoids the possible contribution of effector T cells by the host (Greenberg 1991). The efficacy of 10^7 $CD4^+$ T cells was found to be as effective as an equal number of unseparated spleen cells obtained from specifically immune B6 donors. The efficacy of isodoses of $CD8^+$ T cells in the same model was somewhat less effective, but responsiveness could be completely restored by exogenous supply of rIL-2 5,000 IU daily intraperitoneally (IP) for 6 days starting at the time of adoptive cell transfer (Greenberg 1991). It appears that both T-cell subsets play an essential role in vivo, with $CD4^+$ T cells providing the necessary help to optimize antitumor effects of specifically immune $CD8^+$ T cells. Since most tumor cells bear class I cell-surface Ag, whenever they are immunogenic, antitumor responses by $CD8^+$ T cells represent the final common pathway, provided that IL-2 deficiency is not a limiting factor. This seems true in models of murine leukemias (Greenberg 1986; De Graaf, Horak, and Bookman 1988) as well as in a variety of sarcomas and carcinomas (Yamasaki et al. 1984; Ward et al. 1988; Greenberg 1991) using fresh T cells or in vitro–derived T-cell clones (Dailey, Pillemer, and Weissman 1982; De Graaf et al. 1988), some in association with $CD4^+$ T cells (Schild et al. 1987; Greenberg 1991). In some cases, cell activation could be further augmented by cytokines other than rIL-2, such as interferon-γ (IFN-γ) (De Graaf et al. 1988). TIL are also primarily $CD8^+$ T cells requiring help provided by exogenous rIL-2 (Rosenberg et al. 1988).

Potential Role of B Cells as Mediators of Specific Immunity Against Tumors

B lymphocytes may convey antitumor effects by producing Ab that lyse tumor cells in combination with complement or through antibody-dependent cell-mediated cytotoxicity (ADCC). Since most clinically relevant tumors are nonimmunogenic, naturally occurring Ab do not seem to provide an effective practical approach for eradication of cancer; however, tumor-specific or tumor-associated Ab can eradicate B-cell lymphomas with monoclonal phenotype through the binding specificity of cell-surface idiotopes using anti-idiotypic Ab (Glennie et al. 1988; Campbell et al. 1990). Using the FBL tumor-model system, inoculation of B cells obtained from immune donors did not appear to play an important role in tumor therapy in vivo (Greenberg 1991). Monoclonal Ab with specificity against well-defined cell-surface determinants present on tumor cells were also investigated as possible carriers of cytotoxic chemical compounds or toxins for targeted delivery of anticancer agents, and Ab against tumor cell-surface Ag may serve as homing devices for cytolytic T cells through bispecific Ab or using innovative molecular engineering approaches to guide effector cytotoxic T lymphocytes, the so-called T bodies (Esshar et al. 1993). These modalities are beyond the scope of this chapter (Vitetta 1994).

Antigen Nonspecific Anticancer Effector Cells

Role of Macrophages   Although macrophages can serve as antitumor effector cells, specific reactivity in vivo can be conferred only by the initiators of the antitumor responses, tumor-specific $CD4^+$ T cells (Alexander, Evans, and Grant 1972; Evans and Alexander 1972; Greenberg 1991). Antitumor responses of macrophages may be activated by phorbol myrisate acetate (PMA) (Reed and Lucas 1975) and IL-1 (Foley 1953; Nathan and Cohn 1981; Onozaki et al. 1985). Final effector mechanisms may involve generation of reactive oxygen intermediates, leading to formation of hydrogen peroxide and, most likely, additional free radicals with formation of nitrites inhibiting DNA synthesis (Hibbs, Vavrin, and Taintor 1987). Macrophage-induced antitumor effects were documented in the FBL model as well as in other $CD4^+$-mediated antitumor effector models. Macrophages and other components of the hemopoietic system may play an important role as effector cells against tumor cells opsonized with Ab through binding of Fc portion of the Ab to the Fc receptors of host reticuloendothelial cells, resulting in tumor lysis by ADCC. Based on the above, macrophage-dependent antitumor effects may be amplified by macrophage-activating agents such as phorbol esters, calcium ionophores, a variety of toxins such as lipopolysaccharide (LPS), and adjuvants such as bacille Calmette-Guérin (BCG) and muramyl dipeptide (Drysdale, Agarwal, and Shin 1988; Adams and Hamilton 1984). Conversely, macrophage-dependent antitumor effector cells may be blocked by silica or carageenan (Mule et al. 1985), by Ab against cytokines, or by Ab against macrophages (Paulnock and Lambert 1990).

Role of NK Cells and IL-2–Activated (LAK) Cells   NK cells are characterized as CD3⁻, CD16⁺, CD56⁺ lymphocytes and may be weakly positive for CD2, CD8, and CD7. Immunotherapy with major HC–nonrestricted killing of tumor cells by NK and LAK cells was exploited in experimental animals and humans (Rosenberg and Lotze 1986). Generation of blood LAK cells seems technically simple and reproducible, and antitumor responses can be documented in vitro for both NK-sensitive K562 cells and NK-resistant Daudi cells. There are some in vivo data in experimental animals that suggest that antitumor efficacy of LAK cells may be further amplified by concomitant in vivo activation of effector cells with IL-2 (Rosenberg and Lotze 1986). The antitumor efficacy of NK cells plus in vivo administration of rIL-2 (most likely due to in vivo–activated T cells and possibly NK cells) was previously documented in experimental animals and in patients with leukemia (Slavin and Kedar 1988; Slavin et al. 1990a; Ackerstein et al. 1991; Slavin and Nagler 1991; Weiss, Reich, and Slavin 1992). Cells from patients with measurable disease were shown to respond in vitro to autologous peripheral blood lymphocytes (PBL) activated in vitro or in vivo in response to administration of rIL-2. In these patients, LAK plus rIL-2 therapy resulted in measurable complete response (CR) rates of no more than 10%. Unlike complete cure that can be accomplished with immunogenic tumors by T-cell therapy, complete eradication of disease with NK or LAK cells without coparticipation of T lymphocytes is rare because the effect of NK cells is short term. Due to severe side effects, rIL-2 at doses sufficient to cause effective antitumor effects in vivo cannot be safely administered over a long period. Despite intensive and encouraging clinical trials, the use of rIL-2 for in vivo treatment of cancer is rather limited, with the primary indication being renal cell cancer (Rosenberg and Lotze 1986).

Although many nonimmunogenic tumors may serve as an indication for cell therapy using rIL-2–activated LAK cells, such treatment also activates T cells that contribute to the generation of antitumor effector mechanisms for tumors that are weakly immunogenic. In contrast to results in experimental animals using immunogenic tumors, participation of effector T cells is less likely in clinical situations. NK cells seem to have no major role in cell therapy of experimental models of immunogenic leukemias such as FBL, since elimination of NK1.1$^+$ cells from the pool of lymphocytes obtained from specifically immune donors failed to impair the curative potential of T lymphocytes (Greenberg 1991). It appears that although NK cells or NK cells activated in vivo by cytokines generated in the course of an immune reaction may play a role in immune surveillance against cancer and infectious organisms, their use for specific adoptive immunotherapy seems rather limited, since the overall benefit of immune T cells is by far more effective, continuous, and longlasting, with many clinical benefits as compared with the transient effect of NK cells and LAK cells.

Antitumor reactivity of activated NK cells may be further potentiated in vivo by IFN-α (Slavin and Nagler 1991; Morecki et al. 1992; Nagler et al. 1994), as well as by IFN-γ (Perussia, Santoli, and Trinchieri 1980). Other cytokines may also play a role in further potentiation of the antitumor activity of NK cells such as IL-7 (Perussia et al. 1980).

Although the antitumor effects of NK cells are known to be major HC nonrestricted, recent observations in mice and humans suggest that class I Ag, in particular locus C of the human HLA, may participate in NK cell–mediated alloreactivity and cytolytic activity (Moretta et al. 1993).

■ CELL THERAPY BY ALLOGENEIC LYMPHOCYTES AGAINST NONIMMUNOGENIC TUMORS

Allogeneic T Lymphocytes as Antitumor Effector Cells Following Allogeneic Bone Marrow Transplantation

Allogeneic BMT represents the most effective mode of therapy of resistant leukemias and lymphomas due to the combination of maximal-tolerated doses of chemoradiotherapy and immune-mediated graft-versus-leukemia (GVL) effects induced by donor immunocompetent T cells.

The role of cell-mediated immunotherapy in conjunction with BMT (Chapter 20) is best documented by comparing the rate of relapse of patients undergoing syngeneic and autologous BMT with the rate in patients undergoing allogeneic BMT, both being conditioned by identical chemotherapy (Ringden and Horowitz 1989). The relapse rate in acute and chronic leukemias is negatively correlated with acute and chronic graft-versus-host disease (GVHD) (Weiden, Fluornoy, and Thomas 1979; Apperley et al. 1986; Ringden and Horowitz 1989; Sullivan, Weiden, and Storb 1989; Horowitz et al. 1990). Experimental and clinical data on the negative role of cyclosporine A in MRD were recently published (Weiss, Reich, and Slavin 1990). All of the above suggest that T-lymphocyte–dependent immune effects play a major role in controlling MRD in conjunction with BMT. In view of these findings, it seems reasonable to take advantage of the immune-mediated effector mechanisms to further reduce the risk of relapse following allogeneic as well as autologous BMT (Or et al. 1993, 1995; Slavin et al. 1992d) by allogeneic cell therapy (allo-CT), using potentially alloreactive T lymphocytes and cytokine-activated lymphocytes (Slavin et al. 1992b, c, 1993a, b). (Chapters 24 and 25).

Cell-Mediated Immunotherapy Following Allogeneic Bone Marrow Transplantation

Using the BCL1 model of murine lymphoid leukemia it has been shown that GVL effects can be induced by allogeneic BMT independently of clinical overt GVHD (Slavin et al. 1991). GVL was induced and maintained by donor T lymphocytes, predominantly CD8$^+$ cells (Slavin et al. 1990a; Weiss et al. 1990). Interestingly, although T-cell depletion at the time of BMT resulted in relapse of all mice inoculated with BCL1 prior to or 1 day following BMT, stable GVHD-free chimeras could resist large inocula of BCL1 ($>10^6$ per recipient) (Weiss et al. 1994). These data suggest that relapse following T-cell–depleted BM results from tolerization of newly developing donor T cells by tumor Ag. Introduction of tumor cells in stable chimeras after acquisition of the donor T-cell repertoire did not result in tolerance because mature T cells were more resistant to induction of tolerance to neoantigens compared with newly developing T cells (Weiss et al. 1994). Since complete elimination of all tumor cells before BMT is frequently not possible, an alternative approach to prevent induction of unresponsiveness against TAA involves administration of donor immunocompetent T cells following BMT. Hosts tolerant of donor alloantigens are expected to accept donor lymphocytes and permit induction of GVL after induction of stable chimerism, while induction of chimerism could be safely accomplished with T-cell depletion at BMT (Weiss et al. 1994). It has been previously documented that following induction of chimerism, recipients develop resistance to increments of donor immunocompetent T cells and, if given at sufficiently long time intervals from BMT, GVHD can no longer be induced even in chimeras made across major HC (Slavin et al. 1978). Instead of risking GVHD while inducing GVL, GVL can be safely induced at a second stage following induction of chimerism. The observation was recently confirmed using another model of murine leukemia (Johnson, Drobyski, and Truitt 1993). Induction of potent GVL can be successfully accomplished by administration of allogeneic lymphocytes following initial transplantation with T-lymphocyte–depleted allografts (Weiss et al. 1992; Cohen et al. 1993). Moreover, GVL effects induced by gradual increments of immunocompetent allogeneic lymphocytes given after BMT are significantly potentiated by concomitant administration of a short course of low-dose rIL-2 in vivo (Slavin et al. 1990b, 1992c; Weiss et al. 1992; Vourka-Karussis et al. 1995).

Since GVL operates in close association with GVHD, recognition of effector cells involved in GVL seemed important in view of the desirable goal to be able to separate beneficial GVL effects and harmful GVHD. Effector cells of GVL and GVHD vary, depending on the degree and type of major HC or minor HC disparity as well as strain combinations and the nature of the tumor cells (Slavin et al. 1990c). Effector cells of GVL and GVHD seem to be determined by the type of major HC barrier involved; CD4[+] T cells play the major role against class II positive tumor cells, whereas CD8[+] T cells do so for class I positive, class II negative tumor cells (Horowitz et al. 1990). As shown in various lymphoid malignancies in mice of B- and T-cell origin, the dominant effector T cells mediating the final in vivo antitumor effect are CD8[+] (Sykes, Romick, and Sachs 1990). Similarly to CD8[+] T cells derived from mice specifically immunized against retroviral tumors, alloreactive CD8[+]-mediated reactivity against tumors can be further amplified in vitro and especially in vivo by exogenous supply of rIL-2 (Slavin and Kedar 1988; Slavin et al. 1990a; Ackerstein et al. 1991; Slavin and Nagler 1991; Weiss et al. 1992). CD4[+] T cells were shown to be effective against tumor cells in vivo in either murine system (Korngold, Leighton, and Manser 1994). Alloreactive responses occurring in vivo may generate sufficient amount of help to promote ongoing CD8[+]-mediated antitumor responses until the complete elimination of tumor cells. Unfortunately, GVL across major HC or minor HC may also result in severe, occasionally lethal GVHD, since it has not yet been clearly shown that effector cells of GVL and GVHD can be separated (Slavin et al. 1990c). Several experimental systems, however, suggest that functionally, GVL may be induced in the absence of clinically significant or clinically detectable GVHD (Slavin et al. 1990c) following induction of graft-versus-host tolerance using total lymphoid irradiation (Weiss et al. 1990; Slavin et al. 1981), following other BMT procedures (Okunewick and Meredith 1981; Truitt et al. 1983), and following immunological reconstitution in stable chimeras after induction of tolerance with T-cell–depleted allografts (Weiss et al. 1990). Effective GVL independent of GVHD was successfully accomplished with delayed administration of immunocompetent T cells after establishment of stable chimerism (Slavin et al. 1978), as well as, paradoxically, following administration of a short course of high-dose rIL-2 immediately following allogeneic BMT (Sykes et al. 1990).

Documentation of T-cell clones with specific reactivity against tumor cells and no cytolytic activity against normal syngeneic host blasts (Van Lochem, De Gast, and Goulmy 1992) suggests that effector cells of GVL and GVHD may be separable in principle. Recent analysis from a large series of patients undergoing allogeneic BMT from the International Bone Marrow Transplant Registry confirmed that, indeed, GVL may operate, at least in part, independently of GVHD (Horowitz et al. 1990).

■ CONCLUSIONS AND FUTURE DIRECTIONS

Effective immunotherapy of immunogenic tumor cells by cell therapy can be documented in experimental animals.

Although the final effector cell is Ag-specific CD8$^+$ in the majority of tumor cell systems, CD4$^+$-dependent help or exogenous supply of IL-2 seem mandatory for successful eradication of syngeneic tumor cells. Macrophages and macrophage-activating factors as well as CD4$^+$ cells display an essential role in generation of antitumor responses. NK cells may play a role, too, but their effect is short term and limited.

Antitumor effector cells can be generated and expanded in vitro against immunogenic tumors and used as immunotherapy together with cytokines such as rIL-1, rIL-2, rHuGM-CSF, and IFN-γ to stimulate macrophages and Ag presenting cells.

Unfortunately, a large majority of human tumor cells are nonimmunogenic and, therefore, effective autochtonous antitumor responses cannot be anticipated. Fortunately, recent clinical investigations based on exciting animal data suggest that allo-cell mediated immunities may be used by adoptive transfer of matched or partially mismatched immunocompetent lymphocytes into immunocompromised recipients following allogeneic and even autologous BMT. Successful eradication of MRD and occasionally larger tumor inocula in ongoing clinical studies suggests that various strategies using allo-CMI may be effectively used for patients who have major HC-matched donors available for prevention as well as for treatment of established relapse following BMT (Chapters 24 and 25). Thus, there seems no doubt that allogeneic cell therapy stands out as the most effective anticancer modality for patients relapsing after allogeneic BMT who would normally not be candidates for any alternative curative modality except a second BMT, which is rarely successful.

ACKNOWLEDGMENTS

This work was supported in part by a research grant by Baxter International Healthcare Corporation; a grant from the German Israel Foundation (GIF); and a grant from the Chief Scientist's office, Israel's Ministry of Health (to S. Slavin).

REFERENCES

Ackerstein, A., Kedar, E., and Slavin, S. (1991) Use of recombinant human interleukin-2 in conjunction with syngeneic bone marrow transplantation as a model for control of minimal residual disease in malignant hematological disorders. *Blood*, **78**, 1212–15.

Adams, D.O. and Hamilton, T.A. (1984) The cell biology of macrophage activation. *Annual Review of Immunology*, **2**, 283–318.

Alexander, P., Evans, R., and Grant, C.K. (1972) The interplay of lymphoid cells and macrophages in tumour immunity. *Annals of the Institut Pasteur, Paris*, **122**, 645–58.

Apperley, J.F., Jones, L., Hale, G., and Waldmann, H. (1986) Bone marrow transplantation for patients with chronic myeloid leukaemia: T-cell depletion with Campath-1 reduces the incidence of graft-versus-host disease but may increase the risk of leukaemic relapse. *Bone Marrow Transplantation*, **1**, 53–66.

Archer, T.P., Bretscher, P., and Ziola, B. (1990) Immunotherapy of the rat 137625C mammary adenocarcinoma by vaccinia virus augmentation of tumor immunity. *Clinical and Experimental Metastasis*, **8**, 519–32.

Bashford, E.F. (1904) The transmissibility of malignant new growths from one animal to another. *Scientific Report of the Cancer Research Fund* (later *Imperial Cancer Research Fund*), London, UK, **1**, 11–15.

Baldwin, R.W. (1955) Immunity to methylcholanthrene-induced tumours in inbred rats following atrophy and regression of the implanted tumours. *British Journal of Cancer*, **9**, 652–7.

Baldwin, R.W. (1976) Relevant animal models for tumor immunotherapy. *Cancer Immunology, Immunotherapy*, **1**, 197–8.

Bittner, J.J. (1932) Genetic studies on the transplantation of tumors. III. Interpretations of apparent rhythms. *American Journal of Cancer*, **16**, 1144–52.

Boon, T. (1983) Antigen tumor cell variants obtained with mitogens. *Advances in Cancer Research*, **39**, 121–51.

Boon, T., Van Pel, A., De Plaen, E., et al. (1989) Genes coding for T-cell-defined tum transplantation antigens: point mutations, antigenic peptides, and subgenic expression. *Cold Spring Harbor Symposia on Quantitative Biology*, **1**, 587–96.

Boon, T., Van Pel, A., and De Plaen, E. (1989) Tum- transplantation antigens, point mutations, and antigenic peptides: a model for tumor-specific transplantation antigens? *Cancer Cells*, **1**, 25–8.

Burnet, F.M. (1970) The concept of immunological surveillance. *Progress in Experimental Tumor Research*, **13**, 1–27.

Campbell, M.J., Esserman, L., Byars, N.E., Allison, A.C., and Levy, R. (1990) Idiotype vaccination against murine B cell lymphoma. Humoral and cellular requirements for the full expression of antitumor immunity. *Journal of Immunology*, **145**, 1029–36.

Cheever, M.A., Greenberg, P.D., and Fefer, A. (1980) Specificity of adoptive chemoimmunotherapy of established syngeneic tumors. *Journal of Immunology*, **125**, 711–4.

Cheever, M.A., Greenberg, P.D., and Fefer, A. (1981) Specific adoptive therapy of established leukemia with syngeneic lymphocytes nonspecifically expanded by culture with interleukin 2. *Journal of Immunology*, **126**, 1318–22.

Cheever, M.A., Greenberg, P.D., Fefer, A., and Gillis, S. (1982) Augmentation of the antitumor therapeutic efficacy of long-term cultured T lymphocytes by in vivo administration of purified interleukin 2. *Journal of Experimental Medicine*, **155**, 968–80.

Cohen, P., Vourka-Karussis, U., Weiss, L., and Slavin, S. (1993) Spontaneous and IL-2 induced anti-leukemic and anti-host effects against tumor- and host-specific alloantigens. *Journal of Immunology*, **151**, 4803–10.

Dailey, M.O., Pellemer, E., and Weissman, I.L. (1982) Protection against syngeneic lymphoma by a long-lived cytotoxic T-cell clone. *Proceedings of the National Academy of Sciences of the United States of America*, **79**, 5384–7.

De Graaf, P.W., Horak, E., and Bookman, M.A. (1988) Adoptive immunotherapy of syngeneic murine leukemia is enhanced by the combination of recombinant IFN-gamma and a tumor-specific cytotoxic T cell clone. *Journal of Immunology*, **140**, 2853–7.

Drysdale, B.E., Agarwal, S., and Shin, H.S. (1988) Macrophage-mediated tumoricidal activity: mechanisms of activation and cytotoxicity. *Progress in Allergy*, **40**, 111–61.

Eglitis, M.A., Kantoff, P., Gilboa, E., and Anderson, W.F. (1985) Gene expression in mice after high efficiency retroviral-mediated gene transfer. *Science*, **230**, 1395.

Esshar, Z., Waks, T., Gross, G., and Schindler, D. (1993) Specific activation and targetting of cytotoxic lymphocytes through chimeric single-chain consisting of antibody binding domains and the gamma or zeta subunits of the immunoglobulin and T cell receptor. *Proceedings of the National Academy of Sciences of the United States of America*, **90**, 720–4.

Evans, R. and Alexander, P. (1972) Mechanism of immunologically specific killing of tumour cells by macrophages. *Nature*, **236**, 168–70.

Fidler, I.J. and Schroit, A.J. (1988) Recognition and destruction of neoplastic cells by activated macrophages: discrimination of altered self. *Biochemistry and Biophysics*, **948**, 151–73.

Foa, R., Guarini, A., Cignetti, A., Cronin, K., Rosenthal, F., and Gansbacher, B. (1994) Cytokine gene therapy: a new strategy for the management of cancer patients. *Natural Immunity*, **13**, 65–75.

Foley, E.J. (1953) Antigenic properties of methylcholanthrene-induced tumors in mice of the strain of origin. *Cancer Research*, **13**, 835–7.

Freedman, R.S., Bowen, J.M., Herson, J.H., Wharton, J.T., Edwards, C.L., and Rutledge, F.N. (1983) Immunotherapy for vulvar carcinoma with virus-modified homologous extracts. *Obstetrics and Gynecology*, **62**, 707–14.

Fujiwara, H., Fukuzawa, M., Yoshioka, T., Nakajima, H., and Hamaoka, T. (1984) The role of tumor-specific Lyt-1+2-T cells in eradicating tumor cells in vivo. I. Lyt-1+2-T cells do not necessarily require recruitment of host's cytotoxic T cell precursors for implementation of in vivo immunity. *Journal of Immunology*, **133**, 1671–6.

Furukawa, K., Lotzova, E., Freedman, R.S., et al. (1989) Effect of virus-modified tumor cell extracts, autologous mononuclear cell infusions and interleukin-2 on oncolytic activity of effector cells of patients with advanced ovarian cancer. *Cancer Immunology, Immunotherapy*, **30**, 126–32.

Geiner, J.W., Hand, P.H., Noguchi, P., et al. (1984) Enhanced expression of surface tumor-associated antigens of human breast and colon tumor cells after recombinant leukocyte α-interferon treatment. *Cancer Research*, **44**, 3208.

Giorgio, C. and Guido, F. (1974) Cell reactivity toward syngeneic neoplastic cells in mice hypersensitized to dinitrophenol. *European Journal of Cancer*, **10**, 103–6.

Glennie, M.J., Brennand, D.M., Bryden, F., et al. (1988) Bispecific F(ABγ)$_2$ antibody for the delivery of saporin in the treatment of lymphoma. *Journal of Immunology*, **141**, 3662–70.

Greenberg, P.D. (1986) Therapy of murine leukemia with cyclophosphamide and immune Lyt-2+ cells: cytolytic T cells can mediate eradication of disseminated leukemia. *Journal of Immunology*, **136**, 1917–22.

Greenberg, P.D. (1991) Adoptive T cell therapy of tumors: mechanisms operative in the recognition and elimination of tumor cells. *Advances in Immunology*, **49**, 281–355.

Groopman, J.E. (1987) Neoplasms in the acquired immune deficiency syndrome: the multidisciplinary approach to treatment. *Seminars in Oncology*, **14**, 1–6.

Hanna, N. and Burton, R.C. (1981) Definitive evidence that natural killer (NK) cells inhibit experimental tumor metastasis in vivo. *Journal of Immunology*, **127**, 1754–8.

Hanna, N. and Fidler I.J. (1980) Role of natural killer cells in the destruction of circulating tumor emboli. *Journal of the National Cancer Institute*, **65**, 801–9.

Herberman, R.B., Nunn, M.E., and Lavrin, D.H. (1975) Natural cytotoxic reactivity of mouse lymphoid cells against syngeneic and allogeneic tumors. I. Distribution of reactivity and specificity. *International Journal of Cancer*, **16**, 216–29.

Hewitt, H.B., Blake, E.R., and Walder, A.S. (1976) A critique of the evidence for active host defence against cancer, based on personal studies of 27 murine tumors of spontaneous origin. *British Journal of Cancer*, **33**, 241–59.

Hibbs, J.B., Jr., Vavrin, Z., and Taintor R.R. (1987) L-Arginine is required for expression of the activated macrophage effector mechanism causing selective metabolic inhibition in target cells. *Journal of Immunology*, **138**, 550–65.

Hoover, H.C., Brandhorst, J.S., Peters, L.C., et al. (1993) Adjuvant active specific immunotherapy for human colorectal cancer: 6.5-year median follow up of a phase III prospectively randomized trial. *Journal of Clinical Oncology*, **3**, 390–9.

Horowitz, M., Gale, R.P., Sondel, P.M., et al. (1990) Graft vs. leukemia reactions after bone marrow transplantation. *Blood*, **75**, 555–64.

Iwaki, H., Barnovan, Y., Bash, J., and Wallack, M.K. (1989) Vaccinia virus-infected C-C36 colon tumor cell lysates stimulate cellular responses in vitro and protect syngeneic BALB/C mice from tumor cell challenge. *Journal of Surgical Oncology*, **40**, 90–6.

Jaffee, E.M., Dranoff, G., Cohen, K.L., et al. (1993) High efficiency gene transfer into primary human tumor explants without cell selection. *Cancer Research*, **53**, 2221–6.

Jaffee, H.A., Daniel, C., Longenecker, G., et al. (1992) Adenovirus-mediated in vivo gene transfer and expression in normal rat liver. *Nature Genetics*, **5**, 372–8.

Johnson, B.D., Drobyski, W.R., and Truitt, R.L. (1993) Delayed infusion of normal donor cells after MHC-matched bone marrow transplantation provides an antileukemia reaction without graft-versus-host disease. *Bone Marrow Transplantation*, **11**, 329–36.

Jorge, A., Leon, M., Carolina, G., et al. (1992) Modulation of the antigenic phenotype of human breast carcinoma cells by modifiers of protein kinase C activity and recombinant human interferons. *Cancer Immunology, Immunotherapy*, **35**, 315–24.

June, C.H., Bluestone, J.A., Nadler, L.M., and Thompson, C.B. (1994) The B7 and CD28 receptor families. *Immunology Today*, **15**, 321–31.

Karre, K., Ljunggren, H.G., Piontek, G., and Kiessling, R. (1986) Selective rejection of 11-2-deficient lymphoma variants suggests alternative immune defence strategy. *Nature*, **319**, 675–8.

Klarnet, J.P., Matis, L.A., Kern, D.E., et al. (1987) Antigen-driven T cell clones can proliferate in vivo, eradicate disseminated leukemia and provide specific immunologic memory. *Journal of Immunology*, **138**, 4012–7.

Klein, G. (1978) Commentary and overview. In N.A. Mitchison and M. Landy (Eds.) *Manipulation of the immune response in cancer*, pp. 339–353. London, Academic.

Klein, G., Sjogren, H.O., Klein, E., and Hellstrom K.E. (1960) Demonstration of resistance against methylcholanthrene-induced sarcomas in the primary autochthonous host. *Cancer Research*, **20**, 1561–72.

Klein, J. (1975) *Biology of the mouse histocompatibility-2 complex*, 620 pp. New York, Springer-Verlag.

Korngold, R., Leighton, C., and Manser, T. (1994) Graft-versus-myeloid leukemia responses following syngeneic and allogeneic bone marrow transplantation. *Transplantation*, **58**, 278–87.

Loeb, L. (1906–1907) Further experimental investigations into the growth of tumors. Development of sarcoma and carcinoma after the inoculation of a carcinomatous tumor of the submaxillary gland in a Japanese mouse. *University of Pennsylvania Medical Bulletin*, **19**, 2124–6.

Leon, J.A., Mesa-Tejada, R., Gutierrez, M.C., et al. (1989) Increased surface expression and shedding of tumor associated antigens by human breast carcinoma cells treated with recombinant human interferons or phorbol ester tumor promoters. *Anticancer Research*, **9**, 1639.

Little, C.C. and Tyzzer, E.E. (1915–1916) Further experimental studies on the inheritance of susceptibility to a transplantable tumor, carcinoma (J.W.A.)

of the Japanese waltzing mouse. *Journal of Medical Research*, **33** (New Ser. 28), 393–53.

Matis, L.A., Shu, S., Groves, E.S., et al. (1986) Adoptive immunotherapy of a syngeneic murine leukemia with a tumor-specific cytotoxic T cell clone and recombinant human interleukin 2: correlation with clonal IL-2 receptor expression. *Journal of Immunology*, **136**, 3496–501.

McCune, C.S., O'Donnel, R.W., Marquis, D.M., and Sahasrabudhe, D.M. (1990) Renal cell carcinoma treated by vaccines for active specific immunotherapy: correlation of survival with skin testing by autologous tumor cells. *Cancer Immunology, Immunotherapy*, **32**, 62–66.

Melief, C.J. and Kast, W.M. (1992) Lessons from T cell responses to virus induced tumors for cancer eradication in general. *Cancer Surveys*, **13**, 81–99.

Miller, A.D. (1992) Human gene therapy comes of age. *Nature*, **357**, 455–60.

Mills, C.D. and North, R.J. (1985) Ly-1+2-suppressorT cells inhibit the expression of passively transferred antitumor immunity by suppressing the generation of cytolytic T cells. *Transplantation*, **39**, 202–8.

Moller, G. (Ed.) (1976) Experiments and the concept of immunological surveillance. *Transplantation Review*, **28**, 1–97.

Morecki, S., Revel-Vilk, S., Nabet, C., et al. (1992) Immunological evaluation of patients with hematological malignancies receiving ambulatory cytokine mediated immunotherapy with recombinant human interferon-α2a and interleukin-2. *Cancer Immunology, Immunotherapy*, **35**, 401–11.

Moretta, A., Vitale, M., Bottino, C., et al. (1993) P58 molecules as putative receptors for major histocompatibility complex (MHC) class I molecules in human natural killer (NK) cells. Anti-p58 antibodies reconstitute lysis of MHC class l-protected cells in NK clones displaying different specificities. *Journal of Experimental Medicine*, **178**, 597–604.

Morton, D.L., Foshag, L.J., Hoon, D.S., et al. (1992) Prolongation of survival of metastatic melanoma after active specific immunotherapy with a new polyvalent melanoma vaccine. *Annals of Surgery*, **216**, 463–82.

Mule, J.J., Rosenstein, M., Shu, S., and Rosenberg, S.A. (1985) Eradication of a disseminated syngeneic lymphoma by systemic adoptive transfer of immune lymphocytes is dependent upon a host component(s). *Cancer Research*, **45**, 526–31.

Nagler, A., Ackerstein, A., Barak, V., and Slavin, S. (1994) Treatment of chronic myelogenous leukemia with recombinant human interleukin-2 and interferon-α2a. *Journal of Hematotherapy*, **3**, 75–82.

Naor, D. (1979) Suppressor cells: permitters and promoters of malignancy. *Advances in Cancer Research*, **29**, 45–125.

Nathan, C.F. and Cohn, Z.A. (1981) Antitumor effects of hydrogen peroxide in vivo. *Journal of Experimental Medicine*, **154**, 1539–53.

Okada, H., Wakamiya, N., Okada, N., and Kato, S. (1987) Sensitization of human tumor cells to homologous complement by vaccinia virus treatment. *Cancer Immunology, Immunotherapy*, **25**, 7–9.

Okunewick, J.P. and Meredith, R.F. (1981) *Graft-versus-leukemia in man and animal models*, pp. 1–265. Boca Raton, FL, CRC Press.

Onozaki, K., Matsushima, K., Aggarwal, B.B., and Oppenheim, J.J. (1985) Human interleukin I is a cytocidal factor for several tumor cell lines. *Journal of Immunology*, **135**, 3962–8.

Or, R., Nagler, A., Ackerstein, A., et al. (1995) Allogeneic cell-mediated immunotherapy at the minimal residual disease stage following autologous stem cell transplantation for malignant lymphoma. (Submitted for publication.)

Or, R., Nagler, A., Samuel, S., et al. (1993) Autologous transplantation (AT) using combined bone marrow (EM) + peripheral blood stem cells (PBSC) for patients with malignant lymphomas and solid tumors. *Blood*, **82**, 670.

Outzen, H.C., Custer, R.P., Eaton, G.J., and Prehn, R.J. (1975) Spontaneous and induced tumor incidence in germfree "nude" mice. *Journal of the Reticuloendothelial Society*, **17**, 1–9.

Pardol, D.M. (1993) Cancer vaccines. *Immunology Today*, **14**, 310.

Parr, I. (1972) Response of syngeneic murine lymphoma to immunotherapy in relation to the antigenicity of the tumour. *British Journal of Cancer*, **26**, 174–82.

Paulnock, D.M. and Lambert, L.E. (1990) Identification and characterization of monoclonal antibodies specific for macrophages at intermediate stages in the tumoricidal activation pathway. *Journal of Immunology*, **144**, 765–73.

Perussia, B., Santoli, D., and Trinchieri, G. (1980) Interferon modulation of natural killer cell activity. *Annals of the New York Academy of Sciences*, **350**, 55–62.

Plautz, G.E., Yang, Z.Y., Wu, B.Y., Gao, X., Huang, L., and Nabel, G.J. (1993) Immunotherapy of malignancy by in vivo gene transfer into tumors. *Proceedings of the National Academy of Sciences of the United States of America*, **10**, 4645–9.

Pomer, S., Thiele, R., Riedasch, G., Wiesel, M., Schirrmacher, V., and Staehler, G. (1992) Combined vaccination with autologous tumor material and subcutaneously administered rIL-2 and rIFN-α-2b in the trreatment of renal cell carcinoma. In G. Staehler and S. Pomer (Eds.) *Basic and clinical research in renal cell carcinoma*, pp. 212–20. Berlin, Heidelberg, Springer-Verlag.

Prehn, R.T. and Main, J.M. (1957) Immunity to methylcholanthrene-induced sarcomas. *Journal of the National Cancer Institute*, **18**, 769–78.

Purtilo, D.T. (1984) Biology of disease: defective immune surveillance of viral carcinogenesis. *Laboratory Investigation*, **51**, 373–85.

Reed, W.P. and Lucas, Z.J. (1975) Cytotoxic activity of lymphocytes. V. Role of soluble toxin in macrophage-inhibited cultures of tumor cells. *Journal of Immunology*, **115**, 395–404.

Revesz, L. (1960) Detection of antigenic differences in isologous host-tumor systems by pretreatment with heavily irradiated tumor cells. *Cancer Research*, **20**, 443–51.

Ringden, O. and Horowitz, M.M. (1989) Graft-versus-leukemia reactions in humans. *Transplantation Proceedings*, **21**, 2989.

Rosenberg, S. (1991) Immunotherapy and gene therapy of cancer. *Cancer Research*, **51**(Suppl.), 5074s–9s.

Rosenberg, S.A. and Lotze, M.T. (1986) Cancer immunotherapy using interleukin-2 and interleukin-2-activated lymphocytes. *Annual Review of Immunology*, **4**, 681–709.

Rosenberg, S.A., Packard, B.S., Aebersold, P.M., et al. (1988) Use of tumor-infiltrating lymphocytes and interleukin-2 in the immunotherapy of patients with metastatic melanoma. A preliminary report. *New England Journal of Medicine*, **319**, 1676–80.

Rous, P. (1910) An experimental comparison of transplanted tumor and a transplanted normal tissue capable of growth. *Journal of Experimental Medicine*, **12**, 344–65.

Rygaardc, J. and Povlsen, C.O. (1976) The nude mouse vs. the hypothesis of immunological surveillance. *Transplantation Review,* **28,** 43–61.

Schild, H.J., Kyewski, B., von Hoegen, P., and Schirrmacher, V. (1987) CD4$^+$ helper T cells are required for resistance to a highly metastatic murine tumor. *European Journal of Immunology,* **17,** 1863–6.

Schirrmacher, V. (1989) Immunobiology and immunotherapy of cancer metastases. *Interdisciplinary Science Review,* **14,** 291–303.

Scott, O.C. (1991) Tumor transplantation and tumor immunity: a personal view. *Cancer Research,* **51,** 757–63.

Sendo, F., Aoki, T., Boyse, E.A., and Buafo, C.K. (1975) Natural occurrence of lymphocytes showing cytotoxic activity to BALB/c radiation-induced leukemia RL-male-1 cells. *Journal of the National Cancer Institute,* **55,** 603–29.

Shimizu, Y., Hasumi, K., Masubuchi, K., and Okudairea, Y. (1988) Immunotherapy of tumor-bearing mice utilizing virus help. *Cancer Immunology, Immunotherapy,* **27,** 223–7.

Shoham, J., Hirsch, R., Zakay-Rones, Z., Osband, M.E., and Brennert, H.J. (1990) Augmentation of tumor cell immunogenicity by viruses – an approach to specific immunotherapy of cancer. *Natural Immunology and Cell Growth Regulation,* **9,** 165–72.

Slavin, S., Ackerstein, A., Hardan, I., et al. (1990a) Towards improvement of therapeutic strategies in leukemia by amplification of the immune responses against leukemia. *Hematology and Blood Transfusion,* **33,** 36–40.

Slavin, S., Ackerstein, A., Nagler, A., Naparstek, E., and Weiss, L. (1990b) Cell-mediated cytokine-activated immunotherapy (CCI) of malignant hematological disorders for eradication of minimal residual disease (MRD) in conjunction with conventional chemotherapy or bone marrow transplantation (BMT). *Blood,* **76,** 566a.

Slavin, S., Ackerstein, A., Naparstek, E., et al. (1990c) Hypothesis: the graft-versus-leukemia (GVL) phenomenon: is GVL separable from GVHD? *Bone Marrow Transplantation,* **6,** 155–6l.

Slavin, S., Ackerstein, A., and Weiss, L. (1988) Adoptive immunotherapy in conjunction with bone marrow transplantation – amplification of natural host defence mechanisms against cancer by recombinant IL2. *Natural Immunology and Cell Growth Regulation,* **7,** 180–4.

Slavin, S., Ackerstein, A., Weiss, L., Nagler, A., Or, R., and Naparstek, E. (1992a) Induction of tumor dormancy in BALB/c mice against nonimmunogenic B cell leukemia. In T.H. Stewart and E.F. Wheelock (Eds.) *Cellular immune mechanisms and tumor dormancy,* pp. 99–110. Bota Raton FL, CRC Press.

Slavin, S., Ackerstein, A., Weiss, L., Nagler, A., Or, R., and Naparstek, E. (1992b) Eradication of minimal residual disease (MRD) following autologous (ABMT) and allogeneic bone marrow transplantation (BMT) by cytokine-mediated immunotherapy (CMI) and cell mediated cytokine-activated immunotherapy (CCI) in experimental animals and man. *Blood,* **80,** 535.

Slavin, S., Fuks, Z., Kaplan, H.S., and Strober, S. (1978) Transplantation of allogeneic bone marrow without graft vs. host disease using total lymphoid irradiation. *Journal of Experimental Medicine,* **147,** 963–72.

Slavin S. and Kedar, E. (1988) Current problems and future goals in clinical bone marrow transplantation. *Blood Reviews,* **2,** 259–69.

Slavin, S. and Nagler, A. (1991) New developments in bone marrow transplantation. *Current Opinion in Oncology,* **3,** 254–71.

Slavin, S., Naparstek, E., Nagler, A., Ackerstein, A., Drakos, P., Kapelushnik, Y., Brautbar, C., and Or, R. (1993a) Cell mediated immunotherapy (CMI) for the treatment of malignant hematological diseases in conjunction with autologous bone marrow transplantation (ABMT). *Blood*, **82**, 1152.

Slavin, S., Naparstek, E., Nagler, A., et al. (1993b) Graft vs leukemia (GVL) effects with controlled GVHD by cell mediated immunotherapy (CMI) following allogeneic bone marrow transplantation (BMT). *Blood*, **82**, 1677.

Slavin, S., Or, R., Naparstek, E., et al. (1992c) Immunotherapy of minimal residual disease by immunocompetent lymphocytes and their activation by cytokines. *Cancer Investigation*, **10**, 221–7.

Slavin, S., Weiss, L., Ackerstein, A., et al. (1992d) Establishment of graft vs leukemia (GVL)-like effects in leukemia in conjunction with autologous BMT (ABMT) in experimental animals and man. *European Bone Marrow Transplantation*, 209.

Slavin, S., Weiss, L., Morecki, S., and Weigensberg, M. (1981) Eradication of murine leukemia with histoincompatible marrow grafts in mice conditioned with total lymphoid irradiation (TLI). *Cancer Immunology, Immunotherapy*, **11**, 155.

Sullivan, K.M., Weiden, P.L., and Storb, R. (1989) Influence of acute and chronic graft-versus-host disease on relapse and survival after bone marrow transplantation from HLA-identical siblings as treatment of acute and chronic leukemia. *Blood*, **73**, 1720–6.

Sykes, M., Romick, M. L., and Sachs, D. H. (1990) Interleukin 2 prevents graft-versus-host disease without diminishing the graft-versus-leukemia effect of allogeneic lymphocytes. *Proceedings of the National Academy of Sciences of the United States of America*, **87**, 5633.

Talmadge, J.E., Meyers, K.M., Prieur, D.J., and Starkey, J.R. (1980) Role of natural killer cells in tumor growth and metastasis. C57BL/6 normal and beige mice. *Journal of the National Cancer Institute*, **65**, 929–35.

Tepper, R.I. and Mule, J.J. (1994) Experimental and clinical studies of cytokine gene-modified tumor cells. *Human Gene Therapy*, **5**, 153–64.

Tomita, S., Fujiwara, H., Yamane, Y., et al. (1986) Demonstration of intratumoral infiltration of tumor-specific Lyt-1+2-T cells mediating delayed-type hypersensitivity response and in vivo protective immunity. *Japanese Journal of Cancer Research*, **77**, 182–9.

Townsend, S. and Allison, J.P. (1993) Tumor rejection after direct costimulation of CD8$^+$ T cells by B7 transfected melanoma cells. *Science*, **259**, 367–70.

Truitt, R.L., Shih, C.-Y., Lelevre, A.V., Tempelis, L.D., Andreani, M., and Bortin, M.M. (1983) Characterization of alloimmunization-induced T lymphocytes reactive against AKR leukemia in vitro and correlation with graft-versus-leukemia activity in vivo. *Journal of Immunology*, **131**, 2050.

Tyzzer, E.E. (1909) A study of inheritance in mice with reference to their susceptibility to transplantable tumors. *Journal of Medical Research*, **21** (New Ser. 16), 519–73.

Tyzzer, E.E. (1916) Tumor immunity. *Journal of Cancer Research*, **1**, 125–55.

Van Lochem, E., De Gast, B., and Goulmy, E. (1992) In vitro separation of host specific graft vs host and graft vs leukemia cytotoxic T cell activities. *Bone Marrow Transplantation*, **10**, 181–3.

Vitetta, E.S. (1994) From the basic science of B cells to biological missiles at the bedside. *Journal of Immunology*, **153**, 1407–20.

Vourka-Karussis, U., Karussis, D., Ackerstein, A., and Slavin S. (1994) Enhancement of graft versus leukemia effect (GVL) with recombinant human interleukin 2 (rIL-2) following bone marrow transplantation in a murine model for acute myeloid leukemia in SJL/J mice. *Experimental Hematology*, **23**, 196–201.

Wallack, M.K. and Sivanandham, M. (1993) A randomized prospective trial using VMO for stage II melanoma. *New York Academy of Science*, Washington, DC, Abstract #22.

Ward, B.A., Shu, S., Chou, T., Perry-Lalley, D., and Chang, A.E. (1988) Cellular basis of immunologic interactions in adoptive T cell therapy of established metastases from a syngeneic murine sarcoma. *Journal of Immunology*, **141**, 1047–53.

Weiden, P.L., Fluornoy, N., and Thomas, E.D. (1979) Antileukemic effects of graft versus host disease in human recipients of allogeneic marrow grafts. *New England Journal of Medicine*, **300**, 1068–72.

Weiss, L., Lubin, I., Factorowich, Y., et al. (1994) Effective graft vs leukemia effects independently of graft vs. host disease following T-cell depleted allogeneic bone marrow transplantation in a murine model of B-cell leukemia/lymphoma (BCLl); role of cell therapy and rIL-2. *Journal of Immunology*, **153**, 2562–67.

Weiss, L., Reich, S., and Slavin, S. (1990) Effect of cyclosporine A and methylprednisone on the GVL effect across major histocompatibility transplantation. *Bone Marrow Transplantation*, **6**, 229–33.

Weiss, L., Reich, S., and Slavin, S. (1992) Use of recombinant human interleukin-2 in conjunction with bone marrow transplantation as a model for control of minimal residual disease in malignant hematological disorders. I. Treatment of murine leukemia in conjunction with allogeneic bone marrow transplantation and IL2-activated cell-mediated immunotherapy. *Cancer Investigation*, **10**, 19–26.

Weiss, L., Weigensberg, M., Morecki, S., et al. (1990) Characterization of effector cells of graft vs. leukemia (GVL) following allogeneic bone marrow transplantation in mice inoculated with murine B-cell leukemia (BCLl). *Cancer Immunology, Immunotherapy*, **31**, 236–42.

Wheelock, E.F. (1979) The tumor dormant state. Comparison of L5178Y cells used to establish dormancy with those that emerge after its termination. *Journal of Experimental Medicine*, **149**, 745–57.

Woglom, W.H. (1929) Immunity to transplantable tumours. (1929) *Cancer Reviews*, **4**, 129–14.

Wolf, A. (1969) The activity of cell-free tumour fractions in inducing immunity across a weak histocompatibility barrier. *Transplantation*, **7**, 49–58.

Yamasaki, T., Handa, H., Yanashita, J., Watanabe, Y., Namba, Y., and Hanaoka, M. (1984) Specific adoptive immunotherapy with tumor-specific cytotoxic T-lymphocyte clone for murine malignant gliomas. *Cancer Research*, **44**, 1776–83.

Zhu, N., Leggitt, D., Liu, Y., and Debs, R. (1993) Systemic gene expression after intravenous DNA delivery into adult mice. *Science*, **261**, 209–11.

Hemopoietic Cell Therapy

PART A

Scientific Principles

3

Current and Potential Uses of Defined Cell Populations

MICHAEL LILL AND JUDITH C. GASSON

Defined cell populations may consist of either an enriched population of cells with a common phenotype or the absence of a population of cells with unwanted characteristics. Many of the technologies used to achieve these goals may result in both the enrichment of the desired population and the simultaneous purging of an unwanted fraction of cells. The cells may be separated on the basis of physical characteristics (e.g., density-gradient centrifugation or elutriation). Alternatively, the basis for separation may be immunophenotype such as by fluorescence-activated cell sorting (FACS) analysis or physical separation based on antigen-antibody (Ag-Ab) interactions, (biotinylated Ab and streptavidin column, Ab covalently bound to flasks, magnetic spheres, microspheres, or iron-dextran particles). Separation by immunophenotype may use directly conjugated Ab or an indirect step involving a second Ab.

This chapter will focus mainly on positively selected populations that can be isolated from peripheral blood (PB) and/or bone marrow (BM); however, it is important to note the role of T-cell depletion in allogeneic bone-marrow transplantation (BMT) as well as the role of tumor purging in autologous BMT. There is increasing interest in depletion of specific T-cell subsets, depletion of defined numbers of T cells, or removal with later addition of T cells in an attempt to preserve the graft-versus-leukemia (GVL) effect without graft-versus-host disease (GVHD) (Truitt and Atasoylu 1991a, b; Johnson, Drobyski, and Truitt 1993; Champlin et al. 1990).

The area of tumor purging remains controversial. It is clear that many techniques available in the laboratory and in clinical use are able to purge tumor cells from the BMT product. The clinical significance of tumor purging remains to be proven in clinical trials.

Ideally, these would be prospective randomized studies, but will likely be gene-marking studies. If tumor purging has a significant effect on patient survival, then optimal methods and levels of purging will remain to be resolved.

■ CD34⁺ CELLS

Use in Transplantation

The CD34 (My10) Ag, first described by Civin et al. (1984), is expressed on all hemopoietic progenitor cells including the pluripotent hemopoietic stem cell (HSC). These cells constitute between 0.5% and 2% of BM mononuclear cells (MNC) and fewer then 1% of PB MNC unless they have been mobilized by the use of cytokines, chemotherapy, or a combination of the two (Bender et al. 1994; Brugger et al. 1992; Siena et al. 1992; Brugger et al. 1993a; Kanz, Brugger, and Mertelsmann 1993; Haylock et al. 1990; Ho et al. 1994; Begley et al. 1992; DeLuca et al. 1992; Grigg et al. 1993; Sheridan et al. 1992). Several commercial devices are available for positive selection of CD34⁺ cells. These devices are currently undergoing clinical trials in transplantation (Berenson et al. 1988a, b; Berenson et al. 1990; Berenson et al. 1991; Shpall et al. 1992, 1993, 1994). In general, most of these devices will give a yield of approximately 50% of the starting population of CD34⁺ cells with a purity of 50% to 90% CD34⁺ cells reflecting a 2-log enrichment. Clinical studies have shown that these selected cells are capable of engraftment whether they are derived from the BM or the PB (Shpall et al. 1994). Furthermore, the time to engraftment is the same as for the original unselected product (Shpall et al. 1994). The major clinical advantages to this type of autologous transplantation are a decrease in the total cell volume and, hence, dimethyl sulfoxide (DMSO) infused (with a subsequent reduction in DMSO toxicity) and some degree of tumor purging (see below). Significant side effects including anaphylactoid reactions can be the result of DMSO infusion; however, in our routine clinical practice, these reactions are usually easily manageable by premedication with hydrocortisone and diphenhydramine and slowing the infusion rate.

The major disadvantages of CD34 selection are the added time and cost of the procedure and a reduction in the total number of CD34⁺ cells infused. An interesting potential role for CD34 selection is in allogeneic BMT in which the technique would be used as a form of T-cell depletion. Clinical studies using CD34-selected peripheral blood progenitor cells (PBPC) in allogeneic BMT are currently underway at a number of centers. It is possible that the combination of mobilized PBPC and T-cell depletion may enable haplotype-mismatched allogeneic transplants to be done more safely (Aversa et al. 1994).

Use of CD34 selection results in a 2- to 4-log depletion of tumor cells in patients with breast cancer or myeloma (Shpall et al. 1994; Schiller, Vescio, and Freytes, et al. unpublished data). It is possible that CD34 selection could be coupled with an additional purging step that would further deplete the transplant product of tumor cells. The purging would be more effective because the starting product had a much smaller volume as well as a smaller number of tumor cells present. As mentioned above, the clinical significance of this degree of purging remains to be determined.

Ex Vivo Expansion ("Graft Engineering")

The second role for CD34-selected hemopoietic progenitor cells is in ex vivo expansion (see Chapter 16). There are several potential (and likely conflicting) roles or aims for different ex vivo–expansion programs: to produce a population of almost-mature myeloid cells that would abrogate neutropenia following BMT; to produce a population of almost-mature megakaryocytes that would abrogate thrombocytopenia following BMT; to expand a population of genuinely pluripotent and self-renewing HSC with the aim of either performing multiple transplants or obtaining sufficient stem cells from a 0.5-L aliquot of PB to provide a safe transplant product; and production of natural killer (NK) cells (see also Chapter 13).

The majority of these programs will require an initiating population of CD34$^+$ stem cells. This is partially because of potential inhibitory effects of mature neutrophils and monocytes upon the ex vivo expansion and partially to minimize the volumes of tissue culture medium and subsequent growth factor addition required to obtain an adequate degree of expansion. The cytokines added to the CD34-selected hemopoietic progenitor cells will be chosen to stimulate the progenitor cells to produce the desired cell type.

Production of Myeloid Precursors Our studies have demonstrated that it is possible to obtain a relatively mature, highly expanded population of myeloid cells using a simple liquid-culture system and three growth factors (Fig. 3.1). This system generates functional myeloid cells (as determined by killing of *Staphylococcus aureus*) and can be adapted to serum-free conditions. The degree of expansion and the function of the cells expanded in serum-free conditions can be markedly improved by the addition of 5% autologous

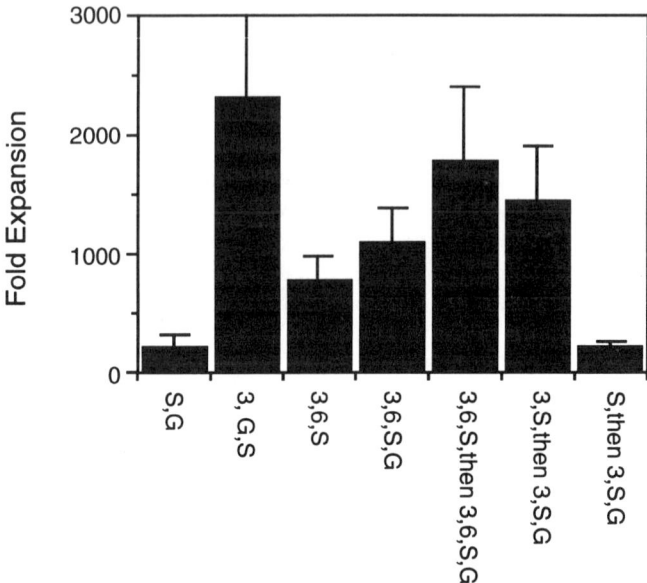

Figure 3.1 Fold expansion of CD34-selected HSC expanded in vitro with combinations of growth factors. All experiments were performed in the presence of fetal bovine serum. All growth factors were present at a concentration of 100 ng/mL. Cells were expanded for 14 days in liquid culture. Fold expansion is calculated as the ratio of total cells on day 14 to the CD34[+] cells on day 0. Data are presented as mean fold expansion ± SE, n = 5 experiments (see Lill et al. 1994 for further details). S = rHuSCF, G = rHuG-CSF, 3 = rHuIL-3, 6 = rHuIL-6.

plasma to the medium (Lill et al. 1994). In our assay system, the addition of interleukin (IL) -6 to the combination of stem cell factor (SCF), IL-3, and granulocyte colony-stimulating factor (G-CSF) did not increase expansion of total cells (Fig. 3.1). The three factors used in this study resulted in a similar degree of expansion to that seen by Haylock et al. (1992) with a six-factor combination. Other authors also have used a variety of different growth factors to demonstrate the feasibility of ex vivo expansion of myeloid precursors (Haylock et al. 1992; To et al. 1992; Brugger et al. 1993b; Mason, Mealiffe, and Ho 1994; Shapiro et al. 1994). It is possible to scale up the expansion using 500-mL gas-permeable Teflon-coated bags, although the degree of expansion is somewhat diminished (Lill et al., unpublished data). Brugger et al. (1994) have shown that ex vivo–expanded cells may be administered to patients without major side effects.

Production of Megakaryocytes   The addition of IL-6 to the combination of IL-3, SCF, and G-CSF results in the production of a number of cells expressing a megakaryocyte immunophenotype (CD61/CD42b$^+$) (Lill, unpublished data). The recent cloning of the c-mpl ligand (MGDF or thrombopoietin), which appears to be the primary growth and differentiation cytokine for megakaryocytes, will probably supersede the use of IL-6 and possibly IL-3 in these ex vivo systems (Bartley et al. 1994; de Sauvage et al. 1994; Kaushansky et al. 1994).

Production of True Hemopoietic Stem Cells   The ultimate goal of graft engineering is the expansion of self-renewing, pluripotent HSC. The major problems in this area are twofold. First, there is no defined assay for the human HSC. All of the current assays are surrogates for the true HSC. Second, most of the true stem cells are in the G_0 phase of the cell cycle and it is possible that any combination of cytokines that can induce one of these cells to proliferate in vitro may result in the inevitable terminal differentiation of the cell. Despite these caveats, there are some interesting animal models that appear to demonstrate that it is possible to transplant mice with an ex vivo–expanded population of murine HSC. The cytokine combinations used have included IL-1 and SCF (Muench, Firpo, and Moore 1993). It is possible that stromal contact is also needed for maintenance of long-term self-renewal capacity, which will require inclusion of stromal elements in the ex vivo–expansion system.

Production of NK Cells   The addition of IL-2 to the culture medium produces large numbers of NK cells in vitro from CD34-selected hemopoietic progenitor cells (Miller, Alley, and McGlave 1994; Miller, Verfaillie, and McGlave 1992a, b) (see Chapter 25). Ex vivo–expanded natural killer (NK) cells may have a role in posttransplantation immunotherapy, and IL-2 therapy has shown some efficacy against leukemia. This may be mediated, at least in part, by lymphocyte-activated killer cells (LAK) derived from NK cells (Boughton, O'Brien, and Simpson 1991). It may also be possible to co-culture the expanded NK cells with irradiated tumor cells and stimulate additional tumor-specific adoptive immunotherapy.

Gene Therapy

An additional role for CD34-selected hemopoietic progenitor cells is that of gene therapy. The major advantage of selecting for CD34$^+$ cells is the reduction in the number of cells and, hence, volume of viral supernatant to be added to the mixture. In the context of CD34$^+$ hemopoietic stem cells there are three major goals of gene therapy.

One is to "replace" missing or defective genes so that a normal protein is expressed in all of the progeny of the CD34$^+$ cells, ideally with some degree of lineage specificity (e.g., hemoglobin should be expressed only in erythrocytes). Most clinical trials of gene therapy in hemopoietic cells have focused on this approach; for example, with adenosine deaminase deficiency (ADA) in children (Culver, Anderson, and Blaese 1991a).

The second major goal is the introduction of therapeutic genes into HSC. Some examples of this approach include the expression of the multidrug resistance (MDR) gene in HSC, to render them relatively resistant to chemotherapy and thereby improve the therapeutic ratio of chemotherapeutic agents. Similarly, one can introduce a sequence-specific gene such as a ribozyme targeted against human immunodeficiency virus type 1 (HIV-1) into HSC, which may then confer immunity against infection by HIV-1 to all the progeny of the transduced HSC.

Problems associated with these approaches include the difficulty of retroviral gene insertion into true pluripotent self-renewing stem cells and reduced expression of the gene after a number of cellular divisions. If these problems prove insurmountable, multiple infusions of transduced cells expanded in vitro could be used. For example, the patient may undergo BM or PB harvesting followed by CD34 selection. The CD34$^+$ cells would be frozen in aliquots, thawed, transduced with viral vectors, and expanded as required. Depending upon the conditions for ex vivo expansion, a transduced population of committed but still primitive cells could be produced that could more precisely target the deficiency.

A third potential goal of gene therapy relies upon the difficulty of transduction of the true HSC with retroviral vectors. Since only committed progenitor cells will be transduced with this approach, expression of gene products by the committed progenitors will be temporary. The use of CD34-selected cells transduced with an IL-2–containing vector that would then produce IL-2 in a high local concentration within the bone marrow can be envisaged. The local production of a potent immune modulatory agent may minimize systemic effects while maximizing local antileukemic paracrine effects of IL-2.

■ T LYMPHOCYTES

T cells have been isolated from PB and transduced with the ADA gene for gene therapy purposes in children with severe combined immunodeficiency (SCID) syndrome, and have expressed the gene of interest in clinically significant quantities (Culver et al. 1991a, b). T cells may be a reasonable target for other aspects of gene therapy. The major problem is that they are terminally differentiated cells that are unlikely to provide long-lasting therapeutic benefit and, hence, may require repeated cycles of harvesting, transduction, and transplantation. A major advantage is that the patients would not require transplantation conditioning before receiving reinfusion of transduced T cells. T-lymphocyte clones with specific reactivity against cytomegalovirus (CMV) may also be selected and expanded in vitro, with potential use in the treatment or prevention of CMV disease in BMT recipients (Santamaria, Bryan, and Barbosa 1990). The expanded CMV-specific clones could be reinfused into the allogeneic recipient who may then possess active cell-mediated immune function against CMV infection. This approach could potentially be generalized to include other viruses. Suicide genes can also be introduced as part of a retroviral vector. Thus, it would be possible to destroy transduced T cells expressing the herpes simplex thymidine kinase gene by treatment of the patient with gancyclovir.

CD8$^+$ T Lymphocytes

Previous observations suggested that patients with HIV and Kaposi's sarcoma (KS) who had higher numbers of CD8 cells had a prolonged survival. There has been some interest in expanding populations of CD8$^+$ T lymphocytes. Mononuclear cells were obtained from patients with HIV-associated KS by leukapheresis. CD8$^+$ cells were isolated by flasks with covalently associated anti-CD8 Ab. The CD8$^+$ cells were then expanded ex vivo with IL-2 as described above and reinfused (Moody et al. 1993). Studies in patients with HIV infection and KS are currently underway and have demonstrated the feasibility of the approach, but have not yet addressed questions of therapeutic benefit.

■ TUMOR-INFILTRATING LYMPHOCYTES

An additional cell population, tumor-infiltrating lymphocytes (TIL) are obtained from within a bulky tumor such as renal cell carcinoma (RCCA) by disrupting the tumor, initially mechanically and then enzymatically. This results in a single-cell suspension containing viable MNC and tumor cells. The suspension is incubated for 2 weeks with IL-2, at the end of which there are no viable tumor cells and a greatly expanded population of TIL. Cells are then expanded an additional 5 to 6 weeks and approximately 10^{11} cells reinfused. A variation on this theme incorporates selection for CD8$^+$ cells after the first 2 weeks in culture. These TIL are believed to have a degree of specificity for the tumor and, hence, may be more efficacious in immunotherapy than LAK cells. Data from UCLA demonstrate a 33% response rate of RCCA to this approach (Pierce et al. 1994). This antitumor effect may potentially be enhanced by the use of gene therapy. In this approach the cells would be transduced with a retroviral vector containing a gene such as interferon-α (IFN-α) or IL-2. The cells would be expanded and reinfused. They would have a defined period of existence within the patient, would home toward and localize in the tumor or tumors, and at that location would have increased cytotoxic activity because of the genes that have been transduced into them.

Many different tumor types are currently under investigation for response to TIL/LAK cells, including melanoma, lung cancer, and head and neck cancer.

■ LYMPHOKINE-ACTIVATED KILLER CELLS

LAK cells are harvested by leukapheresis following treatment with IL-2. They comprise a heterogenous population of cells generated from both NK and T cells. Having obtained a sufficient pheresis product, the cells are expanded ex vivo with high concentrations of IL-2 and are reinfused into the patient with the aim of achieving a significant antitumor immunotherapy effect. A randomized study of IL-2 therapy versus IL-2 and LAK cells in RCCA showed no statistical difference in response rates or survival at 48 months (24% versus 33%, and 25% versus 29%, respectively) (Rosenberg, Lotze, and Yang 1993). This population of cells would be amenable to a similar gene-therapy strategy to that mentioned above for TIL. The advantage of isolating this population of cells is the ease of leukapheresis versus the difficulty of obtaining a large tumor mass and extracting the resident lymphocytes.

■ CONCLUSIONS

Over the last 4 years, there have been a number of major advances in cellular therapy. Perhaps the most important of these has been the ability to select a transplant product based on CD34 expression in a clinically relevant manner with demonstrated safety. CD34-selected cells remain viable after cryopreservation and thawing and are able to reconstitute hemopoiesis at the same rate as unmanipulated marrow or blood.

The major hurdles for cellular therapy in the immediate future are regulatory issues. Currently there is significant disagreement about the licensing of BMT laboratories and which organization should be responsible for accreditation of these laboratories. Both the level of quality control and the type of supervision required for these cell-therapy products remain a source of concern for those working in the field. An additional concern is the demonstration of efficacy for and the definition of success in tumor cell purging. These data will hopefully become available over the next few years.

In the future the two areas of most interest are those of "graft engineering" and gene therapy. Phase I clinical trials are already commencing in both areas and these should progress rapidly to phase II studies. In the longer term, the technology of potentially greatest interest would be the ability to expand and preserve the true pluripotent, self-renewing HSC.

REFERENCES

Aversa, F., Tabilio, A., Terenzi, A., et al. (1994) Succesful engraftment of T-cell depleted haplo-identical "three loci" incompatible transplants in leukemia patients by addition of recombinant human granulocyte colony-stimulating factor mobilized peripheral blood progenitor cells to bone marrow inoculum. *Blood*, **84**, 3948–55.

Bartley, T.D., Bogenberger, J., Hunt, P., et al. (1994) Identification and cloning of a megakaryocyte growth and development factor that is a ligand for the cytokine receptor Mpl. *Cell*, **77**, 1117–24.

Begley, C.G., DeLuca, E., Rowlings, P.A., et al. (1992) G-CSF mobilised progenitor cells in autologous transplantation: in vitro and in vivo aspects. *Journal of Nutritional Science and Vitaminology*, **368**, 368–71.

Bender, J.G., Unverzagt, K., Walker, D.E., et al. (1994) Phenotypic analysis and characterization of CD34$^+$ cells from normal bone marrow, cord blood, peripheral blood, and mobilized peripheral from patients undergoing autologous stem cell transplantation. *Clinical Immunology and Immunopathology*, **70**, 10–18.

Berenson, R.J., Andrews, R.G., Bensinger, W.I., et al. (1988a) Antigen CD34$^+$ marrow cells engraft lethally irradiated baboons. *Journal of Clinical Investigation*, **81**, 951–5.

Berenson, R.J., Andrews, R.G., Bensinger, W.I., et al. (1988b) Autologous marrow transplantation in baboons and man using CD34+ stem cells. *Experimental Hematology*, **16**, 522a.

Berenson, R.J., Bensinger, W.I., Hill, R., et al. (1990) Stem cell selection – clinical experience. *Progress in Clinical and Biological Research*, **333**, 403–10.

Berenson, R.J., Bensinger, W.I., Hill, R.S., et al. (1991) Engraftment after infusion of CD34$^+$ marrow cells in patients with breast cancer or neuroblastoma. *Blood*, **77**, 1717–22.

Boughton, B.J., O'Brien, D., and Simpson, A. (1991) Autologous il2/lak cell therapy for aml in 2nd complete remission. *Haematologica*, **76**, 55a.

Brugger, W., Birken, R., Bertz, H., et al. (1993a) Peripheral blood progenitor cells mobilized by chemotherapy plus granulocyte-colony stimulating factor accelerate both neutrophil and platelet recovery after high-dose VP16, ifosfamide and cisplatin. *British Journal of Haematology*, **84**, 402–7.

Brugger, W., Bross, K., Frisch, J., et al. (1992) Mobilization of peripheral blood progenitor cells by sequential administration of interleukin-3 and granulocyte-macrophage colony-stimulating factor following polychemotherapy with etoposide, ifosfamide, and cisplatin. *Blood*, **79**, 1193–200.

Brugger, W., Mocklin, W., Heimfeld, S., Berenson, R.J., Mertelsmann, R., and Kanz, L. (1993b) Ex vivo expansion of enriched peripheral blood CD34$^+$ progenitor cells by stem cell factor, interleukin-1 beta (IL-1 beta), IL-6, IL-3, interferon-gamma, and erythropoietin. *Blood*, **81**, 2579–84.

Brugger, W., Scheding, S., Heimfeld, S., et al. (1994) Ex vivo expanded peripheral blood CD34$^+$ cells mediate hematopoietic recovery in cancer patients after high dose VP16, ifosfamide, carboplatin and epirubicin. *Blood*, **84**, 1566a.

Champlin, R., Ho, W., Gajewski, J., et al. (1990) Selective depletion of CD8+ T lymphocytes for prevention of graft-versus-host disease after allogeneic bone marrow transplantation. *Blood*, **76**, 418–23.

Civin, C.I., Strauss, L.C., Brovall, C., Fackler, M.J., Schwartz, J.F., and Shaper, J.H. (1984) Antigenic analysis of hematopoiesis. III. A hematopoietic progenitor cell surface antigen defined by a monoclonal antibody raised against KG-1a cells. *Journal of Immunology*, **133**, 157–65.

Culver, K.W., Anderson, W.F., and Blaese, R.M. (1991) Lymphocyte gene therapy. *Human Gene Therapy*, **2**, 107–9.

Culver, K., Cornetta, K., Morgan, R., et al. (1991a) Lymphocytes as cellular vehicles for gene therapy in mouse and man. *Proceedings of the National Academy of Sciences of the United States of America*, **88**, 3155–9.

Culver, K.W., Osborne, W.R., Miller, A.D., et al. (1991b) Correction of ADA deficiency in human T lymphocytes using retroviral-mediated gene transfer. *Transplantation Proceedings*, **23**, 170–1.

DeLuca, E., Sheridan, W.P., Watson, D., Szer, J., and Begley, C.G. (1992) Prior chemotherapy does not prevent effective mobilisation by G-CSF of peripheral blood progenitor cells. *British Journal of Cancer*, **66**, 893–9.

de Sauvage, F.J., Hass, P.E., Spencer, S.D., et al. (1994) Stimulation of megakaryocytopoiesis and thrombopoiesis by the c-Mpl ligand. *Nature*, **369**, 533–8.

Grigg, A., Begley, C.G., Juttner, C.A., et al. (1993) Effect of peripheral blood progenitor cells mobilised by filgrastim (G-CSF) on platelet recovery after high-dose chemotherapy. *Bone Marrow Transplantation*, **2**, 23–9.

Haylock, D.N., To, L.B., Dowse, T.L., Juttner, C.A., and Simmons, P.J. (1992) Ex vivo expansion and maturation of peripheral blood CD34$^+$ cells into the myeloid lineage. *Blood*, **80**, 1405–12.

Haylock, D.N., To, L.B., Dyson, P.G., Niutta, S., and Juttner, C.A. (1990) Analysis of hemopoietic progenitor cells in recovery phase peripheral blood. *Experimental Hematology*, **18**, 716a.

Ho, A.D., Law, P., Maruyama, M., et al. (1994) Harvesting hematopoietic stem cells from normal donors for allogeneic transplantation: mobilization, apheresis and CD34$^+$ cell selection. *Proceedings of the American Association for Cancer Research*, 1145a.

Johnson, B.D., Drobyski, W.R., and Truitt, R.L. (1993) Delayed infusion of normal donor cells after MHC-matched bone marrow transplantation provides an antileukemia reaction without graft- versus-host disease. *Bone Marrow Transplantation*, **11**, 329–36.

Kanz, L., Brugger, W., and Mertelsmann, R. (1993) Haematopoietic growth factors and peripheral blood stem cells as supportive agents in dose intensification. *European Journal of Cancer*, **29A**(Suppl. 5), S23–6.

Kaushansky, K., Lok, S., Holly, R.D., et al. (1994) Promotion of megakaryocyte progenitor expansion and differentiation by the c-Mpl ligand thrombopoietin. *Nature*, **369**, 568–71.

Lill, M., Lynch, M., Fraser, J., et al. (1994) Production of functional myeloid cells from CD34-selected hematopoietic progenitor cells using a clinically relevant ex vivo expansion system. *Stem Cells*, **12**, 626–37.

Mason, J., Mealiffe, M., and Ho, A. (1994) Ex vivo expansion of peripheral blood progenitor cells with interleukin-11. *Proceedings of the American Association for Cancer Research*, 1175a.

Miller, J.S., Alley, K.A., and McGlave, P. (1994) Differentiation of natural killer (NK) cells from human primitive marrow progenitors in a stroma-based long-term culture system: identification of a $CD34^+7+$ NK progenitor. *Blood*, **83**, 2594–601.

Miller, J.S., Verfaillie, C., and McGlave, P. (1992a) The generation of human natural killer cells from $CD34^+$/DR- primitive progenitors in long-term bone marrow culture. *Blood*, **80**, 2182–7.

Miller, J.S., Verfaillie, C.M., and McGlave, P.B. (1992b) The generation of natural killer cells from $CD34^+$/DR- primitive progenitors in human long-term bone marrow culture. *Experimental Hematology*, **20**, 736a.

Moody, D.J., Kremer, A.B., Kahn, J., and Okarma, T.B. (1993) Impact of CD8+ cellular therapy with concomitant IL-2 administration on the peripheral blood lymphocyte composition in AIDS patients with Kaposi's sarcoma. *International Conference on AIDS*, **9**, PO-B28–2162.

Muench, M.O., Firpo, M.T., and Moore, M.A. (1993) Bone marrow transplantation with interleukin-1 plus kit-ligand ex vivo expanded bone marrow accelerates hematopoietic reconstitution in mice without the loss of stem cell lineage and proliferative potential. *Blood*, **81**, 3463–73.

Pierce, W., Beldegrun, A., DeKernion, J., and Figlin, R. (1994) Immunotherapy of patients with metastatic renal cell carcinoma using tumor infiltrating lymphocytes in combination with an outpatient regimen of IL-2 with or without interferon alpha. *Proceedings of the American Society of Clinical Oncology*, **13**, 736a.

Rosenberg, S., Lotze, M., and Yang, J. (1993) Prospective randomized trial of high dose interleukin-2 alone or in conjunction with lymphokine-activated killer cells for the treatment of patients with advanced cancers. *Journal of the National Cancer Institute*, **85**, 622.

Santamaria, P., Bryan, M.K., and Barbosa, J. (1990) Long term expansion of cytomegalovirus-specific T cell lines in the absence of antigen or antigen-presenting cells. Use of monosized polystyrene particles coated with agonistic antibodies. *Journal of Immunological Methods*, **132**, 1–11.

Shapiro, F., Yao, T.-J., Raptis, G., Reich, L., Norton, L., and Moore, M. (1994) Optimization of conditions for ex vivo expansion of $CD34^+$ cells from patients with stage 4 breast cancer. *Blood*, **84**, 3567–74.

Sheridan, W.P., Begley, C.G., Juttner, C.A., et al. (1992) Effect of peripheral-blood progenitor cells mobilised by filgrastim (G-CSF) on platelet recovery after high-dose chemotherapy. *Lancet*, **339**, 640–4.

Shpall, E.J., Jones, R.B., Bearman, S.I., et al. (1993) Positive selection of CD34$^+$ hematopoietic progenitor cells for transplantation. *Stem Cells*, **3**, 48–9.

Shpall, E.J., Jones, R.B., Bearman, S.I., et al. (1994) Transplantation of enriched CD34-positive autologous marrow into breast cancer patients following high-dose chemotherapy: influence of CD34-positive peripheral-blood progenitors and growth factors on engraftment. *Journal of Clinical Oncology*, **12**, 28–36.

Shpall, E.J., Jones, R.B., Johnston, C., et al. (1992) Purified cd34-positive (+) marrow progenitor cells provide effective reconstitution for breast cancer (ca) and non-Hodgkin's lymphoma (nhl) patients receiving high-dose chemotherapy with autologous bone marrow support (hdc/abms): recombinant granulocyte colony-stimulating factor (g-csf) accelerates hematopoietic recovery. *Proceedings of the American Society of Clinical Oncology*, **10**, 61a.

Siena, S., Bregni, M., Brando, B., et al. (1992) Flow cytometry to estimate circulating hematopoietic progenitors for autologous transplantation: comparative analysis of different CD34 monoclonal antibodies. *Research in Experimental Medicine*, **192**, 245–55.

To, L.B., Haylock, D.N., Simmons, P.J., and Juttner, C.A. (1992) Ex vivo expansion of peripheral blood CD34$^+$ cells and their maturation to functional end cells: an adjunct to hemopoietic stem cell transplantation. *Experimental Hematology*, **20**, 753a.

Truitt, R.L. and Atasoylu, A.A. (1991a) Contribution of CD4+ and CD8+ T cells to graft-versus-host disease and graft-versus-leukemia reactivity after transplantation of MHC-compatible bone marrow. *Bone Marrow Transplantation*, **8**, 51–8.

Truitt, R.L. and Atasoylu, A.A. (1991b) Impact of pretransplant conditioning and donor T cells on chimerism, graft-versus-host disease, graft-versus-leukemia reactivity, and tolerance after bone marrow transplantation. *Blood*, **77**, 2515–23.

4

Human Progenitor Cell Assays

C. GLENN BEGLEY

The hemopoietic system is organized in an hierarchical manner and is similar to other tissues that must continually produce a population of mature cells with limited life span. The most primitive cells (stem cells) are also the least frequent cells. Stem cells have several important properties that include the ability to give rise to multiple lineages, the ability to "self-renew" (giving rise to cells with identical or very similar properties), and the capacity for many cell divisions. These cells are responsible for long-term hemopoietic engraftment after hemopoietic cell transplantation procedures; however, assays of their function are cumbersome and time consuming. Although stem cells are of most importance in ensuring sustained hemopoiesis, functional assays quantitating these cells from patient samples remain of little clinical relevance.

Stem cells give rise to committed progenitor cells that have reduced proliferative capacity, limited self-renewal capacity, and ability to generate only a limited number of cell lineages; however, the quantitation of these cells can be performed simply and reliably in clonal cultures. These assays also serve as an essential tool for the experimental hematologist. In addition, they are also being used in many centers to ensure the adequacy of clinical samples collected for transplantation. In this context progenitor-cell assays have demonstrated utility, although they are a surrogate assay for the cells responsible for sustained hemopoietic engraftment despite the time lag involved. Such assays are being widely used in the setting of growth factor– or chemotherapy-mobilized peripheral blood progenitor cells (PBPC) or peripheral blood stem cells (PBSC) and have the advantage of a functional, biological assay when compared with alternative procedures.

59

■ BACKGROUND

The growth of human progenitor cells from bone marrow (BM) and peripheral blood (PB) was first described in 1970 (Pike and Robinson 1970; Chervenick and Boggs 1971; Iscove et al. 1971; Robinson, Kurnick, and Pike 1971). There are two subsets of granulocyte-macrophage colony-forming cells (GM-CFC) evident in human BM that can be separated based on differences in sedimentation velocity (Johnson, Dresch, and Metcalf 1977), lectin binding (Morstyn, Nicola, and Metcalf 1980), and binding of monoclonal antibody (mAB) (Young and Hwang-Chen 1981; Strauss et al. 1984). The most immature cells (day-14 GM-CFC) give rise to day-7 GM-CFC, the progeny of which are cells with even more limited proliferative capacity, the cluster-forming cells (Dresch et al. 1979; Jacobsen et al. 1979; Moore et al. 1980; Begley et al. 1985a). Recently, most attention has been focused on quantitating day-14 GM-CFC, particularly in PBPC populations where day-7 GM-CFC are noticeably diminished (Dührsen et al. 1988; DeLuca et al. 1992). Although referred to as day-14 GM-CFC, as many as 20% of these colonies are eosinophil in type (Metcalf et al. 1986; Burgess et al. 1987).

An analysis of the kinetics of developing erythroid colonies (Gregory 1976; Iscove 1977) and the physical properties of the cells giving rise to these colonies (Heath et al. 1976; Gregory and Eaves 1978) also provided evidence for two subpopulations of progenitor cells: the more primitive committed progenitor (erythroid burst-forming cells [E-BFC]) giving rise to a more mature progenitor population (erythroid colony-forming cells [E-CFC]).

More primitive colony types also can be recognized in human cultures (e.g., multipotential colonies [Fauser and Messner 1981] or blast cell colonies [Nakahata and Ogawa 1982]); however, their clinical usefulness is limited by the low frequency of these colony types and problems associated with their accurate quantitation (e.g., the apparent frequency of multipotential colonies can be spuriously elevated because of colony overlap). Assays of more primitive cells such as pre-CFC (Moore et al. 1980) and longer term cultures of human cells (Gartner and Kaplan 1980; Cicuttini et al. 1992b) have limited clinical application because of the longer time frames involved.

■ PROBLEMS AND PITFALLS

Assays of human progenitor cells are not standardized between laboratories: there is considerable variability in methodologies affecting the scoring procedures used, and the credibility of the reported results. When the results are used to influence clinical decisions or to attempt to validate other assays of progenitor/stem cells (e.g., numbers of $CD34^+$ cells), it is crucial that a rigorous approach be used to generate reproducible and consistent results. The principles and technical aspects of basic methodology have been described in detail elsewhere (Metcalf 1984) and will not be dealt with here. This chapter will focus on specific contentious methodological issues, some of which are peculiar to human samples, and describe our attempts to produce a reliable, reproducible, and validated assay procedure.

Preparing the Cell Sample

It is important to standardize the delivery and handling of the cell sample to the in vitro culture lab. Collection in tubes containing preservative-free heparin is recommended (Metcalf 1984). It is clearly preferable that cells are placed in culture as soon as possible after the sample is taken; however, it is occasionally necessary for samples to be stored overnight. Figure 4.1 shows results of experiments attempting to determine whether overnight storage has a significant impact on GM-CFC levels. GM-CFC levels were compared from cells cultured the same day versus the sample cultured the next day. Samples were stored as collected overnight (maximum of 24 hours) at either 4°C or 25°C. All points represent blood GM-CFC levels per milliliter in patients who had received growth factors (recombinant human granulocyte colony-stimulating factor [rHu-CSF]) alone or rHuG-CSF plus rHu stem cell factor (SCF) to mobilize progenitor/stem cell populations. There was good concordance between levels of GM-CFC from samples that were stored overnight; however, longer periods of storage resulted in increasingly discordant results (not shown). In addition, it appeared that storage at 4°C was somewhat superior to storage at 25°C. Although it is possible that these results were influenced by the continued presence of administered growth factors in the blood, previous work has shown that the majority of human progenitor cells can survive for 24 hours without added factors (Morstyn, Nicola, and Metcalf 1981). Moreover, although the number of progenitor cells quantitated was equivalent, this does not necessarily mean that the same cell was being assayed: the 24-hour time interval could theoretically function as an abbreviated pre-CFC assay (Nicola and Johnson 1982; DeLuca et al. 1992); however, based on these results, it seems reasonable to recommend that, if necessary, samples be stored at 4°C for periods of up to 24 hours before culture.

Ficoll-Paque–gradient separation is used almost universally to obtain mononuclear cells from PB or BM that are enriched for human

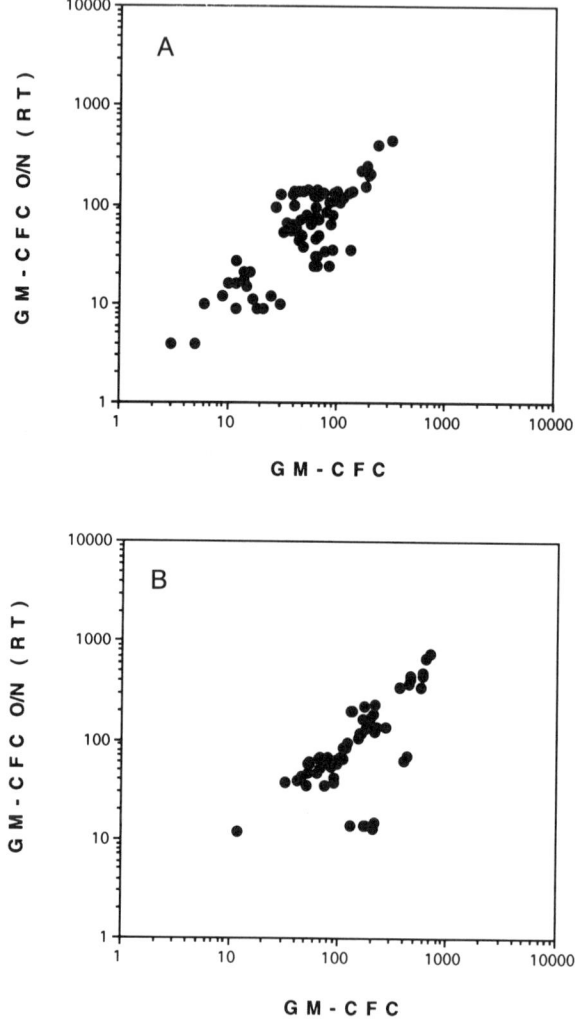

Figure 4.1 Comparison of GM-CFC results per milliliter obtained from fresh blood samples analyzed the same day (*horizontal axis*) versus samples stored and analyzed the next day. *A*, Results for whole blood stored overnight at room temperature: mononuclear cell (MNC) separation was performed the next day. (R^2 = 0.643, slope = 1.413, n = 77). *B*, Results for MNC stored overnight at room temperature in Dulbecco's modified eagles medium (DMEM) and 10% bovine calf serum (BCS) (R^2 = 0.776, slope = 0.847, n = 64).

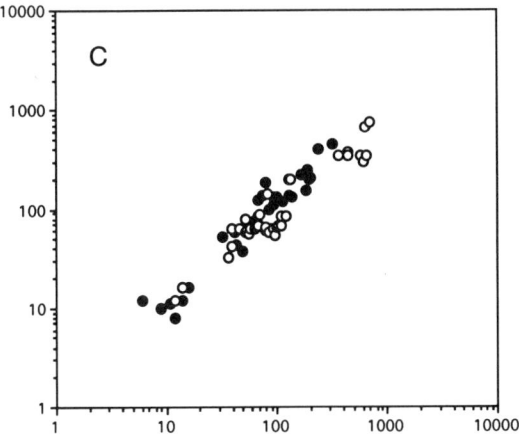

Figure 4.1 *Continued* *C*, Results for samples stored overnight at 4°C either as whole blood with MNC separation being performed the next day (R^2 = 0.873, slope = 1.287, n = 30, ●) or stored as a MNC preparation in DMEM and 10% BCS (R^2 = 0.839, slope = 0.759, n = 40, ○). All samples were obtained from patients with no prior chemotherapy or radiotherapy treatment and normal BM function. PBPC were mobilized either with rHuG-CSF alone or rHuG-CSF plus rHuSCF. All cultures were stimulated with maximal concentrations of rHuG-CSF or rHuGM-CSF plus rHuSCF and examined after 14 days.

progenitor cells. Even this relatively simple technique has proven to be the source of considerable variability between laboratories. Junior staff frequently mistakenly believe that the efficiency of the separation procedure is related to the height of the column of Ficoll-Paque rather than the surface area. Thus, they fail to routinely use a tube with the greatest diameter. Furthermore, clinical samples arriving in the laboratory can vary up to 100-fold in white cell count (WCC) (e.g., blood from normal individuals versus concentrated leukapheresis samples). This can create some difficulty ensuring that equivalent numbers of cells are loaded on the gradient. Moreover, the efficiency of harvesting interface cells can vary greatly from operator to operator. In an attempt to consistently recover all the light-density cells, the entire interface plus all the liquid above the cell pellet is collected. The volume of medium added to wash the cells and the conditions of centrifugation also are standardized. Finally, it is prudent to confirm that Ficoll-gradient separation is an appropriate cell-fractionation procedure for each new mobilization schedule or different disease state: the number of GM-CFC remaining in the pellet after Ficoll separation can be determined directly. Even though considerable numbers of GM-CFC can be lost in the pellet, the procedure remains greater than or equal to 98% efficient for rHuG-CSF–mobilized progenitor cells (DeLuca et al. 1992).

The method for determining the cell count before cell culture is also controversial. Several methods are in common use. These include an automated cell count performed on the PB or BM sample to determine the number of MNC; stains that allow identification of nuclear morphology (e.g., crystal violet stain); or stains that identify viable cells (e.g., eosin) with cell counts being performed manually in the latter two cases. While an automated cell count has the advantage of greater accuracy, extrapolating from an MNC count performed before Ficoll-Paque–gradient fractionation is not reasonable given the assumptions inherent in this approach. Similarly, attempts to enumerate cells based on their morphology (e.g., MNC morphology) are subjective and frequently ignore more differentiated cells that are capable of colony formation in vitro (e.g., promyelocytes and myelocytes) (Begley et al. 1985a; Begley, Metcalf, and Nicola 1988). While counting viable cells is preferred and is most relevant to such an assay, this can be influenced by substantial numbers of contaminating cells that are viable but incapable of proliferation. Such cells are particularly likely to be present in growth factor–mobilized cell samples or artifactually as a result of overloading Ficoll-Paque gradients. The issue of cell counting is an important one as results are typically expressed per 10^5 BM cells, and the calculation of GM-CFC/mL blood is frequently based on the number of GM-CFC enumerated per 10^5 cells. This makes comparisons between laboratories difficult, but can be readily overcome using a volumetric method for the calculation of GM-CFC/mL blood (see below).

Cell-Culture Procedure

The technical details of the cell-culture procedure have been described explicitly elsewhere (Metcalf 1984). The importance of routine checking of incubator function (humidity, temperature, CO_2) and the careful testing and selection of calf serum or serum-free culture medium have been emphasized.

For human samples, there are unique issues that arise and are most evident with growth factor– or chemotherapy-mobilized PBPC samples. The great range in WCC and progenitor cell levels in these samples requires that cultures be set up using at least two cell concentrations. The routine use of cell concentrations of 10^4 cells/mL agar and 10^5 cells/mL agar guarantees that samples in which few progenitor cells are present will be adequately examined (using culture plates with high cell density) and samples rich in progenitor cells will also be adequately examined. Replicate (preferably at least triplicate) cultures should be established without any added growth factors (to examine the production of CSF in the culture dish) and with growth factor combinations suitable for the cell type under study. The combination of optimal concentrations of rHuG-CSF, rHuGM-CSF, and rHuSCF serves as a reliable stimulus for the growth of human GM-CFC (Cicuttini, Begley, and Boyd 1992). In contrast, although rHuGM-CSF, rHuSCF, rHuIL-3 or Multi-CSF, rHuIL-6, and rHuEPO is an appropriate stimulus for the growth of erythroid colonies, this combination is not ideal for enumeration of GM-CFC. Furthermore, although the addition of other growth factors (e.g., *flt*-3 ligand) (Lyman et al. 1993) may further enhance colony growth, it is essential that a normal range and a "therapeutic range" be established for the growth factor combination being used in vitro and that this combination be maintained for the duration of the clinical study. In the absence of purified sources of factors, pretitrated conditioned medium (e.g., human placental conditioned medium [HPCM], U5637 conditioned medium) remains a useful source of combinations of growth factors (Nicola et al. 1979; Nicola, Begley, and Metcalf 1985).

The examination of culture dishes is a tedious, repetitive, but important task that requires considerable training and expertise before consistent results are obtained. This is a potential source of considerable error in the interpretation of progenitor-cell assays. Although it is possible to obtain a high degree of speed and accuracy, there remains a definite variability within cultures even assessed by the same individual (Fig. 4.2). The degree of variability that is reasonable within an individual and between individuals is difficult to define but probably 10% variation is acceptable. The error involved in enumerating colony numbers is greatly increased as the number of colonies increases above approximately 250 per culture dish. Ideally, between 30 and 60 colonies per culture dish ensures accurate, reproducible counts with little likelihood of colonies overlapping: the number of cells placed in culture is deliberately manipulated in an attempt to achieve this result. Thus, using 10^4 and 10^5 cells/mL, one set of cultures will usually either be too sparse or too crowded for reliable results to be generated. The remaining set of cultures are then counted in their entirety. A consistent observation with human blood cells is the nonlinearity in the relationship between colony numbers generated versus the number of cells cultured for some patient samples (To et al. 1983). This is probably due to accessory cell populations that are able to influence colony growth, particularly at higher cell con-

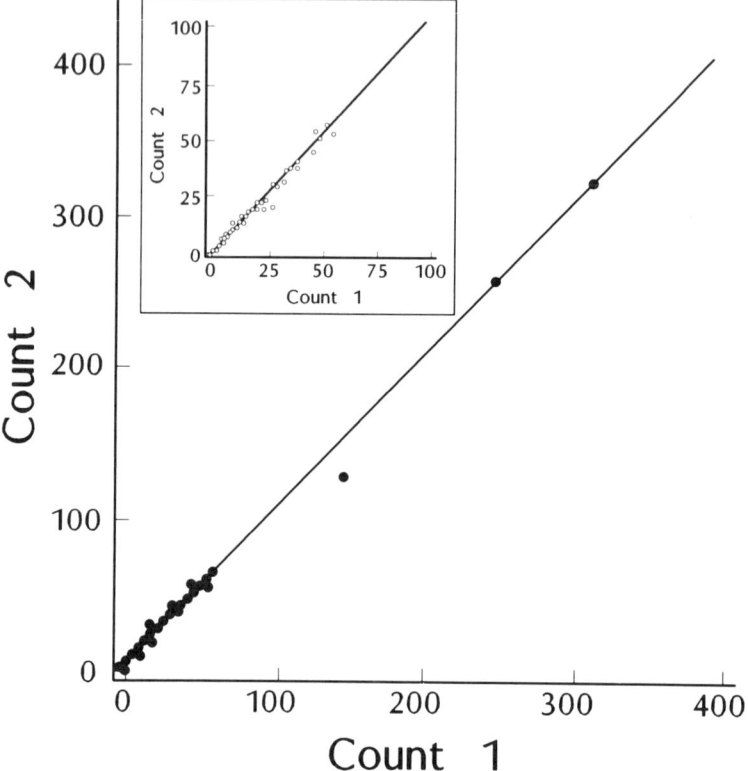

Figure 4.2 Comparison of colony counts performed by one individual. Fifty agar culture dishes were selected that displayed a range in number of colonies. The culture dishes were coded and the investigator examined each culture dish twice while remaining blinded to the code. The number of colonies obtained with the first count is shown compared with results from the second count. The *inset* shows results for culture dishes that were scored as less than 100 colonies. Statistical analysis of cultures with fewer than 100 colonies ($n = 47$) revealed the slope of the regression line was 0.998 and the root mean square error (RMSE, a measure of precision where the larger the RMSE the more variability there is between counts) was 2.2.

centrations (Kannourakis et al. 1988a, b). As the aim with most clinical samples is to enumerate the maximum number of progenitor cells within a sample (regardless of how their growth was stimulated), this phenomenon can usually be ignored. The set of culture plates that generated the greatest number of GM-CFC per cell concentration is reported.

Calculating the Result

Results of cultures of aspirated BM cells are usually expressed as the mean of triplicate cultures per 10^5 Ficoll-Paque–fractionated MNC. Attempts to express results per milliliter of BM are less meaningful given the uncertainty regarding the degree of contamination with PB; however, for PB, the most clinically relevant result is the number of progenitor cells per milliliter. This result can be calculated using two approaches. First, the mean colony number per culture dish is expressed per 10^5 cultured MNC. The number of MNC per milliliter is determined for the sample and used to calculate the number of progenitor cells per milliliter. This approach is critically dependent on accurately determining the MNC count after Ficoll-Paque fractionation (with the inherent problems discussed above). The calculation is also critically dependent on a determination of the MNC count in the sample, which may not be directly related to the MNC count after Ficoll-Paque fractionation (Fig. 4.3*A*). Alternatively, a more simple, accurate procedure is to directly determine the mean colony number per volume. This approach entirely ignores the MNC count (which then simply serves to guarantee approximately 30 to 60 final colonies in the culture dish). The volume of the initial sample loaded onto the Ficoll-Paque is recorded, the cells are washed and resuspended in a second volume (also recorded), and the third volume actually dispensed into the culture dish is also recorded. The mean colony number per volume can be directly related to the volume of the initial sample as it has undergone one concentrating step over Ficoll-Paque. The assumption inherent in this approach is that essentially no progenitor cells are lost during Ficoll-Paque fractionation, an assumption that can be experimentally validated (Fig. 4.3*B*) (DeLuca et al. 1992). Using these procedures, it is possible to achieve reliable and reproducible results: estimates of the coefficient of variation for the progenitor cell assay (when the one sample was fractionated, counted, and assayed ten times) was less than 10% (A. Roberts, unpublished data).

Clinical Utility

Figure 4.4 shows results using this assay to quantitate numbers of progenitor cells in normal BM. BM cells were taken from women before adjuvant chemotherapy for breast cancer. The BM cells were harvested, Ficoll-Paque fractionated, counted with eosin staining, and cultured in agar at cell densities of 10^4 and 10^5 cells/mL. Triplicate cultures stimulated with maximal concentrations of rHuG-CSF and

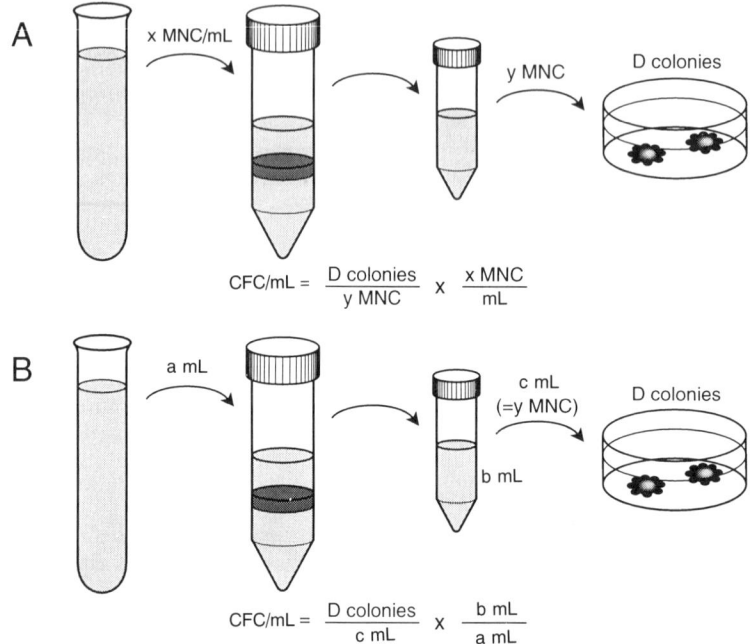

Figure 4.3 Alternative approaches for calculating numbers of CFC per milliliter blood. *A*, Results calculated based on number of colonies expressed per MNC cultured. Problems inherent in accurately quantitating number of MNC after fractionation (y MNC; e.g., 10^4 MNC per culture) and assumptions inherent in MNC counts determined on initial samples (*x*) limit the usefulness of this approach. *B*, Results calculated without reference to MNC counts, and based solely on volume of sample examined in culture (c mL which is equivalent to, e.g., 10^4 MNC.) This volume represents a proportion of the initial sample of blood (a mL) that was concentrated over Ficoll-Paque, washed, and resuspended in a known volume (b mL). See text for details.

rHuGM-CSF were examined after 7 days' incubation for the most mature progenitor cell population, day-7 GM-CFC. This growth factor combination was deliberately chosen to allow direct comparison with previous studies that also examined day-7 GM-CFC (Begley et al. 1985b; Begley, Nicola, and Metcalf 1988). Triplicate cultures stimulated with rHuG-CSF, rHuGM-CSF, and rHuSCF were examined for day-14 GM-CFC and triplicate agar cultures stimulated with maximal concentrations of rHuGM-CSF, rHuIL-3, rHuIL-6, rHuSCF, and r-HuEPO were scored for E-BFC. The results shown in Figure 4.4 are superior to those from earlier studies with a median number of 400 day-7 GM-CFC, 390 day-14 GM-CFC, and 400 E-BFC/10^5 MNC cul-

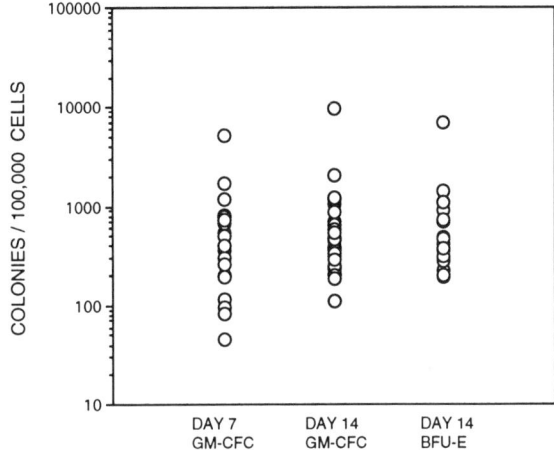

Figure 4.4 Levels of progenitor cells in normal human BM harvests. BM samples were taken from women with breast cancer, who were to receive adjuvant chemotherapy and who had no prior chemotherapy or radiotherapy. Cultures were established at cell concentrations of 10^4 and 10^5 cells/mL and triplicate cultures examined. GM-CFC were enumerated in agar stimulated with maximal concentrations of rHuG-CSF plus rHuGM-CSF and examined after 7 days (day-7 GM-CFC, $n = 22$) or rHuG-CSF, rHuGM-CSF plus rHuSCF and examined after 14 days (day-14 GM-CFC, $n = 31$). E-BFC were quantitated in cultures stimulated with rHuGM-CSF, rHuIL-3, rHuIL-6, rHuSCF, and rHuEPO ($n = 29$).

tured. The most likely explanation for these improved results is the improved quality of the BM aspirate. In this study, the major emphasis in the diagnostic laboratory was to provide a cellular aspirate for quantitation of GM-CFC. In contrast, earlier studies had provided only the remnant of aspirate samples for progenitor cell assays. This notion is supported by results obtained from diagnostic samples provided to the laboratory concurrently, but outside the context of this defined clinical study: the median number day-14 GM-CFC was 165/10^5 MNC (range 40 to 750, $n = 15$). It is noteworthy that day-7 GM-CFC are poorly represented in PBPC samples, indicating some selectivity in the release mechanism (Dührsen et al. 1988; DeLuca et al. 1992); however, it is tempting to speculate that day-7 GM-CFC may be able to generate even more rapid neutrophil recovery if substantial numbers of these cells could be collected.

Additional validation of the assay procedure is provided by comparing GM-CFC and E-BFC assays on blood and leukapheresis samples taken from the same individual on the same day. Figure 4.5 shows

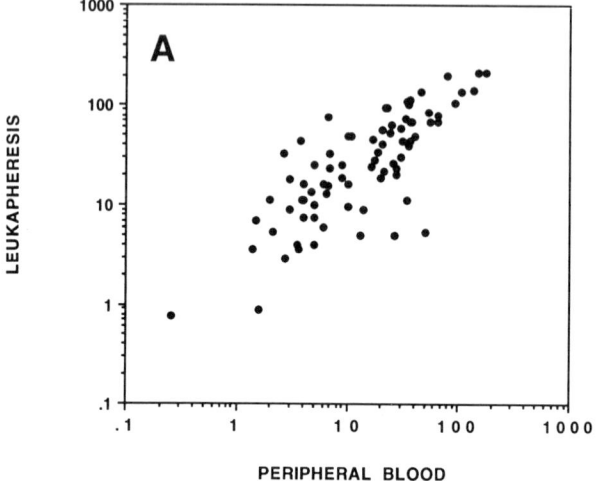

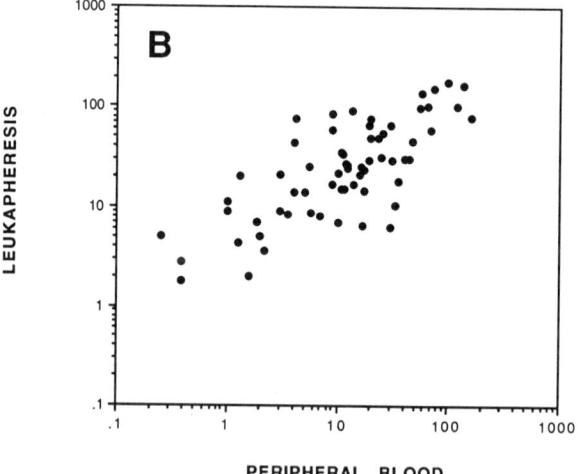

Figure 4.5 Comparison of GM-CFC (*A*) and BFU-E (*B*) levels in blood and leukapheresis products taken from the same individual on the same day. All patients had received prior chemotherapy and/or radiotherapy as treatment for leukemia/lymphoma (Sheridan et al. 1992, 1994). PBPC were mobilized using rHuG-CSF alone. Triplicate cultures were stimulated with rHuG-CSF and rHuGM-CSF and examined after 14 days (for GM-CFC) or with pretitrated HPCM and rHuEPO (for E-BFC). Results are expressed per 10^5 cultured cells to allow direct comparison. Correlation coefficients were: GM-CFC, $R^2 = 0.830$, slope = 1.317 ($n = 78$); BFU-E, $R^2 = 0.878$, slope = 1.661 ($n = 68$).

typical results for patients who had received prior treatment for leukemia or lymphoma as previously described (Sheridan et al. 1992, 1994). Patients then received rHuG-CSF alone to mobilize PBPC. The correlation between GM-CFC and E-BFC assays in the blood and leukapheresis product was good ($R^2 = 0.83$ and $R^2 = 0.88$, respectively). It is of interest that there was a tendency for increased GM-CFC to be observed in leukapheresis compared with blood, perhaps because an inhibitory cell was not harvested by this cell collection procedure (Kannourakis et al. 1988a).

Attempts to correlate levels of progenitor cells with clinical recovery have only been partially successful. This is at least in part because day-14 GM-CFC are only a surrogate for the cells actually responsible for sustained hemopoietic reconstitution and because the number of cells reinfused is considerably greater than the threshold levels required; however, it is very likely that the threshold required for hemopoietic reconstitution is dependent on the PBPC-mobilization strategy used and on the chemotherapy/radiotherapy conditioning regimen. Moreover, the predictive value of assays of $CD34^+$ cells or GM-CFC may or may not also vary with different mobilization strategies and probably should be ascertained directly with each new mobilization protocol. These issues assume greater importance in the context of previously treated patients with poor marrow reserves and when multiple transplant procedures are contemplated. Because current assay procedures vary considerably between laboratories, it is inappropriate to provide specific recommendations on minimum numbers of GM-CFC required for safe transplantation. This threshold should be determined in each institution and for each mobilization schedule; however, although time-consuming, it is possible to establish a reliable, consistent, validated assay procedure as a prerequisite for the accurate quantitation of levels of progenitor cells in clinical samples.

ACKNOWLEDGMENTS

We thank E. DeLuca and R. Mansfield for expert technical assistance and Bill Rich for help with statistical analysis. This work was supported by the National Health and Medical Research Council, Canberra and the Anti-Cancer Council of Victoria. The clinical studies from which these data were derived were supported by Amgen Australia and Amgen Inc., Thousand Oaks, CA, U.S.A.

REFERENCES

Begley, C.G., Lopez, A.F., Vadas, M.A., and Metcalf, D. (1985a) The clonal proliferation in vitro of enriched populations of human promyelocytes and myelocytes. *Blood*, **65**, 951–8.

Begley, C.G., Metcalf, D., Lopez, A.F., and Nicola, N.A. (1985b) Fractionated populations of normal human marrow cells respond to both human colony-stimulating factors with granulocyte-macrophage activity. *Experimental Hematology*, **13**, 956–62.

Begley, C.G., Metcalf, D., and Nicola, N.A. (1988) Binding characteristics and proliferative action of purified granulocyte colony-stimulating factor (G-CSF) on normal and leukemic human promyelocytes. *Experimental Hematology*, **16**, 71–9.

Begley, C.G., Nicola, N.A., and Metcalf, D. (1988) Proliferation of normal human promyelocytes and myelocytes after a single pulse stimulation by purified GM-CSF or G-CSF. *Blood*, **71**, 640–5.

Burgess, A.W., Begley, C.G., Johnson, G.R., et al. (1987) Purification and properties of bacterially synthesized human granulocyte-macrophage colony stimulating factor. *Blood*, **69**, 43–51.

Chervenick, P.A. and Boggs, D.R. (1971) In vitro growth of granulocytic and mononuclear cell colonies from blood of normal individuals. *Blood*, **37**, 131–5.

Cicuttini, F.M., Begley, C.G., and Boyd, A.W. (1992) The effect of recombinant stem cell factor (SCF) on purified CD34-positive human umbilical cord blood progenitor cells. *Growth Factors*, **6**, 31–9.

Cicuttini, F.M., Martin, M., Salvaris, E., et al. (1992b) Support of human cord blood progenitor cells on human stromal cell lines transformed by SV40 large T antigen under the influence of an inducible (metallothionein) promoter. *Blood*, **80**, 102–12.

DeLuca, E., Sheridan, W.P., Watson, D., Szer, J., and Begley, C.G. (1992) Prior chemotherapy does not prevent effective mobilization by G-CSF of peripheral blood progenitor cells. *British Journal of Cancer*, **66**, 893–9.

Dresch, C., Faille, A., Poirier, O., Balitrand, N., and Najean, Y. (1979) Hydroxyurea suicide study of the kinetic heterogeneity of colony forming cells in human bone marrow. *Experimental Hematology*, **7**, 337–44.

Dührsen, U., Villeval, J.L., Boyd, J., Kannourakis, G., Morstyn, G., and Metcalf, D. (1988) Effects of recombinant human granulocyte colony-stimulating factor on hematopoietic progenitor cells in cancer patients. *Blood*, **72**, 2074–81.

Fauser, A.A. and Messner, H.A. (1981) Pluripotent hemopoietic progenitors (CFU-GEMM) in polycythemia vera: analysis of erythropoietin requirement and proliferative activity. *Blood*, **58**, 1224–7.

Gartner, S. and Kaplan, H.S. (1980) Long-term culture of human bone marrow cells. *Proceedings of the National Academy of Sciences of the United States of America*, **77**, 4756–9.

Gregory, C.J. (1976) Erythropoietin sensitivity as a differentiation marker in the hemopoietic system: studies of three erythropoietic colony responses in culture. *Journal of Cellular Physiology*, **89**, 289–301.

Gregory, C.J. and Eaves, A.C. (1978) Three stages of erythropoietic progenitor cell differentiation distinguished by a number of physical and biologic properties. *Blood*, **51**, 527–37.

Heath, D.S., Axelrad, A.A., McLeod, D.L., and Shreeve, M.M. (1976) Separation of the erythropoietin-responsive progenitors BFU-E and CFU-E in mouse bone marrow by unit gravity sedimentation. *Blood*, **47**, 777–92.

Iscove, N.N. (1977) The role of erythropoietin in regulation of population size and cell cycling of early and late erythroid precursors in mouse bone marrow. *Cellular and Tissue Kinetics*, **10**, 323–34.

Iscove, N.N., Senn, J.S., Till, J.E., and McCulloch, E.A. (1971) Colony formation by normal and leukemic human marrow cells in culture: effect of conditioned medium from human leukocytes. *Blood*, **37**, 1–5.

Jacobsen, N., Broxmeyer, H.E., Grossbard, E., and Moore, M.A. (1979) Colony-forming units in diffusion chambers (CFU-d) and colony-forming units in agar culture (CFU-c) obtained from normal human bone marrow: a possible parent-progeny relationship. *Cellular and Tissue Kinetics*, **12**, 213–26.

Johnson, G.R., Dresch, C., and Metcalf, D. (1977) Heterogeneity in human neutrophil, macrophage, and eosinophil progenitor cells demonstrated by velocity sedimentation separation. *Blood*, **50**, 823–31.

Kannourakis, G., Begley, C.G., Johnson, G.R., Werkmeister, J.A., and Burns, G.F. (1988a) Evidence for interactions between monocytes and natural killer cells in the regulation of in vitro hemopoiesis. *Journal of Immunology*, **140**, 2489–94.

Kannourakis, G., Johnson, G.R., Begley, C.G., Werkmeister, J.A., and Burns, G.F. (1988b) Enhancement of in vitro beta-thalassemic and normal hematopoiesis by a noncytotoxic monoclonal antibody, 9.1C3: evidence for negative regulation of hematopoiesis by monocytes and natural killer cells. *Blood*, **72**, 1124–33.

Lyman, S.D., James, L., Johnson, L., et al. (1993) Cloning of the human homologue of the murine flt3 ligand: a growth factor for early hematopoietic progenitor cells. *Blood*, **83**, 2795–801.

Metcalf, D. (1984) *The hemopoietic colony stimulating factors*. Amsterdam, Elsevier.

Metcalf, D., Begley, C.G., Johnson, G.R., et al. (1986) Biologic properties in vitro of a recombinant human granulocyte-macrophage colony-stimulating factor. *Blood*, **67**, 37–45.

Moore, M.A., Broxmeyer, H.E., Sheridan, A.P., Meyers, P.A., Jacobsen, N., and Winchester, R.J. (1980) Continuous human bone marrow culture: Ia antigen characterization of probable pluripotential stem cells. *Blood*, **55**, 682–90.

Morstyn, G., Nicola, N.A., and Metcalf, D. (1980) Purification of hemopoietic progenitor cells from human marrow using a fucose-binding lectin and cell sorting. *Blood*, **56**, 798–805.

Morstyn, G., Nicola, N.A., and Metcalf, D. (1981) Separate actions of different colony stimulating factors from human placental conditioned medium on human hemopoietic progenitor cell survival and proliferation. *Journal of Cellular Physiology*, **109**, 133–42.

Nakahata, T. and Ogawa, M. (1982) Hemopoietic colony-forming cells in umbilical cord blood with extensive capability to generate mono- and multipotential hemopoietic progenitors. *Journal of Clinical Investigation*, **70**, 1324–8.

Nicola, N.A., Begley, C.G., and Metcalf, D. (1985) Identification of the human analogue of a regulator that induces differentiation in murine leukaemic cells. *Nature*, **314**, 625–8.

Nicola, N.A. and Johnson, G.R. (1982) The production of committed hemopoietic colony-forming cells from multipotential precursor cells in vitro. *Blood*, **60**, 1019–29.

Nicola, N.A., Metcalf, D., Johnson, G.R., and Burgess, A.W. (1979) Separation of functionally distinct human granulocyte-macrophage colony-stimulating factors. *Blood*, **54**, 614–27.

Pike, B.L. and Robinson, W.A. (1970) Human bone marrow colony growth in agar-gel. *Journal of Cellular Physiology,* **76**, 77–84.

Robinson, W.A., Kurnick, J.E., and Pike, B.L. (1971) Colony growth of human leukemic peripheral blood cells in vitro. *Blood,* **38**, 500–8.

Sheridan, W.P., Begley, C.G., Juttner, C.A., et al. (1992) Effect of peripheral-blood progenitor cells mobilised by filgrastim (G-CSF) on platelet recovery after high-dose chemotherapy. *Lancet,* **339**, 640–4.

Sheridan, W.P., Begley, C.G., To, L.B., et al. (1994) Phase II study of autologous filgrastim (G-CSF)-mobilized peripheral blood progenitor cells to restore hemopoiesis after high-dose chemotherapy for lymphoid malignancies. *Bone Marrow Transplantation,* **14**, 105–11.

Strauss, L.C., Skubitz, K.M., August, J.T., and Civin, C.I. (1984) Antigenic analysis of hematopoiesis: II. Expression of human neutrophil antigens on normal and leukemic marrow cells. *Blood,* **63**, 574–8.

To, L.B., Haylock, D.N., Juttner, C.A., and Kimber, R.J. (1983) The effect of monocytes in the peripheral blood CFU-C assay system. *Blood,* **62**, 112–27.

Young, N.S. and Hwang-Chen, S.P. (1981) Anti-K562 cell monoclonal antibodies recognize hematopoietic progenitors. *Proceedings of the National Academy of Sciences of the United States of America,* **78**, 7073–7.

5

Flow Cytometric Techniques

DIETHER J. RECKTENWALD AND
EDMUND K. WALLER

In clinical human hemopoietic stem cell work, flow cytometry can be used to count the number of CD34$^+$ cells in cell suspensions and to identify subpopulations based on reactivity with monoclonal antibody (mAB), nucleic acid dyes, and other fluorescent probes.

■ PRINCIPLES OF FLOW CYTOMETRY

Technology

A flow cytometer uses hydrodynamic focusing to align cells from an essentially monodispersed sample in a bulk fluid into a one-dimensional file of particles in a flowing fluid stream. One small spot of the stream is illuminated by a tightly focused light beam typically originating from a laser. Each particle passing through the light beam, at rates of up to 10,000/sec with conventional analysis methods, creates a flash of scattered and fluorescent light. The information in these light flashes is analyzed by angle for scattered light, and by wavelength for fluorescence light intensity. Typical flow cytometers measure two light-scatter intensities and the intensities of at least three different colors of fluorescence.

A minimal intensity requirement for one or more of the signals is used to trigger digitization of all of the signals with at least 8 bits of resolution. The result of the measurement is a list of intensity values for the different signals (parameters) for each of the cells that meet the trigger requirements (list-mode).

For parameters with a very wide intensity range, analog-domain, logarithmic amplifiers with a four-decade range are commonly used. Lately, flow cytometers with software-based logarithmic converters have become available commercially.

Modern flow cytometers measure at least five parameters simultaneously and at least 100 cells should be counted for the smallest population of interest if a better than 10% counting precision is desired and enough cells can be obtained. For very rare populations, such as $CD34^+$ cells in nucleated cell preparations from peripheral blood (PB), this condition requires the collection of 100,000 cells or more.

Flow cytometers have a very low limit of detection for fluorescence; a few hundred molecules of fluorescein per cell can be detected.

Data storage and analysis are performed with microcomputers. One byte is needed per parameter and cell for the storage of 8-bit data; 2 bytes are used for 9- to 16-bit data. Therefore, a sample with 1 million cells and five parameters requires up to 10 megabytes of data storage.

Multiparameter data analysis is performed by specialized software using one- and two-dimensional histogramming. For the simultaneous analysis of more than three parameters, two-dimensional parameter restrictions are placed on some parameter combinations for the analysis of other parameters (gating). Alternatively, multidimensional cluster analysis can be used for the data analysis.

To facilitate the investigation of the relationship between the optical measurements and biological function, many flow cytometers allow the isolation of cells that meet certain optical criteria. Those instruments are called fluorescence-activated cell sorters (FACS) (Herzenberg, Sweet, and Herzenberg 1976). In most cases the sorting is achieved by breaking the fluid stream containing the cells into droplets with 1 or 0 cells each, and by applying an electrostatic charge to droplets to be collected. Other cell sorters use hydrodynamic switching or a capillary activated with a piezocrystal to sort cells in a closed system.

Setup and Calibration

Modern flow cytometers do not require an alignment of the optical system; however, for research applications, the user must ascertain that the number of detectors, the light sources, and the optical filters are adequate for the intended application. For many measurements of progenitor cells and their subsets, excitation with an argon-ion laser at 488 nm and the detection of green, orange, and red fluorescence is sufficient. For those measurements, logarithmic signal amplification spanning four decades of signal intensity (Muirhead, Schmitt, and Muirhead 1983) is used for the fluorescence signals. For the determination of subset fractions, the photomultiplier gains are set to place the fluorescent signal of unstained cells at the lower end of the intensity scale. Light scatter is generally measured on a linear intensity scale and gains are set to show all cell populations of interest on scale. Depending upon the combination of fluorochromes used in a particular application of multicolor fluorescence analysis, compensation can be set to account for the spectral overlap of fluorescent dyes (Lanier and Recktenwald 1991). It is important to note that any change in amplifier-gain setting requires a readjustment of the multicolor fluorescence compensation settings. The adjustment of amplifier and compensation settings can be automated with microspheres and software. With special data analysis software, such as Paint-a-Gate or Attractors, measurements can be easily performed without setting fluorescence compensation. For absolute fluorescence measurements, calibration particles are available commercially for dyes commonly used for immunofluorescence. These particles allow a conversion from relative fluorescence-intensity measurements to an absolute number of fluorophor molecules per cell. Other methods for calibrating cytometers for absolute fluorescence measurements do not require calibration particles and can be done with standard laboratory equipment. Techniques for fluorescence quantitation and their limits can be found in the literature (Hoffman, Recktenwald, and Vogt 1993). It is useful to note that many cytometers are stable enough to use constant-gain settings with only daily performance checks with stable microparticles or known cell preparations.

Verification of Instrument Performance

Instrument performance should be verified at least daily by analyzing particles, either from a known biological sample or from stable, synthetic fluorescent microspheres. The samples are selected to verify the sensitivity of the different detection systems. A loss of sensitivity decreases the distinction between reactive and nonreactive cells and can lead to erroneous results.

For nuclear DNA analysis, the precision of the fluorescence measurement should be checked frequently as well, and a coefficient of variation of less than 2% should be obtained with an appropriate sample.

Rare-Cell Analysis

Until recently, the limit of detection for flow-cytometric cell subset analysis by immunofluorescence was commonly believed to be 1 cell in 10^4 (Ryan 1993), despite the capability of flow cytometry to analyze millions of cells in a relatively short time. Sorting of cells at a lower concentration has been described (Weichel et al. 1985). This limit of detection is very close to the level of about 5 in 10^4 CD34$^+$ cells in normal PB.

In 1993, Gross et al. showed that within a well-defined model system, by carefully controlling factors that can contribute to false-positives in flow cytometry, the limit of detection can be lowered to less than 1 cell in 10^6. This level of sensitivity is not only important for obtaining more precise and accurate CD34$^+$ cell and subset counts, but also should allow the detection of residual malignant cells in bone marrow (BM) or PB after therapy, provided appropriate reagents for identifying the cells of interest are available. The flow-cytometric technique promises better reliability than currently used microscopic techniques (Schlimok et al. 1987; Pantel et al. 1993) that count only approximately 10^6 cells as compared with more than 10^8 cells that have been analyzed from a single blood sample by flow cytometry (Gross et al. 1993). A limit of detection of better than 10^6 also starts to approach the sensitivity needed for validating the removal of malignant cells from therapeutic CD34 cell preparations.

■ ENUMERATION OF CD34$^+$ CELLS BY FLOW CYTOMETRY

Because of commonly used sample preparation protocols that involve several washing steps for a sample with a potential loss of some cells, subset determinations by flow cytometry are generally expressed as fractions of major cell populations such as lymphocytes (i.e., a percentage of CD3$^+$ T cells). This assumes that subset fractions do not change during sample preparation steps, which is probably true within major cell groups such as lymphocytes.

If volumes during sample preparation are carefully controlled or a population of cells or appropriate microspheres are used as a volume standard (Stewart and Steinkamp 1982; Chen et al. 1994), absolute cell counts can be measured by flow cytometry. As with other counting methods, the precision of the counts depends on count statistics and other variables of the sample preparation and the measurement; however, in many cases, the count statistics are the most important contributor to imprecision. Therefore, for a 3% precision, at least,

1,000 particles must be counted for all of the populations used to determine the absolute count. Preferentially, all of the numbers for absolute counts should be determined on the same instrument. The often used practice of using the total white cell count (WCC) and a lymphocyte percentage from hematology counters combined with subset percentages from flow cytometry has been shown to be very imprecise with within-laboratory coefficients of variation of more than 10% and interlaboratory values even higher (J. Kagan, personal communication).

For sample preparation, the red cell lysis technique eliminates an excess of erythrocytes, and cell washing by centrifugation removes less dense cell fragments and, especially, unbound fluorescent reagent. The instrument threshold selects the property that determines whether a particle is measured by the instrument. The fluorescence threshold for the CD34 counting methods 5 and 6 in Table 5.1 ignores red cells and nonfluorescent debris and therefore allows the analysis of samples with many such particles.

More analysis parameters generally define cell populations better and allow the enumeration of smaller subpopulations, provided enough events have been measured.

Several approaches to enumerate CD34 cells routinely were discussed during a recent workshop on the topic.[a] Those methods are summarized in Table 5.1. The use of CD34-FITC combined with a Leukogate/Simulset analysis (Loken et al. 1990) was described by Bonni Hazelton (personal communication). The method relies on only one fluorescein-based immunofluorescence parameter and is, therefore, limited in its sensitivity. For samples high in $CD34^+$, this method combined with the measurement of only 10,000 total cells is acceptable. It should be noted that for the purpose of timing of leukapheresis of PB stem cells, high counts are more relevant and a lower sensitivity should be sufficient.

Ian McNiece (personal communication) reported on a variation of this method, the analysis of a CD34-PE versus side scatter plot, where CD34 binding to neutrophils can be clearly seen. This combination is currently the most commonly used approach for CD34 cell counting. The use of phycoerythrin (PE) instead of fluorescein (FITC) increases the sensitivity of the method due to the more intense fluorescence with PE. Several methods relying on three-parameter fluorescence measurements were also described. Those methods are generally sensitive

[a]"Workshop on definition of CD34+ cell harvest predicting for rapid hematopoietic reconstitution," Chicago, IL, 26 August 1994.

Table 5.1. Methods for CD34 Enumeration (Amgen Data on File)

	Reagents	Preparation	Threshold	Analysis	Source
1	CD34-FITC	Lyse & wash	FSC	Leukogate FSC SSC Fl1	Hazelton
2	CD34-PE	Lyse & wash	FSC	SSC Fl2	McNiece
3	CD45-FITC CD34-PE	Lyse & wash	FSC	FSC SSC Fl1 Fl2	Bender
4	CD14-FITC CD34-PE 7-AAD	Lyse & wash	FSC	FSC SSC Fl1 Fl2 Fl3	Loken
5	TO CD34-PE CD45-PE*CY5	Lyse	Fl1	FSC SSC Fl1 Fl2 Fl3	Terstappen
6	CD15&CD45-FITC CD34-PE LDS751	Wash	Fl3	FSC SSC Fl1 Fl2 Fl3	Recktenwald

FITC = fluorescein; PE = phycoerythrin; 7-AAD = 7-amino-actinomycin-D; TO = thiazole-orange (Lee, Chen, and Chiu 1986); PE*CY5 = phycoerythrin-cyanine5 tandem conjugate (Lanier and Recktenwald 1991); LDS751-red emitting laser dye (Recktenwald 1992).

enough to detect very low concentrations of CD34[+] cells. Details of those methods are described in the legend of Table 5.1. Method 4 of Table 5.1 is optimized for ease of use as described in a separate publication reporting comprehensive test data (Chen et al. 1994). The advantage of this method is that the determination of the CD34 count is done using a real-time analysis of data during the flow cytometric measurement of each blood sample. An accurate measurement of the number of circulating CD34[+] cells in a 100-μL sample of PB can be obtained in 1 hour using commercially available flow-cytometry equipment.

It is likely that the clinical use of CD34[+] cells obtained from the PB of patients will increase in the future, and that accurate methods of enumerating these cells on a routine basis will have widespread clinical application.

■ ISOLATION AND CHARACTERIZATION OF CD34[+] CELLS BY FLOW CYTOMETRY

The CD34 antigen was originally described as a marker present on myeloid leukemia cells, then subsequently recognized as a marker for primitive hemopoietic progenitors (Civin et al. 1984; Civin et al. 1987). Expression of the CD34 antigen is not limited to hemopoietic progenitors; it has also been associated with stromal progenitors isolated from the BM and endothelial cells (Fina et al. 1990; Simmons and Torok-Storb 1991a, b; Udomsakdi et al. 1991; Simmons et al. 1994; Waller et al. 1995).

FACS analysis has been used to delineate the pathways of normal hemopoietic-cell differentiation and maturation in human BM (Loken et al. 1987a, b; Terstappen, Safford, and Loken 1990) and thymus (Terstappen, Huang, and Picker 1992a; Kraft, Weissman, and Waller 1993). In these studies, the differentiation of progenitor cells has been followed by measuring coordinated changes in their light-scatter properties and surface-antigen expression. Differentiation of pluripotent hemopoietic progenitors is associated with down-regulation of CD34 expression and up-regulation of antigens associated with differentiated hemopoietic cell lineages (Loken et al. 1987a, b; Terstappen et al. 1990; Terstappen et al. 1992a; Kraft et al. 1993).

The function of the CD34 molecule in hemopoiesis has not been clearly defined. The CD34 antigen is a mucin molecule that likely functions in cellular adhesion (Majdic et al. 1994). It is also expressed on nonhemopoietic cells, including vascular endothelial cells, and may function as a heterotypic dimer for the adhesion of hemopoietic cells that express the lymphocyte-homing receptor to endothelial cells (Baumheter et al. 1993).

■ CLINICAL APPLICATIONS OF CD34⁺ CELLS

Stem-Cell Transplantation

The use of CD34⁺ peripheral blood progenitor cells (PBPC) for use in stem-cell transplantation has increased at an exponential rate during the past 5 years (Henon 1993; Inwards and Kessinger 1992). Hemopoietic stem cells obtained from the PB either by apheresis alone or following a combination of apheresis and CD34 selection appear to have an equal or superior biologic activity in promoting hematologic recovery following myeloablative therapy compared with BM cells (Kiesel et al. 1989). Current protocols involving CD34⁺ cells obtained from the PB have utilized the preadministration of cytotoxic chemotherapy, hemopoietic growth factors, or a combination of these two agents in order to increase the numbers of circulating stem cells (see Chapters 8 and 9). While either treatment alone can significantly increase the numbers of circulating CD34⁺ cells, a combination of both types of agents may be the more effective in achieving high numbers of circulating CD34⁺ cells in the PB than either administered alone (Gianni et al. 1989; Tarella et al. 1991). Peripheral blood hemopoietic stem cell (PBHSC) preparations obtained in this manner have been used effectively in autologous stem-cell transplantation protocols involving patients with a variety of hemologic and non-hemologic malignancies (Inwards and Kessinger 1992; Henon 1993). The timing of apheresis is often being done empirically, according to changes in the total WCC (Pettengell et al. 1993a, b). The optimal dose and schedule of administration of drugs that mobilize CD34⁺ cells into the peripheral circulation has yet to be determined. Current studies have demonstrated a relatively poor correlation between the measured numbers of CD34⁺ cells in the circulation and laboratory measurements of stem-cell activity such as colony-forming units (CFU) in methylcellulose cultures, or long-term culture-initiating cells (LTC-IC) on stromal monolayers. This is likely due to technical difficulties in accurately measuring the small numbers of PB CD34⁺ cells that are routinely obtained, and to variables affecting progenitor cell assays (see Chapter 3).

Characterization of Subpopulations of CD34⁺ Hemopoietic Stem Cells

The isolation of human hemopoietic stem cells (hHSC) has followed the lead of earlier studies of murine hemopoiesis (Visser et al. 1984; Spangrude, Heimfeld, and Weissman 1988; Uchida and Weissman 1992), and used FACS to characterize and isolate populations of

Color Plates

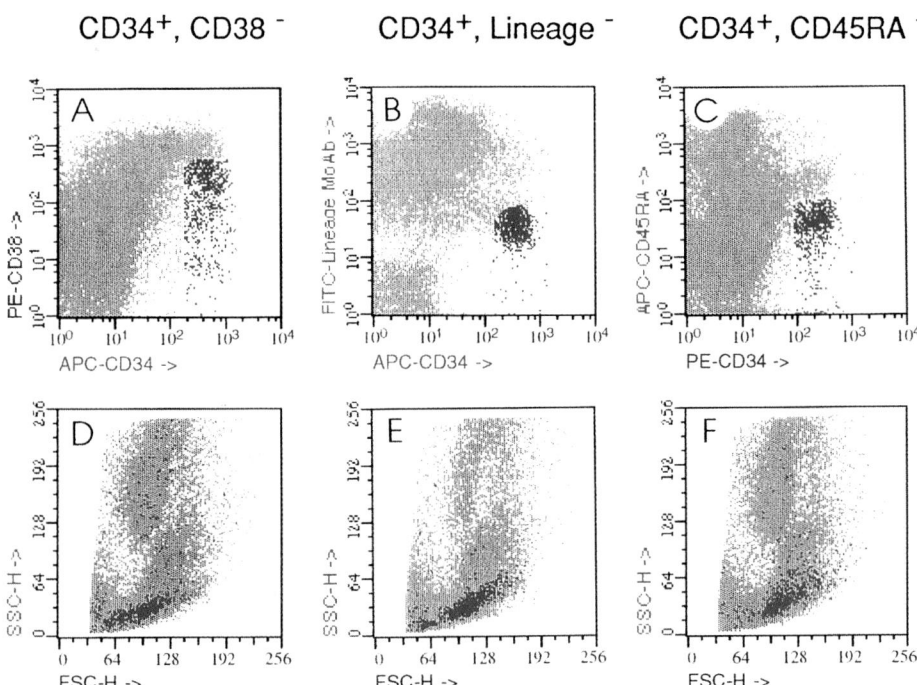

CD34+, CD38 − **CD34+, Lineage −** **CD34+, CD45RA −**

Figure 5.1 FACS analysis of CD34+ cells in normal adult BM. Low-density BM cells from a normal BM donor were separated by centrifugation over a Ficoll-Hypaque step gradient, washed, and stained with three different combinations of mAB. *A* and *D*, CD34-allophycocyanin + CD38-PE, + C45-FITC + HLADR-PerCP. *B* and *E*, CD34-allophycocyanin + Thy 1-PE + a combination of CD4-FITC, CD8-FITC, CD14-FITC, CD15-FITC, CD45RA-FITC, and CD71-FITC + HLA-DR-PerCP. *C* and *F*, CD34-PE + CD45RA-allophycocyanin + CD71-FITC + HLA-DR-PerCP. Three percent of the cells were CD34+ in each case; the 1.4% of CD34+ cells that expressed low to dim levels of a second Ag (shown in the vertical axis in *A* [CD38], *B* [lineage cocktail], or *C* [CD45RA]) were red using Paint-a-Gate^{Plus}. The forward scatter (FSC-H) and side scatter (SSC-H) profiles of the CD34+ cells are shown in *D*, *E*, and *F*.

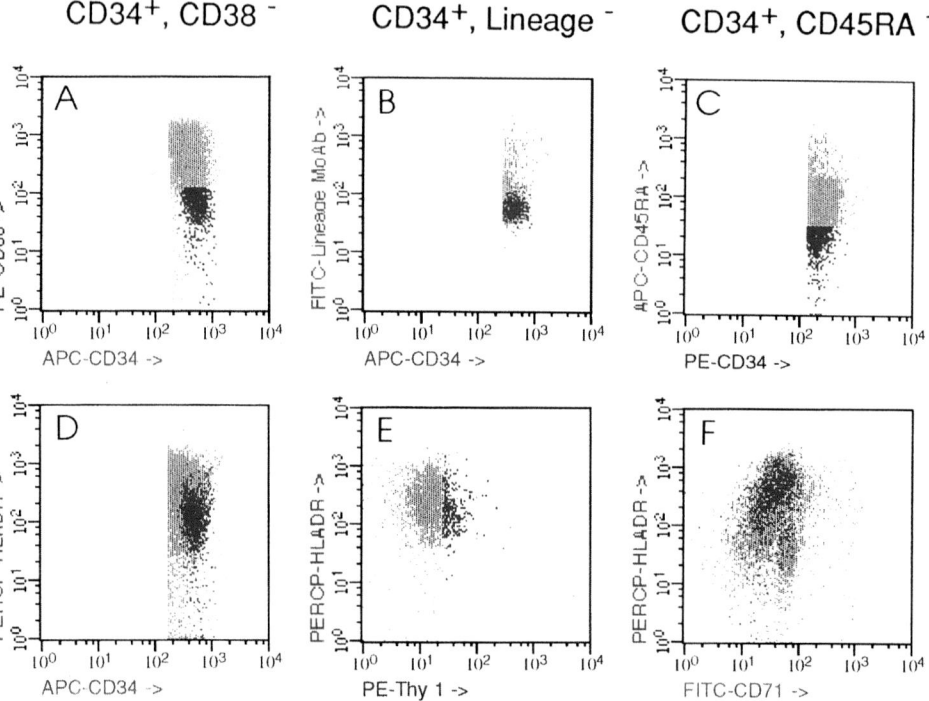

Figure 5.2 The FACS analysis of "gated" CD34⁺ cells in normal adult BM. The same samples analyzed in Figure 5.1 were reanalyzed on a FACScan using an electronic gate so that only data on CD34⁺ cells were collected. The expression of CD34 was compared with three different combinations of lineage specific antigens as described in the legend to Figure 5.1. *A, B,* and *C,* The 10% of CD34⁺ cells that expressed the highest levels of CD34 and the lowest levels of a second antigen(s) were red. *D, E,* and *F,* The expression of HLA-DR (y axis) versus another antigen (*A,* CD38; *E,* Thy-1; *F,* CD71) that has been used to define pluripotent stem cells is shown.

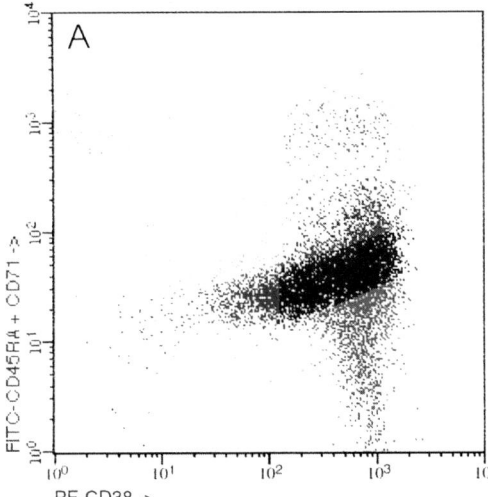

A

PE-CD38 ->

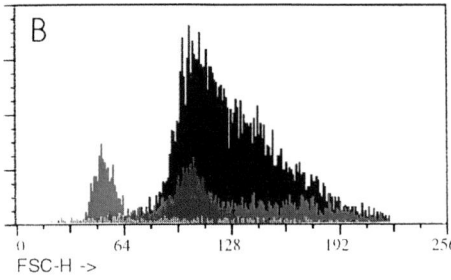

B

FSC-H ->

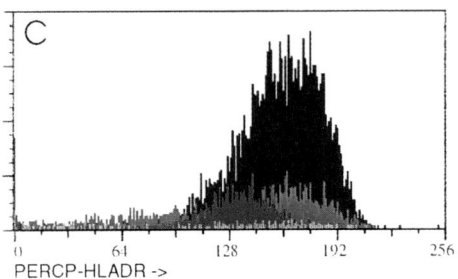

C

PERCP-HLADR ->

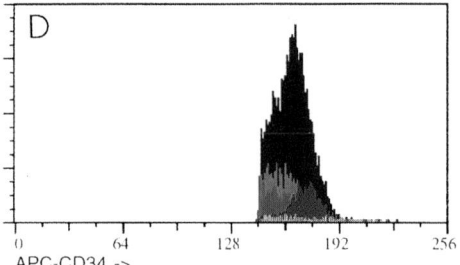

D

APC-CD34 ->

Figure 5.3 A comparison of two different methods of defining the phenotype of pluripotent stem cells by FACS. Low-density BM MNC were stained with a co-mixture of CD-34-allophycocyanin + CD38-PE + CD45RA-FITC + CD71-FITC + HLA-DR-PerCP. *A*, "Gated" data were collected on the total CD34+ (APC+) population which was then subdivided into five different subpopulations using the staining patterns obtained from combination of CD45RA-FITC + CD71-FITC and CD38-PE. The "red" CD38−, CD45RA/CD71^{dim} cells constituted 10% of the CD34+ cells; the "green" CD38+, CD45RA/CD71^{hi} cells constituted 11% of the CD34+ cells; the "purple" CD38+, CD45RA/CD71^{dim} cells constituted 61% of the CD34+ cells; and the "blue" CD38+, CD45RA/CD71− cells constituted 16% of the CD34+ cells. An additional 2% of cells were CD38−, CD45RA/CD71+ and were "yellow." *B*, The histogram for forward scatter (FSC-H) for each colored population is shown. *C*, The histogram for the expression of HLA-DR in each population is shown. *D*, The histogram for the expression of CD34 for each population is shown. Note that the cells colored red have the highest level of CD34 expression, lack expression of CD38, and express "dim" levels of CD45Ra/71 and HLA-DR.

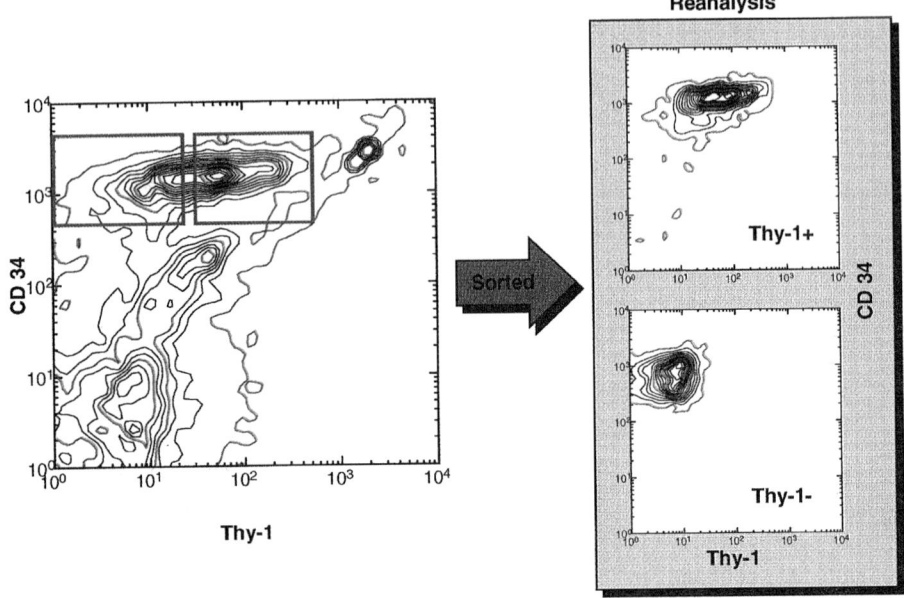

SCID-hu Bone Assay

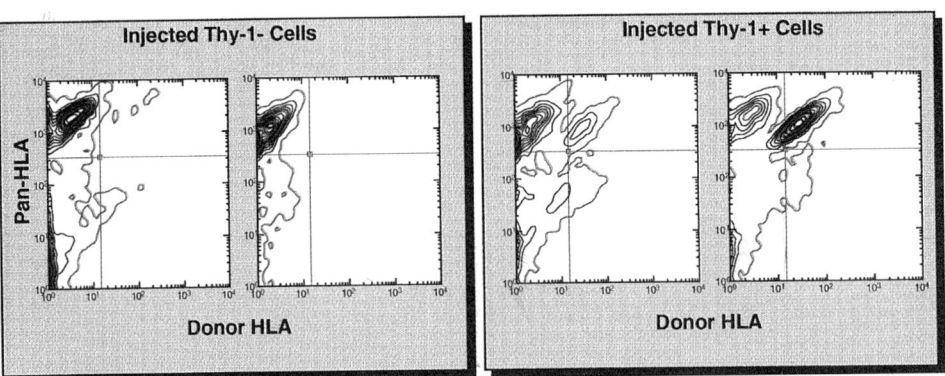

Figure 10.1 Correlation of Thy-1 expression in mobilized PB and engraftment in the SCID-hu bone assay. A mobilized PB sample was analyzed for the presence of Thy-1$^+$ cells within the CD34$^+$Lin$^-$ population. Cells were sorted into Thy-1$^+$ and Thy-1$^-$ populations. 10^4 cells were microinjected into HLA-mismatched SCID-hu bones. BM cells recovered 8 weeks following implantation were analyzed for donor-derived cells by flow cytometry. Representative bone grafts show that the Thy-1$^+$, but not the Thy-1$^-$, population engrafted.

CD34$^+$ candidate stem cells with defined surface phenotypes. Sorted cell populations were then studied in in vitro and in vivo model systems to define their biologic potentials. The phenotype of the putative hHSC has been described either as CD34$^+$, Thy$^+$, Lin$^-$ (Baum et al. 1992); CD34$^+$, HLA-DR$^+$, CD38$^{-/dim}$ (Huang and Terstappen 1992); or CD34$^+$, CD71$^{-/dim}$, CD45RA$^{-/dim}$ (Lansdorp and Dragowska 1992; Fritsch et al. 1993). We performed a comparison of the staining pattern obtained on adult BM cells using these three different methods (shown in Figs. 5.1–5.3). The six panels in Figure 5.1 represent the analysis of three separate aliquots of the same BM sample stained with an allophycocyanin (APC) -conjugated mAB to CD34 and either a PE-conjugated antibody (Ab) to CD38 (Huang and Terstappen 1992) in Figure 5.1*A* (see color plate); an APC-conjugated mAB to CD34 and a cocktail of fluorescein-conjugated Ab to a variety of markers expressed on mature hemopoietic cells (CD4, CD8, CD14, CD15, CD45RA, CD71) (Baum et al. 1992) in Figure 5.1*B*; or a combination of PE-conjugated Ab to CD34 and an APC-conjugated Ab to CD45RA in the upper right panel (Lansdorp and Dragowska 1992) in Figure 5.1*C*. In each case, 3% of the low-density mononuclear cells (MNC) were CD34$^+$, and approximately one-half of these were colored red (1.4% of the total cells) and had undetectable to dim levels of fluorescence in the channel associated with lineage-specific differentiation. These CD34$^+$ fractions consisted of a mixed population of cells that had light-scattering properties similar to those of small to large lymphocytes (Fig. 5.1*D*, *E*, and *F*). In the display of these data (Fig. 5.1), about 720 CD34$^+$ cells were colored red from list-mode files each containing 50,000 events.

In order to isolate and study pluripotent hemopoietic stem cells, the fraction of CD34$^+$ cells that fail to express Ag associated with lineage commitment must be distinguished from the larger population of CD34$^+$ cells that express low to high levels of these same markers. The expression of other Ag on this rare population of cells can then be reliably determined without the confounding presence of lineage-committed CD34$^+$ cells. This analysis requires that large numbers of PB or BM cells be analyzed, since the pluripotent HSC are reported to constitute less than 0.1% (1 cell/1,000) of the total number of BM cells. Therefore, to obtain data on subsets of 1,000 CD34$^+$, lineage dull/negative pluripotent stem cells in BM, a total of 1 million BM cells need to be analyzed; however, list-mode files containing 1 million events consume considerable data storage space, and are unwieldy to analyze. An alternative procedure is to acquire list-mode data only on the CD34$^+$ cells, which constituted about 3% of the total BM cells in this sample. The presence or absence of rare populations of cells with the phenotype(s) ascribed to pluripotent HSC can then be ascertained using the file of "CD34$^+$ gated" data. The CD34$^+$/lineage-negative cell population was identified using each of the three different combinations of mAB, and is shown in Figure 5.2A, B, and C (see color plate). In each case, only those cells expressing high levels of CD34 and low to absent levels of the markers associated with lineage differentiation are "red cells". The red cells represented 10% of the total CD34$^+$ cells, and less than 0.1% of the total MNC (720/1 million cells). The expression of an independent marker, HLA-DR is shown in Figure 5.2D, E, and F. In this case, HLA-DR is expressed at moderate to low levels in the populations defined as CD34$^+$, CD38- (Fig. 5.2D) and CD34$^+$, Thy-1^{low}, lineage-negative (Fig. 5.2E), but is expressed at higher levels in the population defined as CD34$^+$, CD45RA$^-$ (Fig. 5.2F), indicating that there is not an exact correspondence among these three different methods of defining stem cells.

In order to compare directly the definition of HSC as CD34$^+$, CD38$^-$ (Fig. 5.2A) with the definition as CD34$^+$, CD45RA$^-$, CD71$^-$, BM cells were stained with a combination of CD34 (APC), CD38 (PE), CD45RA (FITC), CD71 (FITC), and HLA-DR (PerCP), and are shown in Figure 5.3 (see color plate). Analyzing only the CD34$^+$ cells, collected as a "gated" file during data acquisition, there was heterogeneous expression of CD38 versus the combination of CD45RA plus CD71. There were CD38$^-$ cells that were CD45RA/CD71$^-$ (light blue in Fig. 5.3A) and CD38$^-$ cells that were CD45RA/CD71^{dim} (red in Fig. 5.3A). The majority of CD34$^+$ cells expressed both CD38 as well as moderate levels of one or both of the combination of CD45RA/CD71 (dark blue, Fig. 5.3A), while a few cells were CD38$^+$ and CD45RA/CD71 bright (green, Fig. 5.3A). The forward scatter profiles of these four populations are shown in Figure 5.3B. The cells that were dark blue and the green cells had large forward scatters, suggesting that they were blasts committed to myeloid or erythroid differentiation (Fig. 5.3B). The "red cells" had a forward scatter profile consistent with that of small- to medium-sized lymphocytes, while the light blue cells were smaller (Fig. 5.3B). The levels of HLA-DR expression of these four populations are compared in Figure 5.3C. The "red cell" population was a discrete population with a relatively low level of HLA-DR expression, compared with the cells that were CD38$^+$ and dark blue or green. The level of CD34 expression is shown in Figure 5.3D, and was highest in the "red cell" population, indicating that the CD34$^+$/CD38$^-$, CD45RA/CD71^{dim} subset is likely to be the most primitive hemopoietic progenitor cell. This analysis indicates that the combination of CD34 and CD38 Ab appears to be the most efficient in discriminating the putative pluripotent hemopoietic progenitor cells from other populations of lineage-committed CD34$^+$ cells. CD34 cell enrichment with magnetic microparticles conjugated to CD34 antibody can also be used before subset analysis by immunofluorescence (Kato and Radbruch 1993).

Functional Properties of Isolated Candidate Human Hemopoietic Stem Cells

The ability of the candidate hHSC to differentiate along multiple hemopoietic lineages has been demonstrated by in vitro culture of these cells with the appropriate cocktails of cytokines (Leary et al. 1987; Saeland et al. 1989; Brandt et al. 1990; Bernstein, Andrews, and Zsebo 1991; Briddell et al. 1991; Eaves et al. 1991; Terstappen et al. 1991; Buescher, Nguyen, and Reading 1992a; Hallek et al. 1992; Long et al. 1992; Reddy et al. 1992; Terstappen et al. 1992; Sutherland et al. 1993) and by injecting them into a human thymic or BM microenvironment established using human fetal thymic or bone xenografts in a severe combined immune deficiency (SCID) syndrome mouse model (Baum et al. 1992).

In fetal BM, the hemopoietic progenitor cells are CD34$^+$, CD38$^-$; most of these are HLA-DR$^+$, while a minor fraction are HLA-DR$^-$ (Huang and Terstappen 1994). Both of the HLA-DR$^+$ and the HLA-DR$^-$ fractions of fetal BM have the potential for multilineage differentiation, but the population with the highest initial cloning potential following FACS is within the HLA-DR$^+$ fraction (Huang and Terstappen 1994). In contrast, the expression of HLA-DR on pluripotent HSC population isolated from fetal liver, cord blood (CB), or adult BM is controversial, with some reports claiming that pluripotent hHSC are HLA-DR$^-$ negative (Verfaillie, Blakholmer, and McGlave 1990; Srour et al. l991; Briddell et al. 1992; Srour et al. 1992; Verfaillie 1992), dim (Sutherland et al. 1989, 1990; Udomsakdi et al. 1992; Terstappen and Lund-Johansen 1994), or positive (Greinix et al. 1991; Deeg et al. 1994). Recent studies suggest that CD50 expression in the CD34$^+$, CD38$^-$ cell fraction may be a more reliable marker for hHSC than HLA-DR expression (Waller et al. 1995). Future directions in stem-cell biology will involve further subtyping of the CD34$^+$ population in PB and BM, as well as defining the biologic properties of subpopulations of CD34$^+$ cells that have been isolated by flow cytometry.

REFERENCES

Baum, C.M., Weissman, I.L., Tsukamoto, A.S., Buckle, A.M., and Peault, B. (1992) Isolation of a candidate human hematopoietic stem-cell population. *Proceedings of the National Academy of Sciences of the United States of America*, **89**, 2804–8.

Baumheter, S., Singer, M.S., Henzel, W., et al. (1993) Binding of L-selectin to the vascular sialomucin CD34. *Science*, **262**, 436–8.

Bernstein, I.D., Andrews, R.G., and Zsebo, K.M. (1991) Recombinant human stem cell factor enhances the formation of colonies by CD34+ and CD34+1in- cells, and the generation of colony-forming cell progeny from CD34+1in- cells cultured with interleukin-3, granulocyte colony-stimulating factor, or granulocyte-macrophage colony-stimulating factor. *Blood*, **77**, 2316–21.

Brandt, J., Srour, E.F., Van Besien, K., Bridell, R.A., and Hoffman, R. (1990) Cytokine-dependent long-term culture of highly enriched precursors of hematopoietic progenitor cells from human bone marrow. *Journal of Clinical Investigation*, **86**, 932.

Briddell, R.A., Broudy, V.C., Bruno, E., Brandt, J.E., Srour, E.F., and Hoffman, R. (1992) Further phenotypic characterization and isolation of human hematopoietic progenitor cells using a monoclonal antibody to the c-kit receptor. *Blood*, **79**, 3159–67.

Briddell, R.A., Bruno, E., Cooper, R.J., Brandt, J.E., and Hoffman, R. (1991) Effect of c-kit ligand on in vitro human megakaryocytopoiesis. *Blood*, **78**, 2854–9.

Chen, C.H., Lin, W., Shye, S., et al. (1994) Automated enumeration of CD34+ cells in peripheral blood and bone marrow. *Journal of Hematotherapy*, **3**, 3–13

Civin, C.I., Banquerigo, M.L., Strauss, L.C., and Loken, M.R. (1987) Antigenic analysis of hematopoiesis. IV. Flow cytometric characterization of My-10-positive progenitor cells in normal human bone marrow. *Experimental Hematology*, **15**, 10.

Civin, C.I., Strauss, L.C., Brovall, C., Fackler, M.J., Schwartz, J.F., and Shaper J.H. (1984) A hematopoietic progenitor cell surface antigen defined by a monoclonal antibody raised against KG-1a cells. *Journal of Immunology*, **133**, 157.

Deeg, H.J., Backham C., Huss R., et al. (1994) Rescue from anti-MHC class II antibody-mediated marrow graft failure by c-kit ligand. *Blood*, **83**, 2352–9.

Eaves, C.J., Sutherland, H.J., Cashman, J.D., et al. (1991) Regulation of primitive human hematopoietic cells in long term marrow culture. *Seminars in Hematology*, **28**, 126–31.

Fina, L., Molgaard, H.V., Robertson, D., et al. (1990) Expression of the CD34 gene in vascular endothelial cells. *Blood*, **75**, 2417.

Fritsch, G., Buchinger, P., Printz, D., et al. (1993) Rapid discrimination of early CD34+ myeloid progenitors using CD45RA analysis. *Blood*, **81**, 2301–9.

Gianni, M., Siena, S., Bregni, M., et al. (1989) Granulocyte-macrophage colony-stimulating factor to harvest circulating hematopoietic cells for auto-transplantation. *Lancet*, **2**, 580–5.

Greinix, H.T., Ladiges, W.C., Graham, T.C., et al. (1991) Late failure of autologous marrow grafts in lethally irradiated dogs given anti-class II monoclonal antibody. *Blood*, **78**, 2131–7.

Gross, H.J., Verwer, B., Houck, D., and Recktenwald, D. (1993) Detection of rare cells at a frequency of one/million by flow cytometry. *Cytometry*, **14**, 519–26.

Hallek, M., Druker, B., Lepisto, E.M., Wood, K.W., Ernst, T.J., and Griffin, J.D. (1992) Granulocyte-macrophage colony-stimulating factor and steel factor induce phosphorylation of both unique and overlapping signal transduction intermediates in a human factor-dependent hematopoietic cell line. *Journal of Cellular Physiology*, **153**, 176–86.

Henon, P.R. (1993) Peripheral blood stem cell transplantation: past, present and future. *Stem Cells*, **11**, 154–72.

Herzenberg, L.A., Sweet, R.G., and Herzenberg, L.A. (1976) Fluorescence-activated cell sorting. *Scientific American*, **234**, 108–17.

Hoffman, R.A., Recktenwald, D.J., and Vogt, R.F. (1993) Cell-associated receptor quantitation. In K.D. Bauer, R.E. Duque, and T.V. Shankey (Eds.) *Clinical flow cytometry, principles and application*, pp. 469–77. Baltimore, MD, Williams & Wilkins.

Huang, S. and Terstappen, L.W. (1992) Formation of haematopoietic microenvironment and haematopoietic stem cells from single human bone marrow stem cells. *Nature*, **360**, 745–9.

Huang, S. and Terstappen, L.W. (1994) Lymphoid and myeloid differentiation of single CD34$^+$, HLA-DR$^+$, CD38$^-$ hematopoietic stem cells. *Blood*, **83**, 1515–26.

Inwards, D. and Kessinger, A. (1992) Peripheral blood stem cell transplantation: historical perspective, current status, and prospects for the future. *Transfusion Medicine Reviews*, **6**, 183–90.

Kato, K. and Radbruch, A. (1993) Isolation and characterization of CD34$^+$ hematopoietic stem cells from human peripheral blood by high-gradient magnetic cell sorting. *Cytometry*, **14**, 384–92.

Kiesel, S., Pezzutto, A., Korbling, M., et al. (1989) Autologous peripheral blood stem cell transplantation: analysis of autografted cells and lymphocyte recovery. *Transplantation Proceedings*, **21**, 3084–8.

Kraft, D.L., Weissman, I.L., and Waller, E.K. (1993) Differentiation of CD3-4-8- human fetal thymocytes in vivo: characterization of a CD3-4$^+$8- intermediate. *Journal of Experimental Medicine*, **178**, 265–77.

Lanier, L.L. and Recktenwald, D.J. (1991) Multicolor immunofluorescence and flow cytometry. *Methods*, **2**, 192–9.

Lansdorp, P.M. and Dragowska, W. (1992) Long-term erythropoiesis from constant numbers of CD34$^+$ cells in serum-free cultures initiated with highly purified progenitor cells from the human bone marrow. *Journal of Experimental Medicine*, **175**, 1501–9.

Leary, A.G., Yang, Y.C., Clark, S.C., Gasson, J.C., Golde, D.W., and Ogawa, M. (1987) Recombinant gibbon interleukin 3 supports formation of human multilineage colonies in culture: comparison with recombinant human granulocyte-macrophage colony-stimulating factor. *Blood*, **70**, 1343.

Lee, L.G., Chen, C.H., and Chiu, L.A. (1986) Thiazole orange, a new dye for reticulocyte analysis. *Cytometry*, **7**, 508–17.

Loken, M.R., Brosnan, J.M., Bach, B.A., and Ault, K.A. (1990) Establishing optimal lymphocyte gates for immunophenotyping by flow cytometry. *Cytometry*, **11**, 453–9.

Loken, M.R., Shah, V.O., Datilo, K.L., and Civin, C.I. (1987a) Flow cytometric analysis of human bone marrow: I. Normal erythroid development. *Blood*, **69**, 225.

Loken, M.R., Shah, V.O., Datilo, K.L., and Civin, C.I. (1987b) Flow cytometric analysis of human bone marrow: II. Normal B lymphocyte development. *Blood*, **70**, 1316.

Long, M.W., Briddell, R., Walter, A.W., Bruno, E., and Hoffman, R. (1992) Human hematopoietic stem cell adherence to cytokines and matrix molecules. *Journal of Clinical Investigation,* **90,** 251–5.

Majdic, O., Stockl, J., Pickl, W.F., et al. (1994) Signaling and induction of enhanced cytoadhesiveness via the hematopoietic progenitor cell surface marker CD34. *Blood,* **83,** 1226–34.

Muirhead, K.A., Schmitt, T.C., and Muirhead, A.R. (1983) Determination of linear fluorescence intensities from flow cytometric data accumulated with logarithmic amplifiers. *Cytometry,* **3,** 251–6.

Pantel, K., Izbicki, J.R., Angstwurm, M., et al. (1993) Immunocytological detection of bone marrow micrometastasis in operable non-small cell lung cancer. *Cancer Research,* **53,** 1027–31.

Pettengell, R., Morgenstern, G.R., Woll, P.J., et al. (1993a) Peripheral blood progenitor cell transplantation in lymphoma and leukemia using a single apharesis. *Blood,* **82,** 3770–7.

Pettengell, R., Testa, N.G., Swindell, R., Crowther, D., and Dexter, T.M. (1993b) Transplantation potential of hematopoietic cells released into the circulation during routine chemotherapy for non-Hodgkin's lymphoma. *Blood,* **82,** 2239–48.

Recktenwald, D. (1992) Multicolor immunofluorescence analysis. In A. Radbruch (Ed.) *Flow cytometry and cell sorting,* pp. 47–53. Berlin, Springer Verlag.

Reddy, G.P., Reed, W.C., Deacon, D.H., and Quesenberry, P.J. (1992) Growth factor-dependent proliferative stimulation of hematopoietic cells is associated with the modulation of cytoplasmic and nuclear 68-Kd calmodulin-binding protein. *Blood,* **79,** 1946–55.

Ryan, D.H. (1993) Detection of minimal residual disease by flow cytometry. In K.D. Bauer, R. E. Duque, and T.V. Shankey (Eds.) *Clinical flow cytometry, principles and application,* pp. 479–96. Baltimore, MD, Williams & Wilkins.

Saeland, S., Caux, C., Favre, C., et al. (1989) Combined and sequential effects of human IL-3 and GM-CSF on the proliferation of CD34$^+$ hematopoietic cells from cord blood. *Blood,* **73,** 1195.

Schlimok, G., Funke, I., Holzmann, B., et al. (1987) Micrometastatic cancer cells in bone marrow: in vitro detection with anti-cytokeratin and in vivo labeling with anti-17-1A monoclonal antibodies. *Proceedings of the National Academy of Sciences of the United States of America,* **84,** 8672–6.

Simmons, P.J., Gronthos, S., Zannettino, A., and Graves, S. (1994) Human bone marrow stromal precursors: identification and developmental potential. *Journal of Cellular Biochemistry. Supplement,* **18B,** G022.

Simmons, P.J. and Torok-Storb, B. (1991a) CD34 expression by stromal precursors in normal human adult bone marrow. *Blood,* **78,** 2848–53.

Simmons, P.J. and Torok-Storb, B. (1991b) Identification of stromal cell precursors in human bone marrow by a novel monoclonal antibody, STRO-1. *Blood,* **78,** 55–62.

Spangrude, G.J., Heimfeld, S., and Weissman, I.L. (1988) Purification and characterization of mouse hematopoietic stem cells. *Science,* **124,** 58.

Srour, E.F., Brandt, J.E., Briddell, R.A., Leemhuis, T., Van, B.K., and Hoffman, R. (1991) Human CD34$^+$ HLA-DR- bone marrow cells contain progenitor cells capable of self-renewal, multilineage differentiation, and long-term in vitro hematopoiesis. *Blood Cells,* **17,** 287–95.

Srour, E.F., Zanjani, E.D., Brandt, J.E., et al. (1992) Sustained human hematopoiesis in sheep transplanted in utero during early gestation with fractionated adult bone marrow cells. *Blood*, **79**, 1404–12.

Stewart, C.C. and Steinkamp, J.A. (1982) Quantitation of cell concentration using the flow cytometer. *Cytometry*, **2**, 238–43.

Sutherland, H.J., Eaves, C.J., Eaves, A.C., Dragowska, W., and Lansdorp, P.M. (1989) Characterization and partial purification of human bone marrow cells capable of initiating long-term hematopoiesis in vitro. *Blood*, **74**, 1563.

Sutherland, H.J., Hogge, D.E., Cook, D., and Eaves, C.J. (1993) Alternative mechanisms with and without steel factor support primitive human hematopoiesis. *Blood*, **81**, 1465–70.

Sutherland, H.J., Lansdorp, P.M., Henkelman, D.H., Eaves, A.C., and Eaves C.J. (1990) Functional characterization of individual human hematopoietic stem cells cultured at limiting dilution on supportive marrow stromal layers. *Proceedings of the National Academy of Sciences of the United States of America*, **87**, 3584–8.

Tarella, C., Ferrero, D., Bregni, M., et al. (1991) Peripheral blood expansion of early progenitor cells after high dose cyclophosphamide and rh-GM-CSF. *European Journal of Cancer*, **27**, 22–7.

Terstappen, L.W., Buescher, S., Nguyen, M., and Reading, C. (1992b) Differentiation and maturation of growth factor expanded human hematopoietic progenitors assessed by multidimensional flow cytometry. *Leukemia*, **6**, 1001–10.

Terstappen, L.W., Huang, S., and Picker, L.J. (1992a) Flow cytometric assessment of human T-cell differentiation in thymus and bone marrow. *Blood*, **79**, 666–77.

Terstappen, L.W., Huang, S., Safford, M., Lansdorp, P.M., and Loken, M.R. (1991) Sequential generations of hematopoietic colonies derived from single non-lineage committed CD34+CD38- progenitor cells. *Blood*, **77**, 1218–27.

Terstappen, L.W. and Lund-Johansen, F. (1994) Hematopoietic progenitors in fetal and adult tissue. *Blood Cells*, **20**, 392–6.

Terstappen, L.W., Safford, M., and Loken, M.R. (1990) Flow cytometric analysis of human bone marrow III. Neutrophil maturation. *Leukemia*, **4**, 657–63.

Uchida, N. and Weissman, I.L. (1992) Searching for hematopoietic stem cells: evidence that Thy-1.11O Lin- Sca-1$^+$ cells are the only stem cells in C57BUKa-Thy-1.1 bone marrow. *Journal of Experimental Medicine*, **175**, 175–84.

Udomsakdi, C., Eaves, C.J., Sutherland, H.J., and Lansdorp, P.M. (1991) Separation of functionally distinct subpopulations of primitive human hematopoietic cells using rhodamine-123. *Experimental Hematology*, **19**, 338–42.

Udomsakdi, C., Lansdorp, P.M., Hogge, D.E., Reid, D.S., Eaves, A.C., and Eaves C.J. (1992) Characterization of primitive hematopoietic cells in normal human peripheral blood. *Blood*, **80**, 2513–21.

Verfaillie, C.M. (1992) Direct contact between human primitive hematopoietic progenitors and bone marrow stroma is not required for long-term in vitro hematopoiesis. *Blood*, **79**, 2821–6.

Verfaillie, C.M., Blakholmer, K., and McGlave, P.B. (1990) Purified primitive human hematopoietic progenitors with long term in vitro repopulating capacity adhere selectively to irradiated bone marrow stroma. *Journal of Experimental Medicine*, **172**, 509.

Visser, J.W., Bauman, J.G., Mulder, A.H., Eliason, J.F., and Leeuw, A.M. (1984) Isolation of murine pluripotent hemopoietic stem cells. *Journal of Experimental Medicine*, **59**, 1576.

Waller, E.K., Olweus, J., Lund-Johansen, F.J., et al. (1995) The "common stem cell" hypothesis re-evaluated: human fetal bone marrow contains separate populations of hematopoietic and stromal progenitors. *Blood*, **85**, 2422–35.

Weichel, W., Liesegang, B., Gehrke, K., et al. (1985) Inexpensive upgrading of a FACS I and isolation of rare somatic variants by double-fluorescence sorting. *Cytometry*, **6**, 116–23.

Xiao, M., Leemhuis, T., Broxmeyer, H.E., and Lu, L. (1992) Influence of combinations of cytokines on proliferation of isolated single cell-sorted human bone marrow hematopoietic progenitor cells in the absence and presence of serum. *Experimental Hematology*, **20**, 276–9.

6

Principles of Gene Therapy

DAVID M. BODINE

The concept of correcting genetic disease by introducing a specific gene into cells has been discussed since the demonstration that bacteria could be made resistant to antibiotics by the introduction of exogenous DNA (for a history of gene therapy, see Wolf and Lederberg 1994). The hemopoietic system is especially adaptable to gene-therapy strategies (Anderson 1984), because bone marrow (BM) cells can be cultured ex vivo (Dexter et al. 1978; Sutherland et al. 1990). In addition, the pioneering work of Nobel Laureate Dr. E. Donnal Thomas and others (1975a, b) demonstrated that bone-marrow transplantation (BMT) could successfully reconstitute the entire hemopoietic system of a recipient whose own BM had been destroyed (Thomas et al. 1975a, b). The goal of this chapter is to describe briefly the technology involved in gene transfer into hemopoietic cells, animal models for gene therapy, and the problems that need to be solved before gene therapy for hemopoietic diseases becomes a reality. The references cited are intended to be representative, not complete.

■ RETROVIRUSES

Currently, the delivery of new genetic material to primary hemopoietic cells has been achieved mainly through retroviral vectors (for reviews, see Nienhuis, Walsh, and Liu 1993; Mulligan 1993). Retroviruses have an RNA genome that is reverse transcribed into DNA and integrated into the host-cell genome (Varmus 1982, 1988), the feature upon which gene-therapy strategies depend. The Moloney murine leukemia virus (MoMuLV) has a relatively simple genome and life cycle, and despite the fact that replication-competent MoMuLV causes leukemia in mice, MoMuLV have been adapted for gene therapy (Miller 1992).

The structure of an integrated MoMuLV virus or provirus is shown in Figure 6.1. The transcriptional control sequences, the polyadenylation signal, and the integration sequences are contained within the long terminal repeat (LTR) regions located at the 5' and 3' end of the provirus. The sequence required for packaging the viral genome into a virion is designated "psi," and is located downstream of the 5' LTR (Mann, Mulligan, and Baltimore 1983).

The proteins required for retrovirus packaging and replication are encoded in three distinct regions designated "gag" (for group specific antigens), "pol" (for polymerase), and "env" (for envelope) (Leis et al. 1988). Two RNAs encoding these proteins are transcribed, one RNA encodes the entire genome, and the other is a subgenomic RNA, with the psi and gag/pol sequences spliced out and the env sequences in frame. Both transcripts originate from promoter sequences located in the U5 region of the 5' LTR and terminate in the 3' LTR (Varmus 1982).

Translation of the genomic message yields one of two precursor proteins depending on whether a stop codon at the end of the gag region is suppressed. The $Pr65^{gag}$ precursor is cleaved into four gag proteins. Three of these, p15 matrix, p30 capsid, and p12 nucleocapsid, form the virus particle, while the function of the fourth protein, p12, is not known. The $Pr180^{gag/pol}$ precursor contains the four gag proteins, and three enzymatic activities: p15, a protease; p68, reverse transcriptase; and p32, integrase (Leis et al. 1988). The subgenomic message is translated into a transmembrane precursor protein, $Pr80^{env}$, that is cleaved into two proteins, gp70 and p15e, that form a multimeric complex on the surface of the cell (Hunter and Swanstrom 1990).

Assembly of the virus particle is poorly understood, but the result is an infectious particle containing two complete proviral RNA genomes associated with approximately 3,000 to 4,000 gag region proteins, and 200 to 300 molecules of the pol region proteins (Lever, Richardson, and Harrison 1991). This complex is enveloped in a fragment of the host-cell membrane with a high concentration of the env proteins. The host range of the virus is determined by the gp70 envelope protein, which interacts with specific receptor molecules on the surface of target cells (Hunter and Swanstrom 1990). Ecotropic gp70 binds to a mouse-specific peptide sequence of a cationic amino acid–transport protein (Kim et al. 1991). The gp70 of amphotropic viruses interacts with a different molecule, which is conserved among vertebrates, giving amphotropic viruses a broad host range that in-

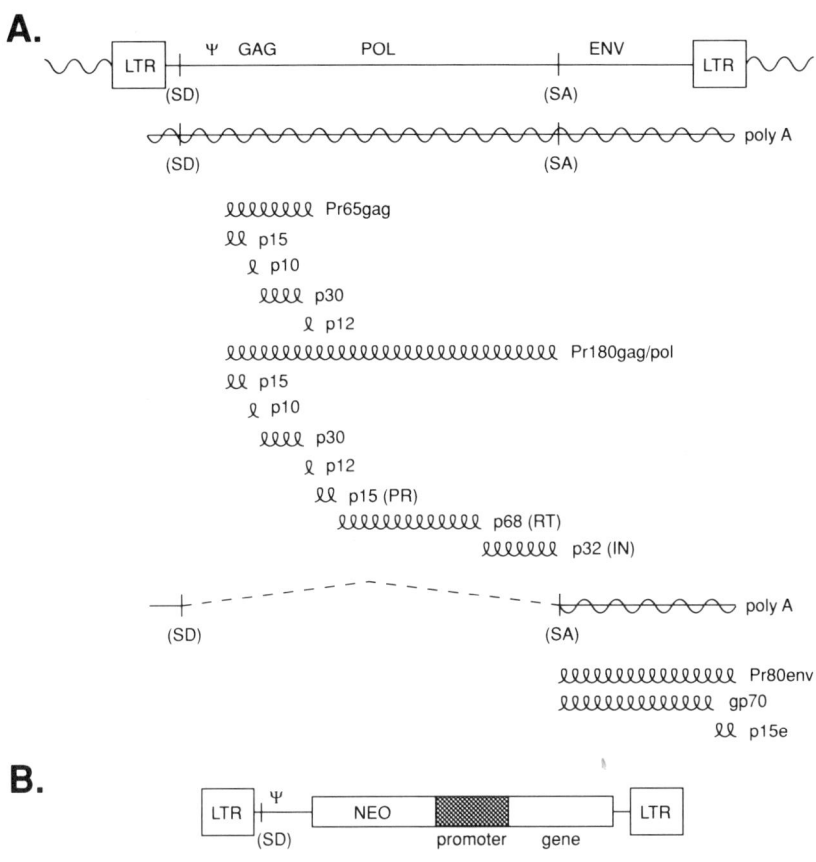

Figure 6.1 Schematic representation of replication-competent and recombinant MoMuLV genomes. *A*, The organization of a replication-competent MoMuLV provirus integrated into genomic DNA. The long terminal repeats (LTR); packaging signal (ψ); splice donor and acceptor (SD and SA) sites; and the regions encoding the group-specific Ag (gag), polymerase (pol), and envelope (env) proteins are indicated. Two viral mRNA molecules are indicated by wavy lines. The coils beneath these lines represent the various precursor proteins and the mature proteins into which they are cleaved. *B*, Schematic representation of a recombinant MoMuLV from which the gag, pol, and env sequences have been removed, and replaced with a neomycin resistance gene (neo) and a second gene fused to an internal promoter.

cludes human cells. Therefore, recombinant amphotropic retroviruses have been adapted for human gene therapy.

After binding of gp70 to its receptor, MoMuLV enter target cells by endocytosis. Fusion of the virus membrane with the endosome releases the nucleocapsid containing the virus RNA genome into the cytoplasm along with the reverse transcriptase and integrase proteins (McClure et al. 1990). A cellular tRNA serves as a primer for reverse transcription of the viral genome (reviewed by Varmus 1988). The product of the reverse transcription is a double-stranded DNA in which the LTR sequences are regenerated on both ends of the molecule. Integration of the virus depends on DNA synthesis in the target cell (Springett et al. 1989; Miller, Adam, and Miller 1990). The viral integrase enzyme generates nicks in the LTRs and the genomic DNA that facilitate integration. The nicks are then repaired by host-cell polymerase (Grandgenett and Mumm 1990; Sandmeyer, Hansen, and Chalker 1990; Bushman and Craigie 1990).

■ RETROVIRUS-MEDIATED GENE TRANSFER

Retrovirus gene-transfer technology is possible because the retroviral sequences required in *cis* for packaging and integration are separable from the sequences which encode the gag, pol, and env proteins. Mann et al. (1983) constructed a MoMuLV that contained a deletion of the packaging signal (psi). The defective virus was transfected into NIH 3T3 cells which then produced gag and pol proteins, and expressed env proteins on their surface. These packaging cells produced virions that contained no viral RNA. A second retrovirus was constructed which preserved the LTRs and the psi sequence, but replaced the gag, pol, and env regions with a dihydrofolate reductase (DHFR) gene. When this vector was introduced into packaging cells, virus particles containing the DHFR gene were produced. These virus particles transduced the DHFR gene into naive NIH 3T3 cells where intact DHFR provirus was detected in the high-molecular-weight DNA (Mann et al. 1983).

The first generation of packaging cell lines (Fig. 6.2*A*) were used to demonstrate the feasibility of retrovirus-mediated gene transfer (Mann et al. 1983; Cone and Mulligan 1984; Miller, Law, and Verma 1985); however, through recombination between the 5′ ends of the recombinant vector and the packaging genome, these cell lines could generate replication-competent virus that can cause leukemia in mice and primates. Concerns about the safety of retrovirus-mediated gene transfer led to a second generation of retrovirus packaging cell lines (Fig. 6.2*B*) which contained two mutations, the psi deletion and replacement of the 3' LTR with the SV40 polyadenylation signal. With these changes, two recombination events are required to generate replication-competent virus. One of these second-generation cell lines, pA317, contains an amphotropic env region, and has been used extensively in human gene-transfer protocols (Miller and Buttimore 1986). The third generation of packaging cell lines (Fig. 6.2*C*) separates the gag/pol region from the env region in the genome. The generation of replication-competent virus from these cell lines requires three separate recombination events, and all but eliminates concern about the safety of retrovirus-mediated gene transfer (Danos and Mulligan 1988; Markowitz, Goff, and Bank 1988a, b).

Improvements and modifications to the vectors used for retroviral gene transfer have kept pace with the modifications of the packaging cell lines. Originally, a dominant selectable marker gene was inserted into a MoMuLV backbone from which the pol and much of the gag and env regions were deleted (Mann et al. 1983; see also Figs. 6.1*B* and 6.3*A*). The expression of the gene in these vectors is under the control of the retroviral promoter elements in the 5' LTR. Concerns about the generation of replication-competent virus prompted further modifications, shown in Figure 6.3*B*. The backbone includes more sequences from the gag region that improve packaging function (Armentano et al. 1987; Bender et al. 1987). Frame-shift or stop-codon mutations introduced into this "gag$^+$" region prevent the generation of replication-competent virus by recombination with the packaging-cell genome, as does the deletion of the remaining env sequences at the 3' end (Miller 1992). In this example, gene expression is under the control of the retroviral LTR; however, a second gene under the control of an internal promoter (or making use of an internal ribosome entry site [Adam et al. 1991; Morgan et al. 1992]) can be inserted 3' to this gene in either the sense (Fig. 6.3*C*) or antisense orientation (Fig. 6.3*D*). The latter strategy allows the transfer of genes with their intron sequences to target cells, since antisense introns are not spliced out prior to packaging (Karlsson et al. 1987; Bender, Miller, and Gelinas 1988; Dzierzak, Papayannopoulou, and Mulligan 1988). Vectors making use of two internal promoters have also been described (Fig. 6.3*E*) (Williams 1990; Miller 1992).

The splice donor site in the retrovirus transcript normally used to generate the subgenomic env message does not have a splice acceptor site in the vectors described above. Some vectors make use of this splice donor by adding the retroviral splice acceptor after the "gag$^+$" sequences (Fig. 6.3*F*) (Ferry et al. 1991). Likewise, an SV40 or other splice acceptor site can be linked to a second gene and inserted 3' to another gene (Fig. 6.3*G*) (Wong et al. 1989). Both of these vectors use

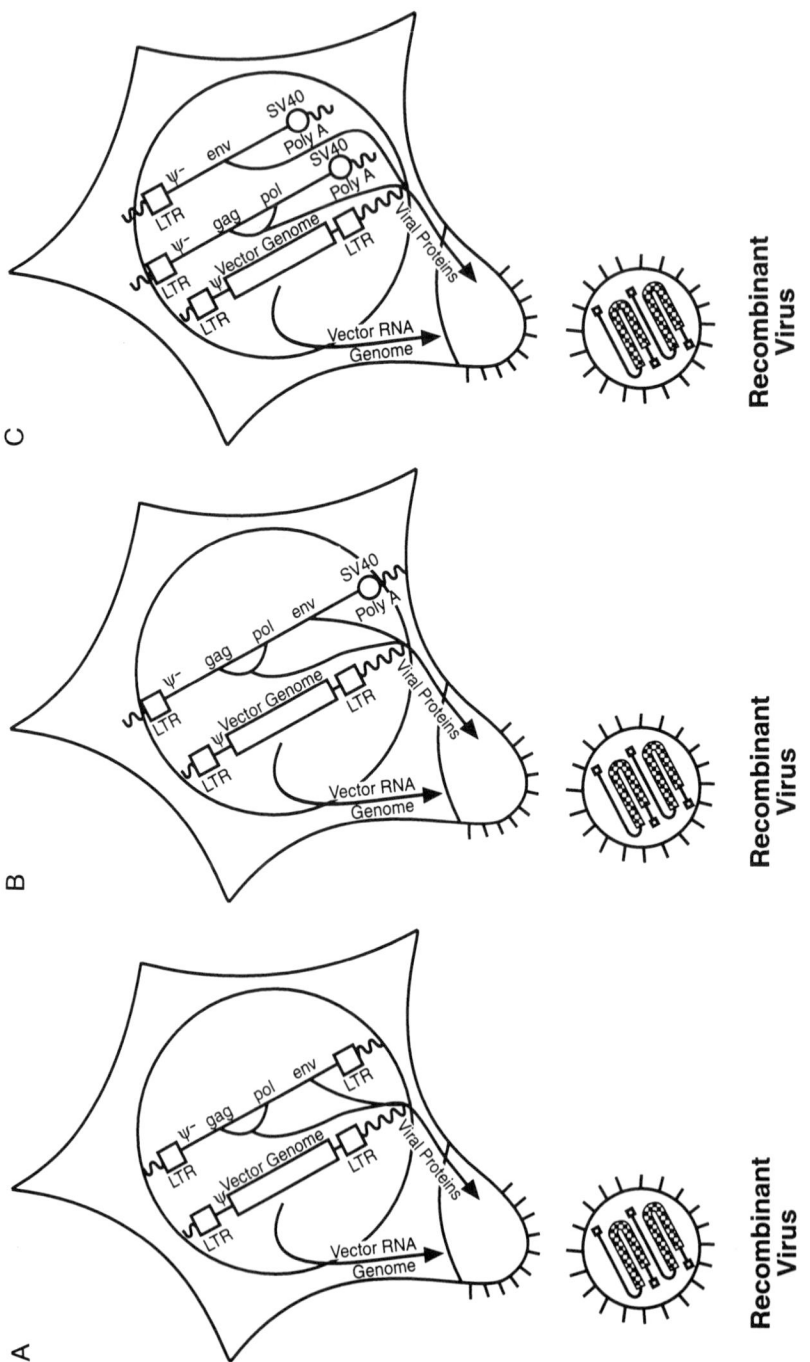

the 5' LTR as a promoter. Finally, a gene can be inserted into the 3' LTR (Fig. 6.3*H*). The duplication of the 3' LTR during the retroviral life cycle generates an integrated provirus with two copies of the gene, one in each of the LTRs. The 5' copy is outside of any retroviral transcriptional control or interference and this may be valuable for obtaining precise gene regulation (Hantzopolous et al. 1989).

At this time there is no consensus regarding the choice of vector or whether to use the LTR promoter or an internal promoter (Williams 1990). Vectors to be used for gene therapy are designed with both safety and gene expression in mind. For example, vectors designed for the treatment of severe combined immunodeficiency (SCID) syndrome containing the adenosine deaminase (ADA) gene driven by either internal promoters or the 5' LTR have been used to express high levels of ADA in the peripheral blood (PB) of mice (Belmont et al. 1988; Lim et al. 1989; Wilson et al. 1990). Similar results have been observed with vectors designed for the treatment of Gaucher disease containing the glucocerebrosidase (GC) gene (Correll et al. 1990; Weinthal et al. 1991). In summary, a wide variety of vector designs have been described, each of which has advantages that may be exploited for gene-therapy protocols.

■ ADENO-ASSOCIATED VIRUS AND GENE TRANSFER

A gene transfer system utilizing the adeno-associated virus (AAV) has been developed and may soon become practical for gene therapy. AAV is a single-stranded DNA virus which, like retroviruses, can integrate into the genomic DNA of target cells. The AAV particle is durable and can be concentrated to extremely high titer on cesium gradients. The virus has never been associated with any human disease despite the fact that antibodies (Ab) to the capsid proteins of AAV are found in 85% of adults, and infectious AAV particles are easily isolated

---

Figure 6.2 The three generations of retrovirus packaging cell lines. *A*, A first-generation cell line with a packaging genome containing a deletion of the packaging signal (ψ^-) with intact LTR and an uninterrupted protein coding region (gag, pol, env). *B*, A cell line containing a modified packaging genome where the 3' LTR is replaced with a polyadenylation signal from the SV40 virus. *C*, A cell line containing further modifications to the packaging genome. The gag/pol coding region is physically separated from the env region.

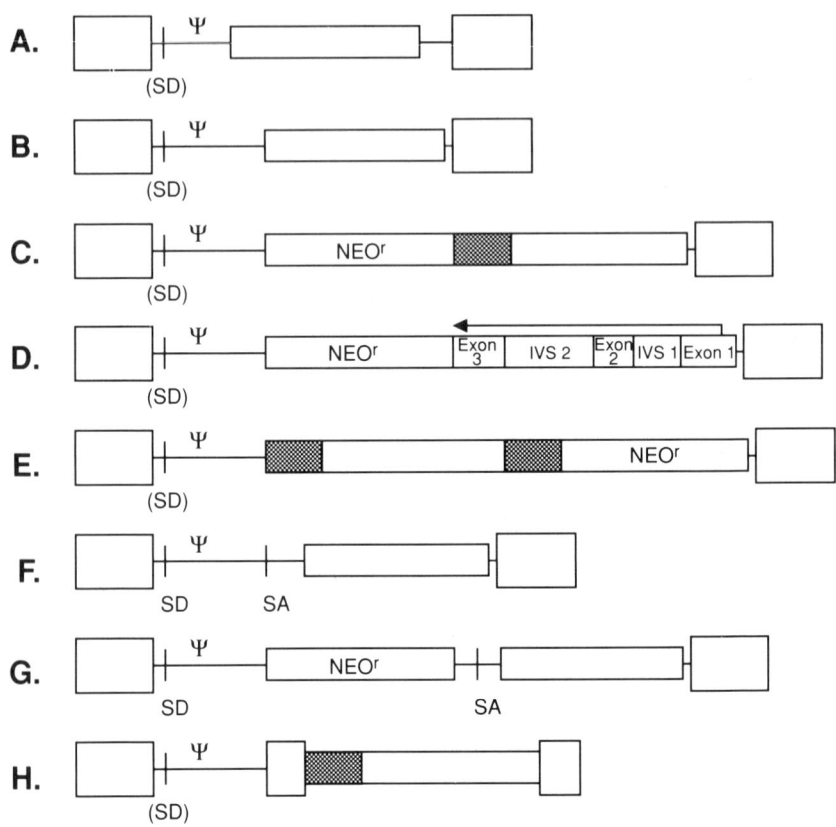

Figure 6.3   Recombinant retroviral vectors. The large rectangles at the ends of the vector represent LTR sequences (a gene is inserted into the right hand LTR in 3H), and the packaging signal (ψ) is shown in each. Open rectangles represent gene sequences, usually cDNAs, except in *D* where a genomic gene is shown. In some cases the neo^r gene is indicated. *Hatched* or *dotted areas* represent promoter sequences. SD and SA sites used for expressing genes are indicated, sites that are not designed to be used are enclosed in *parentheses*.

from patients with adenovirus infections (Blacklow, Hoggan, and Rowe 1968; Hoggan 1970; Berns and Bohenzky 1987).

The AAV genome is depicted in Figure 6.4A. The single DNA strand of 4.6 kb is bounded at the 5' and 3' ends by 145–base pair inverted terminal repeats (ITRs) that contain palindromic sequences that form hairpin structures at the termini which serve as primers for

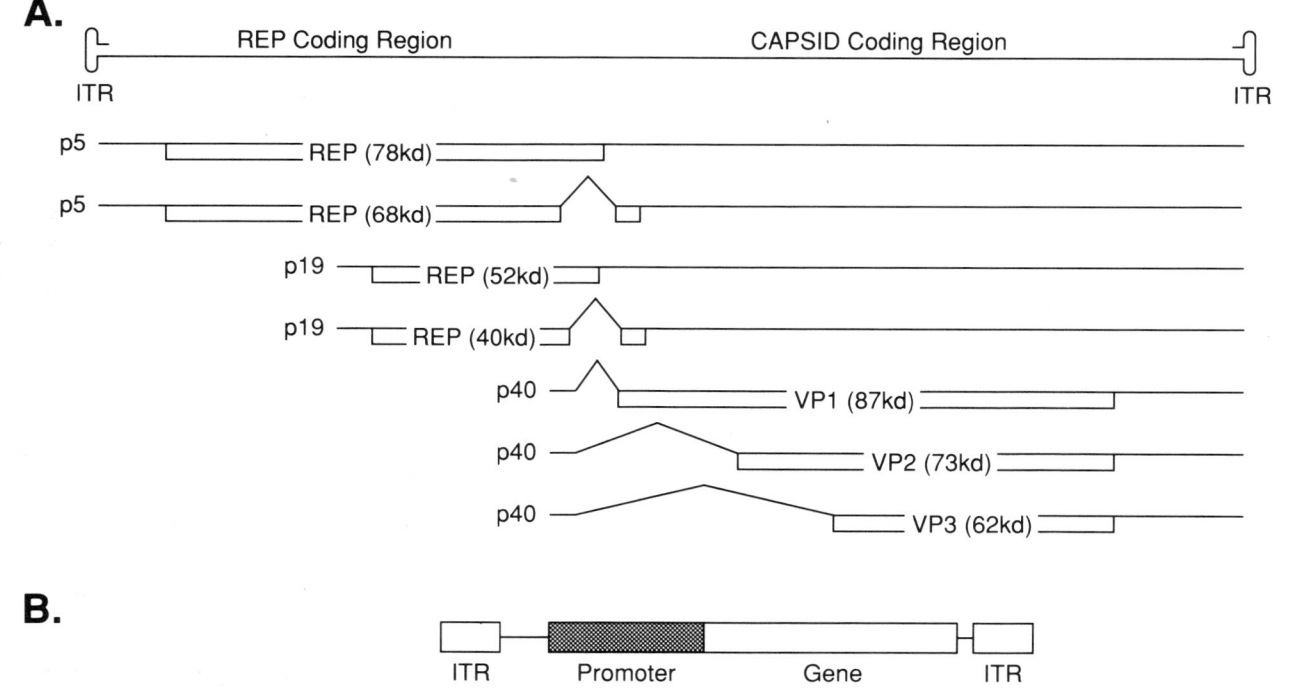

Figure 6.4 Adeno-associated virus. *A,* Wild-type AAV. The single-stranded DNA genome of the virus is represented with the ITR for hairpin structures. The sequences encoding the genes involved in replication (REP coding region) and capsid formation (CAPSID coding region) are indicated. Beneath this genome are shown the seven transcripts encoding individual rep or capsid proteins. *B,* A schematic representation of a recombinant AAV vector. ITR sequences surround a gene (*open box*) attached to a promoter (*hatched box*).

viral replication (Berns and Bohenzky 1987). Seven transcripts with overlapping reading frames initiate at three promoters. The two located near the 5' ITR (p5 and p19) generate RNAs encoding the proteins involved in AAV replication (rep) (Hermonat et al. 1984). The centrally located promoter (p40) generates three transcripts encoding the capsid proteins (Green and Roeder 1980). Cells containing an integrated AAV genome require additional helper functions, which can be provided either by adenovirus or herpes virus. In the absence of one of these viruses, AAV integrates into the genome and enters a stable latent state (Berns et al. 1975).

Recombinant AAV vectors contain the ITR sequences (which are sufficient for integration) separated by the gene to be transferred (Fig. 6.4*B*). Since the ITR sequences do not contain promoter elements, the inserted gene must have an internal promoter (Lebkowski et al. 1988). It is not possible to package genomes larger than 5.0 kb, and genomes smaller than 2.6 kb may be unstable (Walsh et al. 1992). To produce recombinant AAV particles (Fig. 6.5), the recombinant AAV vector is transfected into a cell line permissive for AAV replication (usually HeLa or 293 cells) along with a defective AAV genome consisting of the rep and capsid sequences bounded by ITR from adenovirus which prevents mobilization of this genome. Adenovirus infection of the cells supplies the necessary helper functions for recombinant AAV (rAAV) production (Samulski, Chang, and Shenk 1989). The cells are then lysed, the adenovirus is attenuated by incubating the cell extracts at 56°C, and rAAV is purified and concentrated by CsCl gradient centrifugation. Although AAV vectors have been used to introduce genes into murine, primate, and human progenitor cells, to date no experiments have demonstrated stable integration of rAAV vectors into primitive hemopoietic cells (Laface et al. 1989; Goodman et al. 1994; Walsh et al. 1994; Miller et al. 1994).

■ GENE TRANSFER INTO MURINE HEMOPOIETIC STEM CELLS

The ability of the pluripotent hemopoietic stem cells (HSC) to completely repopulate the entire hemopoietic system following trans-

---

Figure 6.5 Production of adeno-associated virus. Permissive cells are cotransfected with a recombinant AAV plasmid and a defective AAV plasmid (shown at the top of the figure). Helper function is provided by infection of the transfected cells with adenovirus. The recombinant genome is replicated and packaged into virus particles in the nucleus.

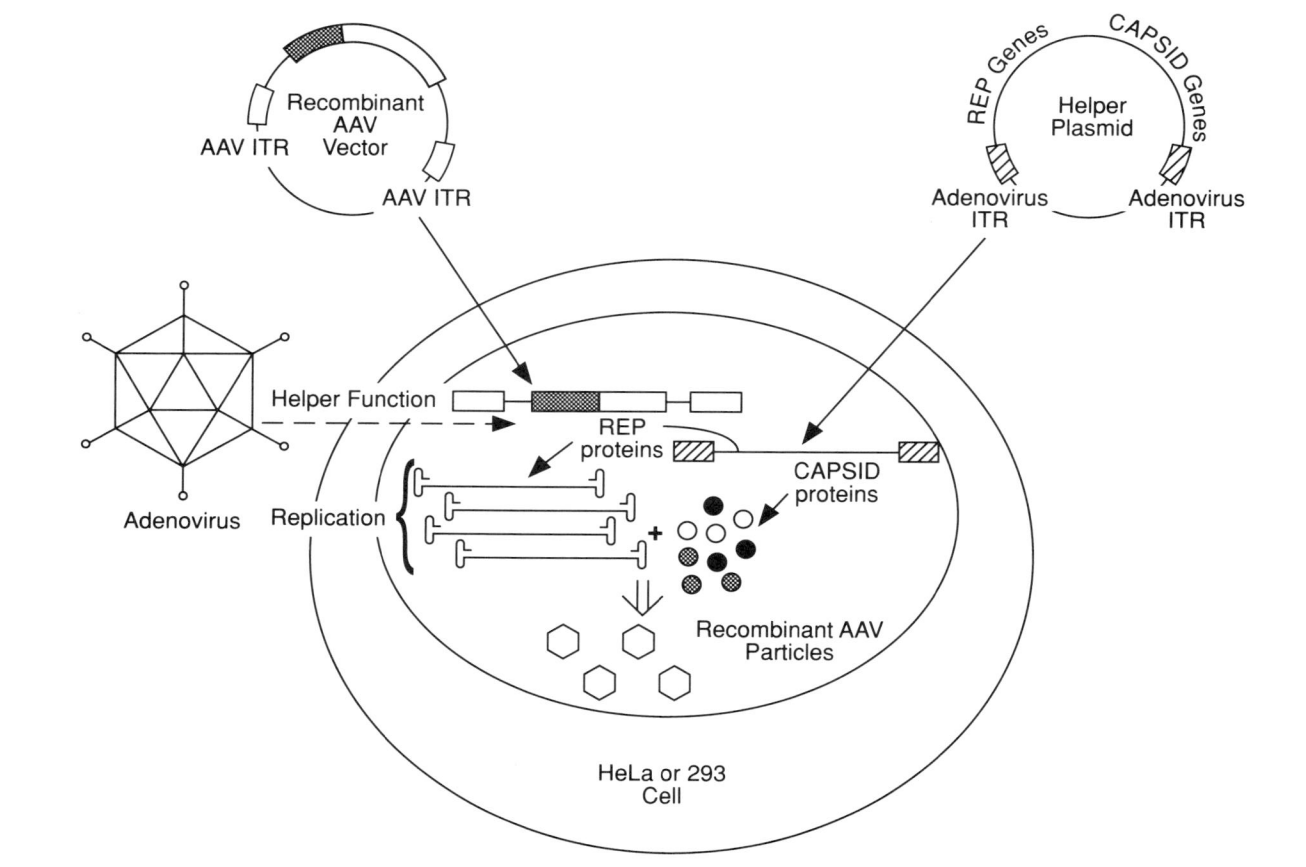

Recombinant
AAV
Vector

AAV ITR

AAV ITR

REP Genes

CAPSID Genes

Helper
Plasmid

Adenovirus
ITR

Adenovirus
ITR

Helper Function

REP
proteins

CAPSID
proteins

Adenovirus

Replication

+

Recombinant AAV
Particles

HeLa or 293
Cell

plantation makes the hemopoietic system a particularly attractive target for gene therapy. Integration of new genetic material into the genome of the HSC ensures that all of the progeny of that cell will also carry the new gene. The ability of the HSC to self-renew without differentiating ensures a continuous supply of modified hemopoietic cells in the transplanted recipient (Anderson 1984).

The initial studies that established the ability of retroviruses to introduce new genes into primitive hemopoietic cells, designated spleen colony-forming cells (S-CFC), were performed in mice. Each S-CFC forms a colony containing mature myeloid cells of all types in the spleen of irradiated mice 8 to 14 days after the injection of normal BM cells and represents the proliferation and differentiation of a single primitive hemopoietic cell. The retroviruses used for these studies contained dominant selectable marker genes, either DHFR or neomycin phosphotransferase (neo^r) rather than genes that would correct inherited deficiencies. BM cells were cultured on a monolayer of virus-producing cells, often in medium conditioned with the hemopoietic growth factor interleukin-3 (IL-3). The cells recovered from these cocultures were then injected into lethally irradiated mice, and the presence of proviral DNA was assayed in DNA extracted from individual spleen foci. The presence of the proviral genome in these foci demonstrated that single primitive progenitor cells had been transduced without losing the ability of those cells to proliferate and differentiate (Williams et al. 1984; Dick et al. 1985; Eglitis et al. 1985). Extensions of these experiments examined mice that had recovered from the BMT. Southern blot analysis of proviral insertion sites in the BM, spleen, and thymus revealed that the HSC that had repopulated these organs contained a provirus in the same site in the genome (Lemischka, Raulet, and Mulligan 1986). Cells containing the unique proviral insertion site persisted in the PB, BM, spleen, and thymus of these mice for periods of 12 months or more, with no changes observed after 90 days (Bodine, Karlsson, and Nienhuis 1989; Bodine et al. 1990b; Jordan and Lemischka 1990). These studies established that single cells could permanently repopulate the lymphoid and myeloid lineages after retrovirus transduction.

In these early studies, the frequency of mice that had long-term persistance of retrovirus-marked cells was less than 1 in 10. In addition, even in the positive mice, 10% or less of the hemopoietic cells contained a provirus (Dzierzak et al. 1988; Bodine et al. 1989). While low levels of transduction were postulated to be sufficient to correct the defect in ADA-deficient SCID patients, for most other inherited hematologic diseases a higher level of transduction would be required. A variety of retroviral vectors have been used to compare protocols for the transduction of the mouse HSC. Although different laboratories use different protocols, the protocols share many common elements. The best results are obtained when the donor animals are treated with 5-fluorouracil (5-FU), a cell cycle–specific drug that is toxic to cycling cells such as hemopoietic progenitor cells (Hodgson and Bradley 1979). The depletion of progenitor cells in the host may induce cycling of their more primitive precursors, improving retroviral integration. Combining IL-3 with other hemopoietic growth factors in the culture medium has been shown to extend the viability of HSC in culture to 6 days or more without significant loss of repopulating ability, and to improve gene transfer (Bodine et al. 1989; Bodine, Crozier, and Clark 1991). Currently, most protocols use stem cell factor (SCF) (for review, see Witte 1990) in combination with IL-6 (Luskey et al. 1992) and IL-3 (Bodine et al. 1992). Some workers substitute IL-11 (Neben et al. 1994) or IL-1 (Jordan and Lemischka 1990) for IL-6. Many protocols include a 48-hour prestimulation of BM cells in medium containing cytokines, before exposure to retrovirus particles (Lim et al. 1989; Bodine et al. 1989). Using the optimum combination of hemopoietic growth factors and culture conditions, several different laboratories have demonstrated that between 20% and 30% of the hemopoietic cells in all transplanted animals contain a provirus.

■ GENE TRANSFER INTO HEMOPOIETIC STEM CELLS FROM LARGER ANIMALS

The initial experiments in mice demonstrated that retroviruses could be used to introduce genes into HSC, and documented the expression of these genes in the differentiated hemopoietic cells. As preclinical models, experiments designed to introduce genes into the HSC of large animals were performed. For these experiments retroviral vectors were generated by amphotropic producer cell lines. Because amphotropic viruses had been used to transduce murine HSC (Osborne et al. 1990), it was felt that the receptor for these viruses would likely be expressed on the HSC of larger animals. Co-culture protocols similar to those used in the transduction of murine PHSC have not been as successful in large-animal models, with an average of less than 2% positive cells present in the best examples (Bodine et al. 1990a; van Beusechem et al. 1992; Bodine et al. 1993). Safety concerns about co-culture of patient BM cells with producer cells were heightened after the discovery that replication-competent virus emerging from producer cells could cause leukemia in severely immunosuppressed rhesus monkeys (Donahue et al. 1992). The use of media that has been collected and stored while tests for replication-competent virus are performed is considered the safest alternative, and several protocols using characterized media conditioned by virus-producing cells have been developed.

In a canine model system, BM cells from the donor were used to establish a long-term bone-marrow culture (LTBMC). These cultures require regular replacement of media, which offers the opportunity for repeated exposure to tested virus-conditioned medium. At the end of 4 weeks in culture, the LTBMC was harvested and the cells used to transplant an irradiated donor. Gene-transfer efficiency using this protocol was as good or better than that observed with co-culture, but less than 2% of the PB and BM cells of the repopulated recipient contained the provirus (Schuening et al. 1989; Carter et al. 1992). An alternative protocol seeded populations of rhesus monkey progenitor cells and HSC (enriched by selection for cells expressing the CD34 antigen) in virus-conditioned medium onto a previously established BM-stromal cell line that expresses membrane-bound SCF. The cells were cultured for 96 hours with a daily change to fresh virus-conditioned medium. The cells were then collected and returned to the irradiated recipient. Eighteen months later, an ADA retrovirus vector transferred with this protocol was present in 2% of all mature PB and BM cells, and was expressed at levels predicted to be curative for ADA-deficient SCID patients (Bodine et al. 1993). In a related study, CD34[+] rhesus monkey BM cells were exposed to medium containing a GC virus for 96 hours in suspension culture without stromal cell support. Again approximately 2% of the PB and BM cells contained the provirus 12 months later, and GC gene expression was detected in all cell types (S. Karlsson, personal communication). In summary, whatever the protocol used, gene-transfer efficiency in large animal models is approximately 10% of that observed in mice.

■ FUTURE DIRECTIONS

Improving the efficiency of gene transfer, particularly in large-animal models, is an important research goal that will transform gene therapy from fiction to reality. Basic research into the biology of the HSC may suggest some new protocols that transfer genes at a higher rate. Retroviral integration is enhanced significantly by DNA synthesis and/or host cell division (Springett et al. 1989; Miller et al. 1990). Unfortunately for gene therapists, the HSC is usually quiescent as evidenced by its resistance to cell cycle–specific drugs such as 5-FU (Lerner and Harrison 1990). The continued evaluation of the effects of novel cytokines on HSC cycling is an important avenue of research that may ultimately solve this problem. Cytokine treatment has been shown to increase both gene transfer and the binding of amphotropic virus to human CD34$^+$ progenitor cells (Crooks and Kohn 1993). These results suggest that increasing the number of amphotropic receptor molecules on the surface of HSC with cytokines or other agents may also improve gene-transfer efficiency. Gene transfer into progenitor cells and murine HSC mobilized into the PB by cytokine treatment is more efficient than gene transfer into their BM counterparts (Cassel et al. 1993; Bodine et al. 1994). Perhaps subsets of HSC, either mobilized by cytokines or separated from populations of BM cells, are more susceptible to virus transduction and would be improved targets for gene therapy. Finally, packaging cell lines utilizing the env region from the gibbon ape leukemia virus (GALV) have been developed. Because the GALV virus is tropic for primate hemopoietic cells, vectors packaged in this envelope may be more capable of transducing human hemopoietic cells, leading to improved human gene therapy applications (Miller et al. 1991).

If the technical obstacles can be overcome, gene therapy will become the treatment of choice for many hematologic diseases. The progress made in the 10 years since the demonstration by Williams et al. (1984) of retrovirus-mediated gene transfer into pluripotent hemopoietic cells allows optimism about the progress to be made during the next decade.

ACKNOWLEDGMENTS

I gratefully acknowledge the longstanding contributions of my colleagues Dr. Arthur W. Nienhuis, Dr. Jane E. Barker, Dr. Donald Orlic, Dr. Cynthia E. Dunbar, and Dr. David A. Williams to my understanding of gene transfer and hemopoiesis.

REFERENCES

Adam, M.A., Ramesh, N., Miller, A.D., and Osborne, W.R. (1991) Internal initiation of translation in retroviral vectors carrying picornavirus 5' nontranslated regions. *Journal of Virology*, **65**, 4985–90.

Armentano, D., Yu, S.F., Kantoff, P.W., von Ruden, T., Anderson, W.F., and Gilboa, E. (1987) Effect of internal viral sequences on the utility of retroviral vectors. *Journal of Virology*, **61**, 1647–50.

Anderson, W.F. (1984) Prospects for human gene therapy. *Science*, **226**, 401–9.

Belmont, J.W., MacGregor, G.R., Wagner-Smith, K., et al. (1988) Expression of adenosine deaminase in murine hematopoietic cells. *Molecular and Cellular Biology*, **8**, 5116–25.

Bender, M.A., Miller, A.D., and Gelinas, R.E. (1988) Expression of the human β-globin gene after retroviral transfer into murine erythroleukemia cells and human BFU-E cells. *Molecular and Cellular Biology*, **8**, 1725–35.

Bender, M.A., Palmer, T.D., Gelinas, R.E., and Miller, A.D. (1987) Evidence that the packaging signal of Moloney murine leukemia virus extends into the gag region. *Journal of Virology*, **61**, 1639–46.

Berns, K.I. and Bohenzky, R.A. (1987) Adeno-associated viruses: an update. *Advances in Virology Research*, **32**, 243–306.

Berns, K.I., Pinkerton, T.C., Thomas, G.F., and Hoggan, M.D. (1975) Detection of adeno-associated virus (AAV) –specific nucleotide sequences in DNA isolated from latently infected Detroit 6 cells. *Virology*, **68**, 556–60.

Blacklow, N.R., Hoggan, M.D., and Rowe, W.P. (1968) Serological evidence for human infection with adeno-associated viruses. *Journal of the National Cancer Institute*, **40**, 319–27.

Bodine, D.M., Crozier, P.S., and Clark, S.C. (1991) Effects of hematopoietic growth factors on the survival of primitive stem cells in liquid suspension culture. *Blood*, **78**, 914–20.

Bodine, D.M., Karlsson, S., and Nienhuis, A.W. (1989) Combination of interleukins 3 and 6 preserves stem cell function in culture and enhances retrovirus-mediated gene transfer into hematopoietic stem cells. *Proceedings of the National Academy of Sciences of the United States of America*, **86**, 8897–901.

Bodine, D.M., McDonagh, K.T., Brandt, S.J., et al. (1990a) Development of a high-titer retrovirus producer cell line capable of gene transfer into rhesus monkey hematopoietic stem cells. *Proceedings of the National Academy of Sciences of the United States of America*, **87**, 3738–42.

Bodine, D.M., McDonagh, K.T., Seidel, N.E., and Nienhuis, A.W. (1990b) Survival and retrovirus infection of murine hematopoietic stem cells in vitro: effects of 5-FU and method of infection. *Experimental Hematology*, **19**, 206–12.

Bodine, D.M., Moritz, T., Donahue, R.E., et al. (1993) Long-term in vivo expression of a murine adenosine deaminase gene in rhesus monkey hematopoietic cells of multiple lineages after retroviral mediated gene transfer into CD34+ bone marrow cells. *Blood*, **82**, 1975–80.

Bodine, D.M., Orlic, D., Burkett, N.C., Seidel, N.E., and Zsebo, K.M. (1992) Stem cell factor increases CFU-S number in vitro in synergy with interleukin-6, and in vivo in *Sl/Sl^d* mice as a single factor. *Blood*, **79**, 913–19.

Bodine, D.M., Seidel, N.E., Gale, M.S., Neinhuis, A.W., and Orlic, D. (1994) Efficient retrovirus transduction of mouse pluripotent hematopoietic stem cells mobilized into the peripheral blood by treatment with granulocyte colony-stimulating factor and stem cell factor. *Blood*, **84**, 1482–91.

Bushman, F.D. and Craigie, R. (1990) Sequence requirements for integration of Moloney murine leukemia virus DNA in vitro. *Journal of Virology*, **64**, 5645–8.

Carter, R.F., Abrams-Ogg, A.C.G., Dick, J.E., et al. (1992) Autologous transplantation of canine long-term marrow culture cells genetically marked by retroviral vectors. *Blood*, **79**, 356–62.

Cassel, A., Cottler-Fox, M., Doren, S., and Dunbar, C.E. (1993) Retroviral-mediated gene transfer into CD-34 enriched human peripheral blood stem cells. *Experimental Hematology*, **21**, 585–91.

Cone, R.D. and Mulligan, R.C. (1984) High efficiency gene transfer into mammalian cells: generation of helper-free recombinant retrovirus with broad mammalian host range. *Proceedings of the National Academy of Sciences of the United States of America*, **81**, 6349–53.

Correll, P.H., Kew, Y., Perry, L.K., Brady, R.O., Fink, J.K., and Karlsson, S. (1990) Expression of human glucocerebrosidase in long-term reconstituted mice following retroviral-mediated gene transfer into hematopoietic stem cells. *Human Gene Therapy*, **1**, 277–83.

Crooks, G.M. and Kohn, D.B. (1993) Growth factors increase amphotropic retrovirus binding to human CD34+ bone marrow progenitor cells. *Blood*, **82**, 3290–7.

Danos, O. and Mulligan, R.C. (1988) Safe and efficient generation of recombinant retroviruses with amphotropic and ecotropic host ranges. *Proceedings of the National Academy of Sciences of the United States of America*, **85**, 6460–4.

Dexter, T.M., Allen, T.D., Lajtha, L.G., Krizsa, F., Testa, N.G., and Moore, M.A.S. (1978) In vitro analysis of self-renewal and commitment of hematopoietic stem cells. In B. Clarkson, P.A. Marks, and J.E. Till (Eds.) *Differentiation of normal and neoplastic hemopoietic cells*, pp. 63–80. Cold Spring Harbor, Cold Spring Harbor Conference on Cell Proliferation, vol. 5.

Dick, J.E., Magli, M.C., Huszar, D., Phillips, R.A., and Bernstein, A. (1985) Introduction of a selectable gene into primitive stem cells capable of reconstitution of the hemopoietic system of W/W^v mice. *Cell*, **42**, 71–9.

Donahue, R.E., Kessler, S.W., Bodine, D., et al. (1992) Helper virus induced T-cell lymphoma in nonhuman primates after retroviral mediated gene transfer. *Journal of Experimental Medicine*, **176**, 1125–35.

Dzierzak, E.A., Papayannopoulou, T., and Mulligan, R.C. (1988) Lineage specific expression of a human β-globin gene in murine bone marrow transplant recipients reconstituted with retrovirus-transduced stem cells. *Nature*, **331**, 35–41.

Eglitis, M.A., Kantoff, P., Gilboa, E., and Anderson, W.F. (1985) Gene expression in mice after high efficiency retroviral-mediated gene transfer. *Science*, **230**, 1395–8.

Ferry, N., Duplessis, O., Houssin, D., Danod, O., and Heard, J.M. (1991) Retroviral-mediated gene transfer into hepatocytes in vivo. *Proceedings of the National Academy of Sciences of the United States of America*, **88**, 8377–81.

Goodman, S., Xiao, X., Donahue, R.E., et al. (1994) Recombinant adeno-associated virus-mediated gene transfer into hematopoietic progenitor cells. *Blood*, **84**, 1492–1500.

Grandgenett, D.P. and Mumm, S.R. (1990) Unraveling retrovirus integration. *Cell*, **60**, 3–4.

Green, M.R. and Roeder, R.G. (1980) Definition of a novel promoter for the major adeno-associated virus mRNA. *Cell*, **22**, 231–43.

Hantzopolous, P.A., Sullenger, B.A., Ungers, G., and Gilboa, E. (1989) Improved gene expression upon transfer of the adenosine deaminase minigene outside the transcriptional unit of a retroviral vector. *Proceedings of the National Academy of Sciences of the United States of America*, **86**, 3519–24.

Hermonat, P.L., Labow, M.A., Wright, R., Berns, K.I., and Muzyczka, N. (1984) Genetics of adeno-associated virus: isolation and preliminary characterization of adeno-associated virus type 2 mutants. *Journal of Virology*, **51**, 329–39.

Hodgson, G.S. and Bradley, T.R. (1979) Properties of haematopoietic stem cells surviving 5-fluorouracil treatment: evidence for a pre CFU-S cell? *Nature*, **281**, 381–2.

Hoggan, M.D. (1970) Adeno-associated viruses. *Progress in Medical Virology*, **12**, 211–39.

Hunter, E. and Swanstrom, R. (1990) Retrovirus envelope glycoproteins. *Current Topics in Microbiology and Immunology*, **157**, 187–253.

Jordan, C.T. and Lemischka, I.R. (1990) Clonal and systemic analysis of long-term hematopoiesis in the mouse. *Genes and Development*, **4**, 220–32.

Karlsson, S., Papayannopoulou, T., Schweiger, S.G., Stamatoyannopoulos, G., and Nienhuis, A.W. (1987) Retroviral-mediated gene transfer of genomic globin genes leads to regulated production of RNA and protein. *Proceedings of the National Academy of Sciences of the United States of America*, **84**, 2411–15.

Kim, J.W., Closs, E.I., Albritton, L.M., and Cunningham, J.M. (1991) Transport of cationic amino acids by the mouse ecotropic retrovirus receptor. *Nature*, **352**, 725–8.

Laface, D., Hermonat, P., Wakeland, E., and Peck, A. (1989) Gene transfer into hematopoietic progenitor cells mediated by an adeno-associated virus vector. *Virology*, **162**, 483–7.

Lebkowski, J.S., McNally, M.M., Okarma, T.B., and Lerch, L.B. (1988) Adeno-associated virus: a vector system for efficient introduction of DNA into a variety of mammalian cell types. *Molecular and Cellular Biology*, **8**, 3988–96.

Leis, J., Baltimore, D., Bishop, J.M., et al. (1988) Standardized and simplified nomenclature for proteins common to all retroviruses. *Journal of Virology*, **62**, 1808–9.

Lemischka, I.R., Raulet, D.H., and Mulligan, R.C. (1986) Developmental potential and dynamic behavior of hematopoietic stem cells. *Cell*, **45**, 917–27.

Lerner, C.P. and Harrison, D.E. (1990) 5-fluorouracil spares hemopoietic stem cells responsible for long-term repopulation. *Experimental Hematology*, **18**, 114–18.

Lever, A.M., Richardson, J.H., and Harrison, G.P. (1991) Retroviral RNA packaging. *Biochemical Society Transactions*, **19**, 963–6.

Lim, B., Apperly, J.F., Orkin, S.H., and Williams, D.A. (1989) Long-term expression of human adenosine deaminase in mice transplanted with retrovirus infected hematopoietic stem cells. *Proceedings of the National Academy of Sciences of the United States of America*, **86**, 8892–6.

Luskey, B.D., Rosenblatt, M., Zsebo, K.M., and Williams, D.A. (1992) Stem cell factor, interleukin-3, and interleukin-6 promote retroviral-mediated gene transfer into murine hematopoietic stem cells. *Blood*, **80**, 396–402.

Mann, R., Mulligan, R.C., and Baltimore, D. (1983) Construction of a retrovirus packaging mutant and its use to produce helper-free defective retrovirus. *Cell*, **33**, 153–9.

Markowitz, D., Goff, S., and Bank, A. (1988a) A safe packaging line for gene transfer: separating viral genes on two different plasmids. *Journal of Virology*, **62**, 1120–4.

Markowitz, D., Goff, S., and Bank, A. (1988b) Construction and use of a safe and efficient amphotropic packaging cell line. *Virology*, **167**, 400–6.

McClure, M.O., Sommerfelt, M.A., Marsh, M., and Weiss, R.A. (1990) The pH independence of mammalian retrovirus infection. *Journal of General Virology*, **71**, 767–73.

Miller, A.D. (1992) Retroviral vectors. *Current Topics in Microbiology and Immunology*, **158**, 1–24.

Miller, A.D. and Buttimore, C. (1986) Redesign of retrovirus packaging cell lines to avoid recombination leading to helper virus production. *Molecular and Cellular Biology*, **6**, 2895–902.

Miller, A.D., Garcia, J.V., von Suhr, N., Lynch, C.M., Wilson, C., and Eiden, M.V. (1991) Construction and properties of retrovirus packaging cells based on gibbon ape leukemia virus. *Journal of Virology*, **65**, 2220–4.

Miller, A.D., Law, M.F., and Verma, I.M. (1985) Generation of helper-free amphotropic retroviruses that transduce a dominant-acting methotrexate-resistant dihydrofolate reductase gene. *Molecular and Cellular Biology*, **5**, 431–7.

Miller, D.G., Adam, M.A., and Miller, A.D. (1990) Gene transfer by retrovirus vectors occurs only in cells that are actively replicating at the time of infection. *Molecular and Cellular Biology*, **10**, 4239–42.

Miller, J.L., Donahue, R.E., Sellers, S.E., Samulski, R.J., Young, N.S., and Nienhuis, A.W. (1994) Recombinant adeno-associated virus (rAAV)-mediated expression of a human γ-globin gene in human progenitor derived erythroid cells. *Proceedings of the National Academy of Sciences of the United States of America*, **91**, 10183–7.

Morgan, R.A., Couture, L., Elroy-Stein, O., Ragheb, J., Moss, B., and Anderson, W.F. (1992) Retroviral vectors containing putative internal ribosome entry sites: development of a polycistronic gene transfer system and applications to human gene therapy. *Nucleic Acids Research*, **20**, 1293–9.

Mulligan, R.C. (1993) The basic science of gene therapy. *Science*, **260**, 926–32.

Neben, S., Donaldson, D., Seiff, C., et al. (1994) Synergistic effects of interleukin-11 with other growth factors in the expansion of murine hematopoietic progenitors and maintenance of stem cells in liquid culture. *Experimental Hematology*, **22**, 353–9.

Nienhuis, A.W., Walsh, C.E., and Liu, J.M. (1993) Viruses as therapeutic gene transfer vectors. In N.S. Young (Ed.) *Viruses and bone marrow*, pp. 353–414. New York, Marcel Dekker.

Osborne, W.R.A., Hock, R.A., Kaleko, M., and Miller, A.D. (1990) Long-term expression of human adenosine deaminase in mice after transplantation of bone marrow infected with amphotropic retroviral vectors. *Human Gene Therapy*, **1**, 31–41.

Samulski, R.J., Chang, L.-S., and Shenk, T. (1989) Helper free stocks of recombinant adeno-associated viruses: normal integration does not require viral gene expression. *Journal of Virology*, **63**, 3822–8.

Sandmeyer, S.B., Hansen, L.J., and Chalker, D.L. (1990) Integration specificity of retrotransposons and retroviruses. *Annual Review of Genetics*, **24**, 491–518.

Schuening, F.G., Storb, R., Stead, R.B., Goehle, S., Nash, R., and Miller, A.D. (1989) Improved retroviral transfer of genes into canine hematopoietic progenitor cells kept in long term marrow culture. *Blood*, **74**, 152–5.

Springett, G.M., Moen, R.C., Anderson, S., Blaese, R.M., and Anderson, W.F. (1989) Infection efficiency of T lymphocytes with amphotropic retroviral vectors is cell cycle dependent. *Journal of Virology*, **63**, 3865–9.

Sutherland, H.J., Lansdorp, P.M., Henkelman, D.H., Eaves, A.C., and Eaves, C.J. (1990) Functional characterization of individual human hematopoietic stem cells cultured at limiting dilution on supportive marrow stromal cells. *Proceedings of the National Academy of Sciences of the United States of America*, **87**, 3584–90.

Thomas, E.D., Storb, R., Clift, R.A., et al. (1975a) Bone marrow transplantation (first of two parts). *New England Journal of Medicine*, **292**, 832–43.

Thomas, E.D., Storb, R., Clift, R.A., et al. (1975b) Bone marrow transplantation (second of two parts). *New England Journal of Medicine*, **292**, 895–902.

van Beusechem, V.W., Kukler, A., Heidt, P.J., and Valerio, D. (1992) Long-term expression of human adenosine deaminase in rhesus monkeys transplanted with retrovirus-infected bone marrow cells. *Proceedings of the National Academy of Sciences of the United States of America*, **89**, 7640–6.

Varmus, H.E. (1982) Form and function of retroviral proviruses. *Science*, **216**, 812–20.

Varmus, H. (1988) Retroviruses. *Science*, **240**, 1427–35.

Walsh, C.E., Liu, J.M., Young, N., Xiao, X., Neinhuis, A.W., and Samulski, R.J. (1992) Regulated high level expression of a human g-globin gene introduced into erythroid cells by a novel adeno-associated virus (AAV) vector. *Proceedings of the National Academy of Sciences of the United States of America*, **89**, 7257–61.

Walsh, C.E., Nienhuis, A.W., Samulski, R.J., et al. (1994) Phenotypic correction of Fanconi anemia in human hematopoietic cells with a recombinant adeno-associated virus vector. *Journal of Clinical Investigation*, **94**, 1440–8.

Weinthal, J., Nolta, J.A., Yu, X.J., Liller, J., Urive, L., and Kohn, D.B. (1991) Expression of human glucocerebrosidase following retroviral vector-mediated transduction of murine hematopoietic stem cells. *Bone Marrow Transplantation*, **8**, 403–12.

Williams, D.A. (1990) Expression of introduced genetic sequences in hematopoietic cells following retroviral mediated gene transfer. *Human Gene Therapy*, **1**, 229–39.

Williams, D.A., Lemischka, I.R., Nathan, D.G., and Mulligan, R.C. (1984) Introduction of new genetic material into pluripotent haematopoietic stem cells of the mouse. *Nature*, **310**, 476–80.

Wilson, J.M., Danos, O., Grossman, M., Raulet, D.H., and Mulligan, R.C. (1990) Expression of human adenosine deaminase in mice reconstituted with retrovirus-transduced hematopoietic stem cells. *Proceedings of the National Academy of Sciences of the United States of America*, **87**, 439–43.

Witte, O.N. (1990) Steel locus defines new multipotent growth factor. *Cell*, **63**, 5–6.

Wolf, J.A. and Lederberg, J. (1994) An early history of gene transfer and therapy. *Human Gene Therapy*, **5**, 469–80.

Wong, P.M.C., Chung, S.-W., Dunbar, C.E., Bodine, D.M., Ruscetti, S., and Nienhuis, A.W. (1989) Retrovirus-mediated transfer and expression of the interleukin-3 gene in mouse hematopoietic cells result in a myeloproliferative disorder. *Molecular and Cellular Biology*, **9**, 798–808.

PART B

Technology of Cell Collection and Preparation

—7—

Sources of Hemopoietic Progenitor Cells for Transplantation

ELIZABETH J. SHPALL, URSULA GEHLING,
PABLO J. CAGNONI, CHRISTOPHER HOGAN,
SCOTT I. BEARMAN, AND ROY B. JONES

High-dose therapy with hemopoietic cell support is effective treatment for selected high-risk patients with hematologic malignancies (Philip et al. 1987) or solid tumors (Shpall, Jones, and Bearman 1994) in whom standard-dose therapy has minimal benefit. Over the past decade, rapid and substantial advances have been made in the procurement and manipulation of hemopoietic progenitor cells for transplantation. Many of these clinical and technological advances are discussed more comprehensively in other chapters of this book. The advances include the development and continued refinement of peripheral blood progenitor cell (PBPC) mobilization regimens using chemotherapy and/or growth factor(s) (Chapters 9 and 10); purging of malignant cells from bone marrow (BM) or peripheral blood progenitor cell (PBPC) fractions (Chapter 16); the isolation of purified hemopoietic cell subpopulations using flow-cytometry (Chapter 11), immunoadsorption (Chapter 12), or immunomagnetic techniques (Chapter 13); and the ex vivo expansion of hemopoietic progenitors using static (Chapter 14) or continuously perfused (Chapter 15) liquid-culture systems.

The major sources of human hemopoietic stem cells (HSC) for clinical transplantation include BM and PBPCs. More recently, umbilical cord blood (CB) has been used as an alternative source of hemopoietic support. Allogeneic transplantation of BM (Thomas et al. 1979), PB (Anasetti et al. 1994), and CB (Broxmeyer et al. 1991) has been performed with cells from both related and unrelated donors. Autologous transplants, where the patient serves as his/her own donor, are typically performed with either BM and/or PBPCs (Peters et al. 1993).

When clinically indicated, patients receive a high-dose therapy regimen followed by infusion of fresh (allogeneic BM or PBPC) or previously cryopreserved (autologous BM and/or PB, allogeneic CB) hemopoietic cells. Within days of high-dose therapy administration, the patients develop profound myelosuppression that is ameliorated by the hemopoietic cell transplant. The time to hemopoietic reconstitution or "engraftment," commonly defined as a granulocyte count of 0.5 x 10^9/L and a platelet count of 20 x10^9/L, can reflect the quality and/or quantity of the infused progenitors.

■ QUALITY CONTROL OF A HEMOPOIETIC GRAFT

What constitutes an adequate hemopoietic product has not been universally defined. The reproducible murine HSC assays such as the colony-forming unit–spleen (CFU-S) (McCullogh and Till 1960) and competitive repopulation studies in lethally irradiated recipients (Phillips 1991) do not exist for the human HSC. The lack of information with any of the available in vitro or in vivo assays to detect and quantitate human hemopoietic cells with long-term, multilineage, in vivo repopulation capacity underscores the difficulty of assessing the reconstitution potential of hemopoietic grafts prior to transplant. Several different variables are currently used as possible surrogate markers of human hemopoietic cell repopulation potential. These include flow-cytometric analysis of CD34$^+$ cell content as discussed in Chapter 5, short- (Rowley et al. 1990) and long-term (Sutherland et al. 1990) tissue-culture assays, and severe combined immunodeficiency (SCID) mouse repopulating assays (Shpall et al. 1994).

Short-Term Tissue-Culture Assay

Short-term methylcellulose-based tissue culture assays are often used to quantitatively assess the content of committed granulocyte-macrophage colony-forming cells (GM-CFC) in culture (Rowley et al. 1987), consisting primarily of myeloid and erythroid progenitors in hemopoietic cell grafts. The CFC typically include GM-CFC, granulocyte-erythroid-megakaryocyte-macrophage (GEMM)-CFC, and G-CFC. A fibrin clot assay (Briddell et al. 1991) can be used to estimate the megakaryocyte (MK)-CFC in the progenitor cell fractions. The obligate 10- to 14-day period required before the cultures can be analyzed make the clinical use of these assays difficult, given the immediate decisions regarding hemopoietic graft quality often necessary for optimal patient care.

Long-Term Tissue-Culture Assay

Sutherland et al. developed the long-term culture-initiating cell (LTC-IC) assay used with increasing frequency in research laboratories to assess a more primitive human hemopoietic progenitor than that represented by the CFU-S (Sutherland et al. 1990). The assay measures cells that give rise to clonogenic progenitors detectable in methylcellulose after a minimum of 5 weeks of culture in the presence of preirradiated stroma. When compared directly in murine experiments, LTC-IC were shown to be more primitive than many CFU-S and to co-purify with long-term, in vivo repopulating cells (Sutherland et al. 1990). Although this assay may be useful in preclinical hemopoietic graft manipulation studies to determine the optimal procedures to be used clinically, the multi-week delay before it can be analyzed makes it impossible to use it clinically for the analysis of specific grafts.

SCID Mouse Assay

The SCID mouse mutant was first described by Bosma and Carroll (1991). By selective breeding, a colony of mice deficient in mature B and T lymphocytes was developed. Because of this immunodeficiency, the SCID mouse was noted to be permissive for the growth of human hemopoietic cells (Bosma and Carroll 1991). Sublethally irradiated SCID mice were transplanted with human BM cells. After transplant, approximately 1% of the hemopoietic cells detected in these mice were of human origin (Lapidot et al. 1992). The administration of human growth factors to the SCID mice following injection significantly enhanced the level of human hemopoietic cell reconstitution to greater than 10% and resulted in the detection of multilineage hemopoiesis. More recently, substantial reconstitution of SCID mice with human CB progenitors, which require no exogenous growth factor support, was reported with a very high fraction (70%) of human cells detected 6 months following transplant (Vormoor et al. 1994; Lowry et al. 1994). Reconstitution in SCID mice is an in vivo assay of repopulating potential that may be of major importance in research laboratories developing new hemopoietic graft manipulation(s) that will ultimately be used clinically; however, given its technical complexity and several months of delay in evaluating the assay, it is obviously not suitable for clinical use.

Future Directions

In clinical studies, time to hemopoietic reconstitution has been shown to correlate with the number of mononuclear cells (MNC)

(Kessinger and Armitage 1991), GM-CFC (Douay et al. 1986; To et al. 1990), and CD34$^+$ cells (Siena et al. 1991) contained in the hemopoietic products. As discussed earlier, in evaluating a clinical graft, neither short-term progenitor cell assays, long-term tissue culture assays, nor reconstitution in SCID mice is practical, given the time delay required before results are analyzed. Because of the current lack of CD34$^+$ cell assay standardization among hemopoietic cell processing laboratories, the total nucleated cell count or MNC is probably the most consistent, although not necessarily the most predictive variable currently in use. Studies have been initiated by the International Society of Hematotherapy and Graft Engineering (ISHAGE) to standardize the flow-cytometric analysis of CD34$^+$ cells in North American hemopoietic cell-processing laboratories. The number of CD34$^+$ cells is likely a better measure of graft quality than the number of cells in the more heterogeneous MNC fraction. Once standardized, flow-cytometric assessment of CD34$^+$ cell number will likely become the standard technique for evaluating hemopoietic graft quality in the next several years.

From the time BM or PBPCs are harvested until they are infused or cryopreserved, the viability of hemopoietic cells declines at a continual rate (Treleaven 1991). Thus, irrespective of quality-control assays, it is generally accepted that the more rapidly a graft can be processed once it has been harvested, the better, with respect to quality of the progenitor cells and patient safety.

■ BONE MARROW

BM has been successfully used to reverse the myelosuppression produced by high-dose chemotherapy since 1957 (Thomas and Storb 1994). The marrow is generally harvested from the posterior iliac crests of the donor or patient under general anesthesia (Peggy and Kemp 1960), and then infused immediately or cryopreserved. A final BM volume of approximately 800 to 2,000 mL is collected. Generally, transplant centers attempt to collect a total of 0.5 to 4.0 × 10^8 MNC/ kg of patient weight, depending upon the additional manipulations planned.

Although reproducible hemopoietic reconstitution is produced with BM, the cells that are actually responsible for either short-term or long-term engraftment are unknown. In murine models, separable progenitor cell subpopulations with either short-term or long-term repopulating potential have been reported (Baum et al. 1992). Baum et al. showed that the Thy1.1^{low} Lin$^-$ Sca-1$^+$ subpopulation of mouse BM cells contained all cells capable of long-term repopulation in lethally irradiated mice (Baum et al. 1992). More recently, their group compared the kinetics of reconstitution using highly purified Thy1.1^{low} Lin$^-$ Sca-1$^+$ cells to that achieved with unfractioned BM containing an equivalent number of the putative stem-cell population (Uchida et al. 1994). Surprisingly, they found that both the early phase (days 7 to 21) and middle phase (days 21 to 35) of hemopoietic reconstitution in lethally irradiated mice was supported by infusion of the highly purified stem-cell fraction. Furthermore, there was no significant difference in the rate of hemopoietic recovery after transplantation of the highly purified (although still heterogeneous) cells, when compared with recipients transplanted with whole BM. These data suggest that this specific subpopulation is responsible for both short-term and long-term repopulating potential. Alternatively, the subpopulation could be heterogeneous, containing cells with different repopulating potential.

In humans, it is commonly believed that a subpopulation of CD34$^+$ pluripotent BM cells is responsible for long-term repopulation, and that a distinct CD34$^+$ subpopulation of more differentiated hemopoietic progenitors can produce an early phase of more rapid hemopoietic recovery. Neither of these assumptions, however, has been formally tested clinically. Whether a highly purified BM subpopulation could produce both short-term and long-term engraftment in patients is unknown. Whether there is a subpopulation that could accelerate the rate of short-term engraftment is also unknown. Similarly, although current evidence suggests that all human long-term repopulating cells express CD34, the possibility that some or even all such cells are CD34$^-$ has not been excluded. With the dramatic advances in hemopoietic graft engineering described throughout this book, the answers to these fundamental questions about human BMT should be forthcoming in the near future.

◼ PERIPHERAL BLOOD PROGENITOR CELLS

PBPCs may soon replace BM as the major source of hemopoietic progenitor cell support in patients receiving high-dose chemotherapy. This trend is due, in part, to the perception that multiple leukapheresis procedures are less morbid than a BM harvest. Additionally, several nonrandomized studies have demonstrated improvements in the rate of platelet recovery for patients who received PBPCs alone (Sheridan et al. 1994) or in combination with BM (Sheridan et al. 1992; Peters et al. 1990) when compared with patients who received BM alone or with posttransplant growth factor support (discussed in Chapters 9 and 10). Initially, a major concern in the transplant community was whether PBPCs as sole hemopoietic support would produce durable long-term engraftment. Several studies with multiyear follow-up have now confirmed the durability of hemopoietic reconstitution produced using only a PBPC graft (Philip et al. 1987; Juttner et al. 1992; Reiffers et al. 1987; Stiff et al. 1983).

Harvesting of Peripheral Blood Progenitor Cells

PBPCs are collected by an outpatient leukapheresis procedure, using a continuous-flow blood cell separator such as the COBE-Spectra or the Fenwall CS-3000. Approximately 9 to 14 L of patient blood is processed, which takes 3 to 4 hours. The vast majority of the processed blood is returned to the patient. A final PBPC volume of approximately 90 to 200 mL is collected and infused (allogeneic) or cryopreserved (autologous/allogeneic). Generally, transplant centers attempt to collect a total of 4.0 to 6.0 $\times$ 10^8 MNC/kg of patient weight (Kessinger et al. 1988). The number of leukaphereses performed depends upon several factors including the patient's disease, amount of prior myelotoxic therapy, extent of tumor involvement in the BM and/or PB, whether the cells are collected from patients in a steady state, or following mobilization from the BM to the PB with growth factors and/or chemotherapy (as discussed, respectively, in Chapters 11 and 12). In the steady state, six or more leukaphereses may be required to reach the target MNC number (Philip et al. 1987; Williams et al. 1990). Because of delayed platelet recovery in patients transplanted with PBPCs collected in the steady state, such collections are now generally reserved for patients who are mobilization failures, due to extensive prior therapy, substantial tumor contamination of the BM, or, rarely, no apparent reason. With mobilized PBPCs, one to four or five leukaphereses may be required, depending upon the mobilization regimen used. Whether tumor cells are also mobilized with chemotherapy and/or growth factors is unknown and requires investigation.

Alteration of the Hemopoietic Cell Source

Can the short- and/or long-term repopulating potential of PBPC harvests be altered and/or directed by the mobilizing regimen administered? Sutherland reported that PBPCs mobilized with cyclophosphamide contained more primitive hemopoietic precursors than PBPCs mobilized with cyclophosphamide plus GM-CSF (Sutherland et al. 1990). Udomsakdi et al. (1992) recently demonstrated that the clonogenic progenitor-producing potential of cells defined as LTC-IC that are present in PBPC harvests collected following mobilization with cyclophosphamide and/or growth factors was significantly lower than that of LTC-IC in normal BM or PB samples. Briddell et al. (in press) have recently demonstrated that PBPCs mobilized with SCF plus G-CSF contained higher numbers of megakaryocyte progenitors (2- to 9-fold more mature MK-CFC, and 10- to 70-fold more primitive burst-forming units [BFU-MK]), than PBPCs mobilized with G-CSF alone. In gene transfer studies both Yan et al. (1994) and Bodine et al. (1994) reported higher transfection rates when they used PBPCs mobilized with SCF plus G-CSF compared with PBPCs mobilized with G-CSF alone. Whether different mobilization regimens will produce PBPC harvests with different repopulating potentials, or unique characteristics suitable for progenitor expansion ex vivo, requires further investigation and will be evaluated in current and future clinical studies.

■ UMBILICAL CORD BLOOD PROGENITORS

Over the past 5 years, umbilical CB has been investigated clinically as an alternative source of hemopoietic progenitors for allogeneic transplantation, in patients lacking an HLA-matched BM donor (Broxmeyer et al. 1991). The relatively early ontologic stage of CB progenitors compared with BM, with less T-cell development, allows for the theoretical possibility that CB transplants will be associated with a lower incidence of severe graft-versus-host disease (GVHD), the major cause of morbidity and mortality in the allogeneic transplant setting (Martin et al. 1994). Immunologic reactivity studies suggest that CB T cells have limited specific cytoxic activity after allogeneic stimulation and rapidly become "tolerant" to induced alloantigen proliferation (Broxmeyer et al. 1994).

Preliminary Clinical Results of Cord Blood Transplant

Between October 1988 and September 1994, CB from 50 donors (44 sibling and 6 unrelated) had been used for hemopoietic support of myeloablative therapy administered to children with malignant (n = 30) and nonmalignant (n = 20) disorders (Wagner et al. 1994). The International Registry of Cord Blood Transplants has been established and collects data on CB transplants. The New York Blood Center has established a Placental Bank, and is cryopreserving CB aliquots for clinical use in patients lacking an adequate BM donor. Table 7.1 summarizes the graft-cell content from reported CB transplants in children with a median weight of 20 kg (Wagner et al. 1994). The en-

Table 7.1. Hemopoietic Cell Content of Cord Blood
Transplants[a]

	Median	Range	Total Cell Content
Volume (mL)	102.5	(42.1–282)	
Nucleated cells	4.3×10^7/kg	$(0.08–33) \times 10^7$/kg	8.0×10^8
GM-CFC	1.9×10^4/kg	$(0.1–25.6) \times 10^4$/kg	4.8×10^5

[a]Data from Wagner, J., Kernan, N.A., Broxmeyer, H.E., and Gluckman, E.
(in press) Transplantation of umbilical cord blood in 50 patients: analysis
of the registry data. *Blood*. Used with permission.

graftment rates for neutrophils (22 days) and platelets (48 days) have
been slower than those typically produced with BM, and 6 of the 50
(12%) patients failed to engraft. Both the delayed engraftment and failure to engraft may occur as a result of transplantation of an inadequate
number of CB progenitors. Alternatively, CB progenitors, being a more
primitive hemopoietic cell population, may require more time than
BM or PB to establish effective hemopoiesis. The progression-free survival rates for recipients of CB transplants appear to be comparable to
results achieved with BM transplants, and there is a suggestion that CB
transplants may produce less GVHD than allogeneic BMT, particularly
in the unrelated donor setting (Wagner et al. 1994). If CB could produce adequate engraftment, with comparable graft-versus-leukemia
(GVL) effects and less GVHD than that associated with BM, this would
be a profound contribution to allogeneic transplant medicine, particularly in the unrelated and mismatched setting where the incidence of
clinically significant and even fatal GVHD can be in excess of 50%
(Wagner et al. 1994). The absolute number of hemopoietic progenitors
contained in a single CB collection, however, may limit its clinical
utility. Whether a CB collection contains sufficient hemopoietic cells
to engraft an unrelated adult is currently unknown. As discussed in
Chapters 16 and 17, several groups are investigating the ex vivo expansion of CB progenitors (Han et al. 1994; Traycoff, Kosak, and Srour
1994). If successful, expanded CB may become a new source of hemopoietic support for large children or adult patients who lack an HLA-
identical allogeneic BM donor.

■ MANIPULATED HEMOPOIETIC PROGENITORS

There has been an explosion in hemopoietic cell graft engineering
technology over the past several years, yet fundamental questions re-

main about the biology of or reconstitution produced by grafts that have been subjected to in vitro manipulations such as CD34 selection, expansion, and/or gene transfer, before their infusion into patients. Many of these unanswered questions are currently being studied: What are the phenotypic and functional characteristics of the subpopulations contained in unfractionated and fractionated hemopoietic cell grafts responsible for long-term repopulation? Are they a different subpopulation than those responsible for short-term repopulation? If so, how consistent is this phenomenon and what are the differential features that might predict such kinetics? The answers to these questions will have enormous clinical implications for both progenitor-cell expansion and gene-transfer technologies, where knowledge of the duration of repopulation and gene expression, respectively, is an essential component of clinical trial design. Careful, comprehensive preclinical and clinical analysis of the manipulated grafts is critical to the future of this field.

Purged Hemopoietic Progenitors

Is the eradication of tumor from a hemopoietic cell graft important? Brenner et al. transferred the neomycin-resistance gene into the normal BM and malignant cells of autologous BM grafts before infusion into children with neuroblastoma or acute leukemia following high-dose therapy administration. In four of five patients who to date have relapsed following transplant, the investigators have unequivocally demonstrated that gene-marked tumor cells are detectable (Rill et al. 1994). These data confirm that tumor cells contained in a hemopoietic graft are at a minimum at least associated with relapse, suggesting that purging or purification of the graft may be necessary for complete eradication of disease.

"Negative" purging methods where hemopoietic cell grafts are treated with immunologic (Gribben et al. 1991) and/or pharmacologic (Rowley et al. 1989; Shpall et al. 1990) agents to remove malignant cells have been shown to play a role in reducing relapse in patients with hematologic malignancies. These negative purging methods can damage or deplete the normal BM progenitors, delaying engraftment and thus increasing the patient's risk of myelosuppressive complications (Shpall et al. 1990). Additionally, the production of specific reagents such as monoclonal antibody (mAB) or active drugs effective for each tumor type is required. This is labor intensive, can be prohibitively expensive, and requires independent standardization for each purging modality used. Because of potential toxicity to the normal progenitors, immunologic or chemical purging of PB progenitors is rarely performed, despite published studies documenting frequent contamination of the PB with tumor cells (Shpall and Jones 1994). These potential drawbacks to negative purging stimulated interest in positive selection techniques for eradication of tumor from hemopoietic grafts.

Positively Selected Hemopoietic Progenitors

The CD34 antigen (Ag) has been found on 1% to 4% of normal BM and approximately 0.2% of normal PB cells (Civin et al. 1984). The CD34 Ag is expressed on all cells that produce colonies of differentiated progeny in methylcellulose cultures, LTC-IC, and also likely to be expressed on cells that can regenerate hemopoiesis following transplantation (Civin et al. 1984). Only a small fraction of the CD34$^+$ hemopoietic cells (perhaps 1%), however, appear likely to have the latter property and more than 90% co-express antigens characteristic of more mature lymphoid, myeloid, erythroid, or megakaryocytic cells. Although expressed on early hemopoietic progenitors, the CD34 Ag is not present on most tumor cell types including breast cancer, lymphoma, and multiple myeloma (Berenson et al. 1991). Thus, hemopoietic cell purification technology is being developed to improve the clinical results of hemopoietic progenitor cell–supported therapy. In the autologous transplant setting, the aim is to eliminate the tumor cells that contaminate the graft, while in allogeneic transplants the aim is to decrease the number of T cells in the graft, thereby decreasing the risk of GVHD (Martin et al. 1994).

The isolation of CD34$^+$ grafts for clinical use is being investigated with several different methods, many of which are discussed in detail in Chapters 13, 14, and 15. All of the methods include a mAB that targets the human CD34 Ag. Several different Ab assigned to the CD34 cluster (Civin et al. 1989) have been raised against the acute myeloid leukemia (AML) –derived KG1 or KG1a cell lines (Civin et al. 1984; Katz et al. 1985; Andrews, Singer, and Bernstein 1986; Watt et al. 1987; Uchanska-Ziegler et al. 1989; Koeffler et al. 1980), and interact with different epitopes on the CD34 Ag. After the hemopoietic cells are incubated with an anti-CD34 Ab, the majority of these methods involve the separation of target cells on immunospecific surfaces including plastic plates (Lebkowski et al. 1992), streptavidin-coated plastic microspheres (Berenson et al. 1991), or magnetic beads or microparticles (Civin et al. 1990; Miltenyi et al. 1990). Sorting of CD34$^+$ cells from small hemopoietic specimens by flow cytometry has been performed successfully to isolate highly purified CD34$^+$ subpopulations, using multiple surface antigens (Uchida et al. 1994).

Depending upon the method, the positively selected hemopoietic fractions can vary from 50% to 99% CD34$^+$. The development of methods to positively select the CD34$^+$ normal progenitors while leaving the tumor cells behind should be effective for eliminating most malignant cell types while overcoming many of the problems associated with negative-purging techniques.

Expanded Hemopoietic Progenitors

Muench et al. showed that hemopoietic progenitor cells cultured ex vivo could successfully engraft lethally irradiated mice (Muench, Schneider, and Moore 1992). In this study, long-term expression of male lymphocytes in female mice was documented 280 days after transplant. If small numbers of human hemopoietic progenitors could be expanded ex vivo to a quantity sufficient for transplantation, then large-volume BM harvesting or multiple leukaphereses could be avoided. Several other important applications of hemopoietic cell expansion are being considered. Long-term culture of BM from patients with leukemia has been shown to differentially support the growth and expansion of normal progenitors while leukemic cells did not survive (Anasetti et al. 1994). Thus, there may be a beneficial purging effect of ex vivo expansion for hematologic malignancies as well as for solid tumors. Sufficient quantities of hemopoietic progenitors could be generated to support multiple cycles of high-dose therapy, a chemotherapeutic strategy being used with increasing frequency. Alternatively, expanded progenitors could be used to supplement a standard autograft, and, perhaps, ablate or markedly shorten the period of absolute neutropenia, that remains approximately 9 days in most major transplant programs using intensive therapy. Ex vivo growth-factor regimens could be used to develop myeloid-rich or megakaryocyte-rich hemopoietic cell fractions, as clinically indicated. Finally, there is substantial interest in developing ex vivo–expansion techniques for use in conjunction with gene-insertion experiments (Bodine et al. 1994; Dunbar et al. 1993).

There are a number of different systems currently being evaluated for the ex vivo expansion of hemopoietic progenitors. A major distinction among the systems is the use of continuous perfusion, typically with BM stroma, versus the use of static culture (typically stroma free). An ex vivo system that could mimic in vivo conditions may have advantages for both the study of hemopoietic cell biology, as well as the expansion of progenitors for clinical use (Verfaillie 1992; Koller and Palsson 1993). Dexter-type murine long-term BM cultures (LTBMC) developed in the mid-1970s appeared to fulfill these requirements by producing a stable ex vivo hemopoietic system for months (Shpall et al. 1994). Human LTBMC, first developed in the 1980s, typically exhibits an exponential decrease in numbers of total and progenitor cells, rendering the cultures unsuitable for cell expansion. Lack of perfusion in static cultures makes support of high cell densities difficult, and probably contributes to the lack of documented expansion of progenitors with long-term repopulating potential. The addition of recombinant growth factors ameliorates the decline and now continuously perfused and static culture systems have been shown to be effective at maintaining or expanding human hemopoietic progenitors as discussed, respectively, in Chapters 14 and 15.

In a previously reported clinical trial, prompt engraftment was demonstrated in all patients who received CD34$^+$ PBPCs as sole hemopoietic support (Shpall et al. 1994). Those patients received an average total of 9.8×10^6 GM-CFC, which were collected in three to four leukapheresis procedures. PBPC from a single leukapheresis donated by four breast cancer patients for research, was purified and cultured ex vivo in Teflon-coated bags with defined media and an SCF-based growth factor regimen (Purdy et al. 1995). As shown in

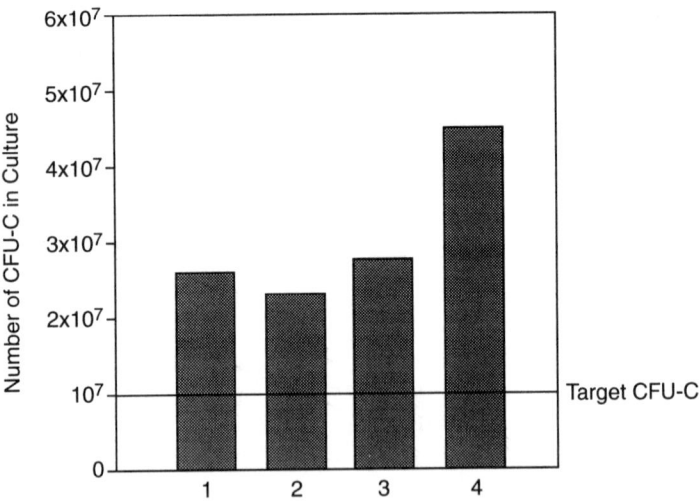

Figure 7.1 Expansion of hemopoietic cells after 10 days of culture in IL-3, IL-6, SCF, and G-CSF (100 ng/mL) in plasma-free medium (Amgen-defined medium). CD34$^+$-enriched PBPCs were cultured in Teflon-coated bags at a starting cell density of 2×10^4 cells/mL; each bar represents total number of cells at the end of the culture for an individual experiment (From Purdy et al. 1995).

Figure 7.1, the number of GM-CFC generated was five times higher than the target number of 9.8×10^6, and we postulate, that if this product were to be infused, it should produce prompt engraftment. All four of these patients had breast cancer cells detected in their $CD34^+$ graft prior to culture. Following culture, rare malignant cells were still detected in one specimen, while no breast cancer cells were detected in the other three. The rate and durability of reconstitution produced with cultured cells remain to be determined and will be evaluated prospectively in a clinical trial.

REFERENCES

Anasetti, C., Martin, P.J., Storb, R., and Hansen, J.A. (1994) Engraftment of allogeneic hemopoietic stem cells in patients conditioned only with anti-CD3 monoclonal antibody BC3 plus methylprednisolone. *Blood*, **84**, 249a (980).

Andrews, R.G., Singer, J.W., and Bernstein, I.D. (1986) Monoclonal antibody 12.8 recognizes a 115-kd molecule present on both unipotent and multipotent colony-forming cells and their precursors. *Blood*, **67**, 842.

Baum, C.M., Weissman, I.L., Tsukamoto, A.S., Buckle, A.M., and Peault, B. (1992) Isolation of a candidate human hemopoietic stem cell population. *Proceedings of the National Academy of Sciences of the United States of America*, **89**, 2804–8.

Berenson, R., Bensinger, W.I., Hill, R.S., et al. (1991) Engraftment after infusion of CD34$^+$ marrow cells in patients with breast cancer or neuroblastoma. *Blood*, **77**, 1717–22.

Bodine, D.M., Seidel, N.E., Gale, M.S., and Neinhuis, A. (1994) Efficient retroviral transduction of mouse pluripotent hemopoietic stem cells mobilized into peripheral blood by treatment with granulocyte colony stimulating factor and stem cell factor. *Blood*, **84**, 1482–91.

Bosma, M.J. and Carroll, A.M. (1991) The SCID mouse mutant: definition, characterization, and potential uses. *Annual Review of Immunology*, **9**, 323–50.

Briddell, R., Stoney, G., Glaspy, J., et al. (in press) Peripheral blood progenitor cells (PBPC) from breast cancer patients mobilized with stem cell factor (rhSCF) plus filgrastim (rhG-CSF) demonstrate typical in vitro growth factor responsiveness. *Blood*.

Briddell, R.A., Bruno, E., Cooper, R.J., et al. (1991) Plasma clot assay for the evaluation of megakaryocyte progenitor cells. *Blood*, **78**, 2854–9.

Broxmeyer, H.E., Kurtzerg, J., Gluckman, E., et al. (1991) Umbilical cord blood hemopoietic stem and repopulating cells in human clinical transplantation. *Blood Cells*, **17**, 313.

Broxmeyer, H.E., Lu, L., Risdon, G., et al. (1994) Cord blood transplantation: an update. *Experimental Hematology*, **22**, 677.

Civin, C.I., Lewis, C., Strauss, C., et al. (1990) Positive stem cell selection: basic science. In A. Gee (Ed.) *Bone marrow purging and processing*, pp. 387–402. New York, Alan R. Liss, Inc.

Civin, C.I., Strauss, L.C., Brovall, C., Fackler, M.J., Schwartz, J.F., and Shaper, J.H. (1984) Antigenic analysis of hemopoiesis III. A hemopoietic progenitor cell surface antigen defined by a monoclonal antibody raised against KG1a cells. *Journal of Immunology,* **133**, 157.

Civin, C.I., Trischman, T., Fackler, M.J., et al. (1989) Summary of CD34 cluster workshop section. In W. Knapp et al. (Ed.) *Leucocyte typing IV,* pp. 818– 25. Boston, Oxford University Press.

Dexter, T.M., Allen, T.D., and Lajtha, L.G. (1977) Conditions controlling the proliferation of hemopoietic stem cell in vitro. *Journal of Cellular Physiology,* **91**, 335–44.

Douay, L., Gorin, N., Mary, J., et al. (1986) Recovery of CFU-GM from cryopreserved marrow and in vivo evaluation after autologous bone marrow transplantation are predictive of engraftment. *Experimental Hematology,* **14**, 358–65.

Dunbar, C., Nienhuis, A., Stewart, F.M., et al. (1993) Genetic marking with retroviral vectors to study the feasibility of stem cell gene transfer and the biology of hemopoietic reconstitution after autologous transplantation in multiple myeloma, chronic myelogenous leukemia, or metastatic breast cancer. *Human Gene Therapy,* **4**, 205–22.

Gribben, J.C., Freedman, A.S., Neuberg, D., et al. (1991) Immunologic purging of marrow assessed by PCR with autologous bone marrow transplantation for B-cell lymphoma. *New England Journal of Medicine,* **325**, 1525–33.

Han, C.S., Dugan, M.J., Verfaille, C.M., Wagner, J.E., and McGlave, P.B. (1994) In vitro expansion of umbilical cord blood committed and primitive hemopoietic progenitors. *Experimental Hematology,* **22**, 723.

Juttner, C.A., To, L.B., Roberts, M.M., et al. (1992) Comparison of hematologic recovery, toxicity, and supportive care of autologous PBSC, autologous BM, and allogeneic BM transplants. *International Journal of Cell Cloning,* **10**, 160.

Katz, F., Tindle, R.W., Sutherland, D.R., and Greaves, M.F. (1985) Identification of a membrane glycoprotein associated with hemopoietic progenitor cells. *Leukemia Research,* **9**, 191.

Kessinger, A. and Armitage, J.O. (1991) The evolving role of autologous peripheral stem cell transplantation following high-dose therapy for malignancies. *Blood,* **77**, 211–13.

Kessinger, A., Armitage, J.O., Landmark, J.D., Smith, D.M., and Weisenburger, D. (1988) Autologous peripheral hemopoietic stem cell transplantation restores hemopoietic function following marrow ablative therapy. *Blood,* **71**, 723–7.

Koeffler, H.P., Billing, R., Lusis, J., Sparkles, R., and Golde, D.W. (1980) An undifferentiated variant derived from human acute myelogenous leukemia cell line (KG1). *Blood,* **56**, 265.

Koller, M.R. and Palsson, B.O. (1993) Tissue engineering: reconstitution of human hemopoiesis ex vivo. *Biotechnology and Bioengineering,* **42**, 909– 30.

Lapidot, T., Pflumio, F., Doedens, M., Murdoch, B., Williams, D.E., and Dick, J.E. (1992) Cytokine stimulation of multilineage hemopoiesis from immature human cells engrafted in SCID mice. *Science,* **255**, 1137.

Lebkowski, J.S., Schain, L.R., Okrongly, D., Levinsky, R., Harvey, M.J., and Okarma, T.B. (1992) Rapid isolation of human CD34 hemopoietic stem cells-purging of human tumor cells. *Transplantation,* **53**, 1011–19.

Lowry, P.A., Schultz, L.D., Greinier, D., et al. (1994) Human hemopoietic progenitor engragraftment into NOD-scid/scid mice does not require cytokine support. *Experimental Hematology,* **22**, 803.

Martin, A., Pamphilon, D., Cornish, J., and Oakhill, A. (1994) A comparison of HLA-matched and mismatched unrelated donor (UD) BMT in children with ALL. *Experimental Hematology*, **22**, 693.

McCullogh, E. and Till, J. (1960) The radiation sensitivity of normal mouse bone marrow cells, determined by quantitative marrow transplantation into irradiated mice. *Radiation Research*, **13**, 15–125.

Miltenyi, S., Muller, W., Weichel, W., and Radbruch, A. (1990) High-gradient magnetic cell separation with MACS. *Cytometry*, **11**, 231–6.

Muench, M., Schneider, J., and Moore, M.A. (1992) Interactions among colony-stimulating factors, IL-1 beta, IL-6, and Kit-ligand in the regulation of primitive murine hemopoietic cells. *Experimental Hematology*, **20**, 339–49.

Peggy, D. and Kemp, N. (1960) Collection, storage, and administration of autologous bone marrow. *Lancet*, **2**, 1426–8.

Peters, W.P., Davis, R., Shpall, E.J., et al. (1990) Adjuvant chemotherapy involving high-dose combination CPA/BCNU/cDDP with bone marrow support for stage II/II breast cancer involving ten or more lymph nodes (CALGB 8782): a preliminary report. *Proceedings of the American Society of Clinical Oncology*, **31**, 22.

Peters, W.P., Ross, M., Vredenburgh, J.J., et al. (1993) High-dose chemotherapy and autologous bone marrow support as consolidation after standard-dose adjuvant therapy for high-risk primary breast cancer. *Journal of Clinical Oncology*, **11**, 1132–43.

Philip, T., Armitage, J.O., Spitzer, G., et al. (1987) High-dose therapy and autologous bone marrow transplantation after failure of conventional chemotherapy in adults with intermediate-grade or high-grade non-Hodgkin's lymphoma. *New England Journal of Medicine*, **316**, 1493–8.

Phillips, R.A. (1991) Hemopoietic stem cells: concepts, assays, and controversies. *Seminars in Immunology*, **3**, 337–41.

Purdy, M.H., Hogan, C., Hami, L., et al. (1995) Large volume ex vivo expansion of CD34 positive hemopoietic progenitor cells for transplantation. *Journal of Hematotherapy*.

Reiffers, J., Castaigne, S., Tilly, H., et al. (1987) Hemopoietic reconstitution after autologous blood stem cell transplantation. A report of 46 cases. *Plasma Therapy and Transfusion Technology*, **8**, 360–4.

Rill, D.R., Santana, V.M., Roberts, W.M., et al. (1994) Direct demonstration that autologous bone marrow transplantation for solid tumors can return a multiplicity of tumorigenic cells. *Blood*, **84**, 380–3.

Rowley, S., Jones, R.J., Piantadosi, S., et al. (1989) Efficacy of ex vivo purging for autologous bone marrow transplantation in the treatment of acute nonlymphoblastic leukemia. *Blood*, **74**, 501–96.

Rowley, S., Sharkis, S., Hattenburg, C., and Sensenbrenner, L. (1987) Culture from human bone marrow of blast progenitor cells with and extensive proliferative capacity. *Blood*, **69**, 804–8.

Sheridan, W., Begley, C.G., Juttner, C.A., et al. (1992) Effect of peripheral blood progenitor cells mobilized by filgrastim (G-CSF) on platelet recovery after high-dose chemotherapy. *Lancet*, **i**, 640–4.

Sheridan, W.P., Begley, C.G., To, L.B., et al. (1994) Phase II study of autologous filgrastim (G-CSF)-mobilised peripheral blood progenitor cells to restore hemopoiesis after high dose chemotherapy for lymphoid malignancies. *Bone Marrow Transplantation*, **14**, 105–11.

Shpall, E.J., Anderson, I.C., Bast, R.C., et al. (1990) Immunopharmacologic purging of breast cancer from bone marrow for autologous bone marrow transplantation. *Progress in Clinical Biological Research*, **333**, 321–36.

Shpall, E.J. and Jones, R.B. (1994) Release of tumor cells from bone marrow. *Blood*, **83**(3), 623–5.

Shpall, E.J., Jones, R.B., and Bearman, S.I. (1994) High-dose therapy with autologous bone marrow transplantation for the treatment of solid tumors. *Current Science*, **6**, 135–8.

Shpall, E.J., Jones, R.B., Franklin, W., et al. (1994a) Transplantation of enriched CD34 positive ($^{+}$) autologous marrow into breast cancer patients following high-dose chemotherapy: influence of CD34^{+} peripheral blood progenitors and growth factors on engraftment. *Journal of Clinical Oncology*, **12**, 28–36.

Shpall, E.J., Stemmer, S.M., Hami, L., et al. (1994b) Amifostine (WR-2721) shortens the engraftment period of 4-hydroperoxy-cyclophosphamide–purged bone marrow in breast cancer patients receiving high-dose chemotherapy with autologous bone marrow support. *Blood*, **83**, 3132–7.

Siena, S., Bregni, M., Brando, B., et al. (1991) Flow-cytometry for clinical estimation of circulating hemopoietic progenitors for autologous transplantation in cancer patients. *Blood*, **77**, 400–6.

Stiff, P.J., Murgo, A.J., Wittes, R.E., et al. (1983) Quantification of peripheral blood colony forming unit-culture rise following chemotherapy: could leukocytaphereses replace bone marrow for autologous transplantation? *Transfusion*, **23**, 500–3.

Sutherland, H.J., Lansdorp, P.M., Henkelmean, D.H., Eaves, A.C., and Eaves, C.J. (1990) Functional characterization of individual human hemopoietic stem cells cultured at limiting dilution on supportive marrow stromal layers. *Proceedings of the National Academy of Sciences of the United States of America*, **87**, 3584–8.

Thomas, E.D., Buckner, C.D., Clift, R.A., et al. (1979) Marrow transplantation for acute nonlymphoblastic leukemia in first remission. *New England Journal of Medicine*, **301**, 597–9.

Thomas, E.D. and Storb, R. (1994) The scientific foundation of marrow transplantation based on animal studies. In S. Forman, K. Blume, and E.D. Thomas (Eds.) *Bone marrow transplantation*, pp. 3–11. Boston, Blackwell Scientific Publications.

To, L.B., Shepperd, K.M., Haylock, D.N., et al. (1990) Single high doses of cyclophosphamide enable the collection of high numbers of stem cells from the peripheral blood. *Experimental Hematology*, **18**, 442.

Traycoff, C.M., Kosak, S., and Srour, E.F. (1994) Assessment of the ex vivo expansion potential of umbilical cord blood and bone marrow long-term hemopoietic culture-initiating cells. *Experimental Hematology*, **22**, 723.

Treleaven, J. (1991) Bone marrow harvesting and reinfusion. In A. Gee (Ed.) *Bone marrow processing and purging, a practical guide*, pp. 31–38. Boca Raton, FL, CRC Press.

Uchanska-Ziegler, B., Petrasch, S., Michel, J., and Ziegler, A. (1989) Characterization of the CD34-specific monoclonal antibody TUK3. *Tissue Antigens*, **33**, 230.

Uchida, N., Aguila, H.L., Fleming, W.H., Jerabek, L., and Weissman, I.L. (1994a) Rapid and sustained hemopoietic recovery in lethally irradiated mice transplanted with purified Thy-1.1^{lo}Lin-Sca-1^{+} hemopoietic stem cells. *Blood*, **83**, 3758–79.

Uchida, N., Combs, A., Conti, S., et al. (1994b) The in vivo hemopoietic population of a rhodamine 123 low population of human marrow. *Experimental Hematology*, **22**, 755.

Udomsakdi, C., Eaves, C.J., Swolin, B., Reid, D., Barnet, J.M., and Eaves, A.C. (1992) Rapid decline of chronic myeloid leukemic cells on long-term culture due to a defect at the leukemic stem cell level. *Proceedings of the National Academy of Sciences of the United States of America*, **89**, 6192–6.

Verfaillie, C.M. (1992) Direct contract between human primitive hemopoietic progenitors and bone marrow stroma is not required for long-term in vitro hemopoiesis. *Blood*, **70**, 2821–6.

Vormoor, J., Lapidot, T., Pflumio, F., et al. (1994) Immature human cord blood progenitors engraft and proliferate to high levels in severe combined immunodeficient mice. *Blood*, **83**, 2489–97.

Wagner, J., Kernan, N.A., Broxmeyer, H.E., and Gluckman, E. (in press) Transplantation of umbilical cord blood in 50 patients: analysis of the registry data. *Blood*.

Watt, S.M., Karhi, K., Gatter, K., et al. (1987) Distribution and epitope analysis of the cell membrane glycoprotein (HPCA-1) associated with human haemopoietic progenitor cells. *Leukaemia*, **1**, 417.

Williams, S.F., Bitran, J.D., Richards, J.M., et al. (1990) Peripheral blood-derived stem cell collections for use in autologous transplantation after high dose chemotherapy: an alternative approach. *Bone Marrow Transplantation*, **5**, 129–33.

Yan, X.Q., Briddell, R., Hartley, C., Stoney, G., Samal, B., and McNiece, I. (1994) Mobilization of long-term hemopoietic reconstituting cells in mice by the combination of stem cell factor and granulocyte colony stimulating factor. *Blood*, **84**, 795–9.

— 8

Chemotherapy-Based Approaches to Mobilization of Progenitor Cells

LUEN BIK TO, DAVID HAYLOCK, PAMELA DYSON, PAUL SIMMONS, AND CHRISTOPHER JUTTNER

The occurrence of high levels of peripheral blood progenitor cells (PBPC) during recovery from myelosuppressive chemotherapy was first described in the 1970s (Richman, Weiner, and Yankee 1976; Lohrmann et al. 1979); however, mobilization of PBPC by chemotherapy for hemopoietic rescue following high-dose therapy did not occur for almost another decade (To et al. 1984; Juttner et al. 1985; Korbling et al. 1986; Reiffers et al. 1986a) except for a report in a patient with chronic myeloid leukemia (CML) (Korbling et al. 1981). The levels of progenitor during the period when the leukocyte and platelet counts are recovering rapidly from their nadirs may be 50-fold or greater than in normal subjects in steady-phase hemopoiesis, although lesser increases are more common (To et al. 1984, 1989). Such high levels may persist for up to 1 week and leukapheresis performed then yields several times the number of myeloid progenitor cells (e.g., granulocyte-macrophage colony-forming cells [GM-CFC]) or CD34$^+$ cells compared with that of a bone marrow (BM) harvest. There were initial doubts whether PB cells were capable of hemopoietic reconstitution (HR) based on conflicting animal data (Micklem, Anderson, and Ross 1975; Storb et al. 1977; Abrams et al. 1981; Chertkov, Gurevitch, and Udalov 1982) and early case reports (Hershko et al. 1979; Abrams et al. 1980). This developmental phase of PB mobilization using chemotherapeutic agents has been reviewed recently (To and Juttner 1993).

■ TYPES OF MOBILIZING CHEMOTHERAPY

Initial studies of PBPC mobilization by chemotherapy were mostly performed as part of induction, consolidation, or intensifica-

130

tion. The general consensus is that chemotherapy that produces a severe and prolonged neutropenia such as less than 0.5×10^9/L for 5 days or more is likely to be more effective than chemotherapy that is less myelosuppressive such as consolidation chemotherapy for acute myeloid leukemia (AML) and cyclophosphamide, doxorubicin, vincristine, and prednisone (CHOP) (To et al. 1984; Reiffers et al. 1986b). Patients who received etoposide 600 mg/m^2 as well as cyclophosphamide 4 gm/m^2 have higher GM-CFC and CD34$^+$ cell levels than those receiving cyclophosphamide alone (Schwartzberg et al. 1992). Moreover, 56% of those receiving etoposide and cyclophosphamide achieved the mononuclear cell (MNC) target of greater than 4×10^8/kg and GM-CFC target greater than 20×10^4/kg compared with 16% of those receiving cyclophosphamide alone.

The administration of high-dose cyclophosphamide (4 to 7 gm/m^2) specifically for mobilization was first reported by Korbling et al. (1986) and subsequently studied in detail by a number of groups (Gianni et al. 1989; To et al. 1989; Rowlings et al. 1992; Kotasek et al. 1993). Tumor cytoreduction is an important additional benefit, but the particular advantage of such a protocol is that PBPC mobilization can be achieved in diseases where conventional treatment is not sufficiently myelosuppressive. Being a more uniform protocol, this also reduces but does not eliminate the unpredictability and logistic problems of recovery-phase PBPC harvesting.

■ LIMITATIONS OF MOBILIZATION BY CHEMOTHERAPY

Neutropenic sepsis and bleeding diathesis are the main toxicity of the myelosuppressive chemotherapy used for PBPC mobilization. In a series of 60 patients who received high-dose cyclophosphamide, hospitalization for parenteral antibiotics was required in 44% to 100%, platelet transfusion in 18%, and septic deaths were reported in 3% (Rowlings et al. 1992). Since yield is related to the severity of myelosuppression, it is unlikely that more effective mobilization protocol using chemotherapy alone can be identified that has less toxicity.

Another limitation is the progenitor cell yield of mobilization by chemotherapy. Published data suggest that the yield is usually sufficient for single, but not for multiple, rescues (Rowlings et al. 1992; Schwartzberg 1993).

■ MOBILIZATION BY CHEMOTHERAPY AND HEMOPOIETIC GROWTH FACTORS

The most significant development in PBPC mobilization by myelosuppressive chemotherapy is the incorporation of hemopoietic growth factors (HGF) as part of the mobilization stimulus.

Some of the HGF have been shown to have the unexpected property of mobilizing PBPC (Chapter 9), either on their own (singly or in combination) or by enhancing mobilization with chemotherapy (Duhrsen et al. 1988; Geissler et al. 1990; Sheridan et al. 1992; To 1994). When used alone recombinant human granulocyte colony-stimulating factor (rHuG-CSF) has the highest activity (Duhrsen et al. 1988; Sheridan et al. 1992, 1994), which seems to be enhanced by combination with rHuSCF (Begley et al. 1984; de Revel et al. 1994), while rHu interleukin (IL)-3, rHu granulocyte-macrophage (GM)-CSF, and rHu stem cell factor (SCF) seem relatively inactive; however, when combined with chemotherapy, rHuG-CSF, rHuGM-CSF, and rHuIL-3 all seem to enhance mobilization by chemotherapy.

Chemotherapy plus rHuG-CSF

There are numerous reports describing the efficacy and safety of chemotherapy and rHuG-CSF for PBPC mobilization (Schwartzberg et al. 1992; Fukuda et al. 1992; Pettengell et al. 1993; Haas et al. 1994); however, the largest study comparing this strategy with chemotherapy alone is that of a series of 382 patients with various malignancies undergoing mobilization with cyclophosphamide (HDC, 4 gm/m^2), cyclophosphamide and etoposide (600 mg/m^2) (HDCE), HDCE with rHuG-CSF (6 μg/kg/day), and HDCE with rHuG-CSF and cisplatin (105 mg/m^2) (Schwartzberg 1993). Both dose escalation and addition of rHuG-CSF were associated with increased CD34$^+$ cell yields. The regimens with rHuG-CSF were associated with a doubling of MNC yield but also a mean four- to sixfold increase in CD34$^+$ cell yield from 1.4 $\times$ 10^6/kg (HDCE) to 6.6 $\times$ 10^6/kg (HDCE+rHuG-CSF) and 8.6 $\times$ 10^6/kg (HDCEP+rHuG-CSF). Moreover, over half of the patients mobilized with HDCEP+rHuG-CSF achieve the desired target level after one leukapheresis while only 40% of HDC-treated patients reached the target number after six aphereses. Thus the combination of dose escalation and the addition of rHuG-CSF led to a higher yield with fewer aphereses. In an earler study, Schwartzberg et al. (1992) reported that leukocyte recovery occurred 3 days earlier in the group receiving rHuG-CSF. Moreover, the incidence of hospitalization due to toxicity is 33% with chemotherapy alone and 8% to 20% with chemotherapy plus rHuG-CSF.

The dose of rHuG-CSF used with chemotherapy is in the range of 3 to 6 μg/kg/day (Schwartzberg et al. 1992; Haas et al. 1994), considerably lower than that of 12 to 16 μg/kg/day when used alone (Sheridan et al. 1992; Weaver et al. 1993). The total cost, however, is similar because the duration of administration is 10 to 14 days compared with 6 days when used alone. Whether even lower doses would be effective has not been reported. Both continuous intravenous (IV) infusions and subcutaneous (SC) injections have been used. The latter route seems more convenient and just as effective. The mobilization ability of the two common formulations of rHuG-CSF does not seem to differ and rHuG-CSF is usually started the day following chemotherapy. Whether a delayed start, with its savings in cost, is also effective for both mobilization and prophylaxis of febrile neutropenia has not been reported.

Chemotherapy plus rHuGM-CSF

Recombinant HuGM-CSF was the first HGF shown to enhance PBPC mobilization by chemotherapy while reducing hematologic toxicity (Gianni et al. 1989, 1990), although it has little activity when used alone (Haas et al. 1990); rHuGM-CSF has more side effects than rHuG-CSF, but its potentiation effect seems comparable. The same group also showed that starting rHuGM-CSF 5 days after chemotherapy was just as effective for mobilization as starting on day 1, but starting 7 or 10 days after chemotherapy may be less effective.

The dose of rHuGM-CSF used with chemotherapy is usually 5 μg/kg/day or 250 μg/m^2/day. Continuous IV infusions were used initially, although the SC route seems just as effective and more convenient. Higher doses are associated with more side effects so are rarely used. Whether lower doses are just as effective has not been tested.

Chemotherapy plus rHuIL-3/rHuGM-CSF

Brugger et al. (1992) reported that sequential rHuIL-3 and rHuGM-CSF following chemotherapy gives higher yield of PBPC compared with rHuGM-CSF following chemotherapy or chemotherapy alone. Both rHuIL-3 (days 1 to 5) and rHuGM-CSF (days 6 to 14) were used at 250 μg/m^2/day. Alternative dose and administration schedules similar to those reported without chemotherapy (To et al. 1993) have not been studied.

Chemotherapy plus PIXY321

Preliminary data suggest that PIXY321 (GM-CSF/IL-3 fusion protein) 500 to 1,000 μg/m^2 following chemotherapy also enhances mobilization (Weinthal et al. 1994) and that 6 to 10 $\times$ 10^6/kg CD34$^+$ cells could be harvested with one to two aphereses following cyclophosphamide 4 gm/m^2 and PIXY321 375 μg/m^2 (Bitran et al. 1994).

Other cytokines such as IL-1 and IL-11 (Fibbe et al. 1992; Hastings et al. 1994) have also been tested in experimental animals, but no human data are available. It is also important to note that in spite of the prevalent opinion that HGF enhance PBPC mobilization by chemotherapy, no phase III studies comparing chemotherapy alone with chemotherapy plus HGF have been reported. A multicenter phase III study comparing cyclophosphamide with and without rHuGM-CSF is nearing completion, and results should be available soon.

■ LEUKAPHERESIS SCHEDULE

Leukaphereses are usually started when the leukocyte count reaches 1 $\times$ 10^9/L for mobilization with chemotherapy alone (To et al. 1989). Other groups have used increasing platelet counts or monocytosis as the starting criterion, although they generally occur simultaneously. The recommendation to begin leukapheresis so early poses a logistic problem because it requires daily blood count monitoring, often starting on weekends. It was based partly on the need to maximize yield and partly on the uncertainty that there were no data to indicate whether primitive progenitors were mobilized at the same time as the more mature progenitors that are measurable by GM-CFC assay. Consequently, aphereses were scheduled throughout the recovery phase. Several studies have now shown that long-term culture-initiating cells (LTC-IC) were present throughout the recovery phase (Bender et al. 1992b; Neben, Marous, and Minch 1993; Pettengell et al. 1993; Sutherland et al. 1994b); therefore, it is probably not vital to start so early.

In chemotherapy plus HGF mobilization, the more rapid increase in PBPC and their higher levels means that it is even less critical to start leukapheresis early. Several groups have elected to start when the leukocyte count is 2 to 5 $\times$ 10^9/L and one report recommends not starting until the leukocyte count is greater than 10 $\times$ 10^9/L (Fukuda et al. 1992).

■ LEUKAPHERESIS TARGETS

Leukaphereses are continued until a specific MNC or CD34$^+$ cell target is reached. Leukapheresis targets vary among laboratories and may range from 3 to 8 $\times$ 10^8 MNC/kg and 1 to 8 $\times$ 10^6 CD34$^+$ cells/kg. An MNC target was used during the earlier years even though it is a relatively insensitive indicator of progenitor cell content because GM-CFC results take 2 weeks and therefore are not available at the time of leukapheresis. More recently, real-time $CD34^+$ cell measurements have been used. Increasing evidence now demonstrates a close correlation between GM-CFC and $CD34^+$ cell levels and that a $CD34^+$ cell dose greater than or equal to 2×10^6/kg is associated with increasingly rapid HR, although there may also be an upper threshold effect at 5 to 8×10^6/kg, above which further increases in cell dose may not substantially further hasten recovery (Siena et al. 1991; Bender et al. 1992a; To et al. 1994b). Flow cytometric measurement by whole blood lysis and labeling with directly conjugated CD34 antibody (Ab) was pioneered by Siena et al. (1989) and markedly improves the rapidity and accuracy of the assay. Several refinements have been proposed such as improved gating and quantitation using fluorescent beads (Chen et al. 1994; Sutherland et al. 1994a). For laboratories without ready access to a flow cytometer, the APAAP technique may be used instead (Dyson et al. 1994). Standardization of the $CD34^+$ cell measurement to make data from different laboratories comparable is an area of intense effort and will contribute to a better defined target; however, it is worth noting that CD34 measurement identifies a heterogeneous population of late and primitive progenitors, while HR following transplant is probably polyphasic (i.e., the early and late phase of HR are mediated by different progenitors) (Jones et al. 1989) so that measurement of $CD34^+$ maturation subsets may provide a more accurate assessment of engraftment potentials. Furthermore, lineage subsets of $CD34^+$ cells may provide more specific indicators of individual lineage reconstitution.

■ FACTORS INFLUENCING YIELD

Several factors have been identified that influence the degree of mobilization with chemotherapy alone or with hemopoietic growth factors. The dose of chemotherapy, the severity of the preceding myelosuppression, and the rate of increase of the leukocyte count correlate positively with yield following chemotherapy (Reiffers et al. 1986a; To et al. 1989; Rowlings et al. 1992; Kotasek et al. 1993). The degree of BM involvement, previous wide-field irradiation, and the amount of previous chemotherapy correlate negatively with yield even when HGF are added (To et al. 1989; Brugger et al. 1992; Gianni et al. 1993; Haas et al. 1994).

Table 8.1 shows a comparison of $CD34^+$ cell and GM-CFC yields between the various mobilization protocols used in the authors' institution. Notwithstanding the heterogeneity in patient groups in re-

Table 8.1. A Comparison of Cell Yields in Different Stem Cell Harvest Protocols in Royal Adelaide Hospital

	Nucleated Cell Yield[b] ($\times 10^8$/kg)	CD34$^+$ Cell Yield[b] ($\times 10^6$/kg)	GM-CFC Yield[b] ($\times 10^4$/kg)
Autologous BM	2.1 ± 0.1 (133)	0.8 ± .01 (23)	11 ± 1 (131)
Allogeneic BM	3.0 ± 0.1 (78)	1.4 ± 0.2 (11)	17 ± 2 (62)
G-CSF mobilized PB[a]			
1. Previously treated (14)	8.3 ± 1.1	0.9 ± 0.3 (3)	37 ± 9.9
2. No prior chemotherapy (15)	9.3 ± 1.3	7.3 ± 1.1	137 ± 17
Chemotherapy mobilized PB			
1. Cyclophosphamide 4 gm/m^2 (68)	3.1 ± 0.2	ND	34 ± 5
2. Cyclophosphamide 7 gm/m^2 (35)	5.8 ± 1.9	3.6 ± 2.5 (11)	44 ± 11
Chemotherapy + G-CSF mobilized PB (14)	5.7 ± 1.2	7.9 ± 3.8	77 ± 35
IL-3/GM-CSF mobilized PB (24)	6.2 ± 0.9	1.5 ± 0.4	24 ± 5
Chemotherapy + GM-CSF mobilized PB (12)	5.3 ± 0.9	13.2 ± 6.8	152 ± 55

[a]Numbers in parentheses represent the number of subjects. [b]Cell yields are expressed as mean ± SE.

lation to their disease type, BM involvement, or previous chemoradiotherapy, the data indicate that chemotherapy plus HGF appear to provide a higher number of progenitors compared with chemotherapy alone. While use of G-CSF alone gives high yields in patients with breast cancer who have had no prior chemotherapy, in previously treated patients the yield with G-CSF alone is little better than chemotherapy alone.

In conclusion, chemotherapy plus HGF appears to be the method of choice for PBPC mobilization in most cancer patients. Tumor cytoreduction is achieved while PBPC is mobilized. PBPC yield is enhanced, myelotoxicity is minimized, and the number of leukaphereses is reduced compared with chemotherapy alone. The adverse effect of prior chemoradiotherapy on yield underscores the importance of incorporating PBPC mobilization as part of planned treatment rather than as part of salvage for resistant disease (Moore 1992; To et al. 1993). Mobilization with rHuG-CSF may provide a comparable yield, especially in previously untreated patients. The avoidance of myelosuppression is an advantage but there is no antitumor effect. Other HGF combinations such as rHuG-CSF plus rHuSCF or rHuIL-3 plus rHuG-CSF are still being evaluated.

▉ NEW QUESTIONS

The rapid improvement in PBPC mobilization by chemotherapy plus HGF enables the harvest of target numbers of progenitors in the majority of patients, and therefore safer transplants. A number of new questions now face clinical investigators for the next phase of development: the quality of PBPC collections, the mechanism of mobilization, and specific targets for different clinical programs.

The Biological Characterization of Mobilized Progenitors

The clinical and hematologic effects of chemotherapy plus HGF (i.e., myelosuppression followed by recovery) are quite different from HGF alone and yet both strategies result in PBPC mobilization. Do they produce qualitatively different mobilized PBPC? In both the normal hemopoietic compartment as well as in the malignant compartment, any differences may have important clinical implications.

Mobilized $CD34^+$ cells from a variety of mobilization protocols (chemotherapy alone, chemotherapy plus rHuG-CSF, chemotherapy plus rHuGM-CSF, and rHuG-CSF alone) were recently shown to be similar to one another in their expression of lineage- and stage-specific phenotypic markers, quiescent cycling status, and in their ability to generate GM-CFC in liquid culture (To et al. 1994a). The presence of LTC-IC has also been shown (Sutherland et al. 1994a) and results in mice show the same pattern (Neben et al. 1993). These similarities are remarkable in view of the different stimuli employed and suggest that there is a final common pathway for mobilization.

The Mobilization of Malignant Progenitors

In patients with CML, Korbling et al. (1981) first reported the mobilization of Philadelphia chromosome–negative (Ph⁻) progenitors during recovery from chemotherapy. Carella et al. (1993) have reported an impressive series of intensive chemotherapy (ICE) and rHuG-CSF with mobilization of Ph⁻, *bcr/abl*⁻ PB cells and achievement of a Ph⁻ remission following autologous transplantation. Hence, both chemotherapy and chemotherapy plus rHuG-CSF mobilize Ph⁻ progenitors but not Ph⁺ progenitors in a proportion of patients in the chronic phase of CML. Whether HGF alone can achieve such a differential mobilization is not yet known.

In lymphoma, myeloma, breast cancer, and neuroblastoma, cells bearing clonal or phenotypic markers seen on malignant cells have been identified in PBPC mobilized with chemotherapy and/or HGF (Sharp et al. 1992; Nagafuji et al. 1993; Brugger et al. 1994; Craig et al. 1994; Moss et al. 1994a; Pantel et al. 1994; Ross et al. 1993; Vora et al. 1994). There were some suggestions that the levels of malignant cells are lower in mobilized PBPC than in BM, but assay sensitivity and specificity remain major hurdles (Moss, To, and Pantel 1994b; Pantel et al. 1994).

The Mechanism of Mobilization

The large variety of mobilization stimuli reported (To 1994) suggests complex interactions; however, the final common pathway through which different stimuli act is most probably that of progenitor/stromal adherence. Papayannopoulou and Nakamoto (1993) described mobilization of progenitors in primates treated with anti–VLA₄ integrin. Since VLA₄ integrin is known to be expressed on primitive hemopoietic progenitors (Simmons et al. 1994), modulation of the progenitor/stromal adherence mechanism may be a more direct means of progenitor mobilization.

The down-modulation of *c-kit* on mobilized CD34⁺ cells is another important observation (To et al. 1994a). The *c-kit*/SCF ligand pair probably plays a significant role in progenitor/stromal interaction

(Simmons et al. 1994) and in addition SCF has been shown to potentiate mobilization by G-CSF (Basser et al. 1993; de Revel et al. 1994). Of particular interest is a preliminary analysis that shows a significant correlation between the level of *c-kit* on CD34$^+$ cells and the number of progenitors mobilized (Simmons et al. 1994). Studies of other adhesion molecules have already identified modulation of the expression of $\alpha 4\beta 1$ and $\alpha 5\beta 1$ integrins, leukocyte integrins $\alpha L\beta 2$ and the $\beta 2$ chain itself (CD18), and LFA-3 (CD58) (Simmons et al. 1994). In all cases, the levels of these molecules on mobilized CD34$^+$ cells were reduced relative to that on steady-phase BM CD34$^+$ cells. Further functional studies may lead to the development of more direct strategies for mobilization.

Specific Targets for Different Clinical Programs

There is clear interest in PBPC harvest protocols that require only a single leukapheresis or even a one-unit venesection (Pettengell et al. 1993; Jones et al. 1994). The reduction of costs and inconvenience to patients are worthwhile objectives. This may also result in a lower tumor-cell load infused, although whether this bears a significant bearing on disease outcome is still to be determined; however, there are several considerations, such as the risks of microbial contamination or other technical mishaps in cell processing, which would potentially render the patient vulnerable by dependence on a single leukapheresis product. Additional leukaphereses may also provide cells for a second transplant or as a back-up for graft failure (fortunately rare). There are also anecdotal experiences of patients who experienced incomplete HR when rescued with cells collected late in the recovery phase that had adequate numbers of GM-CFC (To and Juttner 1993). This raises doubts as to whether CD34$^+$ cell or GM-CFC measurement provides sufficiently specific information on the content of long-term as well as short-term marrow repopulating cells.

Further significant developments in high-dose therapy that influence how we set mobilization targets include the trend towards multiple high-dose therapy (Basser et al. 1993; Tepler et al. 1993) and various ex vivo manipulations such as purging (Gribben et al. 1994), stem cell selection (Berenson et al. 1991; Broun et al. 1994), and ex vivo expansion (Haylock et al. 1992). These techniques obviously require more cells either because several rescues are required or because allowance has to be made for cell loss during manipulation. It is therefore important to identify appropriate targets for individual clinical programs so that sufficient progenitors are harvested with the minimum number of procedures.

ACKNOWLEDGMENTS

The authors thank T. Rawling, C. Rawling, J. Bayly, D. Leavesley, and M. Huxtable for their expert assistance.

REFERENCES

Abrams, R.A., Glaubiger, D., Appelbaum, F.R., and Deisseroth, A.B. (1980) Result of attempted hematopoietic reconstitution using isologous, peripheral blood mononuclear cells: a case report. *Blood,* **56,** 516–20.

Abrams, R.A., McCormack, K., Bowles, C., and Deisseroth, A.B. (1981) Cyclophosphamide treatment expands the circulating hematopoietic stem cell pool in dogs. *Journal of Clinical Investigation,* **67,** 1392–9.

Basser, R., To, L.B., Green, M., et al. (1993) Rapid hematopoietic reconstitution following three cycles of high dose chemotherapy with filgrastim (G-CSF) mobilized peripheral blood progenitor cells (PBPC) and filgrastim in patients with high risk breast cancer. *Blood,* **82,** 233a.

Begley, C.G., Basser, R., Mansfield, R., et al. (1994) Randomized prospective study demonstrating a prolonged effect of SCF with G-CSF (filgrastim) on PBPC in untreated patients: early results. *Blood,* **84,** 25a.

Bender, J.G., To, L.B., Williams, S., and Schwartzberg, L.S. (1992a) Defining a therapeutic dose of peripheral blood stem cells. *Journal of Hematotherapy,* **1,** 329–42.

Bender, J.G., Unverzagt, K.L., Walker, D.E., et al. (1992b) Characterization of CD34$^+$ cells mobilized to the peripheral blood during the recovery from cyclophosphamide chemotherapy. *International Journal of Cell Cloning,* **10,** 23–5.

Berenson, R.J., Bensinger, W.I., Hill, R.S., et al. (1991) Engraftment after infusion of CD34+ marrow cells in patients with breast cancer or neuroblastoma. *Blood,* **77,** 1717–22.

Bitran, J.D., Hanauer, S., Johnson, L., Martinec, J., and Klein, L. (1984) "Mobilized" peripheral blood progenitor cell harvests utilizing cyclophosphamide and PIXY321. *Blood,* **84,** 733a.

Broun, E.R., Traycoff, C., Graves, V., et al. (1994) A comparison of engraftment following high dose chemotherapy with autologous bone marrow transplantation with either full bone marrow or CD34$^+$ cells isolated with the Baxter Isolex 300. *Experimental Hematology,* **22,** 773.

Brugger, W., Bross, K., Frisch, J., et al. (1992) Mobilization of peripheral blood progenitor cells by sequential administration of interleukin-3 and granulocyte-macrophage colony-stimulating factor following polychemotherapy with etoposide, ifosfamide, and cisplatin. *Blood,* **70,** 1193–200.

Brugger, W., Bross, K.J., Glatt, M., Weber, F., Mertelsmann, R., and Kanz, L. (1994) Mobilization of tumour cells and hematopoietic progenitor cells into peripheral blood of patients with solid tumours. *Blood,* **83,** 636–40.

Carella, A.M., Podesta, M., Frassoni, F., et al. (1993) Collection of "normal" blood repopulating cells during early hemopoietic recovery after intensive conventional chemotherapy in chronic myelogenous leukaemia. *Bone Marrow Transplantation,* **12,** 267–71.

Chen, C.H., Lin, W., Shye, S., et al. (1994) Automated enumeration of CD34$^+$ cells in peripheral blood and bone marrow. *Journal of Hematotherapy,* **3,** 3–13.

Cherktov, J.L., Gurevitch, O.A., and Udalov, G.A. (1982) Self maintenance ability of circulating hemopoietic stem cells. *Experimental Hematology*, **10**, 90–7.

Craig, J.I., Langlands, K., Parker, A.C., and Anthony, R.S. (1994) Molecular detection of tumor contamination in peripheral blood stem cell harvests. *Experimental Hematology*, **22**, 898–902.

de Revel, T., Appelbaum, F.R., Storb, R., et al. (1994) Effects of granulocyte colony-stimulating factor and stem cell factor, alone and in combination, on the mobilization of peripheral blood cells that engraft lethally irradiated dogs. *Blood*, **83**, 3795–9.

Duhrsen, U., Villeval, J.L., Boyd, J., Kannourakis, G., Morstyn, G., and Metcalf, D. (1988) Effects of recombinant human granulocyte-colony stimulating factor on hemopoietic progenitor cells in cancer patients. *Blood*, **72**, 2074–81.

Dyson, P.G., Ho, J.Q., Dowse, T.L., Haylock, D.N., Juttner, C.A., and To, L.B. (1994) The use of the APAAP technique as a rapid indicator of peripheral blood progenitor cell levels. *Pathology*, **26**, 296–300.

Fibbe, W.E., Hamilton, M.S., Laterveer, L.L., et al. (1992) Sustained engraftment of mice transplanted with IL-1 primed blood-derived stem cells. *Journal of Immunology*, **148**, 417–21.

Fukuda, M., Kojima, S., Matsumoto, K., and Matsuyama, T. (1992) Autotransplantation of peripheral blood stem cells mobilized by chemotherapy and recombinant human granulocyte colony-stimulating factor in childhood neuroblastoma and non-Hodgkin's lymphoma. *British Journal of Haematology*, **80**, 327–31.

Geissler, K., Valent, P., Mayer, P., et al. (1990) Recombinant human interleukin-3 expands the pool of circulating hematopoietic progenitor cells in primates and synergism with recombinant granulocyte/macrophage colony-stimulating factor. *Blood*, **75**, 2305–10.

Gianni, A.M., Bregni, M., Siena, S., et al. (1990) Recombinant human granulocyte-macrophage colony-stimulating factor reduces hematologic toxicity and widens clinical applicability of high-dose cyclophosphamide treatment in breast cancer and non-Hodgkin's lymphoma. *Journal of Clinical Oncology*, **8**, 768–78.

Gianni, A.M., Bregni, M., Siena, S., et al. (1993) Clinical usefulness and optimal harvesting of peripheral blood stem cells mobilized by high dose cyclophosphamide and recombinant human GM-CSF. In E.W. Wunder and P.R. Henon (Eds.) *Peripheral blood stem cell autografts*, pp. 145–54, Heidelberg, Springer-Verlag.

Gianni, A.M., Siena, S., Bregni, M., et al. (1989) Granulocyte-macrophage colony-stimulating factor to harvest circulating hemopoietic stem cells for autotransplantation. *Lancet*, **2**, 580–5.

Gribben, J.C., Newberg, D., Barber, M., et al. (1994) Detection of residual lymphoma cells by polymerase chain reaction in peripheral blood is significantly less predictive for relapse than detection in bone marrow. *Blood*, **83**, 3800–7.

Haas, R., Ho, A.D., Bredthauer, U., et al. (1990) Successful autologous transplantation of blood stem cells mobilized with recombinant human granulocyte-macrophage colony-stimulating factors. *Experimental Hematology*, **18**, 94–8.

Haas, R., Mohle, R., Fruhauf, S., et al. (1994) Patient characteristics associated with successful mobilizing and autografting of peripheral blood progenitor cells in malignant lymphoma. *Blood*, **83**, 3787–94.

Hastings, R., Kaviani, M.D., Schlerman, F., Hitz, S., Bree, A., and Goldman, S.J. (1994) Mobilization of hematopoietic progenitors by rhIL-11 and rhG-CSF in non-human primates. *Blood*, **84**, 23a.

Haylock, D.N., To, L.B., Dowse, T.L., Juttner, C.A., and Simmons, P.J. (1992) Ex vivo expansion and maturation of peripheral blood CD34$^+$ cells into the myeloid lineage. *Blood*, **89**, 1405–12.

Hershko, C., Ho, W.G., Gale, R.P., and Cline, M.J. (1979) Cure of aplastic anaemia in paroxysmal nocturnal hemoglobulinuria by marrow transfusion from identical twin: failure of peripheral leucocyte transfusion to correct marrow aplasia. *Lancet*, **1**, 945–7.

Jones, R.J., Celano, P., Sharkis, S.J., and Sensenbrenner, L.L. (1989) Two phases of engraftment established by serial bone marrow transplantation in mice. *Blood*, **73**, 397–401.

Jones, H.M., Jones, S.A., Watts, M.J., et al. (1994) Development of a simplified single leukapheresis approach for peripheral blood progenitor cell transplantation in previously treated patients with lymphoma. *Journal of Clinical Oncology*, **12**, 1693–702.

Juttner, C.A., To, L.B., Haylock, D.N., Branford, A., and Kimber, R.J. (1985) Circulating autologous stem cells collected in very early remission from acute non-lymphoblastic leukaemia produce prompt but incomplete hemopoietic reconstitution after high dose melphalan or supralethal chemoradiotherapy. *British Journal of Haematology*, **61**, 739–45.

Korbling, M., Burke, P., Braine, H., Elfenbein, G., Santos, G.W., and Kaizer, H. (1981) Successful engraftment of blood derived normal hemopoietic stem cells in chronic myelogenous leukemia. *Experimental Hematology*, **9**, 684–90.

Korbling, M., Dorken, B., Ho, A.D., Pezzuto, A., Hunstein, W., and Fliedner, T.M. (1986) Autologous transplantation of blood derived hemopoietic stem cells after myeloablative therapy in a patient with Burkett's lymphoma. *Blood*, **67**, 629–32.

Kotasek, D., Sage, R.E., Dale, B.M., Norman, J.E., and Bolton, A. (1993) High dose chemotherapy and autologous transplantation with peripheral blood stem cells (PBSC) mobilized using cyclophosphamide (CY) with and without granulocyte colony-stimulating factor (G-CSF). *Third International Symposium on Peripheral Blood Stem Cell Autografts*. Bordeaux, France, October 11–13, abstract.

Lohrmann, H.P., Schreml, W., Fliedner, T.M., and Heimpel, H. (1979) Reaction of human granulopoiesis to high dose cyclophosphamide therapy. *Blut*, **38**, 9–16.

Micklem, H.S., Anderson, N., and Ross, R. (1975) Limited potential of circulating hemopoietic stem cells. *Nature*, **256**, 41–3.

Moore, M.A.S. (1992) Does stem cell exhaustion result from combining hematopoietic growth factors with chemotherapy? If so, how do we prevent it? *Blood*, **80**, 3–7.

Moss, T.J., Cairo, M., Santana, V.M., Weinthal, J., Hurvitz, C., and Bostrom, B. (1994a) Clonogenicity of circulating neuroblastoma cells: implications regarding peripheral blood stem cell transplantation. *Blood*, **83**, 3085–9.

Moss, T.J., To, L.B., and Pantel, K. (1994b) Evaluation of grafts for occult tumor cells. *Journal of Hematotherapy*, **3**, 163–4.

Nagafuji, K., Harada, M., Takamatsu, Y., et al. (1993) Evaluation of leukaemic contamination in peripheral blood stem cell harvests by reverse transcriptase polymerase chain reaction. *British Journal of Haematology*, **85**, 578–83.

Neben, S., Marous, K., and Minch, P. (1993) Mobilization of hematopoietic stem and progenitor cell populations from marrow to the blood of mice following cyclophosphamide and/or granulocyte colony-stimulating factor. *Blood*, **81**, 1960–7.

Pantel, K., Schlimok, G., Angstwurm, M., et al. (1994) Methodological analysis of immunocytochemical screening for disseminated epithelial tumor cells in bone marrow. *Journal of Hematotherapy*, **3**, 165–73.

Papayannopoulou, T. and Nakamoto, B. (1993) Peripheralization of hemopoietic progenitors in primates treated with anti-VLA$_4$ integrin. *Proceedings of the National Academy of Sciences of the United States of America*, **90**, 9374–8.

Pettengell, R., Morgenstern, G.R., Wall, P.J., et al. (1993) Peripheral blood progenitor cell transplantation in lymphoma and leukaemia using a single leukapheresis. *Blood*, **82**, 3770–7.

Reiffers, J., Bernard, P., David, B., et al. (1986a) Successful autologous transplantation with peripheral blood hemopoietic cells in a patient with acute leukaemia. *Experimental Hematology*, **14**, 312–5.

Reiffers, J., Bernard, P.H., Marit, G., et al. (1986b) Collection of blood derived hemopoietic stem cells and applications for autologous transplantation. *Bone Marrow Transplantation*, **1**, 371–2.

Richman, C.M., Weiner, R.S., and Yankee, R.A. (1976) Increase in circulating stem cells following chemotherapy in man. *Blood*, **47**, 1031–9.

Ross, A.A., Cooper, B.W., Lazarus, H.M., et al. (1993) Detection and viability of tumour cells in peripheral blood stem cell collections from breast cancer patients using immunocytochemical and clonogenic assay techniques. *Blood*, **82**, 2605–10.

Rowlings, P.A., Rawling, C.A., To, L.B., Bayly, J.L., and Juttner, C.A. (1992) A comparison of peripheral blood stem cell mobilization after chemotherapy with cyclophosphamide as a single agent in doses of 4 g/m^2 or 7 g/m^2 in patients with advanced cancer. *Australian and New Zealand Journal of Medicine*, **22**, 660–4.

Schwartzberg, L.S. (1993) Peripheral blood stem cell mobilization in the outpatient setting. In E.W. Wunder and P.R. Henon (Eds.) *Peripheral blood stem cell autografts*, pp. 177–84. Heidelberg, Springer-Verlag.

Schwartzberg, L.S., Birch, R., Hazelton, B., et al. (1992) Peripheral blood stem cell mobilization by chemotherapy with and without recombinant human granulocyte colony-stimulating factor. *Journal of Hematotherapy*, **1**, 317–27.

Sharp, J.G., Kessinger, A., Vaughan, W.P., et al. (1992) Detection and clinical significance of minimal tumor cell contamination of peripheral stem cell harvests. *International Journal of Cell Cloning*, **10**, 92–4.

Sheridan, W.P., Begley, C.G., Juttner, C.A., et al. (1992) Effect of peripheral blood progenitor cells mobilized by filgrastim (G-CSF) on platelet recovery after high dose chemotherapy. *Lancet*, **339**, 640–4.

Sheridan, W.P., Begley, C.G., To, L.B., et al. (1994) Phase II study of autologous filgrastim (G-CSF)-mobilized peripheral blood progenitor cells to restore hemopoiesis after high dose chemotherapy for lymphoid malignancies. *Bone Marrow Transplantation*, **14**, 105–11.

Siena, S., Bregni, M., Brando, B., Ravagnani, F., Bonadonna, G., and Gianni, A. (1989) Circulation of CD34$^+$ hematopoietic stem cells in the peripheral blood of high dose cyclophosphamide treated patients: enhancement by intravenous recombinant human GM-CSF. *Blood*, **74**, 1905–14.

Siena, S., Bregni, M., Brando, B., et al. (1991) Flow cytometry for clinical estimation of circulating hematopoietic progenitors for autologous transplantation in cancer patients. *Blood*, **77**, 400–9.

Simmons, P.J., Leavesley, D.I., Levesque, J.-P., et al. (1994) The mobilization of primitive hemopoietic progenitors into the peripheral blood. *Stem Cells*, **12**(Suppl. 1), 187–202.

Simmons, P.J., Zannettino, A., Gronthos, S., and Leavesley, D. (1994) Potential adhesion mechanisms for localization of hemopoietic progenitors to bone marrow stroma. *Leukemia and Lymphoma*, **12**, 353–63.

Storb, R., Graham, T.C., Epstein, R.B., Sale, G.E., and Thomas, E.D. (1977) Demonstration of hemopoietic stem cells in the peripheral blood of baboons by cross-circulation. *Blood*, **50**, 537–42.

Sutherland, D.R., Keating, A., Nayar, R., Anania, S., and Stewart, A.K. (1994a) Sensitive detection and enumeration of CD34$^+$ cells in peripheral and cord blood by flow cytometry. *Experimental Hematology*, **22**, 1003–10.

Sutherland, H.J., Eaves, C.J., Lansdorp, P.M., Phillips, G.L., and Hogge, D.E. (1994b) Kinetics of committed and primitive blood progenitor mobilization after chemotherapy and growth factor treatment and their use in autotransplants. *Blood*, **83**, 3808–14.

Tepler, I., Cannistra, S.A., Frei, E., III, et al. (1993) Use of peripheral blood progenitor cells abrogates the myelotoxicity of repetitive outpatient high dose carboplatin and cyclophosphamide chemotherapy. *Journal of Clinical Oncology*, **11**, 1583–91.

To, L.B. (1993) Is our current strategy in manipulating hemopoiesis in autologous transplantation correct? *Stem Cells*, **11**, 283–9.

To, L.B. (1994) Mobilizing and collecting blood stem cells. In R.P. Gale, C.A. Juttner, and P. Henon (Eds.) *Peripheral blood stem cell autografts*, pp. 56–74. New York, Cambridge University Press.

To, L.B., Haylock, D.N., Dowse, T., et al. (1994a) A comparative study of the phenotype and proliferative capacity of peripheral blood (PB) CD34$^+$ cells mobilized by four different protocols and those of steady-phase PB and bone marrow CD34$^+$ cells. *Blood*, **84**, 2930–9.

To, L.B., Haylock, D.N., Kimber, R.J., and Juttner, C.A. (1984) High levels of circulating hemopoietic stem cells in very early remission from acute non-lymphoblastic leukaemia and their collection and cryopreservation. *British Journal of Haematology*, **58**, 399–410.

To, L.B. and Juttner, C.A. (1993) Stem cell mobilization by myelosuppressive chemotherapy. In E.W. Wunder and P.R. Henon (Eds.) *Peripheral blood stem cell autografts*, pp. 132–44. Heidelberg, Springer-Verlag.

To, L.B., Rawling, C., Andary, C., et al. (1993) The efficacy of sequential/combined IL-3/GM-CSF administration in peripheral blood (PB) progenitor mobilization. *Blood*, **82**, 319.

To, L.B., Roberts, M.M., Rawling, C.M., et al. (1994b) Establishment of a clinical threshold cell dose: correlation between CFU-GM and duration of aplasia. In *Hematopoietic stem cells: the Mulhouse manual*, pp. 15–20. AlphaMed Press.

To, L.B., Sheppard, K.M., Haylock, D.N., et al. (1989) Single high doses of cyclophosphamide enable the collection of high numbers of hemopoietic stem cells from the peripheral blood. *Experimental Hematology*, **18**, 442–7.

Vora, A.J., Toh, C.H., Peel, J., and Greaves, M. (1994) Use of granulocyte colony-stimulating factor (G-CSF) for mobilizing peripheral blood stem cells:

risk of mobilizing clonal myeloma cells in patients with bone marrow infiltration. *British Journal of Haematology*, **86**, 180–2.

Weaver, C.H., Buckner, C.D., Longin, K., et al. (1993) Syngeneic transplantation with peripheral blood mononuclear cells collected after the administration of recombinant human granulocyte colony-stimulating factor. *Blood*, **82**, 1981–4.

Weinthal, J., Blazar, B., Garrison, L., et al. (1994) PIXY321 induces circulating hematopoietic progenitors, inflammatory cytokines, and receptor modulation in children with recurrent solid tumors following ICE chemotherapy. *Blood*, **84**, 27a.

9

Cytokine-Only Approaches to Mobilization of Progenitor Cells

WILLIAM SHERIDAN

The presence of hemopoietic stem cells (HSC) in the peripheral blood (PB) was first described in mice by Goodman and Hodgson (1962). Subsequent experiments showed that marrow function could be restored after lethal irradiation by infusion of PB leukocytes in guinea pigs (Malinin et al. 1965), dogs (Cavins et al. 1964; Storb et al. 1967), and baboons (Storb et al. 1977). Initial clinical attempts to make use of this source of hemopoietic progenitor cells failed, as in the case of an identical-twin transplant (Hershko, Ho, and Gale 1979). The low frequency of progenitor cells in the blood of unstimulated donors required very large numbers of leukapheresis collections in order to obtain sufficient cells for transplantation (Kessinger et al. 1988), and this technique was at first reserved for patients in whom bone marrow (BM) could not be collected because of damage from radiation or tumor infiltration. The discovery by Richman, Winer, and Yankee (1976) that the perturbation of marrow homeostasis by cytotoxic chemotherapy increased the number of circulating colony-forming cells in humans stimulated the investigation of chemotherapy-mobilized peripheral blood progenitor cell (PBPC) transplantation (reviewed in Chapter 8), and this was the only practical way of increasing the blood content of hemopoietic progenitors until the introduction of the colony-stimulating factors (CSF) into clinical medicine in 1987. The activity of CSF in mobilizing PBPC was first observed in the phase I clinical trials of recombinant human granulocyte (rHuG)-CSF (Bronchud et al. 1988; Dührsen et al. 1988; Gabrilove et al 1988a) and recombinant human granulocyte-macrophage (rHuGM)-CSF (Socinski et al. 1988; Villeval et al. 1990) in cancer patients. This chapter will focus on the mobilization of PBPC by the hemopoietic growth factors (Tables 9.1 and 9.2) in the absence of chemotherapy, and the use of mobilized PBPC in supportive care of patients undergoing high-dose chemotherapy.

146

Table 9.1. Hemopoietic Growth Factors: Classic Colony-Stimulating Factors

Factor	Principal Actions on Hemopoiesis on Colony-Forming Cells	
	In Vitro	In Vivo
G-CSF	Stimulation of G-CFC	Neutrophilia
GM-CSF	Stimulation of GM-CFC, G-CFC, M-CFC, Eo-CFC	Neutrophilia, monocytosis, eosinophilia
M-CSF	Stimulation of M-CFC	Monocytosis
Multi-CSF, IL-3	Stimulation of GM-CFC, G-CFC, M-CFC, Eo-CFC, Mast-CFC, MK-CFC	Neutrophilia, monocytosis, eosinophilia, mild thrombocytosis
Eo-CSF, IL-5	Stimulation of Eo-CFC	Eosinophilia
EPO	Stimulation of E-BFC, E-CFC	Erythrocytosis
MPL ligand	Stimulation of MK-CFC	Thrombocytosis

G-CFC = granulocyte colony-forming cell; GM-CFC = granulocyte-macrophage colony-forming cell; M-CFC = macrophage colony-forming cell; Eo-CFC = eosinophil colony-forming cell; MK-CFC = megakaryocyte colony-forming cell; M-CSF = macrophage colony-stimulating factor; E-BFC = erythrocyte blast-forming cell; EPO = erythropoietin.

Table 9.2. Hemopoietic Growth Factors: Other Identified Hemopoietic Growth Factors

Factor	Principal Actions on Hemopoiesis	
	On Colony-Forming Cells In Vitro	In Vivo
SCF	Synergistic augmentation of specific colony-stimulating activity of all other CSFs and HGFs; stimulation of Mast-CFC	PBPC mobilization, mast-cell hyperplasia
LIF	Stimulation of MK-CFC	Mild thrombocytosis
FL	Synergistic augmentation of specific colony-stimulating activity of other CSFs (except EPO)	Unknown
IL-1	Synergistic activity with other CSFs	Neutrophilia, delayed thrombocytosis
IL-2	Inhibits GM-CFC	Lymphocytosis
IL-6	Stimulation of G-CFC, GM-CFC, MK-CFC	Mild thrombocytosis, mild neutrophilia
IL-9	Stimulates E-CFC, Mast-CFC	NR
IL-11	Stimulates MK-CFC, Mast-CFC	Mild thrombocytosis, mild neutrophilia
IL-12	Synergistic activity with SCF or FL on G-CFC	Anemia, neutropenia

SCF = stem cell factor; LIF = leukemia-inhibiting factor; FL = flt^2/flk^3 ligand; IL = interleukin; CSF = colony-stimulating factor; HGF = hemopoietic growth factor; NR = not reported.

■ GRANULOCYTE COLONY-STIMULATING FACTOR

Animal Models

Rodents Molineux, Podja, and Dexter (1990a) gave rHuG-CSF to male and female B6D2F$_1$ mice at 250 μg/kg/d (a dose that produces a maximum degree of neutrophilia) for 4 days, and observed an increase in spleen colony-forming cells (S-CFC) in both the spleen and the blood. The degree of increase in blood S-CFC and GM-CFC was greater in splenectomized mice, and in both normal and splenectomized mice rHuG-CSF treatment decreased marrow cellularity, S-CFC content, and GM-CFC content. Further work by others (Bungart et al. 1990; Briddell et al. 1993; Roberts and Metcalf 1994; Yan et al. 1994) has confirmed the potent effect of rHuG-CSF in mice of inducing release of primitive and committed hemopoietic progenitor cells.

Using sex-mismatched transplants (male donor into female recipient) and a molecular probe for Y-chromosome–specific DNA sequences, the Manchester group also showed that blood cells from rHuG-CSF–treated mice were capable of reconstituting the hemopoietic system (Molineux et al. 1990b). The cells in as little as 10 μL of blood from rHuG-CSF–treated mice contained sufficient repopulating cells to ensure survival of 98% of irradiated recipients, whereas the cell content of 3,000 μL of normal blood (1.5 times the mouse blood volume) was required to achieve similar survival. The pattern of Y-chromosome expression in female recipients, in the BM, spleen, blood, and thymus, indicated that reconstitution of hemopoiesis by very primitive cells had occurred; S-CFC were 100% donor in origin.

The reduction of femoral GM-CFC observed by Molineux et al. (1990a) was not seen in the experiments of Bungart et al. (1990). Female C57/bl6 mice were given subcutaneous (SC) glycosylated rHuG-CSF for 6 days at a dose of 150 μg/kg/d (a dose producing plateau neutrophilia) and GM-CFC increased in femoral BM, spleen, and PB. The different results of these studies may represent variation in response to G-CSF among different mouse strains. In addition, the detailed analysis of Roberts and Metcalf (1994) of the effect of rHuG-CSF in intact *Balb/c* mice clearly indicates that the decrease in femoral progenitor-cell content varies with the duration of therapy and is more than offset by the increase in splenic hemopoiesis. The effect of G-CSF on PB CFC content was dose dependent over the range tested, approximately 4 to 400 μg/kg/d (Fig. 9.1) (Roberts and Metcalf 1994), and although G-CFC, GM-CFC, M-CFC, Eo-CFC, BL-CFC, and MK-

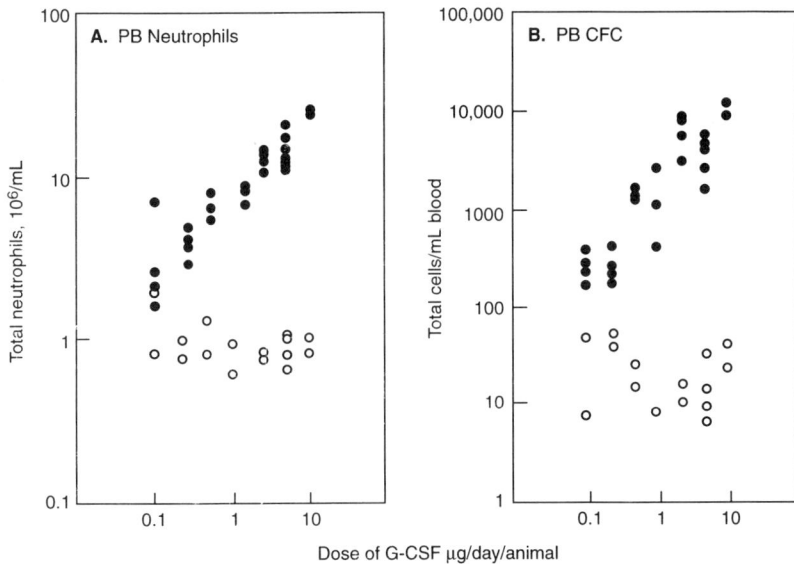

Figure 9.1 The effect of 5 days of SC rHG-CSF (*solid symbols*) or saline (*open symbols*) on the peripheral blood neutrophil count (*A*) and clonogenic progenitor cell content (*B*) in *Balb/c* mice. Each point represents a single animal. (Adapted from Roberts, A.W. and Metcalf, D. [1994] Granulocyte colony-stimulating factor induces selective elevations of progenitor cells in the peripheral blood of mice. *Experimental Hematology,* **22,** 1156–63.)

CFC were all elevated, the effect of G-CSF on mobilizing MK-CFC was disproportionately greater.

Of interest is the diminished response of mice deficient in either stem-cell factor (SCF) (steel phenotype, *Sl/Sl*d) or c-*kit* (white-spotting phenotype, *W/W*v) to G-CSF, when compared with their normal littermates (Cynshi et al. 1991).

Dogs   Recombinant canine G-CSF (rcG-CSF) (10 μgmg/kg/d for 7 days) was administered to five beagles by de Revel et al. (1994). PB GM-CFC levels increased 5.7-fold over baseline and erythroid burst-forming cells (E-BFC) increased 5.4-fold. PB was collected by phlebotomy on day 8 and 10^8/kg mononuclear cells (MNC) from the buffy coat fraction cryopreserved. After radiation (920 cGy) and autologous PBPC infusion, all five dogs recovered hemopoiesis that was sustained up to at least 6 months, compared with no recovery in three control dogs not given rcG-CSF–mobilized progenitor cells.

Primates   Baboons (*Papio cynocephalus*) given rHuG-CSF also display the phenomenon of hemopoietic progenitor-cell mobilization. Recombinant HuG-CSF induces a dose-dependent leukocytosis in baboons, with the dose limited by effects of hyperleukocytosis. Even though rHuG-CSF was not given at doses known to induce plateau neutrophilia, at a dose of 100 μg/kg/d for 14 days, mobilization of GM-CFC, E-BFC, and MK-CFC was elicited (Andrews et al. 1994).

Clinical Studies of rHuG-CSF Mobilization

The phenomenon of mobilization of hemopoietic progenitor cells by rHuG-CSF was first recognized in phase I clinical trials in cancer patients (Fig. 9.2) (Dührsen et al. 1988; Gabrilove et al. 1988a). These laboratory studies were done as a precaution in case rHuG-CSF treatment led to depletion of progenitor cells, as seen in in vitro studies of the action of rHuG-CSF (Dührsen et al. 1988).

Mobilization by rHuG-CSF in Normal Individuals   Studies of the response of normal individuals to rHuG-CSF have confirmed that the wide range of response seen in cancer patients (Dührsen et al. 1988; Gabrilove et al. 1988a; De Luca et al. 1992; Sheridan et al. 1992c) is at least partly due to physiologic variation (Matsunaga et al. 1993; Dreger et al. 1994; Sato et al. 1994; Tjonnfjord et al. 1994; Weaver et al. 1993; 1994; Lane et al. 1995). The kinetic characteristics of the mobilization response to rHuG-CSF identified in the initial studies (Dührsen et al. 1988; Gabrilove et al. 1988a; De Luca et al. 1992; Sheridan et al. 1992c) have also been seen in normal subjects, with peak blood levels of clonogenic progenitor cells and CD34$^+$ cells on day 5 or 6 of rHuG-CSF administration even if only a single dose of 15 μg/kg (Schwinger et al. 1993) or low doses (2 μg/kg/d for 5 days) (Sato et al. 1994) are given. Side-effects of rHuG-CSF reported in these studies have been limited to musculoskeletal pain.

The interindividual variation in PBPC mobilization response to rHuG-CSF may be partly explained on the basis of age. Dreger et al. (1994) reported that in ten normal donors aged 18 to 67 years given 10 μg/kg/d ($n = 6$) or 5 to 6 μg/kg/d ($n = 4$) rHuG-CSF there was an inverse correlation of the peak PB CD34$^+$ cell level with age ($r = -0.934$). In this study, leukapheresis collections were done for allogeneic transplantation, and the yield of CD34$^+$ cells per 10 L of blood volume apheresed was also inversely correlated with age ($r = -0.956$). Compared with five allogeneic BM harvests, these PBPC collections contained 3 times more CD34$^+$ cells, 7 times more T cells, and 20 times more natural killer (NK) cells. The markedly higher lymphocyte

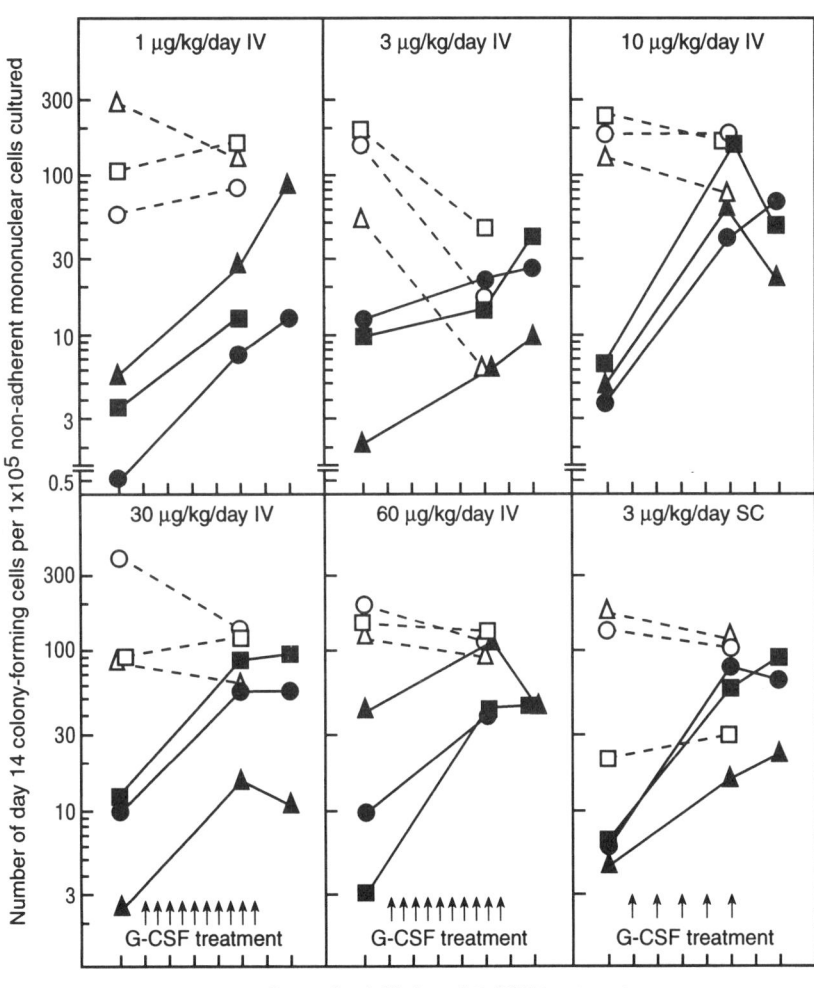

Figure 9.2 Frequency of day-14 colony-forming cells (CFC) in peripheral blood (*closed symbols*) and bone-marrow (*open symbols*) of cancer patients before, during, and after treatment with different doses of rHuG-CSF. In each panel, the different symbols (*circles, squares, triangles*) represent an individual patient at the dose/route. (Adapted from Dührsen, U., Villeval, J.L., Boyd, J., Kannourakis, G., Morstyn, G., and Metcalf, D. [1988] Effects of recombinant granulocyte colony-stimulating factor on hemopoietic progenitor cells in cancer patients. *Blood*, **72**, 2074–81.)

content of rHuG-CSF mobilized PBPC harvests compared with standard BM harvests has been confirmed in the autologous setting (Weaver et al. 1994). A decline in mobilization response with age is supported by results of a recent normal volunteer study of rHuG-CSF (Chatta et al. 1994). After 5 days of 300 μg/d rHuG-CSF, PB levels of GM-CFC were approximately 60% less in the elderly group compared with the young group ($p = 0.03$).

DOSE RESPONSE IN NORMAL INDIVIDUALS Dose-response studies in normal subjects have been limited. Yield of CD34$^+$ cells was superior in the six subjects of Dreger et al. (1994) given 10 μg/kg/d compared with the three subjects given 5 or 6 μg/kg/d (6.6 $\times$ 10^6/kg versus 3 $\times$ 10^6/kg; Table 9.3). A dose of 16 μg/kg/d rHuG-CSF for 5 days was used by the Seattle group in four syngeneic donors (Weaver et al. 1993) and also in eight allogeneic donors (Bensinger et al. 1995) aged 12 to 47 years. The total yield in the identical-twin donors ranged from 47 to 211 $\times$ 10^4/kg GM-CFC and 1.6 to 12.6 $\times$ 10^6/kg CD34$^+$ cells from one leukapheresis, and in the allograft donors the yield of CD34$^+$ cells was a median of 13.1 $\times$ 10^6/kg from two leukaphereses. It is difficult to make direct comparisons to Dreger's results, however, because of the nature of rare-event flow cytometry (Chapter 5) and possible differences in apheresis technique. Other investigators have studied 5 μg/kg/d for 5 days ($n = 9$; Fritsch et al. 1994), 10 μg/kg/d for 7 days ($n = 6$; Tjonnfjord et al. 1994) or 4 days ($n = 8$; Lane et al. 1995), 30 μg/d ($n = 14$) versus 300 μg/d ($n = 14$) (Chatta et al. 1994), 3 μg/d versus 5 μg/d versus 10 μg/d ($n = 6$ each) (Hoglund et al. 1994), and 10 μg/kg/d ($n = 11$) versus 24 μg/kg/d ($n = 11$) (Zeller et al. 1994). In the only randomized study reported to date (Chatta et al. 1994), both a higher dose of rHuG-CSF (300 μg/d versus 30 μg/d) and youth were associated with higher PB GM-CFC levels ($p < 10^{-5}$ and $p = 0.03$, respectively).

Mobilization by rHuG-CSF in Cancer Patients Studies of mobilization of PBPC by rHuG-CSF in cancer patients have concentrated on patients with lymphoid malignancies or solid tumors. The work of Dührsen et al. (1988), which demonstrated striking increases in a variety of clonogenic hemopoietic progenitor cells on the fifth day of rHuG-CSF treatment, has been confirmed in subsequent studies. The kinetics of PBPC mobilization has a characteristic pattern of a wave reaching clinically useful levels on days 4 through 8 and peaking on day 5 or 6 (Fig. 9.3) (Dührsen et al. 1988; De Luca et al. 1992; Sheridan et al. 1992c) and follows a different kinetic profile compared with that of the neutrophilia induced by rHuG-CSF. The characteristic time

Table 9.3. Dose of G-CSF and Yield of Progenitor Cells in Normal Donors

Authors	n	Dose of G-CSF/Day & Schedule	Number of Apherses, median (range)	Yield of GM-CFC, 10^4/kg median (range) or mean $\pm$ SEM	Yield of CD34[+] Cells, 10^6/kg median (range) or mean $\pm$ SEM
Weaver et al. 1993	5	16 μg/kg	2[a]	113 (47–211)	9.6 (1.6–12.6)
Bensinger et al. 1995	8	16 μg/kg	2	ND	13.6 (6.9–21.6)
Dreger et al. 1994	3	5 μg/kg or 6 μg/kg $\times$ 5 days	1–3	13 (7–19)	3 (1.5–6.6)
	6	10 μg/kg $\times$ 5 days	1–3	41 (12–100)	6.6 (2.2–21.3)
Lane et al. 1995	8	10 μg/kg $\times$ 4 days	1	NR	119 $\pm$ 65[b]

[a]One of five donors had one apheresis.
[b]10^6 total CD34 cells, not per kilogram.
NR = not reported; SEM = standard error of the mean; ND = not determined.

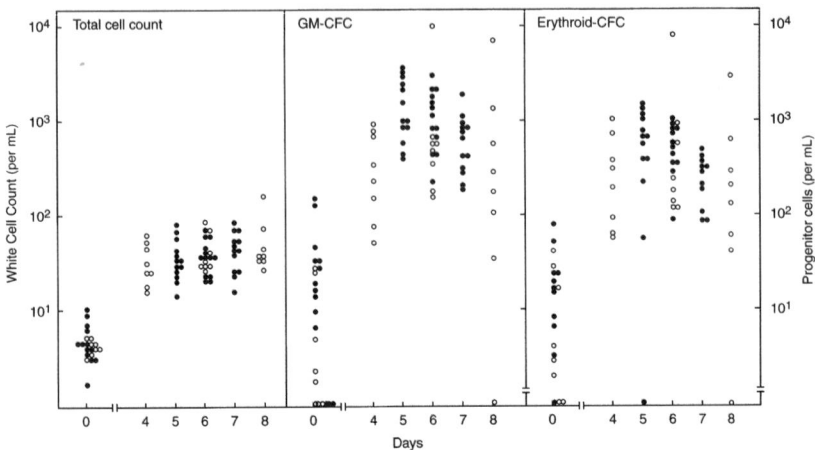

Figure 9.3 Total white cell counts and peripheral blood progenitor cell levels determined in 21 patients receiving 12 μg/kg/d SC infusion of rHuG-CSF. Each point represents mean values from replicate cultures stimulated with either rHuGM-CSF or rHuG-CSF. Blood and leukapheresis samples were obtained on days 0, 4, 6, and 8 (n = 8, *open symbols*) or days 0, 5, 6, and 7 (n = 13, *closed symbols*). (Used with permission, adapted from De Luca, E., Sheridan, W.P., Watson, D., Szer, J., and Begley, C.G. [1992] Prior chemotherapy does not prevent effective mobilisation by G-CSF of peripheral blood progenitor cells. *British Journal of Cancer*, **66**, 893–9.)

course of neutrophilic leukocytosis induced by rHuG-CSF is an acute but transient decrease due to margination followed by an increase to supra-normal levels within hours (Morstyn et al. 1988; Gabrilove et al. 1988b), due to release from the mature granulocyte pool in the marrow (Lord et al. 1989). The neutrophil level continues to increase for several days and then plateaus, remaining elevated due to new neutrophil generation from committed precursors, until rHuG-CSF treatment is ceased (Morstyn et al. 1988; Lord et al. 1989).

The observation of substantial interindividual variation in the peak levels of progenitor cells after rHuG-CSF treatment was first ascribed to the variation in the extent of prior treatment with radiation and chemotherapeutic agents, which damage marrow function and reduce the number of stem cells (Sheridan et al. 1992c). Subsequent studies have confirmed that marrow damage with radiation or chemotherapy significantly reduces PBPC yield after rHuG-CSF (p = 0.004 and p = 0.008, respectively; Bensinger et al. 1994). Of interest is the existence of a similar degree of variation in PBPC response to rHuG-

CSF in cancer patients before the use of radiation or chemotherapy (Basser et al. 1994) and in normal donors (Weaver et al. 1993; Bensinger et al. 1995; Chatta et al. 1994; Dreger et al. 1994; Tjonnfjord et al. 1994), which indicates that this range of response between individuals is a normal physiologic phenomenon. In contrast, data from limited numbers of patients given rHuG-CSF on more than one occasion, with no intervening chemotherapy, show that the response to rHuG-CSF within individual patients is highly reproducible (De Luca et al. 1992).

DOSE RESPONSE IN CANCER PATIENTS No formal randomized dose-response studies have so far been performed in cancer patients. The initial data suggested that although the activity of rHuG-CSF in increasing the levels of circulating progenitor cells was seen at doses as low as 0.3 μg/kg/d, consistently large fold increases were observed with doses of greater than or equal to 10 μg/kg/d (Dührsen et al. 1988). In sequential studies of lymphoma patients who were unsuitable for autologous BM harvest, Nadamanee et al. (1994) collected PBPC until a target of 10^9/kg MNC were obtained. Treatment with 10 μg/kg/d of rHuG-CSF resulted in higher yields of CD34$^+$ cells compared with treatment with 5 μg/kg/d (6.2 versus 3.4 $\times$ 10^6/kg, p = 0.04). In this report, the superiority of PBPC harvest after rHuG-CSF treatment compared with unmobilized harvests was confirmed (Table 9.4) with higher yields of CD34$^+$ cells obtained using fewer leukapheresis procedures (ten leukaphereses for no G-CSF versus seven for 5 μg/kg G-CSF versus six for 10 μg/kg G-CSF).

It is not yet clear whether substantial further increases are observed at doses higher than 10 to 12 μg/kg/d. Sheridan et al. (1992a) examined doses of 12 μg/kg/d (n = 30) and 24 μg/kg/d (n = 6) and although GM-CFC yields were higher in the group of patients treated with the higher dose (21 versus 47.5 $\times$ 10^4/kg; Tables 9.3 and 9.4), this difference was not statistically significant. The higher baseline levels of PB GM-CFC in the 24-μg/kg/d group (43 versus 25/mL) (Sheridan et al. 1992b) may indicate that apparently higher yields associated with the higher dose were, in fact, due to random physiologic differences. The mild to moderate bone pain reported as the most frequent adverse effect of rHuG-CSF is seen more frequently when rHuG-CSF is given during steady-state hemopoiesis compared with administration after high-dose chemotherapy in the same patients (22 of 29 versus 10 of 29; p = 0.03) (Sheridan et al. 1994), and the frequency of more severe bone pain may increase with higher doses of rHuG-CSF. An additional practical concern is that most physicians monitor the white cell count (WCC) and reduce the dose of rHuG-

Table 9.4. Dose of G-CSF and Yield of Progenitor Cells in Cancer Patients

Authors	n	Dose & Schedule of G-CSF, μg/kg/d	Number of Apherses, median (range)	Yield of GM-CFC, 10^4/kg, median (range) or mean ± SEM	Yield of CD34+ Cells, 10^6/kg median (range) or mean ± SEM
Sheridan et al. 1992c	17	12	3	33 ± 5.7	NR
Sheridan et al. 1992a	30[a]	12 SC × 7 days	3	21 (0.5–89)	NR
	6	24 SC × 7 days	3	48 (1.3–87)	NR
	6	12 SC × 7 days + 12 IV × 3 days	3	31 (9.6–105)	NR
Peters et al. 1993	14	6 IV × 8 days	3	12.9 ± 6	8.6 ± 1.7
Chao et al. 1993	32	None	9 (7–14)	4.4 (0–11)	NR
	20	10	4 (2–11)	9.4 (0–48)	NR
Bolwell et al. 1993	49	5	3	NR	187[b] (0–748)
Bensinger et al. 1993	12	16	NR (2–5)	20.5 (2.4–98)	8.6 (1.6–14.6)
Bensinger et al. 1994	54[c]	16	3 (2–6)	39.3 (1–178)	5.1 (0.1–33)
Nadamannee et al. 1994	30	None	10 (5–19)	NR	1.2 (0–41)
	26	5	7 (3–24)	NR	3.4 (0.5–15)
	39	10	6 (3–12)	NR	6.2 (1.9–31.7)
Faucher et al. 1994	16	10	3 (2–5)	25[d] (8.8–105)	5.8[d] (1.4–13.5)

[a]Series includes 14 patients reported in Sheridan et al. 1992c.
[b]Total, not per kilogram.
[c]Series includes 12 patients reported in Bensinger et al. 1993.
[d]Mean.
SEM = standard error of the mean; NR = not reported.

CSF if the WCC is greater than or equal to 75 to 100 × 10^9/L, and this is more likely to occur when higher doses are used. It is also difficult to draw conclusions from comparisons of mobilization results across studies when the clonogenic progenitor cell assays or flow cytometry assays for $CD34^+$ cells are performed in different laboratories using different methods. Until there is clear-cut evidence of a clinical advantage of using higher doses of rHuG-CSF, it seems reasonable to recommend a dose of approximately 10 μg/kg/d for mobilization of PBPC.

In Vitro Biological Characteristics of rHuG-CSF–Mobilized Peripheral Blood Cells

The variety of progenitor cells mobilized by rHuG-CSF includes G-, GM-, Eo-, MK-, and MIX-CFC (Dührsen et al. 1988; Sheridan et al. 1992c) and also more primitive cells capable of generating 14-day colonies in semisolid media after a preliminary 5-day liquid culture (De Luca et al. 1992). Studies of long-term culture-initiating cells (LTC-IC) have not been reported. Clinical transplantation studies leave little doubt, however, that adequate numbers of the most primitive HSC capable of supporting long-term hemopoiesis are also mobilized by rHuG-CSF (see below).

Circulating progenitor cells observed under unstimulated conditions differ from marrow progenitor cells in several characteristics. These include a higher proportion of day-14 CFC to day-5 CFC (Dührsen et al. 1988), a higher proportion of rhodamine 123^{low} staining cells, a lower proportion of $CD71^+$ cells (To et al. 1994), and a markedly lower proportion of S-phase cells (Roberts and Metcalf 1995). These differences compared with normal marrow progenitors persist or become more prominent after treatment with rHuG-CSF. There are a number of potential explanations for this: the mobilization phenomenon itself could favor the types of progenitor cells that normally circulate; rHuG-CSF may induce phenotypic changes in marrow progenitor cells associated with egress into the circulation; the loss of signals normally present in the marrow microenvironment may induce phenotypic changes; or the primary effect may be proliferation of the progenitor cell populations that normally circulate. The latter hypothesis is unlikely, as this would require mitogenic responsiveness to rHuG-CSF in a broad range of different hemopoietic cells, which has not been observed in vitro, and is inconsistent with the observation of very low proportion of S-phase PB progenitor cells after G-CSF therapy (Roberts and Metcalf 1995). It is not currently known whether the apparently more efficient mobilization of MK-CFC compared with other types of CFC observed in mice (Roberts and Metcalf 1994) is also the case in humans.

The proportions of different CD34$^+$ cell subsets present before and after rHuG-CSF treatment has been difficult to study because of inherent problems associated with rare-cell analysis by flow cytometry. This difficulty is not as acute in the situation of mobilization by chemotherapy and cytokines because when the peak mobilization response occurs, the WCC is still low in comparison with rHuG-CSF–only mobilization and the ratio of CD34$^+$ cells to CD34$^-$ cells is higher. The proportion of rHuG-CSF–mobilized CD34$^+$ PB cells that are also CD38$^+$ appears to be lower than in the BM, and c-*kit* expression is markedly lower (To et al. 1994). The proportion of CD34$^+$ cells expressing CD38 or HLA-DR is lower for rHuG-CSF–only mobilized cells compared with cells mobilized by chemotherapy alone (To et al. 1994) or chemotherapy and rHuG-CSF (To et al. 1994; Mohle et al. 1994); however, the number of these more primitive progenitors mobilized by the combination approach appears to be greater (Mohle et al. 1994). The clinical significance of these findings is unknown.

Therapeutic Use of rHuG-CSF–Mobilized Cells in Transplantation

Autologous Transplantation The cardinal clinical feature associated with transplantation of rHuG-CSF–mobilized PBPC is rapid hematologic recovery (Table 9.5, Fig. 9.4). This has been confirmed in numerous investigations (Sheridan et al. 1992c; Bensinger et al. 1993; Bolwell et al. 1993; Chao et al. 1993; Peters et al. 1993; Faucher et al. 1994; Nademanee et al. 1994; Sheridan et al. 1994). Recombinant HuG-CSF–mobilized PBPC were combined with standard autologous BM in the initial studies (Sheridan et al. 1992c; Bolwell et al. 1993; Peters et al. 1993), but subsequently the ability of mobilized PB cells to support hemopoietic recovery without BM was demonstrated (Bensinger et al. 1993; Chao et al. 1993; Faucher et al. 1994; Nademanee et al. 1994; Sheridan et al. 1994).

The pattern of hematologic recovery is biphasic in a proportion of patients, with an initial period of platelet production followed by a brief decline in platelet counts and spontaneous recovery (Sheridan et al. 1994). This kinetic pattern is also seen in chemotherapy-mobilized PBPC transplantation for acute myeloid leukemia (AML) (To et al. 1990) and may possibly be due to polyphasic hemopoiesis (Jones et al. 1989). Long-term hemopoiesis appears to be stable after rHuG-CSF–mobilized PBPC transplantation (Sheridan et al. 1994).

Table 9.5. Hematologic Recovery After High-Dose Chemotherapy and Autologous Transplantation of G-CSF–Mobilized PBPC Collected by Leukapheresis

Authors	n	Median (range) GM-CFC 10^4/kg	Median (range) CD34$^+$ 10^6/kg	Chemotherapy Regimen	ANC >0.5×10^9/L	ANC >1×10^9/L	PLT >20×10^9/L	PLT >50×10^9/L
						Median Days To:		
Sheridan et al. 1992	14	33 ± 5.7	NR	Bu/Cy[a]	9 (8–21)	NR	NR	15 (10–62)
Chao et al. 1993	20	9.4 (0–48)	NR	VP16/Cy/ ±BCNU±TBI	10 (7–14)	NR	13 (7–39)	NR
Bolwell et al. 1993	49	NR	187 (0–748)[b]	Various	10	NR	16	NR
Bensinger et al. 1993	12	20.5	8.6	By/Cy	13 (10–15)	14 (11–16)	10 (7–49)	NR
		2.4–98)	(1.6–14.6)					
Sheridan et al. 1994	29	21 (1–198)	NR	Bu/Cy	10 (8–13)	NR	11 (9–136)	15 (8–314)
Bensinger et al. 1994	54[c]	39.3 (1–178)	5.1 (0.1–33)	Various	12 (7–16)	12 (8–22)	10 (7–60)	NR
Ossenkoppele et al. 1994	6	4.5[d] (0.5–44.5)	NR	Mel 140 mg/m²	12 (10–35)	14 (12–55)	23 (15–115)	NR
Nademanee et al. 1994	26[e]	NR	3.4 (0.5–15)	VP16/Cy ±BCNU or FTBI	10 (9–15)	NR	17 (19–117)	NR
	39[f]	NR	6.2 (1.9–39.7)	VP16/Cy ±BCNU or FTBI	10 (7–40)	NR	15.5 (7–63)	NR
Faucher et al. 1994	16	25[g] (8.8–105)	5.8[g] (1.4–13.5)	BEAM or Cy/Mel/Mtox	10.5 (8–13)	NR	14.5 (10–26)	16.5 (12–35)

[a]Bu = busulphan; Cy = cyclophosphamide; VP16 = etoposide; BCNU = carmustine; TBI = total body irradiation; Mel = melphalan; FTBI = fractionated TBI; BEAM = BCNU, etoposide, cytosine arabinoside, and melphalan; Mtox = mitoxantrone; NR = not reported; ANC = absolute neutrophil count; PLT = platelets.
[b]Total, not per kilogram.
[c]Series includes patients reported in Bensinger et al. 1993.
[d]PBPC collection done by a single 1-L phlebotomy, not leukapheresis.
[e]Mobilized with 5 μg/kg/d.
[f]Mobilized with 10 μg/kg/d.
[g]Mean.

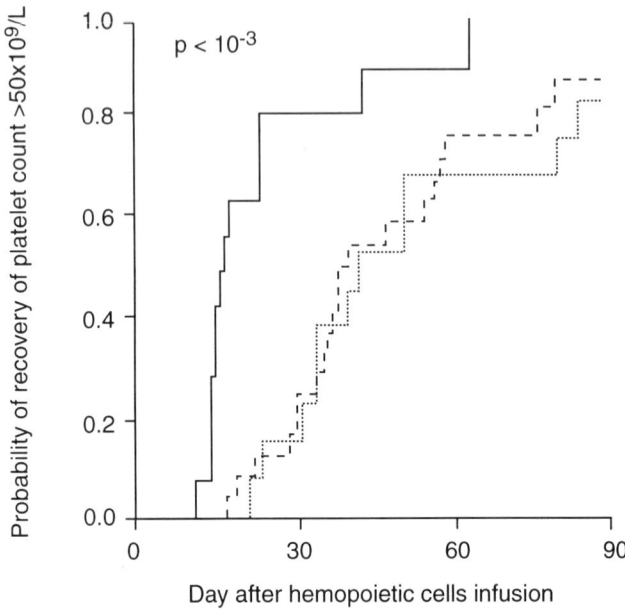

Figure 9.4 Probability of recovery of the platelet count to at least 50 × 10⁹/L after high-dose chemotherapy with busulfan and cyclophosphamide and infusion of autologous hemopoietic cells. Patients received either G-CSF-mobilized PBPC plus bone marrow and postinfusion G-CSF (*solid line, n = 14*), bone marrow and postinfusion G-CSF (*dashed line, n = 25*), or bone marrow without postinfusion G-CSF (*dotted line, n = 13*). (Adapted from Sheridan, W.P., Begley, C.G., Juttner, C.A., et al. [1992c] Effect of peripheral-blood progenitor cells mobilised by filgrastim [G-CSF] on platelet recovery after high-dose chemotherapy. *Lancet*, **339**, 640–4.)

The degree of clinical benefit associated with rHuG-CSF–mobilized PBPC has been estimated by comparisons with historical control patients receiving either standard autologous BM infusion (Sheridan et al. 1992c; Bensinger et al. 1993; Bolwell et al. 1993; Peters et al. 1993), unmobilized PBPC (Chao et al. 1993; Nademanee et al. 1994), or no hemopoietic cells (Ossenkoppele et al. 1994). In all of these historically controlled studies, neutrophil and platelet recovery was superior in the patients receiving rHuG-CSF–mobilized PBPC. This consistent observation has led to widespread adoption of PBPC mobilized by rHuG-CSF (with or without chemotherapy) for support of high-dose chemotherapy. A preliminary report of a randomized trial of rHuG-CSF–mobilized PBPC transplantation versus standard auto-logous BM transplantation was presented recently (Schmitz et al.

1994). The full report of this study is expected to formally confirm the degree of clinical benefit, including reduced duration of hospitalization, associated with rHuG-CSF–mobilized PBPC transplant (N. Schmitz, personal communication).

The rapid tempo of hematologic recovery after rHuG-CSF–mobilized PBPC infusion has been attributed to the large number of hemopoietic progenitor cells infused (Sheridan et al. 1992c). This hypothesis has been supported by the observation of more rapid hematologic recovery in patients receiving higher numbers of PBPC as measured by either GM-CFC ($\geq$30 $\times$ 10^4/kg versus <30 $\times$ 10^4/kg [Fig. 9.5]; Sheridan et al. 1994); or CD34$^+$ cells ($\geq$5 $\times$ 10^6/kg versus <5 $\times$ 10^6/kg [Fig. 9.6]; Bensinger et al. 1994).

The infusion of rHuG-CSF–mobilized PBPC has generally been followed by rHuG-CSF administration in order to accelerate neutrophil recovery (Sheridan et al. 1992c). Use of rHuG-CSF after autologous BM transplantation (BMT) markedly accelerates recovery of marrow neutrophil production (Sheridan et al. 1989; Taylor et al. 1989; Diaz Mediavilla et al. submitted; van der Wall et al. submitted; Schwartzberg data on file), but even in the presence of this powerful stimulus to neutrophil granulopoiesis, use of mobilized PBPC appears to convey additional benefit in further shortening the period of severe neutropenia (Sheridan et al. 1992c). Conversely, omission of rHuG-CSF after PBPC infusion significantly lengthens the period of severe neutropenia (Schwartzberg et al. 1994). This synergy between infusion of large numbers of progenitor cells and a specific lineage-restricted CSF suggests that the specific platelet-lineage factor MGDF (c-*mpl* ligand) (Bartley et al. 1994; De Sauvage et al. 1994; Kaushansky et al. 1994; Lok et al. 1994; Kato et al. in press) should also be tested after rHuG-CSF–mobilized PBPC infusion.

Syngeneic and Allogeneic Transplantation Although in animals it has been clear since 1990 that G-CSF is able to mobilize long-term repopulating cells (Molineux et al. 1990b), clinical use of PBPC mobilized by rHuG-CSF for allogeneic transplantation has been limited. The first published reports were of individual cases (Dreger et al. 1993; Russell et al. 1993; Arseniev 1994), but recently reports of small series of identical-twin transplants (Weaver et al. 1993) and allogeneic transplants (Bensinger et al. 1995; Schmitz et al. 1995) have appeared. The delay in initiation of transplant studies utilizing rHuG-CSF–mobilized PBPC from normal donors was due to a combination of reluctance to administer a hemopoietic cytokine to normal individuals and the unsatisfactory results of limited animal (Storb et al. 1967) and human (Anasetti et al. 1988) studies of unmobilized allogeneic leu-

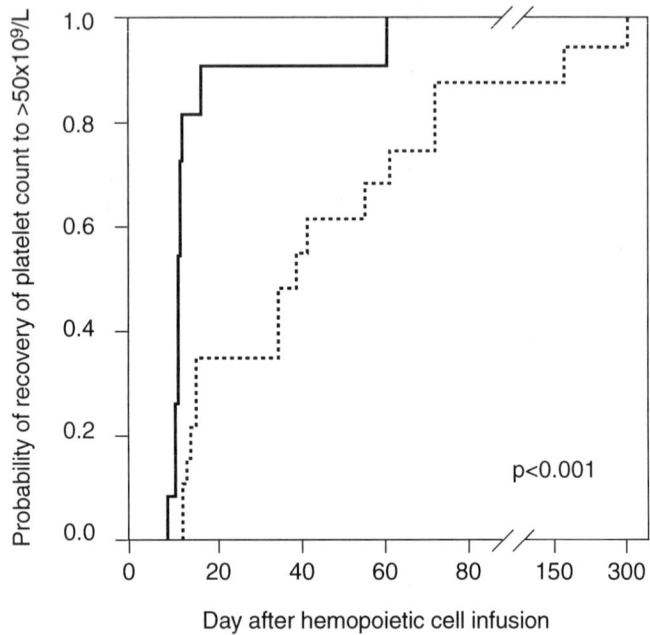

Figure 9.5 Probability of recovery of the platelet count to at least 50 x 10⁹/L after high-dose busulfan and cyclophosphamide and infusion of autologous hemopoietic cells. *Solid line*, 11 patients with PB GM-CFC harvest ≥30 x 10⁴/kg (who received rHuG-CSF mobilized PBPC only); *dashed line*, 18 patients with PB GM-CFC harvest <30 x 10⁴/kg (who received both rHuG-CSF–mobilized PBPC and bone marrow). (Adapted from Sheridan, W.P., Begley, G.C., To, L.B., et al. [1994] Phase II study of autologous filgrastim [G-CSF] -mobilized peripheral blood progenitor cells to restore hemopoiesis after high dose chemotherapy for lymphoid malignancies. *Bone Marrow Transplantation*, **14**, 105–11.)

kocyte transplants. These studies showed an apparent high frequency of severe acute graft-versus-host disease (GVHD), but used prophylactic regimens for GVHD that are now superseded (single-agent methotrexate). Recent human studies (Bensinger et al. 1995; Schmitz et al. 1995) of rHuG-CSF–mobilized allogeneic PBPC transplants have used one of the current standards for GVHD prophylaxis: cyclosporine plus short-course methotrexate (Storb et al. 1989) or cyclosporine plus corticosteroids, and the incidence of severe acute GVHD has not been alarming. Follow-up has so far been short, so there is no information available on the incidence of chronic GVHD.

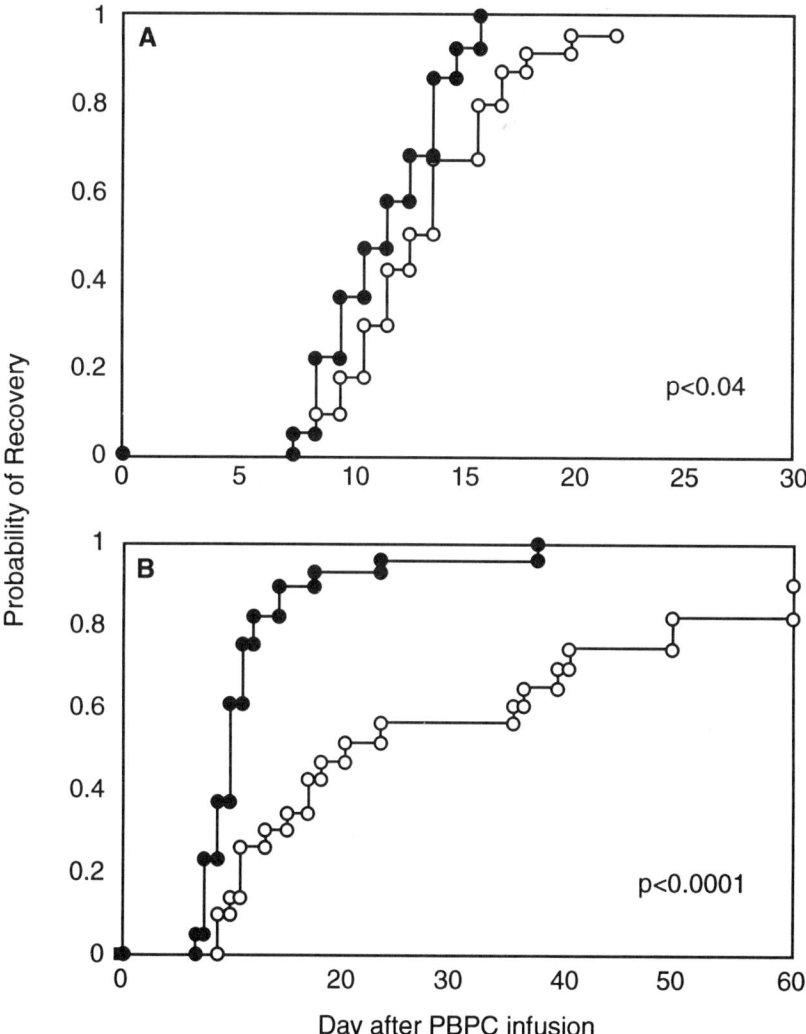

Figure 9.6 Recovery of granulocytes (*upper panel*) and platelets (*lower panel*) in 54 patients receiving G-CSF mobilized PBPC after high-dose chemotherapy. *Closed circles*, CD34$^+$ cell harvest >5.0 × 10^6/kg; *open circles*, CD34$^+$ cell harvest <5.0 × 10^6/kg. (Adapted from Bensinger, W.I., Longin, K., Appelbaum, F., et al. [1994] Peripheral blood stem cells [PBSCs] collected after recombinant granulocyte colony stimulating factor [rhG-CSF]: an analysis of factors correlating with the tempo of engraftment after transplantation. *British Journal of Haematology*, **87**, 825–31.)

Although the pathophysiology of acute GVHD clearly involves donor T-cell proliferation, as evidenced by the results of prophylaxis with either T-cell depletion of the graft or conventional immunosuppression (Chapter 24), it does not necessarily follow that infusion of larger than normal T-cell numbers will increase the incidence of GVHD (Schmitz et al. 1995). There may in fact be advantages in providing tenfold more T cells and natural killer (NK) cells, such as faster reconstitution of cell-mediated immunity and a more potent graft-versus-leukemia (GVL) effect. There is a clear need for properly designed clinical trials of adequate size to address the potential risks and benefits of rHuG-CSF–mobilized allogeneic PBPC transplantation; the European Group for Blood and Marrow Transplantation (EBMT) has recently commenced a randomized study of allogeneic PBPC transplant versus BMT in patients with good-risk leukemia.

■ GRANULOCYTE-MACROPHAGE COLONY-STIMULATING FACTOR

Recombinant HuGM-CSF has a broader range of activity on hemopoietic cells both in vitro and in vivo (Tables 9.1 and 9.2) (Lieschke and Burgess 1992a, b) compared with rHuG-CSF. As with rHuG-CSF, the effect of rHuGM-CSF on mobilization of marrow progenitor cells to the PB was identified in early phase I and phase II studies in cancer patients (Socinski et al. 1988; Villeval et al. 1990) and was later also seen in studies in normal volunteers (Lane et al. 1995). Further clinical investigation of rHuGM-CSF as a mobilizing agent has predominantly been in the setting of rHuGM-CSF administration after chemotherapy (Chapter 8).

Socinski et al. (1988) studied doses of 4 μg/kg/d up to 64 μg/kg/d given by continuous intravenous (IV) infusion for up to 7 days in a group of 12 patients with sarcoma. PB levels of GM-CFC increased a median 18-fold from a baseline of 36 ± 15/mL to 469 ± 144/mL, with 9 of 12 patients showing statistically significant increases. E-BFC levels also increased, from 68 ± 40/mL to 242 ± 103/mL. A dose-response relationship was not apparent in this study. In another study 37 patients were treated with 0.3 μg/kg/d up to 30 μg/kg/d SC or 0.3 to 20 μg/kg/d IV short infusion, for up to 10 days (Villeval et al. 1990). The level of blood GM-CFC was significantly elevated after 4 to 5 days of treatment with rHuGM-CSF, and there was a clear effect of higher doses (Fig. 9.7). The highest increase observed was 50-fold in a patient treated with 20 μg/kg/d. Various subtypes of hemopoietic progenitor cells were evaluated and elevations of G-, GM-, M-, Eo-, E-, Mix-, and MK-CFC were detected. The magnitude of the rise in MK-CFC was about half that for the day-14 GM-CFC.

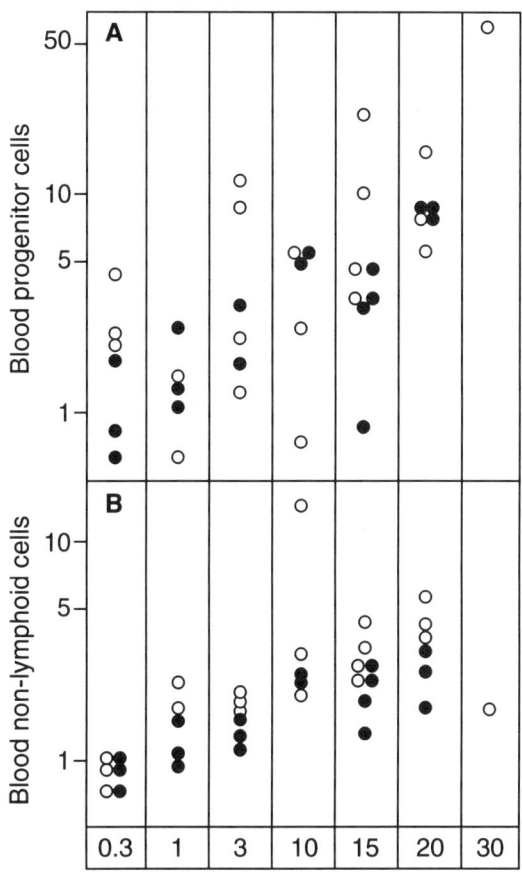

Dose of GM-CSF, µg/kg/d

Figure 9.7 Increases over baseline in peripheral blood clonogenic progenitor cells (*A*) and mature nonlymphoid cells (*B*) in 37 patients treated with rHuGM-CSF. *Open symbols*, subcutaneous injection; *closed symbols*, intravenous short infusion. (Adapted from Villeval, J.-L., Dührsen, U., Morstyn, G., and Metcalf, D. [1990] Effect of recombinant human granulocyte-macrophage colony stimulating factor on progenitor cells in patients with advanced malignancies. *British Journal of Haematology*, **74**, 36–44.)

There have been several clinical reports of mobilization and harvest of PBPC using GM-CSF alone (Table 9.6) and the use of these cells for transplantation after high-dose chemotherapy (Table 9.7) (Haas et al. 1990; Kritz et al. 1993; Peters et al. 1993; Bishop et al. 1994). A dose of 250 $\mu g/m^2/d$ of GM-CSF appears to be superior to 125 $\mu g/m^2/d$ in non-Hodgkin's lymphoma (NHL) or Hodgkin's disease (HD) patients unsuitable for marrow harvest, but the median number of leukaphereses required remains large (Bishop et al. 1994).

Although these studies confirm the feasibility of using GM-CSF in PBPC mobilization, the results generally seem to be no better than or inferior to those obtained with rHuG-CSF, for measures of both mobilization efficiency (e.g., yield of harvested GM-CFC or CD34$^+$ cells) and hemopoietic recovery after transplantation. In addition, rHuGM-CSF administration is associated with a broader range of side effects compared with rHuG-CSF, including a first-dose effect, fever, skin reactions, serositis, and musculoskeletal pain (Lieschke et al. 1989, 1990; Lieschke and Burgess 1992a, b). These effects are most likely due to stimulation of monocytes and macrophages with secondary cytokine release. One further problem that may be seen with rHuGM-CSF is an increased incidence of catheter thrombosis during PBPC collection (Stephens et al. 1993). In this study rHuGM-CSF was given by continuous IV infusion (250 $\mu g/m^2/d$) through the apheresis catheter and 20 of 37 catheters had thrombotic occlusions versus 1 of 29 catheters of patients undergoing unmobilized PBPC collection ($p < 0.0001$).

Although no randomized comparisons of rHuG-CSF versus r-HuGM-CSF have been reported, the available data would appear to indicate that rHuG-CSF is superior to rHuGM-CSF for cytokine-only mobilization (Peters et al. 1993; Lane et al. 1995).

■ STEM CELL FACTOR

One of the outstanding biologic properties of SCF (c-*kit* ligand) is amplification of the effects of a wide range of hemopoietic growth factors. In addition, SCF is necessary for the migration and survival of germ cells and melanoblasts in the developing embryo and is the most important CSF for the mast-cell lineage (reviewed in Galli, Zsebo, and Geissler 1994).

The effects of SCF on mobilization of hemopoietic stem and progenitor cells have been studied in mice, dogs, and baboons, and in clinical studies. Although SCF is capable of mobilizing repopulating cells and more mature progenitor cells when used as a single agent

Table 9.6. Dose of GM-CSF and Yield of Progenitor Cells in Cancer Patients

Authors	n	Dose of GM-CSF/Day & Schedule	Number of Apherses, median (range)	Yield of GM-CFC, 10^4/kg median (range) or mean ± SEM	Yield of CD34$^+$ Cells, 10^6/kg median (range) or mean ± SEM
Haas et al. 1990	10	250 μg/m^2	6 (3–9)	30 (10–169)[a]	NR
Kritz et al. 1993	13	10 μg/kg × 11 days	4	NR	NR
Peters et al. 1993	17	8 μg/kg IV × 8 days	3	12.5 ± 5.7[b]	1.6 ± 0.5[b]
	8	16 μg/kg IV × 8 days	3	6 ± 1.6[b]	5.4 ± 1.5[b]
	7	16 μg/kg IV × 4 days	3	2.1 ± 0.5[b]	0.5 ± 1[b]
Bishop et al. 1994	86	None	9 (6–18)	0.7 (0.04–30)	NR
	34	125 μg/m^2	7 (6–17)	3.6 (0.7–58)	NR
	24	250 μg/m^2	7 (6–15)	8.8 (0.6–104)	NR

[a]Per apheresis, not per kilogram.
[b]Mean (± SEM).
SEM = standard error of the mean; NR = not reported.

Table 9.7. Hematologic Recovery After High-Dose Chemotherapy and Autologous Transplantation of GM-CSF-Mobilized PBPC Collected by Leukapheresis

Authors	n	Median (range) GM-CFC Infused 10^4/kg	Median (range) CD34$^+$ Infused 10^6/kg	Chemotherapy Regimen	Median Days To:			
					ANC >0.5×10^9/L	ANC >1×10^9/L	PLT >20×10^9/L	PLT >50×10^9/L
Haas et al. 1990	6	30.1[a] (10–169)	NR	Cy/TBI[b] or CBV	28 (14–42)	NR	39 (18–49)	NR
Kritz et al. 1993	13	NR	NR	CEP	15 (11–24)	NR	14 (11–34)	17 (12–37)
Bishop et al. 1994	34[c]	3.6 (0.7–58)	NR	Various CBV	23 (12–49)	NR	24 (7–102)	NR
	24[d]	8.8 (0.6–104)	NR	programs	18 (10–46)	NR	15 (8–41)	NR

[a]Total collected, not per kilogram.
[b]Cy/TBI = cyclophosphamide, total body irradiation; CBV = cyclophosphamide, lomustine, etoposide; CEP = cyclophosphamide, etoposide, cisplatin; NR = not reported; ANC = absolute neutrophil count; PLT = platelet.
[c]Mobilized by 125 μg/m^2/d.
[d]Mobilized by 250 μg/m^2/d.

(Briddell et al. 1993; Andrews et al. 1992), the doses required are large. In early clinical trials, the dose of SCF that could be safely administered was limited by mast-cell–mediated adverse effects (Crawford et al. 1993; Demetri et al. 1993), so further clinical studies of SCF for PBPC mobilization have used low doses of SCF (together with prophylactic antihistamines) plus rHuG-CSF. This combination has been further explored in animal models.

In mice, there were greater than additive increases in circulating low-density mononuclear cells (LDMNC), GM-CFC, and high-proliferative-potential colony–forming cells (HPP-CFC) when the combination of recombinant rat SCF (rrSCF) and rHuG-CSF were used compared with rrSCF or rHuG-CSF alone (Briddell et al. 1993; McNiece et al. 1994; Yan et al. 1994). The combination of rcSCF and rcG-CSF dramatically increases the PB levels of GM-CFC in dogs (de Revel et al. 1994). PB MNC mobilized by either rHuG-CSF or SCF plus rHuG-CSF were able to rescue lethally irradiated dogs while an equal number of PB MNC from animals not given CSF were not. Low doses of SCF, which cause no change in the WCC when administered alone to baboons, were found to significantly increase the PB levels of hemopoietic progenitor cells of multiple lineages, including MK-CFC, when given with rHuG-CSF (Andrews et al. 1994). Cells collected after combination treatment engraft more rapidly in irradiated baboons than cells collected after G-CSF alone (Andrews et al. 1995).

Clinical studies of the effects of rHuSCF plus rHuG-CSF on the mobilization of PBPC are in progress (Basser et al. 1994; Glaspy et al. 1994; Moskowitz et al. 1994). In breast cancer patients receiving rHuG-CSF (10 μg/kg/d) or rHuG-CSF plus SCF (5 to 20 μg/kg/d), there were three- to fourfold greater numbers of harvested GM-CFC and E-BFC with the combination of rHuG-CSF plus 10 or more μg/kg/d rHuSCF (Briddell et al. 1994) compared with rHuG-CSF alone. These patients also had threefold greater mobilization of CD34[+] cells and increases in MK-CFC and MK-BFC in comparison to patients receiving filgrastim alone.

■ OTHER HEMOPOIETIC GROWTH FACTORS

Several other hemopoietic growth factors are known to mobilize BM progenitor cells in vivo, including erythropoietin (EPO) (Stockenhuber et al. 1990; Pettengell et al. 1994), M-CSF (Eto et al. 1994), IL-1α (Fibbe et al. 1992), IL-1β (Gasparetto et al. 1994), and IL-3 (Geissler et al. 1990; Ottmann et al. 1992). Clinical evaluation of the mobilization efficacy for most of these cytokines has been limited. IL-3 has been studied alone (Ottmann et al. 1992) and in combination with or prior to GM-CSF (To et al. 1993), and to date the available data do not indicate a significant advantage over rHuG-CSF. The extent of mobilization by EPO (Stokenhuber et al. 1990; Pettengell et al. 1994), M-CSF (in combination with chemotherapy) (Eto et al. 1994), or IL-3 (Geissler et al. 1990; Ottmann et al. 1992) is weak in comparison with rHuG-CSF. IL-1 suffers from the disadvantage of causing a wide range of adverse clinical side effects including local reactions, fever, chills, rigors, hypotension, headache, hallucinations, abdominal pain, and dyspnea (Furman et al. 1994; Wilson et al. 1993), which will probably limit its clinical use. Of interest is the apparently very different kinetic pattern of mobilization with IL-1 compared with that seen with rHuG-CSF or rHuGM-CSF. After administration of a single dose of IL-1, the increase of progenitor cell levels in the blood peaks within hours (Fibbe et al. 1992), an acute response similar in timing to the systemic effects of IL-1. The activity of the newly described c-*mpl* ligand (Bartley et al. 1994; De Sauvage et al. 1994; Kaushansky et al. 1994; Lok et al. 1994; Kato et al. in press) in progenitor cell mobilization has not been reported.

■ MECHANISMS OF PERIPHERAL PROGENITOR CELL MOBILIZATION BY CYTOKINES

The mechanisms involved in hemopoietic stem and progenitor cell migration, homing, and mobilization are poorly understood and are likely to be complex (reviewed in Liesveld, DiPersio, and Abboud 1994; Turner 1994). Both the CD34 sialomucin (Baumheuter et al. 1993) and c-*kit* (Kodama et al. 1994) could participate in these related processes by functioning as receptors on the plasma membrane of hemopoietic cells for L-selectin and SCF expressed on endothelial and stromal cells, respectively. CD34$^+$ cells may also express an additional ligand for L-selectin other than CD34 (Oxley and Sackstein 1994). Primitive CD34$^+$ cells also express a variety of recognized adhesion receptors such as CD18, CD11a, CD49b, CD44, ICAM-1, and ICAM-3 (reviewed in Liesveld et al. 1994). BM microvessels and cultured endothelial cell monolayers (BMEC) express CD34, PECAM, and thrombospondin, and incubation of BMEC with marrow mononuclear cells results in selective adhesion of CD34$^+$ cells and megakaryocytes. The CD34 molecule may also function as a switch for up-regulating adhesion in some hemopoietic cells, such as the KG-1a cell line (Majdic et al. 1994).

Several lines of evidence suggest that the interaction of membrane-bound SCF and its receptor, c-*kit*, may function as part of the repertoire of cell-adhesion interactions between hemopoietic progenitor cells and BM microenvironmental cells. Mobilization of progenitor cells by rHuG-CSF in SCF- or c-*kit*–deficient mice is less efficient than in wild-type mice (Cynshi et al. 1991). G-CSF–mobilized CD34$^+$ cells have lower expression of c-*kit* compared with BM CD34$^+$ cells, indicating that c-*kit* is down-modulated during PBPC mobilization (To et al. 1994). In addition, there is experimental evidence for SCF/c-*kit*– mediated cell adhesion in the case of both mast cell lines (Kinashi and Springer 1994) and the hemopoietic cell line MO7E. Interestingly, in the case of M07E cells, modulation of the avidity of cell surface integrins appears to be biphasic (Kovach et al. 1995). Finally, adhesion of normal murine stem cells to stromal cells is inhibited by anti–c-*kit* antibodies (Ab) (Kodama et al. 1994).

A more thorough understanding of these processes could lead to improvements in clinical PBPC mobilization and transplantation and could also be important for optimizing ex vivo applications of mobilized cells.

■ OPTIMIZATION OF CYTOKINE-ONLY MOBILIZATION

Mobilization of PBPC by rHuG-CSF, and to a lesser extent rHuGM-CSF, has been rapidly adopted into the clinical practice of high-dose chemotherapy for malignancy, and the success of CSF mobilization has been a key factor in the growth of PBPC transplantation (Eaves 1993; Gale et al. 1994). Attempts at improving and extending the utility of PBPC mobilization with cytokines have examined alterations of leukapheresis technique, combinations of cytokines (Glaspy et al. 1994), use of higher doses of rHuG-CSF (Sheridan et al. 1992a; Bensinger et al. 1994; Zeller et al. 1994), combination with cytotoxic chemotherapy (Chapter 8), chemical or immunologic removal of contaminating tumor cells (Chapter 15), and positive selection of CD34$^+$ cells (Chapters 11 and 12).

Most of the published data on chemotherapy-plus-cytokine PBPC mobilization suggest that use of either rHuG-CSF or rHuGM-CSF increases the levels of PB progenitors over that seen with chemotherapy alone. There have been few published studies that address the reverse question of whether addition of chemotherapy increases PBPC levels compared with use of cytokines alone. Recently, Mohle et al. (1994) reported the results of mobilization first by rHuG-CSF alone then by rHuG-CSF following chemotherapy (ifosfamide 5 gm/m^2 plus epirubicin 100 mg/m^2) in seven patients with myeloma; the median PB CD34$^+$ cell levels were higher in the combination group (Fig. 9.8). Chemotherapy-based approaches to PBPC mobilization are not appli-

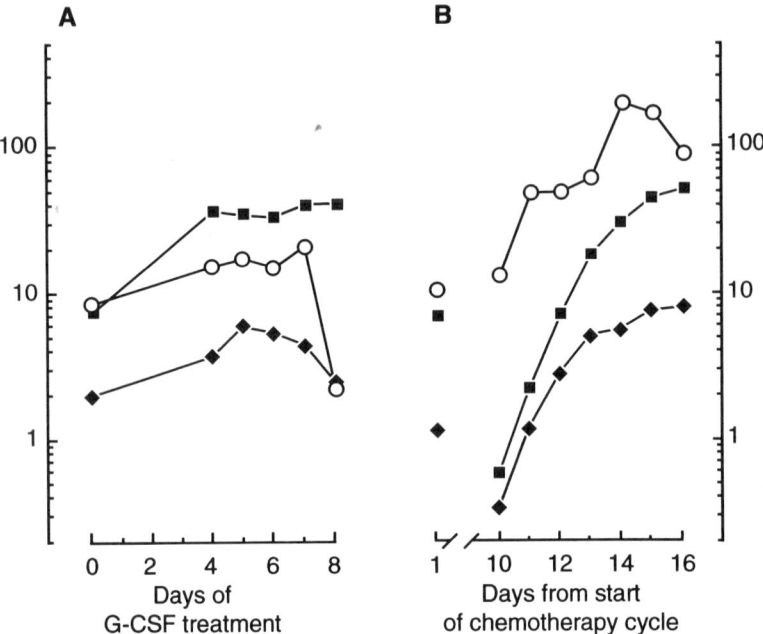

Figure 9.8 Mean levels of peripheral blood CD34$^+$ cells/μL (*open circles*), WBC (10^9/L) (*squares*), and mononuclear cells (10^9/L) (*diamonds*) in seven patients treated first with rHuG-CSF alone (*A*) and then with rHuG-CSF following chemotherapy with ifosfamide and epirubicin given on days 1 to 3 (*B*). (Adapted from Mohle, R., Pforisch, M., Fruehauf, S., Witt, B., Kramer, A., and Haas, R. [1994] Filgrastim post-chemotherapy mobilizes more CD34$^+$ cells with a different antigenic profile compared with use during steady-state hemopoiesis. *Bone Marrow Transplantation*, **14**, 827–32.)

cable in the allograft setting. A comparison of the differences between various sources of hemopoietic cells is given in Table 9.8. Some of the clinical variables that might influence the choice of mobilizing tool are tumor type, remission status, and timing of PBPC collection in relation to the course of the underlying disease.

The most immediately useful improvements in the clinical practice of cytokine-mobilized PBPC transplantation would be in the fields of rare-event flow cytometry for CD34$^+$ cells and CD34$^+$ subsets; predictive modeling of PBPC mobilization and hematologic recovery; and development of sensitive and reproducible techniques for measurement of tumor-cell contamination. Each of these areas is also im-

Table 9.8. Comparison of Various Sources of Hemopoietic Progenitor Cells for Clinical Use

	Bone Marrow	Unmobilized Peripheral Blood	Cytokine-Mobilized Peripheral Blood	Chemotherapy plus Cytokine-Mobilized Peripheral Blood	Umbilical Cord Blood
Relative number of progenitor cells in harvests	++	+	++++	+++++	++
Collection by venesection feasible	No	No	Yes	Probably	Yes
Collection by leukapheresis	No	Yes	Yes	Yes	No
Utility for autologous transplants	High	Low	High	High	Unknown
Utility for allogeneic transplants	High	Low	High	None	High
Utility for multiple-harvest protocols	None	None	High	Moderate	None
Rapid hematologic recovery after high-dose chemotherapy	No	No	Yes	Yes	No

portant in the emerging techniques involving selection and manipulation of CD34$^+$ cells such as ex vivo expansion of hemopoietic progenitors (Chapter 13) and gene therapy (Chapters 6 and 21).

■ CONCLUSIONS

The introduction of the colony stimulating factors into the clinical practice of hematology and oncology is in the process of transforming the field. The recognition of the mobilization effect and its utility for supportive care of patients receiving high-dose chemotherapy procedures has accelerated testing of the dose-response hypothesis in medical oncology, and it appears that PBPC mobilization will remain a useful tool in all clinical applications for which large numbers of hemopoietic stem and progenitor cells are required.

ACKNOWLEDGMENTS

My thanks to R. M. Fox, G. Morstyn, C. G. Begley, and C. Juttner for their advice and collaboration in clinical studies in the PBPC field.

REFERENCES

Anasetti, C., Storb, R., Longton, G., et al. (1988) Donor buffy coat cell infusion after marrow transplantation for aplastic anemia. *Blood*, **72**, 1099–100.

Andrews, R.G., Bensinger, W.I., Knitter, G.H., et al. (1992) The ligand for c-kit, stem cell factor, stimulates the circulation of cells that engraft lethally irradiated baboons. *Blood*, **80**, 2715–20.

Andrews, R.G., Briddell, R.A., Knitter, G.H., et al. (1994) In vivo synergy between recombinant human stem cell factor and recombinant human granulocyte colony-stimulating factor in baboons: enhanced circulation of progenitor cells. *Blood*, **84**, 800–10.

Andrews, R.G., Briddell, R.A., Knitter, G.H., Rowley, S.D., Appelbaum, F.R., and McNiece, I.K. (1995) Rapid engraftment by peripheral blood progenitor cells mobilized by recombinant human stem cell factor and recombinant human granulocyte colony-stimulating factor in nonhuman primates. *Blood*, **85**, 15–20.

Arseniev, L., Tischler, H.J., Battmer, K., Suedmeier, I., Casper, J., and Link, H. (1994) Treatment of poor marrow graft function with allogeneic CD34$^+$ cells immunoselected from G-CSF-mobilized peripheral blood progenitor cells of the marrow donor. *Bone Marrow Transplantation*, **14**, 791–7.

Bartley, T.D., Bogenberger, J., Hunt, P., et al. (1994) Identification and cloning of a megakaryocyte growth and development factor that is a ligand for the cytokine receptor Mpl. *Cell*, **77**, 1117–24.

Basser, R., Begley, G.C., Maher, D., et al. (1994) The use of peripheral blood progenitor cells (PBPC) mobilized by stem cell factor (SCF) and filgrastim (G-CSF) to support multiple cycles of high-dose chemotherapy in untreated women with poor prognosis breast cancer. *British Journal of Haematology*, **87**, 91a.

Baumheuter, S., Singer, M.S., Henzel, W., et al. (1993) Binding of L-selectin to the vascular sialomucin CD. *Science*, **262**, 327–67.

Bensinger, W., Singer, J., Appelbaum, F., et al. (1993) Autologous transplantation with peripheral blood mononuclear cells collected after administration of recombinant granulocyte stimulating factor. *Blood*, **81**, 3158–63.

Bensinger, W.I., Longin, K., Appelbaum, F., et al. (1994) Peripheral blood stem cells (PBSCs) collected after recombinant granulocyte colony stimulating factor (rhG-CSF): an analysis of factors correlating with the tempo of engraftment after transplantation. *Britsh Journal of Haematology*, **87**, 825–31.

Bensinger, W.I., Weaver, C.H., Appelbaum, F.R., et al. (1995) Transplantation of allogeneic peripheral blood stem cells mobilized by recombinant human granulocyte colony-stimulating factor (rh-G-CSF). *Blood*, **85**, 1655–8.

Bishop, M.R., Anderson, J.R., Jackson, J.D., et al. (1994) High-dose therapy and peripheral blood progenitor cell transplantation: effects of recombinant human granulocyte-macrophage colony-stimulating factor on the autograft. *Blood*, **83**, 610–6.

Bolwell, B.J., Fishleder, A., Andresen, S.W., et al. (1993) G-CSF primed peripheral blood progenitor cells in autologous bone marrow transplantation: parameters affecting bone marrow engraftment. *Bone Marrow Transplantation*, **12**, 609–14.

Briddell, R.A., Hartley, C.A., Smith, K.A., and McNiece, I.K. (1993) Recombinant rat stem cell factor synergizes with recombinant human granulocyte colony-stimulating factor in vivo in mice to mobilize peripheral blood progenitor cells that have enhanced repopulating potential. *Blood*, **82**, 1720–3.

Briddell, R., Glaspy, J., Shpall, E.J., LeMaistre, F., Menchaca, D., and McNiece, I. (1994) Recombinant human stem cell factor (rhSCF) and filgrastim (rhG-CSF) synergize to mobilize myeloid, erythroid and megakaryocyte progenitors in patients with breast cancer. *British Journal of Haematology*, **87**, 92a.

Bronchud, M.H., Potter, M.R., Morgenstern, G., et al. (1988) In vitro and in vivo analysis of the effects of recombinant human granulocyte colony-stimulating factor in patients. *British Journal of Cancer*, **58**, 64–9.

Bungart, B., Loeffler, M., Goris, H., Dontje, B., and Nijhof, W. (1990) Differential effects of recombinant human colony stimulating factor (rhG-CSf) on stem cells in marrow, spleen, and peripheral blood in mice. *Bone Marrow Transplantation*, **76**, 174–9.

Cavins, J.A., Scheer, S.C., Thomas, E.D., and Ferrebee, J.W. (1964) The recovery of lethally irradiated dogs given infusions of autologous leukocytes preserved at −80°C. *Blood*, **23**, 38–43.

Chao, N.J., Schriber, J.R., Grimes, K., et al. (1993) Granulocyte colony-stimulating factor "mobilized" peripheral blood progenitor cells accelerate granulocyte and platelet recovery after high-dose chemotherapy. *Blood*, **81**, 2031–5.

Chatta, G.S., Price, T.H., Allen, R.C., and Dale, D. C. (1994) Effects of in vivo recombinant methionyl human granulocyte colony-stimulating factor on the neutrophil response and peripheral blood colony-forming cells in healthy young and elderly adult volunteers. *Blood*, **84**, 2923–9.

Crawford, J., Lau, D., Erwin, R., Rich, W., McGuire, B., and Meyers, F. (1993) A phase I trial of recombinant methionyl human stem cell factor (SCF) in patients with advanced non-small cell lung carcinoma (NSCLC). *Proceedings of the American Society of Clinical Oncology*, **12**, 135a.

Cynshi, O., Satoh, K., Shimonaka, Y., et al. (1991) Reduced response to granulocyte colony-stimulating factor in W/W^v and Sl/Sl^d mice. *Leukemia*, **5**, 75–7.

De Luca, E., Sheridan, W.P., Watson, D., Szer, J., and Begley, C.G. (1992) Prior chemotherapy does not prevent effective mobilisation by G-CSF of peripheral blood progenitor cells. *British Journal of Cancer*, **66**, 893–9.

de Revel, T., Appelbaum, F.R., Storb, R., et al. (1994) Effects of granulocyte colony-stimulating factor and stem cell factor, alone and in combination, on the mobilization of peripheral blood cells that engraft lethally irradiated dogs. *Blood*, **83**, 3795–9.

Demetri, G., Costa, J., Hayes, D., et al. (1993) A phase I trial of recombinant human methionyl human stem cell factor (SCF) in patients with advanced breast carcinoma pre- and post-chemotherapy (chemo) with cyclophosphamide (C) and doxorubicin (A). *Proceedings of the American Society of Clinical Oncology*, **12**, 142a.

De Sauvage, F.J., Hass, P.E., Spencer, S.D., et al. (1994) Stimulation of megakaryocytopoiesis and thrombopoiesis by the c-Mpl ligand. *Nature*, **369**, 533–8.

Dreger, P., Suttorp, M., Haferlach, T., Loffler, H., Schmitz, N., and Schroyens, W. (1993) Allogeneic granulocyte colony-stimualting factor-mobilized peripheral blood progenitor cells for treatment of engraftment failure after bone marrow transplantation. *Blood*, **81**, 1404–7.

Dreger, P., Haferlach, T., Eckstein, V., et al. (1994) G-CSF-mobilized peripheral blood progenitor cells for allogeneic transplantation: safety, kinetics of mobilization, and composition of the graft. *British Journal of Haematology*, **87**, 609–13.

Dührsen, U., Villeval, J.L., Boyd, J., Kannourakis, G., Morstyn, G., and Metcalf, D. (1988) Effects of recombinant granulocyte colony-stimulating factor on hemopoietic progenitor cells in cancer patients. *Blood*, **72**, 2074–81.

Eaves, C.J. (1993) Peripheral blood stem cells reach new heights. *Blood*, **82**, 1957–9.

Eto, T., Takamatsu, Y., Harada, M., et al. (1994) Effects of macrophage colony-stimulating factor (M-CSF) on the mobilization of peripheral blood stem cells. *Bone Marrow Transplantation*, **13**, 125–9.

Faucher, C., Le Corroller, A.G., Blaise, D., et al. (1994) Comparison of G-CSF-primed peripheral blood progenitor cells and bone marrow auto transplantation: clinical assessment and cost-effectiveness. *Bone Marrow Transplantation*, **14**, 895–901.

Fibbe, W.E., Hamilton, M.S., Laterveer, L.L., et al. (1992) Sustained engraftment of mice transplanted with IL-1-primed blood-derived stem cells. *Journal of Immunology*, **148**, 417–21.

Fritsch, G., Fischmeister, G., Haas, O.A., et al. (1994) Peripheral blood hemopoietic progenitor cells of cytokine-stimulated healthy donors as an alternative for allogeneic transplantation. *Blood*, **83**, 3420–1.

Furman, W., Fairclough, D., Garrison, L., et al. (1994) A phase I/II trial of subcutaneous (SC) interleukin-1α (rhuIL-1α) administered pre-chemotherapy in pediatric patients with malignant solid tumors. *Proceedings of the American Society of Clinical Oncology*, **12**, 410a.

Gabrilove, J.L., Jakubowski, A., Fain, K., et al. (1988a) Phase I study of granulocyte colony-stimulating factor in patients with transitional cell carcinoma of the urothelium. *Journal of Clinical Investigation*, **82**, 1454– 61.

Gabrilove, J.L., Jakubowski, A., Scher, H., et al. (1988b) Effect of granulocyte colony-stimulating factor on neutropenia and associated morbidity due to chemotherapy for transitional-cell carcinoma of the urothelium. *New England Journal of Medicine*, **318**, 1414–22.

Gale, R.P., Reiffers, J., and Juttner, C.A. (1994) What's new in blood progenitor cell autotransplants? *Bone Marrow Transplantation*, **14**, 343–6.

Galli, S.J., Zsebo, K.M., and Geissler, E.N. (1994) The kit ligand, stem cell factor. *Advances in Immunology*, **55**, 1–96.

Gasparetto, C., Smith, C., Gillio, A., Stoppa, A., Moore, M.A., and O'Reilly, R. J. (1994) Enrichment of peripheral blood stem cells in a primate model following administration of a single dose of rh-IL-1β. *Bone Marrow Transplantation*, **14**, 717–23.

Geissler, K., Valent, P., Mayer, P., et al. (1990) Recombinant human interleukin-3 expands the pool of circulating hemopoietic progenitor cells in primates – synergism with recombinant human granulocyte/macrophage colony-stimulating factor. *Blood*, **75**, 2305–10.

Glaspy, J., McNiece, I., LeMaistre, F., et al. (1994) Effects of stem cell factor (rhSCF) and filgrastim (rhG-CSF) on the mobilization of peripheral blood progenitor cells (PBPC) and hematological recovery post transplant: preliminary phase I/II study results. *British Journal of Haematology*, **87**, 156a.

Goodman, J.W., and Hodgson, G.S. (1962) Evidence for stem cells in the peripheral blood of mice. *Blood*, **19**, 702–14.

Haas, R., Ho, A.D., Bredthauer, U., et al. (1990) Successful autologous transplantation of blood stem cells mobilized with recombinant human granulocyte-macrophage colony-stimulating factor. *Experimental Hematology*, **18**, 94–8.

Hershko, C., Ho, W.G., and Gale, R.P. (1979) Cure of aplastic anaemia in paroxysmal nocturnal haemoglobinuria by marrow transfusion from identical twin: failure of peripheral leukocyte transfusion to correct marrow aplasia. *Lancet*, **1**, 945–7.

Höglund, M., Bengtsson, M., Simonsson, B., Smedmyr, B., and Tötterman, T. (1994) Leukapheresis with peripheral blood progenitor cell (PBPC) harvest in healthy volunteers receiving different doses of Lenograstim – evidence of a dose response effect. *Blood*, **84**, 1377a.

Jones, R.J., Celano, P., Sharkis, S.J., and Sensenbrenner, L.L. (1989) Two phases of engraftment established by serial bone marrow transplantation in mice. *Blood*, **73**, 397–401.

Kato, T., Ogami, K., Shimada, Y., et al. (1995) Purification and characterization of thrombopoietin. *Journal of Biochemistry*, **118**, 229–36.

Kaushansky, K., Lok, S., Holly, R.D., et al. (1994) Promotion of megakaryocyte progenitor expansion and differentiation by the c-Mpl ligand thrombopoietin. *Nature*, **369**, 568–71.

Kessinger, A., Armitage, J.O., Landmark, J.D., Smith, D.M., and Weisenburger, D.D. (1988) Autologous peripheral haematopoietic stem cell transplantation restores function following marrow ablative therapy. *Blood*, **71**, 723–7.

Kinashi, T., and Springer, T.A. (1994) Steel factor and c-kit regulate cell-matrix adhesion. *Blood*, **83**, 1033–8.

Kodama, H., Nose, M., Niida, S., Nishikawa, S., and Nishikawa, S.-I. (1994) Involvement of the c-kit receptor in the adhesion of hemopoietic stem cells to stromal cells. *Experimental Hematology*, **22**, 979–84.

Kovach, N.L., Lin, N., Yednock, T., Harlan, J.M., and Broudy, V.C. (1995) Stem cell factor modulates avidity of $\alpha_4\beta_1$ and $\alpha_5\beta_1$ integrins expressed on hematopoietic cell lines. *Blood*, **85**, 159–67.

Kritz, A., Crown, J.P., Motzer, R.J., et al. (1993) Beneficial impact of peripheral blood cells in patients with metastatic breast cancer treated with high-dose chemotherapy plus granulocyte-macrophage colony-stimulating factor. A randomized trial. *Cancer*, **71**, 2515–21.

Lane, T.A., Law, P., Maruyama, M., et al. (1995) Harvesting and enrichment of hematopoietic progenitor cells mobilized into the peripheral blood of normal donors by granulocyte-macrophage colony-stimulating factor (GM-CSF) or G-CSF: potential role in allogeneic marrow transplantation. *Blood*, **85**, 275–82.

Lieschke, G.J., Maher, D., Cebon, J., et al. (1989) Effects of bacterially synthesized recombinant human granulocyte-macrophage colony-stimulating factor in patients with advanced malignancy. *Annals of Internal Medicine*, **110**, 357–64.

Lieschke, G.J., Maher, D., O'Connor, M., et al. (1990) Phase I study of intravenously administered bacterially synthesized granulocyte-macrophage colony-stimulating factor and comparison with subcutaneous administration. *Cancer Research*, **50**, 606–14.

Lieschke, G.J., and Burgess, A.W. (1992a) Granulocyte colony-stimulating factor and granulocyte-macrophage colony-stimulating factor (1). *New England Journal of Medicine*, **327**, 28–35.

Lieschke, G.J., and Burgess, A.W. (1992b) Granulocyte colony-stimulating factor and granulocyte-macrophage colony-stimulating factor (2). *New England Journal of Medicine*, **327**, 99–106.

Liesveld, J.L., DiPersio, J.F., and Abboud, C.N. (1994) Integrins and adhesive receptors in normal and leukemic CD34$^+$ progenitor cells: potential regulatory checkpoints for cellular traffic. *Leukemia and Lymphoma*, **14**, 19–28.

Lok, S., Kaushansky, K., Holly, R.D., et al. (1994) Cloning and expression of murine thrombopoietin cDNA and stimulation of platelet production in vivo. *Nature*, **369**, 565–8.

Lord, B.I., Bronchud, M.H., Owens, S., et al. (1989) The kinetics of human granulopoiesis following treatment with granulocyte colony-stimulating factor in vivo. *Proceedings of the National Academy of Sciences of the United States of America*, **86**, 9499–503.

Majdic, O., Stöckl, J., Pickl, W.F., et al. (1994) Signaling and induction of enhanced cytoadhesiveness via the hemopoietic progenitor cell surface molecule CD. *Blood*, **83**, 1226–34.

Malinin, T.I., Perry, V.P., Kerby, C.C., and Dolan, M.F. (1965) Peripheral leukocyte infusion into lethally irradiated guinea pigs. *Blood*, **25**, 693–702.

Matsunaga, T., Sakamaki, S., Kohgo, Y., Ohi, Y., Hirayama, Y., and Niitsu, Y. (1993) Recombinant human granulocyte colony-stimulating factor can mobilize sufficient amounts of peripheral blood stem cells in healthy volunteers for allogeneic transplantation. *Bone Marrow Transplantation*, **11**, 103–8.

McNiece, I.K., Briddell, R.A., Yan, X.-Q., et al. (1994) The role of stem cell factor in mobilization of peripheral blood progenitor cells. *Leukemia and Lymphoma*, **15**, 405–9.

Mohle, R., Pforisch, M., Fruehauf, S., Witt, B., Kramer, A., and Haas, R. (1994) Filgrastim post-chemotherapy mobilizes more CD34$^+$ cells with a different antigenic profile compared with use during steady-state hemopoiesis. *Bone Marrow Transplantation,* **14**, 827–32.

Molineux, G., Podja, Z., and Dexter, T.M. (1990a) A comparison of hemopoiesis in normal and splenectomized mice treated with granulocyte colony-stimulating factor. *Blood,* **75**, 563–9.

Molineux, G., Pojda, Z., Hampson, I.N., Lord, B.I., and Dexter, T.M. (1990b) Transplantation potential of peripheral blood stem cells induced by granulocyte colony-stimulating factor. *Blood,* **76**, 2153–8.

Morstyn, G., Campbell, L., Souza, L.M., et al. (1988) Effect of granulocyte colony stimulating factor on neutropenia induced by cytotoxic chemotherapy. *Lancet,* **1**, 667–72.

Moskowitz, C., Stiff, P., Gordon, M., et al. (1994) The influence of extensive prior chemotherapy on the mobilization of peripheral blood progenitor cells (PBPC) using stem cell factor (rhSCF) and filgrastim (rmetHuG-CSF) and on hematologic recovery post cyclophosphamide, BCNU, and VP-16 (CBV) in patients (pts) with relapsed non-Hodgkin's lymphoma (NHL): an interim analysis. *Blood,* **84**, 107a.

Nademanee, A., Sniecinski, I., Schmidt, G.M., et al. (1994) High-dose therapy followed by autologous peripheral-blood stem-cell transplantation for patients with Hodgkin's disease and non-Hodgkin's lymphoma using unprimed and granulocyte colony-stimulating factor-mobilized peripheral-blood stem cells. *Journal of Clinical Oncology,* **12**, 2176–86.

Ossenkoppele, G.J., Jonkhoff, A.R., Huijgens, P.C., et al. (1994) Peripheral blood progenitors mobilised by G-CSF (filgrastim) and reinfused as unprocessed autologous whole blood shorten the pancytopenic period following high-dose melphalan in multiple myeloma. *Bone Marrow Transplantation,* **13**, 37–41.

Ottmann, O.G., Brucher, J., Geissler, G., et al. (1992) Effect of sequential interleukin-3 (rhIL-3) and granulocyte-macrophage colony stimulating factor (rhGM-CSF) on circulating GM-CFC. *International Journal of Cell Cloning,* **10**, 65–7.

Oxley, S.M., and Sackstein, R. (1994) Detection of an L-selectin ligand on hemopoietic progenitor cell line. *Blood,* **84**, 3299–306.

Peters, W.P., Rosner, G., Ross, M., et al. (1993) Comparative effects of granulocyte-macrophage colony-stimulating factor (GM-CSF) and granulocyte colony-stimulating factor (G-CSF) on priming peripheral blood progenitor cells for use with autologous bone marrow after high-dose chemotherapy. *Blood,* **81**, 1709–19.

Pettengell, R., Woll, P.J., Chang, J., Coutinho, L., Testa, N.G., and Crowther, D. (1994) Effects of erythropoietin on mobilization of haemopoietic progenitor cells. *Bone Marrow Transplantation,* **14**, 125–30.

Richman, C.M., Winer, R.S., and Yankee, R.A. (1976) Increase in circulating stem cells following chemotherapy in man. *Blood,* **47**, 1031–9.

Roberts, A.W., and Metcalf, D. (1994) Granulocyte colony-stimulating factor induces selective elevations of progenitor cells in the peripheral blood of mice. *Experimental Hematology,* **22**, 1156–63.

Roberts, A. and Metcalf, D. (1995) Non-cycling state of peripheral blood cells mobilized by granulocyte colony-stimulating factor and other cytokines. *Blood,* **86**, 1600–5.

Russell, N.H., Hunter, A., Rogers, S., Hanley, J., and Anderson, D. (1993) Peripheral blood stem cells as an alternative to marrow for allogeneic transplantation. *Lancet*, **341**, 1482.

Sato, N., Sawada, K., Takahashi, T.A., et al. (1994) Time course study for optimal harvest of peripheral blood progenitor cells by granulocyte colony-stimulating factor in healthy volunteers. *Experimental Hematology*, **22**, 973–8.

Schmitz, N., Linch, D.C., Dreger, P., et al. (1994) Randomized phase III study of filgrastim-mobilized peripheral blood progenitor cell transplantation (PBPCT) in comparison with autologous bone marrow transplantation (ABMT) in patients with Hodgkin's disease (HD) and non-Hodgkin's lymphoma (NHL). *Blood*, **84**, 204a.

Schmitz, N., Dreger, P., Suttorp, M., et al. (1995) Primary transplantation of allogeneic peripheral blood progenitor cells mobilized by filgrastim (granulocyte colony-stimulating factor). *Blood*, **85**, 1666–72.

Schwartzberg, L., Birch, B., Weaver, C., and West, W. (1994) The effect of varying durations of granulocyte colony stimulating factor (G-CSF) on neutrophil engraftment and supportive care following peripheral blood progenitor cell (PBPC) infusion. *Blood*, **84**, 91a.

Schwartzberg, L. Data on file. Amgen Inc.

Schwinger, W., Mache, C., Urban, C., Beaufort, F., and Töglhofer, W. (1993) Single dose of filgrastim (rhG-CSF) increases the number of hemopoietic progenitors in the peripheral blood of adult volunteers. *Bone Marrow Transplantation*, **11**, 489–92.

Sheridan, W.P., Morstyn, G., Wolf, M., et al. (1989) Granulocyte colony-stimulating factor and neutrophil recovery after high-dose chemotherapy and autologous bone marrow transplantation. *Lancet*, **2**, 891–5.

Sheridan, W., Begley, G., Juttner, C., et al. (1992a) Effect of different doses and schedules of r-metHuG-CSF (filgrastim) on mononuclear cell and PBPC collections and haematopoietic recovery after high dose chemotherapy (HDC) and infusion of r-metHuG-CSF mobilized peripheral blood progenitor cells (PBPC) without bone marrow. *Blood*, **80**, 331a.

Sheridan, W., Begley, G., Juttner, C., et al. (1992b) The impact of r-metHuG-CSF (filgrastim) dose on the mobilisation of mononuclear and progenitor cells in peripheral blood in patients with malignancy. *Blood*, **80**, 420a.

Sheridan, W.P., Begley, C.G., Juttner, C.A., et al. (1992c) Effect of peripheral-blood progenitor cells mobilised by filgrastim (G-CSF) on platelet recovery after high-dose chemotherapy. *Lancet*, **339**, 640–4.

Sheridan, W.P., Begley, G.C., To, L.B., et al. (1994) Phase II study of autologous filgrastim (G-CSF) -mobilized peripheral blood progenitor cells to restore hemopoiesis after high dose chemotherapy for lymphoid malignancies. *Bone Marrow Transplantation*, **14**, 105–11.

Socinski, M.A., Cannistra, S.A., Elias, A., Antman, K.H., Schnipper, L., and Griffin, J. D. (1988) Granulocyte-macrophage colony-stimulating factor expands the circulating haemopoietic progenitor cell compartment in man. *Lancet*, **1**, 1194–8.

Stephens, L.C., Haire, W.D., Schmit-Pokorny, K., Kessinger, A., and Kotaluk, G. (1993) Granulocyte macrophage colony stimulating factor: high incidence of apheresis catheter thrombosis during peripheral stem cell collection. *Bone Marrow Transplantation*, **11**, 51–4.

Stockenhuber, F., Kurz, R.W., Geissler, K., et al. (1990) Recombinant human erythropoietin activates a broad spectrum of progenitor cells. *Kidney International*, **37**, 150–6.

Storb, R., Epstein, R.B., Radge, H., Bryant, J., and Thomas, E.D. (1967) Marrow engraftment by allogeneic leukocytes in lethally irradiated dogs. *Blood*, **30**, 805–11.

Storb, R., Graham, T.C., Epstein, R.B., Sale, G.E., and Thomas, E.D. (1977) Demonstration of hemopoietic stem cells in the peripheral blood of baboons by cross circulation. *Blood*, **50**, 537–42.

Storb, R., Deeg, H.J., Pepe, M., et al. (1989) Methotrexate and cyclosporine versus cyclosporine alone for prophylaxis of graft-versus-host disease in patients given HLA-identical marrow grafts for leukemia: long-term follow-up of a controlled trial. *Blood*, **73**, 1729–34.

Taylor, K.M., Jagannath, S., Spitzer, G., et al. (1989) Recombinant human granulocyte colony-stimulating factor hastens granulocyte recovery after high-dose chemotherapy and autologous bone marrow transplantation in Hodgkin's disease. *Journal of Clinical Oncology*, **7**, 1791–9.

Tjonnfjord, G.E., Steen, R., Evensen, S.A., Thorsby, E., and Egeland, T. (1994) Characterization of CD34$^+$ peripheral blood cells from healthy adults mobilized by recombinant human granulocyte colony-stimulating factor. *Blood*, **84**, 2795–801.

To, L.B., Haylock, D.N., Dyson, P.G., Thorp, D., Roberts, M.M., and Juttner, C.A. (1990) An unusual pattern of hemopoietic reconstitution in patients with acute myeloid leukemia transplanted with autologous recovery phase peripheral blood. *Bone Marrow Transplantation*, **6**, 109–14.

To, L.B., Rawling, C., Andary, C., et al. (1993) The efficacy of sequential/combined IL-3/GM-CSF administration in peripheral blood (PB) progenitor mobilization. *Blood*, **82**, 83a.

To, L.B., Haylock, D N., Dowse, T., et al. (1994) A comparative study of the phenotype and proliferative capacity of peripheral blood (PB) CD34$^+$ cells mobilized by four different protocols and those of steady-phase PB and bone marrow CD34$^+$ cells. *Blood*, **84**, 2930–9.

Turner, M.L. (1994) Regulation of hemopoietic progenitor cell migration, mobilization, and homing. *Stem Cells*, **12**, 227–9.

van der Wall, E., Richel, D., Holtkamp, M., et al. (1994) Bone marrow reconstitution after high dose chemotherapy and autologous peripheral blood progenitor cells: effect of graft size. *Annals of Oncology*, **5**, 795–802.

Villeval, J.-L., Dührsen, U., Morstyn, G., and Metcalf, D. (1990) Effect of recombinant human granulocyte-macrophage colony stimulating factor on progenitor cells in patients with advanced malignancies. *British Journal of Haematology*, **74**, 36–44.

Weaver, C.H., Buckner, C.D., Longin, K., et al. (1993) Syngeneic transplantation with peripheral blood mononuclear cells collected after the administration of recombinant human granulocyte colony-stimulating factor. *Blood*, **82**, 1981 4.

Weaver, C.H., Longin, K., Buckner, C.D., and Bensinger, W. (1994) Lymphocyte content in peripheral blood mononuclear cells collected after the administration of recombinant human granulocyte colony-stimulating factor. *Bone Marrow Transplantation*, **13**, 411–5.

Wilson, W.H., Bryant, G., Fox, M., et al. (1993) Interleukin-1α administered before high-dose ifosfamide (I), CBDCA (C), and etoposide (E) (ICE) with autologous bone marrow rescue shortens neutrophil recovery: a phase I/II study. *Proceedings of the American Society of Clinical Oncology*, **12**, 289a.

Yan, X.-Q., Briddell, R., Hartley, C., Stoney, G., Samal, B., and McNiece, I. (1994) Mobilization of long-term hemopoietic reconstituting cells in mice by the combination of stem cell factor plus granulocyte colony-stimulating factor. *Blood*, **84**, 795–9.

Zeller, W., Cassens, U., Stockschlader, M., et al. (1994) Higher dose of G-CSF increases yield of mobilized CD34$^+$ cells. *Blood*, **84**, 413a.

—10

Characterization and Isolation of Mobilized Peripheral Blood Stem Cells Using a High-Speed Cell Sorter

ANN TSUKAMOTO, DENNIS SASAKI,
BENJAMIN P. CHEN, AND RONALD HOFFMAN

Acceleration of engraftment and increased disease-free survival following autologous hemopoietic cell transplantation of patients with a variety of neoplastic diseases is a target of many clinical investigators. To address these issues, recent studies have focused on the use of specific growth factors and mobilized peripheral blood progenitor cells (PBPC) as an alternative to bone marrow (BM) cells, to accelerate hemopoietic recovery following transplantation. Additionally, the use of purified $CD34^+$ cells to provide tumor-cell–depleted grafts has been explored recently (Berenson et al. 1991; Shpall et al. 1992, 1994) (see Chapters 7 and 11).

Technological advances in stem-cell phenotypic analysis and fractionation procedures permit the isolation of purified hemopoietic stem-cell (HSC) populations. Because of the primitive nature of the HSC, some investigators have hypothesized that the use of purified HSC as a graft would result in unacceptable delays in time to hemopoietic engraftment. The premise by which these highly purified HSC populations would provide rapid and sustained engraftment is based upon recent studies in the mouse. In these studies, purified mouse stem cells (MSC) consisting of $Thy-1.1^{low}Lin^-Sca^+$ cells infused into lethally irradiated mice led to neutrophil and platelet recovery with a similar rate and degree of hemopoietic reconstitution as seen following transplantation of whole BM cells containing the same number of nonpurified MSC (Uchida et al. 1994). These results suggest that early as well as long-term engraftment results from the infusion of cells contained within the enriched mouse BM stem-cell population. For this reason and with hope of providing disease-free grafts, an extensive amount of research has focused on characterization and purification of human

183

HSC that will be used as grafts during allogeneic and autologous transplantation.

Numerous studies have demonstrated that the CD34 antigen (Ag) is expressed on both progenitor cells and stem cells. Further characterization of stem cells has been achieved by defining subpopulations of CD34$^+$ cells. Studies patterned after those in the mouse system have further characterized the human HSC as a subfraction of CD34$^+$ cells negative for lineage markers, but which express c-*kit* and Thy-1 and retain small quantities of the vital dye rhodamine 123 (reviewed in Watt and Visser 1992; Spangrude 1994). In previous work from this group, Thy-1 has been shown to subset the CD34$^+$ fraction of fetal BM and to be a marker expressed by fetal BM stem cells (Baum et al. 1992). This analysis has recently been extended to adult BM (Murray et al. 1994). In these studies, Thy-1 was shown to be expressed by about 25% of the BM CD34$^+$ population. The CD34$^+$Thy-1$^+$Lin$^-$ population has multilineage differentiation capacity as shown by its ability to produce both B cells and myeloid cells in vitro and to generate T, B, and myeloid cells in vivo in the SCID-hu mouse assay system (Murray et al. 1994; Tsukamoto et al. in press; Uchida et al. 1994). These studies have also demonstrated the expansion potential of the CD34$^+$Thy-1$^+$Lin$^-$ cells by their ability to produce CD34$^+$ progenitors continuously in both in vitro and in vivo assays (Murray et al. 1994, 1995).

Peripheral blood (PB) autografts are increasingly becoming the standard cell source of progenitor cells and HSC for autologous grafts; however, studies that demonstrate true long-term multilineage engrafting potential of such grafts are limited. Evidence from animal studies (Molineux et al. 1990; Fibbe et al. 1992; Andrews et al. 1993, 1994; Briddell, et al. 1993; Fleming et al. 1993; De Revel et al. 1994; Yan et al. 1994) indicates the mobilization of HSC into peripheral circulation following cytokine administration. In humans, numerous clinical studies suggest the existence of long-term repopulating cells in PBPC grafts (reviewed in Juttner et al. 1992). Transplantation studies using peripheral blood stem cells (PBSC) in conjunction with cytokine administration have demonstrated significant shortening of the time to neutrophil and platelet recovery compared with bone-marrow transplantation (BMT) (Chapters 8 and 9). More recent gene-marking studies have revealed that PBPC grafts do indeed contain cells that are capable of giving rise to detectable T, B, and myeloid cells in patients after transplantation and therefore contain cells that resemble stem cells. Although treatment of patients who have solid tumors associated with BM involvement with PBPC grafts may result in the infusion of fewer tumor cells than BMT, these PBSC are not entirely free of tumor cells. Gene-marking studies have shown that residual tumor cells present in such grafts are capable of contributing to disease relapse (Brenner et al. 1993; Deisseroth et al. 1994). Thus, purification of the short- and long-term engrafting cells, free of residual disease in such grafts, might be useful in the treatment of many malignancies. Since the CD34 Ag marks both stem cells and progenitor cells of normal and malignant stem cells in some hematologic malignancies, isolation using solely a CD34-selection variable may not be sufficient for isolating a disease-free graft. In addition, even where CD34 does not mark malignant cells, the purity of such grafts must be high to ensure the absence of residual tumor cells. Therefore, isolation of purified stem cells from PB may provide a superior graft for autologous BMT when used for the treatment of many malignant disorders. This review will focus on the characterization and isolation of stem cells from mobilized PB using a novel high-speed cell sorter.

■ CHARACTERIZATION OF PERIPHERAL BLOOD STEM CELLS

Studies of human BM have indicated that the HSC is $CD34^+$, Thy-1^+, c-kit^+, HLA-DR^-, $CD38^-$ and rhodamine 123^{low} (reviewed in Watt and Visser 1992; Tsukamoto et al. in press). Each of these phenotypic characteristics has been used to enrich for human HSC populations.

To demonstrate the biological activity of mobilized PB HSC, $CD34^+Lin^-$ cells were separated into Thy-1^+ and Thy-1^- subsets isolated by fluorescence-activated cell sorting (FACS). Biological activities of these two populations have been tested in both in vitro and in vivo assays. In vitro, the cobblestone area–forming cell (CAFC) frequencies are enriched in the Thy-1^+ subset compared with the Thy-1^- fraction. Work from our laboratories has demonstrated the equivalence of CAFC frequencies at 5 to 6 weeks with long-term culture-initiating cell (LTC-IC) frequencies. These assay systems represent the best presently available means of quantifying HSC in vitro. In these analyses, PB-derived $CD34^+Thy-1^+Lin^-$ cells grown on a xenogeneic mouse BM stromal cell line, *SyS1*, in the presence of human leukemia-inhibiting factor (LIF) (50 ng/mL), IL-6 (10 ng/mL), and IL-3 (10 ng/mL) produce CAFC frequencies ranging from 1:14 to 1:41 compared with 1:67 to 1:161 for the Thy-1^- fraction (Reading et al. 1994; Murray et al. 1995). This in vitro culture assay also showed the potential of Thy-1^+ cells to differentiate into $CD19^+$ cells (B cells), and $CD33^+$ cells (immature myeloid cells), and maintain a $CD34^+Lin^-$ progenitor cell population. These results are similar to those obtained for fetal and adult BM-derived $CD34^+Thy-1^+Lin^-$ cells.

The in vivo potential of the mobilized PB CD34$^+$Thy-1$^+$Lin$^-$ cells was assessed in the SCID-hu assay for T-cell–repopulating ability and marrow-repopulating ability. These SCID-hu assays serve as allogeneic transplant models for detecting engraftment and differentiation potentials of putative stem-cell populations. These studies require the ability to distinguish donor-derived cells from host cells based on human leukocyte antigen (HLA) markers. In published work, the T-cell progenitor content of adult BM and mobilized PB CD34$^+$Lin$^-$ cells were compared in the SCID-hu thymus assay and shown to be qualitatively identical (Galy et al. 1994). In more recent studies, the ability to generate donor-derived thymocytes was found to be a property of both the Thy-1$^+$ and Thy-1$^-$ subsets of the CD34$^+$Lin$^-$ cells. Both populations produced double-positive CD4$^+$CD8$^+$ immature-cortical thymocytes as well as CD3$^+$CD1$^+$ mature thymocytes. These T cells display the phenotype of cells normally found in human thymus (Terstappen, Huang, and Picker 1992).

The marrow-repopulating ability of the Thy-1 subsets of CD34$^+$Lin$^-$ cells was analyzed in the SCID-hu bone system. Upon injection of Thy-1$^+$ cells into SCID mice implanted with human fetal bone fragments, donor-derived long-term human B-cell and myeloid-cell production was observed. Little or no donor engraftment was seen when Thy-1$^-$ cells were injected. Moreover, donor CD34$^+$Lin$^-$ progenitor cells were also detected from bone fragments injected with Thy-1$^+$ cells, implying the maintenance of an early cell capable of sustained hemopoiesis. The reduced ability of Thy-1$^-$ cells to engraft in the SCID-hu bone assay, coupled with their ability to produce T cells in the thymus assay, suggests the possibility of a T-cell progenitor present within the Thy-1$^-$ population (A. Galy, unpublished data). The clear demonstration of the lymphoid potential of PB Thy-1$^+$ cells has major relevance for clinical BMT. These observations eliminate any concern about the ability of pure HSC transplantation to result in both T- and B-cell reconstitution.

These studies indicate that CD34$^+$Thy-1$^+$Lin$^-$ cells from mobilized PB are phenotypically and functionally similar to CD34$^+$Thy-1$^+$Lin$^-$ BM cells.

■ MOBILIZATION OF HEMOPOIETIC STEM CELLS

Steady-state PB has previously been used as an alternative to BM, in patients receiving high-dose chemotherapy/radiation therapy for a number of malignancies, including Hodgkin's disease (HD) and non-Hodgkin's lymphoma (NHL), characterized by BM involvement (Kessinger et al. 1989). A major limitation of steady-state PBSC grafts is the time required and the number of leukapheresis sessions needed to obtain an adequate cell dose to ensure engraftment. The range of cell numbers required to ensure engraftment in these studies has been estimated either by monitoring the dose of mononuclear cells (MNC) per kilogram, granulocyte-macrophage colony-forming cells (GM-CFC) per kilogram, or $CD34^+$ cells per kilogram within the graft; however, there is no indication of which cells within these heterogeneous populations are responsible for rapid and sustained engraftment. Moreover, these variables are not good indicators of the long-term self-renewal potential of cells within these leukapheresis products.

In basal PB, circulating levels of $CD34^+$ cells are very low. Pretreatment of an individual with mobilizing agents such as cytokines or chemotherapy has been shown to increase CD34 cell numbers in the circulation. Cytokines such as rHuG-CSF or rHuGM-CSF alone (Chapter 9) or in combination with high-dose chemotherapy agents (Chapter 8) have been used as mobilizing agents (Dührsen et al. 1988; Gianni et al. 1989). High-dose cyclophosphamide, in particular, has been shown to increase PB CD34 levels (Siena et al. 1989; To et al. 1989).

Since the $CD34^+$ population includes committed progenitors, primitive progenitors, and stem cells, it is important to characterize the subclasses of $CD34^+$ cells mobilized using different chemotherapy and/or cytokine regimens. Since $CD34^+$ cells constitute a heterogeneous population, it is difficult to assess the quality of the graft by measuring this single variable. Wide variations in times to neutrophil and platelet recovery have been observed in patients receiving $CD34^+$ grafts, variations which could be due to the presence of different CD34 subsets, to genetic variability, or to stem-cell damage from prior chemotherapy. Thus, detailed knowledge of PBPC/PBSC released during mobilization may allow us to better predict both rapid and long-term engraftment.

As for BM cells, mobilized PB $CD34^+$ cells can be further fractionated by use of antibodies (Ab) to Thy-1. In contrast to BM, however, the proportion of Thy-1^+ cells varies greatly among mobilized PB samples. Levels of Thy-1 expression in the PB $CD34^+$ population of multiple myeloma (MM) patients mobilized with cyclophosphamide (6 gm/m^2) and GM-CSF (250 mg/m^2) (Uchida et al. 1993; Murray et al. 1995) have ranged from approximately 1% to 60% (Table 10.1).

As can be seen in Table 10.1, the $CD34^+Lin^-$ and $CD34^+Thy$-1^+Lin^- content of individual grafts varies from specimen to specimen. Analysis of more than 40 patients treated under the same mobilization regimen has defined the kinetics of mobilization of $CD34^+$ and $CD34^+Thy$-1^+Lin^- cells.

Table 10.1. Content of Leukapheresis Products[a]

Patient Number	Leukapheresis Day	% CD34+Lin−	% Thy-1+ (of CD34+Lin−)[b]
1	1	5.86	36.00
	2	2.06	6.80
	3	2.39	2.93
	4	1.78	1.69
	5	1.50	9.33
	6	0.95	3.16
2	1	2.99	40.47
	2	1.77	9.04
	3	1.67	5.98
	4	0.65	3.08
	5	1.09	24.77
3	1	15.00	14.67
	2	9.00	10.56
	3	5.00	5.20
	4	3.80	16.19
	5	1.77	7.91
	7	2.00	1.00
4	1	15.90	22.45
	2	27.20	57.10
	6	5.05	1.39
	7	2.17	1.84
5	1	3.72	18.55
	2	2.93	22.87
	3	1.31	23.66
	4	1.10	20.00
	5	1.70	4.71

[a]Leukapheresis collections were initiated when whole blood cell count (WBC) rose to >0.5 × 10^9/L. Samples were analyzed by flow cytometry using values of CD34+Lin− reported as a percentage of the size-gated and dead cell–gated whole sample. Values for Thy-1 are the percentage of CD34+Lin− cells that stain above isotype control values using a Thy-1 antibody.
[b]Percentage of Thy-1% cells within CD34+Lin− fraction of mobilized PB samples.

From extensive analysis of fetal and adult BM cells, the population that consistently repopulates allogeneic fetal bone in the SCID-hu assay has been identified and has been shown to reside within the Thy-1+ subset of CD34+Lin− cells (Baum et al. 1992; Murray et al. 1994). In mobilized PB samples there is also a correlation between Thy-1 expression and engraftment potential in the SCID-hu bone assay. In

Figure 10.1 (see color plate), a mobilized PB sample obtained on day 2 of leukapheresis is separated into Thy-1$^+$ and Thy-1$^-$ subsets. Marrow-repopulating activity was found in the CD34$^+$Thy-1$^+$Lin$^-$ fraction, whereas little to no activity was found in the Thy-1$^-$ fraction. These results show the consistency of Thy-1 expression on primitive cells in mobilized PB as well as fetal and adult BM cells.

These cells fulfilled the functional criteria of HSC as defined by their ability to undergo multilineage differentiation and self-renewal in both in vitro and in vivo assays. Of 28 patient samples analyzed for levels of CD34$^+$, CD34$^+$Lin$^-$ cells, and CD34$^+$Thy$^+$Lin$^-$, only eight patients showed an obvious peak of mobilization of Thy-1$^+$ cells into the circulation, where peak values were observed between days 2 to 5 of leukapheresis (days following cyclophosphamide ranged from day 16 to day 21). In the example shown (Fig. 10.2), the percentage of Thy-1$^+$ cells present within the CD34$^+$ cell population increased from 38% on day 1 to 52% on day 2 followed by a rapid decline to below 20% thereafter. Thus, analysis of a single sample of a patient's mobilized PB may or may not demonstrate a large number of Thy-1$^+$

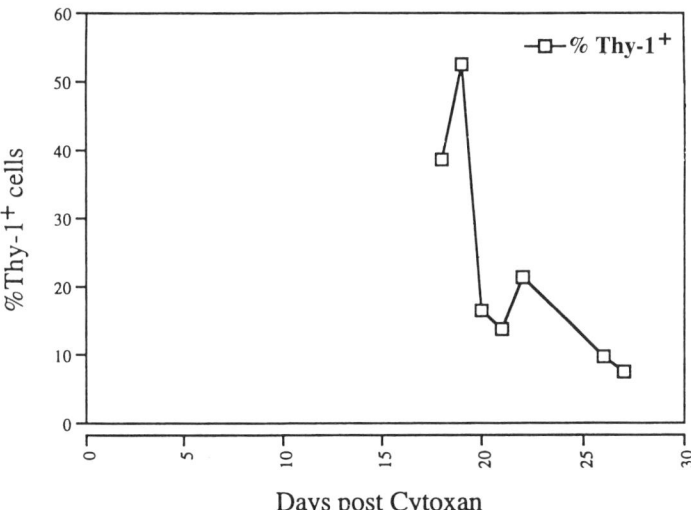

Days post Cytoxan

Figure 10.2 Kinetic analysis of the mobilization of Thy-1$^+$ cells. Flow cytometric analysis of leukapheresis products obtained on sequential days following treatment with cyclophosphamide (6 gm/m^2) and GM-CSF (0.25 mg/m^2). Apheresis was started the day following a WBC count greater than 0.5 × 10^9/L. (Samples were depleted for red cells.) Samples were stained with Ab to CD34, CD2, CD10, CD14, CD15, CD19, glycophorin A (Lin$^-$), and Thy-1.

cells, and may merely reflect a snapshot of the kinetics of HSC mobilization.

■ HIGH-SPEED CELL SORTING

There are numerous methods to enrich for hemopoietic cells based on their physical properties. Density-gradient centrifugation, velocity sedimentation, and elutriation are processes that separate cells based on cell size and buoyant density. Immunologic selection techniques, in particular positive selection, generally accomplish a greater degree of enrichment and take advantage of the expression of specific antigens on the cell surface. The demonstration of the presence of the CD34 Ag on HSC has led to a number of selection systems (Chapters 11 and 12), which use monoclonal antibodies (mAB) to purify HSC (reviewed in Berenson, Bensinger, and Kalamasz 1986; Berenson et al. 1987; Civin et al. 1990; Hardwick et al. 1992; Lebkowski et al. 1992; Okarma 1992; Okarma et al. 1992; Sutherland et al. 1992; Hardwick et al. 1993; Law et al. 1993; Auditore-Hargereaves, Heimfeld, and Berenson 1994). A solid-phase immunoaffinity column using biotin-avidin interaction has been widely studied (Berenson et al. 1991; Shpall et al. 1992, 1994), for enrichment of CD34$^+$ cells for use as hemopoietic grafts. These methods result in a limited enrichment of HSC, and the applicability of such devices is restricted to isolation based on a single variable.

FACS may be used to isolate HSC from a heterogeneous population of cells and offers the advantage of allowing multiparameter measurements such as a cocktail of mAB to various cell-surface markers in conjunction with intracellular properties indicating cellular function using supravital dyes (propidium iodide [cell viability], rhodamine 123 [p-glycoprotein], and Hoechts 33342 [cell cycle]).

There are several potential advantages of multiparameter selection of HSC. First, a more enriched population of cells can be obtained using additional positive or negative markers using GMP-manufactured mAB, and second, use of combinatorial assortments of markers allows for HSC selection in a multitude of malignancies as long as the selection variables are not co-expressed by the malignant cells. Previously, one criticism of using flow cytometry for HSC isolation has been the untenable length of time required for processing the whole BM harvest or PB leukapheresis product. The estimated time for processing such large specimens on commercially available cell sorters is greater than 400 hours at a throughput rate of 2,500 to 5,000 cells/sec. Through the development of a presorting protocol to deplete the starting material of mature granulocytes and erythrocytes, and the development of a high-speed cell sorter (HSCS), the sample processing time can now be reduced to an 8- to 12-hour time period.

Development of multiparameter high-speed cell sorting has been described by several groups (Hiebert, Jett, and Salzman 1981; Peters et al. 1985; Herweiger, Stokdijk, and Visser, 1988; van den Engh and Stokdijk 1989) over the years. This technology has been used for isolation of chromosomes for the creation of genomic libraries. The HSCS, developed at SyStemix on initial license from Lawrence Livermore National Laboratory, has three main components that provide for high-speed sorting capabilities while ensuring sample sterility. The parallel-pulse processing unit used for data acquisition is a digitally synchronized unit that handles multiple input channels. The processing electronics have a cycle time of 4 μs or less and an extremely low rate of error (1 in 10^8 events). This ensures an improved rate of cell identification and recovery. The optical bench, composed of the illumination stage, detector stage, and sample stations, operates under 40 psi and generates droplets at a frequency of 60 kHz; this is four times the average performance of commercial systems. Viable cells have been sorted at rates as high as 40,000 cells/sec using a sorter jet velocity of 20 m/sec. Last, the optical bench and sample collection station are enclosed to ensure maximum integrity and sterility of the sorted cells for later infusion into patients.

A potential pitfall of sorting at high speed is the need for increased sheath pressure (>10 psi), necessary to obtain higher droplet-generation frequencies, and its effect on cell viability and function. The effect of increased pressure on cell viability following HSCS was examined by measuring the viability of freshly thawed, fragile PB lymphocytes. Initially, 89% of these cells were viable. The cells were run through the sorter at various operational sheath pressures from 10 psi to 60 psi. Following each test, cell viability was determined and found to range from 73% to 84%, indicating no deleterious effects resulting from increased operational pressure. Mobilized PB samples also were tested for viability and biological activity following purification by high-speed cell sorting. In three experiments, viability of mobilized PB cells after transit through the high-speed cell sorter ranged from 96% to 99%. These cells also contained assayable GM-CFC, E-BFC, and MIX-CFC colonies (D. Sasaki and R. Tushinski, personal communication). In additional experiments, mobilized PB cells were sorted with the HSCS for CD34$^+$Thy-1$^+$Lin$^-$ cells for analysis of CAFC activity while adult BM CD34$^+$Thy-1$^+$Lin$^-$ cells were sorted and analyzed in the SCID-hu bone assay, as measures of HSC content. In seven experiments, the CAFC frequency in long-term bone-marrow culture (LTBMC) of cells sorted on the HSCS ranged from 1:11.8 to 1:

Table 10.2. Functional Activity of CD34$^+$Thy-1$^+$Lin$^-$ Cells Sorted on the High-Speed Cell Sorter (HSCS)

Tissue ID	HSCS		Vantage FACS	
	CAFC High-Speed Frequency[a]	95% Confidence Limits	CAFC Frequency	95% Confidence Limits
7687	1/24.4	1/18.1–1/37.2	1/47.7	1/34.5–1/77.2
7772	1/11.8	1/9.4–1/15.8	1/14.7	1/11.7–1/19.6
7807	1/26.6	1/19.7–1/41.2	1/9.8	1/7.8–1/13.2
7864	1/42.2	1/33.3–1/57.6	1/46.3	1/36.7–1/62.8
7893	1/18.2	1/14.6–1/23.8	1/19.9	1/16.0–1/26.3
7897	1/20.5	1/14.9–1/32.4	1/17.5	1/14.0–1/23.2
7912	1/12.0	1/9.6–1/15.8	1/15.0	1/11.3–1/22.6

[a]Mobilized PB CD34$^+$Thy-1$^+$Lin$^-$ cells were plated at limiting dilution into long-term *SyS1* co-cultures in the presence of leukemia-inhibiting factor (LIF) (50 ng/mL), IL-3, and IL-6 (10 ng/mL). At week 6, CAFC were enumerated and their frequencies calculated using a linear-regression analysis. CAFC Frequency = frequency of cobblestone area–forming cells in CD34$^+$Thy-1$^+$Lin$^-$ cell fraction.

42. These numbers are comparable to CAFC frequencies obtained for the same mobilized PB sample sorted on a Becton-Dickinson FACS Vantage (1:9.8 to 1:47.7) (Table 10.2). In five experiments, the engraftment potential of adult BM CD34$^+$Thy-1$^+$Lin$^-$ cells sorted with the HSCS was assessed in the SCID-hu bone assay. Cells sorted with the HSCS were able to engraft with 88% success. Table 10.3 and Figure 10.3 show the CAFC frequencies, marrow repopulating potential, and multilineage differentiation potential of these Thy-1$^+$ cells isolated on the HSCS.

As discussed above, selection of cells using a combinational assortment of markers, absent on malignant cells, but present on primitive HSC, should allow the purification of cell populations highly enriched for HSC free of malignant cells. This has recently been tested with the processing of clinical samples from MM patients. Autotransplantation for MM patients is an increasingly popular modality of therapy; however, the large majority of these patients ultimately relapse. Recent gene-marking experiments in a number of cancers have demonstrated the contribution of reinfused tumor cells to relapse, indicating the importance of providing tumor-free autografts. Isolation of CD34$^+$Thy-1$^+$Lin$^-$ cells from mobilized PB products of myeloma patients has been shown to be an effective way of removing

Table 10.3. Functional Analysis of Bone Marrow HSC Sorted on the High-Speed Cell Sorter

	SYS1 Co-Culture	SCID-hu Bone Assay	
Sample ID	Cobblestone Area–Forming Cell Frequency[a]	No. of Cells Injected[b] per Bone Graft	Engraftment Success
7679	1/8	10,000	6/7
7701	1/74	10,000	8/8
	1/74	20,000	4/4

[a]CD34$^+$Thy-1$^+$Lin$^-$ cells sorted on the high-speed cell sorter from normal BM aspirates were plated at limiting dilutions onto LT-BMC *SyS1* cells in the presence of growth factors (LIF 25 ng/mL and IL-6 10 ng/mL). Wells were analyzed for CAFC at 6 weeks. The frequency of the wells with CAFC (% responding cells) was calculated.
[b]CD34$^+$Thy-1$^+$Lin$^-$ cells were injected into fetal bone grafts in the SCID-hu bone assay at the indicated concentrations. Engraftment success was scored as positive in any bone graft demonstrating greater than 1% donor-derived cells.

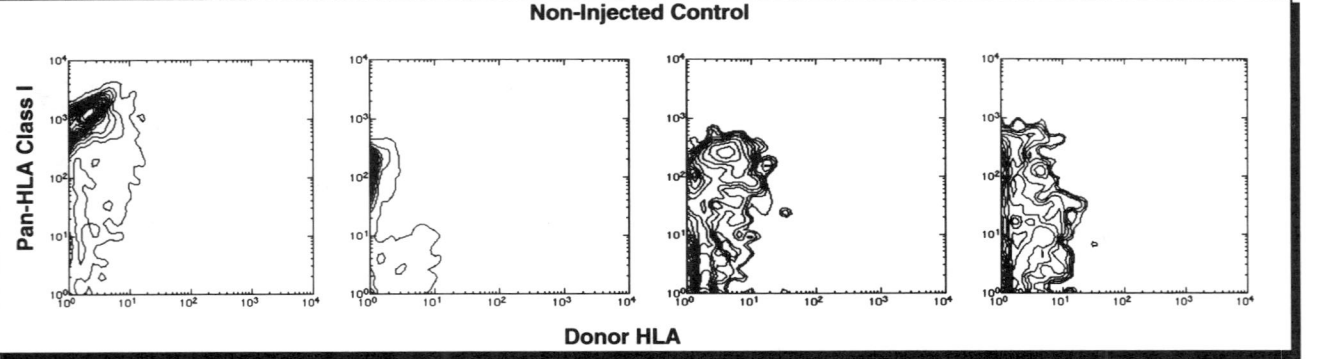

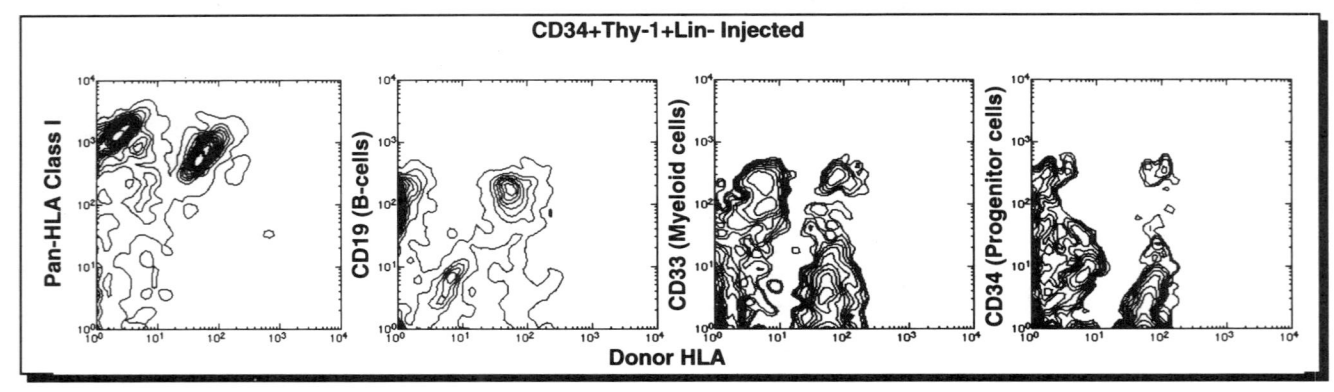

Figure 10.3 Biological activity of ABM CD34⁺Thy-1⁺Lin⁻ cells sorter on the high-speed cell sorter. 1 to 2 × 10⁴ Thy-1⁺ were microinjected into HLA-mismatched SCID-hu bones and BM cells recovered 8 weeks following implantation were analyzed by flow cytometry for the presence of donor cells. Representative bone grafts showed that the Thy-1⁺ cells engrafted and produced CD19, CD33, and CD34 progeny cells. Engraftment rates were more than 85% successful for biological activity as analyzed by CAFC formation in LT-BMC and in vivo engraftment in the SCID-hu bone assay.

myeloma cells (Gazitt et al. 1994; G. Tricot et al., personal communication).

■ CONCLUSIONS

The demonstration that mobilized PB samples contain $CD34^+Thy-1^+Lin^-$ cells that have biological properties analogous to BM $CD34^+Thy-1^+Lin^-$ cells suggest that these cells are true long-term repopulating stem cells. Although some differences may exist between these two populations, their functional properties are basically identical. The ability to purify these cells, depleted of residual tumor cells, has been accomplished with leukapheresis products obtained from patients with MM (Gazitt et al. 1994; G. Tricot et al., personal communication). The marrow repopulating potential of such HSC grafts will be tested clinically in the near future. Moreover, the utility of such HSC grafts will be further evaluated in clinical allogeneic and in utero transplantation studies.

ACKNOWLEDGMENTS

The authors wish to thank Kari Phillips and Sue Puryear for administrative support. Special thanks to the Cell Biology, FACS, Experimental Cell Therapy and the Comparative Medicine Group at SyStemix for their hard work and dedication.

REFERENCES

Andrews, R.G., Briddell, R.A., Knitter, G.H., et al. (1993) Low dose recombinant human stem cell factor (SCF) has a synergistic interaction with recombinant human granulocyte colony-stimulating factor (G-SCF) in vivo for stimulating the circulation of progenitor cells of multiple types in peripheral blood of baboons. *Blood*, **82**(Suppl. 1), 232a.

Andrews, R.G., Briddell, R.A., Knitter, G.H., et al. (1994) In vivo synergy between recombinant human stem cell factor and recombinant human granulocyte colony-stimulating factor in baboons: enhanced circulation of progenitor cells. *Blood*, **84**, 800–10.

Auditore-Hargreaves, K., Heimfeld, S., and Berenson, R.J. (1994) Selection and transplantation of hematopoietic stem and progenitor cells. *Bioconjugate Chemistry*, **5**, 287–300.

Baum, C.M., Weissman, I.L., Tsukamoto, A.T., et al. (1992) Isolation of a candidate human hematopoietic stem cell population. *Proceedings of the National Academy of Sciences of the United States of America*, **89**, 2804–08.

Berenson, R.J., Bensinger, W.I., Hill, R.S., et al. (1991) Engraftment after infusion of $CD34^+$ marrow cells in patients with breast cancer or neuroblastoma. *Blood*, **77**, 1717–22.

Berenson, R.J., Bensinger, W.I., and Kalamasz, D. (1986) Possible selection of viable cell populations using avidin-biotin immunoadsorption. *Journal of Immunological Methods*, **91**, 11–19.

Berenson, R.J., Bensinger, W.I., Kalamasz, D., Schuening, F., Deeg, H.J., and Storb, R. (1987) Avidin-biotin immunoadsorption: a technique to purify cells and its potential applications. In R.P. Gale and R. Champlin (Eds.) *Progress in bone marrow transplantation*, pp. 423–8. New York, Alan R. Liss.

Brenner, M.K., Rill, D.R., Moen, R.C., et al. (1993) Gene-marking to trace origin of relapse after autologous bone-marrow transplantation. *Lancet*, **341**, 85–6.

Briddell, R.A., Hartley, C.A., Smith, K.A., and McNiece, I.K. (1993) Recombinant rat stem cell factor synergizes with recombinant human granulocyte colony-stimulating factor in vivo in mice to mobilize peripheral blood progenitor cells that have enhanced repopulating potential. *Blood*, **82**, 1720a.

Civin, C.I., Strauss, L.C., Fackler, M.J., Trischmann, T.M., Wiley, J.M., and Loken, M.R. (1990) Positive stem cell selection – basic science. In S. Gross, A.P. Gee, and D.A. Worthington-White (Eds.) *Bone marrow purging and processing*, pp. 387–402. New York, Alan R. Liss.

De Revel, T., Appelbaum, F.R., Storb, R., et al. (1994) Effects of granulocyte colony stimulating factor and stem cell factor, alone and in combination on the mobilization of peripheral blood cells that engraft lethally irradiated dogs. *Blood*, **83**, 3795–9.

Deisseroth, A.B., Zu, Z., Claxton, D., et al. (1994) Genetic marking shows that Ph+ cells present in autologous transplants of chronic myelogenous leukemia (CML) contribute to relapse after autologous bone marrow in CML. *Blood*, **83**, 3068–76.

Dührsen, U., Villeval, J.L., Boyd, J., Kannourakis, G., Morstyn, G., and Metcalf, D. (1988) Effects of recombinant human granulocyte colony stimulating factor on hematopoietic progenitor cells in cancer patients. *Blood*, **72**, 125–38.

Fibbe, W.E., Hamilton, M.S., Laterveer, L.L., et al. (1992) Sustained engraftment of mice transplanted with IL-1-primed blood-derived stem cells. *Journal of Immunology*, **148**, 417.

Fleming, W.H., Alpern, E.J., Uchida, N., Ikuta, K., and Weissman, I.L. (1993) Steel factor influences the distribution and activity of murine hematopoietic stem cells in vivo. *Proceedings of the National Academy of Sciences of the United States of America*, **90**, 3760.

Galy, A.H.M., Webb, S., Cen, D., et al. (1994) Generation of T cells from cytokine-mobilized peripheral blood and adult bone marrow CD34[+] cells. *Blood*, **84**, 104–10.

Gazitt, Y., Reading, C., Stefanova, R., et al. (1994) Myeloma cells can be effectively depleted from mobilized peripheral blood mononuclear cells by selecting CD34[+], Thy-1+, Lin[−] stem cells. *Experimental Hematology*, **22**, 802.

Gianni, A.M., Siena, S., Bregni, M., et al. (1989) Granulocyte-macrophage colony-stimulating factor to harvest circulating hematopoietic stem cells for autotransplantation. *Lancet*, **ii**, 580–5.

Hardwick, R.A., Kulcinski, D., Mansour, V., Ishizawa, L., Law, P., and Gee, A.P. (1993) Design of large-scale separation systems for positive and negative immunomagnetic selection of cells using superparamagnetic microspheres. *Journal of Hematotherapy*, **1**, 379–86.

Hardwick, R.A., Law, P., Mansour, V., Kulcinski, D., Ishizawa, L., and Gee, A.P. (1992) Development of a large-scale immunomagnetic separation system for harvesting CD34-positive cells from bone marrow. In D.A. Worthington-White, A.P. Gee, and S. Gross (Eds.) *Advances in bone marrow purging and processing*, pp. 583–9. New York, Wiley-Liss.

Herweijer, H., Stokdijk, W., and Visser, J. (1988) High-speed photodamager cell selection using bromodeoxyuridine/Hoechts 33342 photosensitized cell killing. *Cytometry*, **9**, 143–9.

Hiebert, R.D., Jett, J.H., and Salzman, G.C. (1981) Modular electronics for flow cytometry and sorting: the LACEL system. *Cytometry*, **1**, 337–41.

Juttner, C.A., To, L.B., Roberts, M.M., et al. (1992) Comparison of hematological recovery, toxicity and supportive care of autologous PBSC, autologous BM and allogeneic BM transplants. *International Journal of Cell Cloning*, **10**, 160.

Kessinger, A., Armitage, J.O., Smith, D.M., Landmark, J.D., Bierman, P.J., and Weisenberger, D.D. (1989) High-dose therapy and autologous peripheral blood stem cell transplantation for patients with lymphoma. *Blood*, **74**, 1260–5.

Law, P., Ishizawa, L., van de Ven, C., et al. (1993) Immunomagnetic positive selection and colony culture of CD34+ cells from blood. *Journal of Hematotherapy*, **2**, 247–50.

Lebkowski, J.S., Schain, L.R., Okrongly, D., Levinsky, R., Harvey, M., and Okarma, T.B. (1992) Rapid isolation of human CD34 hemopoietic stem cells: purging of human tumor cells. *Transplantation*, **53**, 1011–19.

Molineux, G., Migdalska, A., Szmitkowski, M., Zsebo, K., and Dexter, T.M. (1991) The effects on hematopoiesis of recombinant stem cell factor (ligand for c-kit) administered in vivo to mice either alone or in combination with granulocyte colony-stimulating factor. *Blood*, **78**, 961–5.

Molineux, G., Pojda, Z., Hampson, I.N., and Dexter, T.M. (1990) Transplantation potential of peripheral blood stem cells induced by granulocyte colony-stimulating factor. *Blood*, **76**, 2153.

Murray, L., Chen, B., Chen, S., et al. (1994) Analysis of human hematopoietic stem cell populations. *Blood Cells*, **20**, 364–70.

Murray, L., Chen, B., Galy, A., et al. (1995) Enrichment of human hematopoietic stem cell activity in the CD34$^+$Lin$^-$Thy-1$^+$ subpopulation from mobilized peripheral blood. *Blood*, **85**, 368–78.

Okarma, T.B. (1992) Stem cell selection for autologous bone marrow transplantation. *Seminars in Hematology*, **29**(Suppl. 1), 9–20.

Okarma, T., Lebkowski, J., Schain, L., et al. (1992) The AIS Cellector: a new technique for stem cell purification. In D.A. Worthington-White, A.P. Gee, and S. Gross (Eds.) *Advances in bone marrow purging and processing*, pp. 449–59. New York, Wiley-Liss.

Peters, D., Branscomb, E., Dean, P., et al. (1985) The LLNL high-speed sorter: design features, operational characteristics, and biological utility. *Cytometry*, **6**, 290–301.

Reading, C., Tricot, G., Dietz, I., et al. (1994) Evaluation of in vitro and in vivo assays of human hematopoietic stem cells. *Experimental Hematology*, **22**, 786.

Shpall, E.J., Jones, R.B., Franklin, W.A., et al. (1994) Transplantation of enriched CD34-positive autologous marrow into breast cancer patients following high-dose chemotherapy: influence of CD34+ peripheral blood progenitors and growth factors on engraftment. *Journal of Clinical Oncology*, **12**, 28–36.

Shpall, E.J., Jones, R.B., Franklin, W., et al. (1992) CD34+ marrow and/or peripheral blood progenitor cells (PBPCs) provide effective hematopoietic reconstitution of breast cancer patients following high-dose chemotherapy with autologous hematopoietic progenitor cell support. *Blood,* **80**(Suppl. 1), 24a.

Siena, S., Bregni, M., Brando, B., Ravagnani, F., Bonadonna, B., and Gianni, A.M. (1989) Circulation of CD34+ hematopoietic stem cells in the peripheral blood of high-dose cyclophosphamide-treated patients: enhancement by intravenous recombinant human granulocyte-macrophage colony-stimulating factor. *Blood,* **74**, 1905–14.

Spangrude, G.J. (1994) Biological and clinical aspects of hematopoietic stem cells. *Annual Review of Medicine,* **45**, 93–104.

Sutherland, D.R., Marsh, J.C.W., Davidson, J., Barker, M.A., Keating, A., and Mellors, A. (1992) Differential sensitivity of CD34 epitopes to cleavage by *Pasturella hemolytica* glycoprotease: implications for purification of CD34-positive progenitor cells. *Experimental Hematology,* **20**, 590.

Terstappen, L.W.M.M., Huang, S., and Picker, L.J. (1992) Flow cytometric assessment of human T-cell differentiation in thymus and bone marrow. *Blood,* **79**, 666.

To, L.B., Haylock, D.N., Thorp, D., et al. (1989) The optimization of collection of peripheral blood stem cells for autotransplantation in acute myeloid leukemia. *Bone Marrow Transplantation,* **4**, 41–47.

Tsukamoto, A., Chen, B., DiGiusto, D., et al. Phenotypic and functional analysis of hematopoietic stem cells in mouse and human. In: D. Levitt and R. Mertelsmann (Eds.) *Hematopoietic stem cells: biology and therapeutic applications,* New York: Marcel Dekker, Inc.; 1995:85–124.

Uchida, N., Aguila, H.L., Fleming, W.H., Jerabek, L., and Weissman, I.L. (1994) Rapid and sustained hematopoietic recovery in lethally irradiated mice transplanted with purified Thy-1.1^{lo} Lin$^-$ Sca-1$^+$ hematopoietic stem cells. *Blood,* **83**, 3758–79.

Uchida, N., Murray, L., Altenhofen, J., et al. (1993) Kinetic analysis and isolation of CD34+Thy-1+Lin- cells from mobilized peripheral blood of multiple myeloma patients. *Blood,* **82**, 84a.

Van den Engh, G., and Stokdijk, W. (1989) Parallel processing data acquisition system for multilaser flow cytometry and cell sorting. *Cytometry,* **10**, 282–93.

Watt, S.M., and Visser, J.W. (1992) Recent advances in the growth and isolation of primitive hematopoietic progenitor cells. *Cell Proliferation,* **25**, 263–97.

Yan, X.-Q., Briddell, R., Hartley, G., Stoney, G., Samal, B., and McNiece, I. (1994) Mobilization of long-term hematopoietic reconstituting cells in mice by the combination of stem cell factor plus granulocyte colony-stimulating factor. *Blood,* **84**, 795–9.

11

Hemopoietic Stem Cell Selection Using Monoclonal Antibodies

KAREN AUDITORE-HARGREAVES,
MONICA KRIEGER, SHELLY HEIMFELD, AND
RONALD J. BERENSON

In the autologous transplant setting, there are two primary reasons for stem-cell selection. The first is to reduce the tumor-cell burden in a marrow or leukapheresis product. Gene-marking studies have now shown conclusively that reinfusion of tumor cells can contribute to relapse (Brenner et al. 1993). The second reason is to reduce the infusional toxicities associated with transplant. These are related to the volume of dimethyl sulfoxide (DMSO) used to cryopreserve the bone marrow (BM) (Kligman 1965; Shlafer, Matheny, and Karow 1976; O'Donnell et al. 1981; Hameroff et al. 1983; Samoszuk, Reid, and Toy 1983; Davis et al. 1990; Stroncek et al. 1991; Styler et al. 1992), and to cellular debris arising from the failure of mature, nonengrafting cells to survive the freeze-thaw cycle (Fisch, Feigenbaum, and Bowas 1964; Smith et al. 1987; Pinski and Maloney 1990; Stroncek et al. 1991).

In the allogeneic transplant setting, the primary rationale for stem-cell selection is to reduce the incidence and severity of graft-versus-host disease (GVHD), mediated by T cells present in the graft that respond to histocompatibility differences between donor and patient. The pool of potential donors will be markedly expanded if it is demonstrated that GVHD can be prevented through stem-cell selection, without adversely affecting engraftment success.

Studies in mice have shown that hematologic recovery is optimal when both committed progenitor cells and more primitive, pluripotent stem cells are transplanted (Jones et al. 1989, 1990). The presumed reason is that committed progenitors are responsible for rapid, short-term recovery, while true stem cells are required for sustained recovery. What is necessary, then, for optimal treatment of the patient is a marker that identifies both populations of cells, but is not expressed on most malignant cells or on mature blood cells. Equally important is a method that enables rapid isolation of large quantities of stem cells and progenitor cells without compromising their biological activity.

At present, the best-studied marker for hemopoietic engrafting capacity is the CD34 antigen (Ag). CD34 is a 115-kDa type-I, integral membrane glycoprotein that marks both human stem cells and more committed progenitor cells (Civin and Loken 1987; Sutherland and Keating 1992; Civin and Gore 1993). Using an antibody (Ab) designated "12.8" that cross-reacts with the nonhuman primate homologue of CD34 (Andrews, Singer, and Bernstein 1986), Berenson and colleagues showed that the CD34$^+$ cell population in BM can restore trilineage hemopoiesis in lethally irradiated baboons (Berenson et al. 1988). These studies paved the way to clinical studies, some of which will be reviewed here.

■ CD34$^+$ CELL-SELECTION TECHNOLOGY

We developed a continuous-flow affinity chromatography system, called the CEPRATE Stem Cell Concentration System, for selection of CD34$^+$ cells from BM or peripheral blood (PB). In this system, a marrow buffy coat is incubated with biotinylated Ab to CD34. The resultant mixture is then perfused through a disposable column packed with approximately 120 mL avidin-coated polyacrylamide beads. CD34$^+$ cells are retained on the column by virtue of the high-affinity binding of biotin to avidin, while CD34$^-$ cells are washed away. The captured cells are then eluted by mechanically agitating the contents of the column with a magnetically driven stirring bar (Fig. 11.1). The system is computer controlled and is capable of processing up to 100 billion cells in as little as 2 hours.

The avidin-biotin interaction used to capture the CD34$^+$ cells in the CEPRATE SC system has an extremely high dissociation constant ($K_d = 10^{-15}$ M^{-1}), approaching the strength of a covalent bond. This high-affinity interaction has two important advantages for cell selection. First, the selection step can be performed under conditions of continuous medium flow through the column, which is believed to minimize nonspecific binding of cells to the beads. Second, mechanical agitation of the column bed results in disruptions of the bonds attaching the cells to the solid phase predominantly at the chain's weakest link, namely, between Ab and Ag, rather than between avidin and biotin. Hence, bound cells are eluted from the column largely free of Ab. No human anti–mouse Ab (HAMA) response has been seen in the more than 300 patients transplanted to date with CEPRATE-

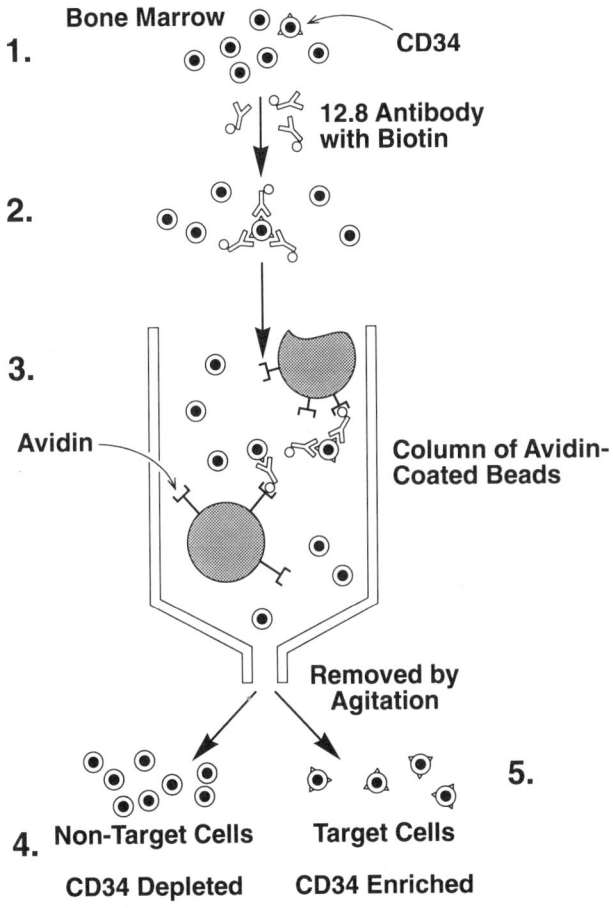

Figure 11.1 A buffy coat is prepared from bone marrow (step 1), and the resulting cell suspension is incubated with a biotinylated, mouse mAB to the CD34 Ag (step 2). The cell suspension is then passed through a column containing polyacrylamide beads to which avidin has been covalently attached (step 3). CD34$^+$ cells adhere to the beads via the biotinylated antibody with which they are labeled, while CD34$^-$ cells flow through the column without binding (step 4). The contents of the column are agitated with a magnetic stirring bar to release the bound CD34$^+$ cells from the beads, and these cells are washed out of the column and collected (step 5).

enriched CD34[+] cells (unpublished data). These results suggest that it will be possible to use immunoselected CD34[+] cells to provide hematologic support to patients undergoing multiple cycles of high-dose chemotherapy, without significant risk of their mounting an immune response to murine Ab used in the selection process.

After elution from the column, the CD34[+]-enriched cells can be stained with fluorescent-labeled anti-CD34 Ab, indicating that there is still immunoreactive Ag expressed at the cell surface. This may be important if the CD34 Ag plays a role in homing of cells to the BM.

■ AUTOLOGOUS TRANSPLANTATION OF CD34[+]-SELECTED CELLS

We have recently completed a prospective, randomized, multicenter phase III study in patients with advanced breast cancer, in which we compared the rate and pattern of hematologic recovery between patients transplanted with autologous CD34[+]-selected cells with patients transplanted with unselected marrow buffy coat (Shpall et al. 1993). The primary objectives of this study were to demonstrate that engraftment was equivalent in both groups and that the cardiovascular side effects of BM infusion were less in the group that received CD34[+]-selected cells.

Ninety-two eligible patients were randomized after BM harvest to receive either an infusion of unselected buffy coat or an infusion of CD34[+] cells. All patients received recombinant human granulocyte colony-stimulating factor (rHuG-CSF) 10 μg/kg/d following transplant. Engraftment, defined as absolute neutrophil count (ANC) above 0.5 x 10^9/L by day 20 following transplant, was equivalent in both groups in the study. Toxicity, as measured by specific cardiovascular endpoints, was significantly decreased in the CD34[+]-selected group (Shpall et al., manuscript in preparation).

Transplantation of stem and progenitor cells enriched from PB is an attractive alternative to bone-marrow transplantation (BMT). One to three leukapheresis collections can yield sufficient CD34[+] cells from mobilized PB for transplantation of an average 70-kg adult. As shown in Table 11.1, the number of CD34[+] cells obtained by leukapheresis varies, depending on the mobilization regimen used. In general, the combination of chemotherapy and growth-factor mobilization appears to be superior to rHuG-CSF alone. Of particular interest are the large yields of CD34[+] cells obtained by Schiller and Berenson, who used cyclophosphamide, rHuG-CSF, and prednisone to mobilize multiple myeloma (MM) patients. Presently, it is unclear whether this phenomenon is due to underlying patient differences, such as the

Table 11.1. CD34$^+$ Peripheral Blood Progenitor Cell Transplantation Trials[a]

Investigator (Site)	Disease	Mobilization (No. Aphereses)	CD34$^+$ Cells ($\times 10^6$/kg)	Days to Neutrophils >0.5$\times 10^9$/L	Days to Platelet Recovery
Shpall (Colorado) n=34	Breast	rHuG-CSF (3)	1.6 (0.4–3.9)	12 (10–14)	14 (10–156+)
Spitzer (St. Louis) n=6	Breast	rHuG-CSF (3)	1.3 (0.9–9.8)	10 (9–12)	10 (8–15)
Somlo (City of Hope) n=10	Breast	rHuG-CSF (3)	1.1 (0.3–3.9)	11 (8–17)	14 (6–20)
Brugger, Kanz (Freiberg) n=15	Breast, lung, lymphoma	VIP + rHuG-CSF (1)	2.2 (0.3–9.5)	12 (8–16)	15 (9–24)
Schiller, Berenson (UCLA) n=42	Multiple myeloma	Cy + Steroids + rHuG-CSF (2)	4.2 (1.2–23.3)	13 (11–15)	12 (9–52+)
Watts, Linch (London) n=4	Lymphoma	Cy + rHuG-CSF (1)	>1.0	13 (12–22)	14 (9–21)

[a]Results from five clinical sites in the United States and Europe using the CEPRATE SC to harvest CD34$^+$ PBPC from leukapheresis products. The table shows the principal investigators at each site, the disease for which transplantation is being performed, the mobilization regimen, the number of CD34$^+$ cells per kilogram, and the median days to neutrophil and platelet engraftment for each site. VIP = etoposide, Cy = cyclophosphamide.

extent of pretreatment, or to the inclusion of a steroid in the mobilization scheme.

Recent data suggest that hematologic recovery may be faster in patients transplanted with CD34[+]-selected peripheral blood progenitor cells (PBPC) than in patients transplanted with CD34[+]-selected cells derived from BM (Shpall et al. 1992; Heimfeld et al. 1993; Shpall et al. 1994b). Median time to neutrophil engraftment was approximately the same (10 to 11 days) in patients who received rHuG-CSF after transplant and either PB CD34[+] cells (seven patients) or BM CD34[+] cells (ten patients). Median time to platelet recovery, however, was significantly shorter in the cohort that received CD34[+] PBPC (10 days) versus the cohort that received BM CD34[+] cells (23 days) (Shpall et al. 1994b). This is consistent with the accelerated platelet recovery reported for unselected rHuG-CSF–mobilized PBPC compared with that of unselected BM (see Chapter 8).

A significant concern in autologous transplantation is the contamination of BM and PBPC harvests with tumor cells (Berendsen et al. 1988; Cote et al. 1988; Porro et al. 1988; Moss et al. 1990, 1991; Sharp et al. 1992; Ross et al. 1993). In at least one study, the level of contamination was reported to increase following mobilization of patients with cytotoxic drugs and rHuG-CSF (Brugger et al. 1994).

Wilbur Franklin and his colleagues at the University of Colorado devised an immunocytochemical method of detection for breast cancer cells in BM and PB that is sensitive to one tumor cell in 1 million (Shpall et al. 1994a). Using this assay, Franklin found that approximately 28% of BM specimens and 15% of PBPC collections from women with advanced breast cancer contain tumor cells. Among those patients with detectable tumor, the tumor burden was approximately ten times greater in BM than in PB. In these same patients, CD34[+] selection, using the CEPRATE SC, depleted tumor cells to less than the assay's limit of detection in 83% (10 of 12) of PBPC harvests and 19% (4 of 21) of BM harvests. Of chief importance, however, was the finding that disease-free survival was prolonged in those patients whose BM or PBPC harvests were successfully purged, versus those patients whose harvests still contained detectable tumor cells after CD34[+] selection (Shpall et al. 1994a).

■ ALLOGENEIC TRANSPLANTATION OF CD34[+]-SELECTED CELLS

Allogeneic BMT is generally regarded as the treatment of choice for most serious hematologic malignancies; however, its application is limited by the inability to transplant across a major histocompatibility complex (HC) barrier. When matched unrelated donors or mismatched related donors are used, there is a significant risk of graft failure (Anasetti et al. 1989) and of severe GVHD (Beatty et al. 1985, 1988, 1993; Anasetti et al. 1990). Depletion of T cells from the graft has been shown to reduce the risk of grade III/IV GVHD in several studies (Ash et al. 1990, 1991; Kernan et al. 1993).

Andrews et al. (1992) demonstrated in an animal model that selection of CD34[+] progenitor cells from BM results in a substantial degree of T-cell depletion without compromising engraftment. Five baboons received CD34[+]-selected allogeneic cells; each animal also received cyclosporine as prophylaxis for GVHD. All five animals showed cytogenetic evidence of engraftment. None of the animals developed serious GVHD, and two of the animals survived long term.

To date, 12 patients at three sites have been transplanted with CD34[+] cells selected using the CEPRATE SC system from donor BM or PB (unpublished data). As can be seen in Table 11.2, a median of 2.8 logs of T-cell depletion was obtained in these patients, regardless of the source of progenitor cells. Accordingly, the number of T cells infused into the patient is quite small, probably on the order of 10^5 cells/kg. It is too early yet to determine the incidence and severity of GVHD in these patients. Likewise, longer follow-up and additional patients will be required before conclusions can be drawn regarding engraftment, graft failure, and disease relapse.

Table 11.2. CD34[+] Cell and T-Cell Content After CD34[+] Selection of Donor Cells for Allogeneic Transplantation

	CD34[+] Cells		CD3[+] Cells		
CD34[+] Selected Cell Fraction	%	$\times 10^6$/kg	%	$\times 10^5$/kg	T-Cell (Log Depletion)
rHuG-CSF mobilized aphereses (total of 2) n=7	78 (68–79)	3.1 (1.6–5.6)	6 (4–13)	2.1 (1.2–7.2)	2.8 (2.5–3.2)
Bone marrow n=5	83 (77–88)	3.5 (1.0–6.5)	2 (1–2)	0.7 (0.2–0.8)	2.8 (2.5–3.5)

[a]PB and/or BM was collected from ten donors for CD34[+] selection and allotransplantation at three clinical sites (Vancouver General Hospital, University of Utah, and University of Rochester). The table shows the percentage and number of CD34[+] and CD3[+] (T) cells for seven donors who underwent leukapheresis twice, and for five donors who provided BM. Two of the BM donors also donated PB.

Elutriation is another possible method of T-cell depletion (Noga et al. 1986a, b). Unfortunately, the majority of CD34[+] progenitor cells elute in the lymphocyte-enriched small-cell fractions that are normally discarded in this procedure. Accordingly, hematologic recovery, especially of platelets, is typically delayed in patients receiving elutriated BM. In collaboration with Steven Noga and Richard Jones at Johns Hopkins University, we have studied the ability of the CEPRATE SC system to recover CD34[+] cells from the small-cell fractions obtained by BM elutriation (Noga et al. 1994b). The CD34[+]-selected cells are infused into the patient with the large-cell (T-depleted) fraction. Median time to hematologic recovery was shorter in patients receiving elutriated and CD34[+]-selected BM than in patients transplanted with unfractionated BM or elutriated, unsupplemented BM. Platelet recovery (defined as days to >50 $\times$ 10^9/L) was 24 days in the elutriated plus CD34[+]-selected group, versus 30 to 48 days in the latter two groups (Noga et al. 1994a).

■ EX VIVO STEM-CELL EXPANSION

The ability to select CD34[+] cells from BM or PB makes it feasible to expand these cells in culture. Previously, the presence of inhibitory accessory cells in BM or PB limited the degree of expansion in the progenitor compartment that could be attained ex vivo. Figure 11.2 shows that a higher degree of expansion, in terms of both total cell number and number of GM-CFC, is possible when CD34[+]-selected cells, rather than whole BM cells, are cultured ex vivo. There are also practical advantages to the use of CD34[+]-selected cells as the starting material for expansion, such as ease of handling and savings in the amount of medium and growth factors consumed by the culture.

We have found expansion to be optimal when stem-cell factor (SCF), interleukin-1α (IL-1α), IL-3, and IL-6 are included in the expansion medium (Fig. 11.3). We have also observed that cell density is a critical factor in the expansion of progenitor cells. Starting concentrations of CD34[+] cells at or below 10^4/mL are required for maximal expansion (data not shown). Using these conditions, we can obtain a 50- to 150-fold expansion of progenitor cells in 7 to 14 days of culture, without refeeding (Fei et al. 1994; Heimfeld et al. 1994).

Stem-cell expansion is of interest for a number of reasons. The most obvious is that it should be possible to achieve an engrafting dose of cells from a much smaller initial harvest. More importantly, however, transplantation of ex vivo–expanded cells may lead to faster hematologic recovery because of the higher content of committed progenitor cells in the graft. Mice transplanted with BM that was ex-

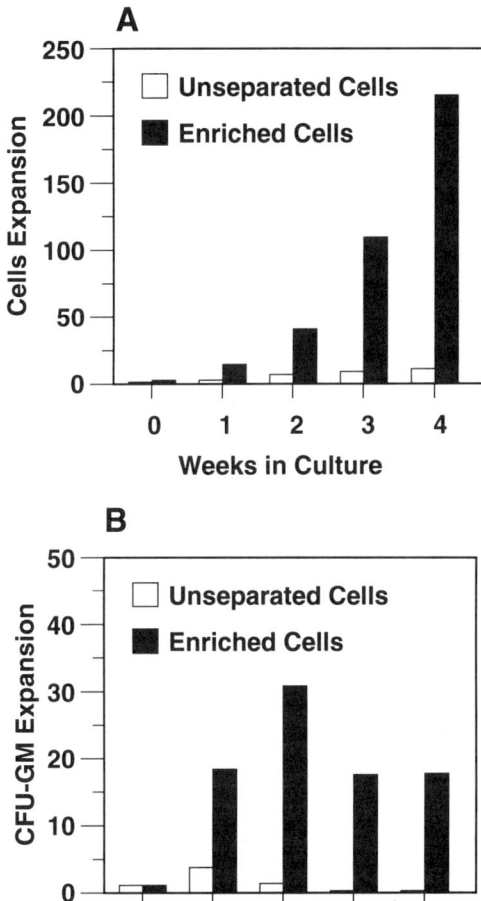

Figure 11.2 Comparison of unseparated BM with CD34$^+$ cells enriched from BM using the CEPRATE SC stem cell concentration system for ex vivo expansion potential. Panel *A* shows the increase in total cell numbers after 1 to 4 weeks in culture, while panel *B* shows the increase in CFU-GM. All cultures contained 10% human serum plus IL-1α, IL-3, IL-6, and SCF.

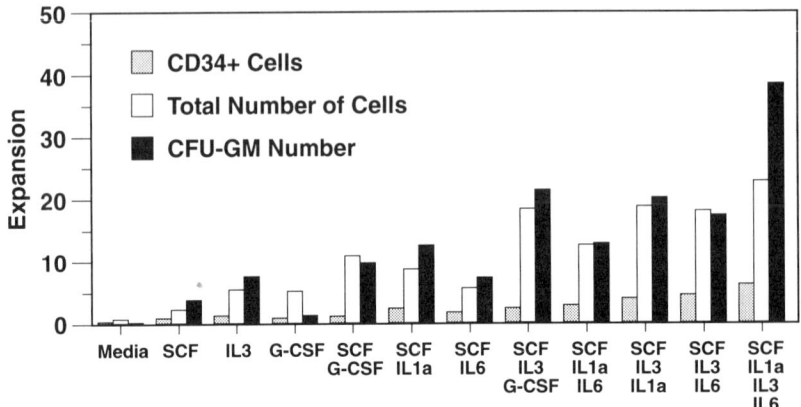

Figure 11.3 The effects of different cytokine combinations on increase in total cells, CD34$^+$ cells, and colony-forming unit–granulocyte-macrophage (CFU-GM) during ex vivo expansion of CD34$^+$-selected cells. All cultures were initiated with CD34$^+$ cells enriched from BM using the CEPRATE SC and contained 10% human serum, in addition to the growth factors listed.

panded ex vivo recovered PB counts more rapidly than animals transplanted with BM that had not been expanded, and fewer expanded cells were necessary for engraftment than unexpanded cells (Muench and Moore 1992).

Stem-cell expansion is also potentially important in gene therapy, both for the initial transfection and subsequently for the selection of transfected cells. Gene transfer using viral vectors occurs more readily in cells that are cycling than in noncycling cells. Even at high efficiencies of transfection, there will inevitably be some cells that have not taken up the gene. A posttransfection selection for those cells that have taken up the gene, followed by ex vivo expansion of this population, may improve the outcome of gene therapy by increasing the likelihood that the BM will be functionally repopulated with stem cells expressing the introduced gene.

■ SUMMARY

The ability to select CD34$^+$ stem cells from BM and PB represents a first step toward engineering the cellular composition of hemopoietic grafts. By judicious choice of markers, it is possible to selectively enrich the graft for one subset of cells and simultaneously deplete it of other subsets, such as T cells and tumor cells, without losing BM-repopulating activity. Thus, hemopoietic stem-cell (HSC) transplants are finding application in both the autologous and allogeneic settings, where tumor depletion and T-cell depletion, respectively, are important.

The exploitation of PBPC for transplant is likely to lead to an increase in the number of autologous procedures, as well as to a change in location where they are performed. Once exclusively the province of tertiary care centers, autologous transplants are now being done in community hospitals and may eventually be done in out-patient clinics. A key to making this transition smoothly will be a reduction in the complications associated with transplantation. Stem-cell selection will be important in reducing the volume of material to be transfused and, hence, the incidence and severity of infusional toxicity. Likewise, the potential to shorten engraftment times by using PBPC or ex vivo–expanded cells will facilitate this transition.

REFERENCES

Anasetti, C., Amos, D., Beatty, P.G., et al. (1989) Effect of HLA compatibility on engraftment of bone marrow transplants in patients with leukemia or lymphoma. *New England Journal of Medicine*, **320**, 197–204.

Anasetti, C., Beatty, P.G., Storb, R., et al. (1990) Effect of HLA incompatibility on graft versus host disease, relapse, and survival after marrow transplantation for patients with leukemia or lymphoma. *Human Immunology*, **29**, 79–91.

Andrews, R.G., Bryant, E.M., Bartelmez, S.H., et al. (1992) CD34$^+$ marrow cells, devoid of T and B lymphocytes, reconstitute stable lymphopoiesis and myelopoiesis in lethally irradiated allogeneic baboons. *Blood*, **80**, 1693–1701.

Andrews, R.G., Singer, J.W., and Bernstein, I.D. (1986) Monoclonal antibody 12-8 recognizes a 115-kd molecule present on both unipotent and multipotent hemopoietic colony-forming cells and their precursors. *Blood*, **67**, 842–5.

Ash, R.C., Casper, J.T., Chitambar, C.R., et al. (1990) Successful allogeneic transplantation of T-cell depleted bone marrow from closely HLA-matched unrelated donors. *New England Journal of Medicine*, **322**, 485–94.

Ash, R.C., Horowitz, M.M., Gale, R.P., et al. (1991) Bone marrow transplantation from related donors other than HLA-identical siblings: effect of T cell depletion. *Bone Marrow Transplantation*, **7**, 443–52.

Beatty, P.G., Anasetti, C., Hansen, J.A., et al. (1993) Marrow transplantation from unrelated donors for treatment of hematologic malignancies: effect of mismatching for one HLA locus. *Blood*, **81**, 249–53.

Beatty, P.G., Clift, R.A., Mickelson, E.M., et al. (1985) Marrow transplantation from related donors other than HLA-identical siblings. *New England Journal of Medicine*, **313**, 765–71.

Beatty, P.G., Hansen, J.A., Longton, G.M., et al. (1988) Marrow transplantation from HLA-matched unrelated donors for treatment of hematologic malignancies. *Transplantation*, **45**, 714–18.

Berendsen, H.H., De Leij, L., Postmus, P.E., Ter Haar, J.G., Poppmea, S., and The, H.H. (1988) Detection of small cell lung cancer metastases in bone marrow aspirates using monoclonal antibody directed against neuroendocrine differentation antigen. *Journal of Clinical Pathology*, **41**, 273–6.

Berenson, R.J., Andrews, R.G., Bensinger, W.I., et al. (1988) Antigen CD34$^+$ marrow cells engraft lethally irradiated baboons. *Journal of Clinical Investigation*, **81**, 951–5.

Brenner, M.K., Rill, D.R., Moen, R.C., et al. (1993) Gene marking to trace origin of relapse after autologous bone marrow transplantation. *Lancet*, **341**, 85–6.

Brugger, W., Bross, K.J., Glatt, M., Weber, F., Mertelsmann, R., and Kanz, L. (1994) Mobilization of tumor cells and hemopoietic progenitor cells into peripheral blood of patients with solid tumors. *Blood*, **83**, 636–40.

Civin, C.I., and Gore, S.D. (1993) Antigenic analysis of hematopoiesis: a review. *Journal of Hematotherapy*, **2**, 137–44.

Civin, C.I., and Loken, M.R. (1987) Cell surface antigens on human marrow cells: dissection of hematopoietic development using monoclonal antibodies and multiparameter flow cytometry. *International Journal of Cell Cloning*, **5**, 267–88.

Cote, R.J., Rosen, P.P., Hakes, T.B., et al. (1988) Monoclonal antibodies detect occult breast carcinoma metastases in the bone marrow of patients with early stage disease. *American Journal of Surgical Pathology*, **12**, 333–40.

Davis, J.M., Rowley, S.D., Braine, H.G., et al. (1990) Clinical toxicity of cryopreserved bone marrow graft infusion. *Blood*, **75**, 781–6.

Fei, R., Heimfeld, S., Xu, Z., et al. (1994) Ex-vivo expansion of human CD34$^+$ hematopoietic progenitor cells. *Experimental Hematology*, **22**, 726.

Fisch, C., Feigenbaum, H., and Bowas, J.A. (1964) Non-paroxysmal A-V nodal tachycardia due to potassium. *American Journal of Cardiology*, **14**, 357–61.

Hameroff, S.R., Otto, C.W., Kanel, J., et al. (1983) Acute cardiovascular effects of dimethylsulfoxide. *Annals of the New York Academy of Sciences*, **411**, 94–9.

Heimfeld, S., Fei, R., Xu, Z., et al. (1994) Ex vivo expansion of human bone marrow cord blood CD34$^+$ progenitor cells. *British Journal of Haematology*, **87**, 97.

Heimfeld, S., Shpall, E.J., Jones, R.B., and Berenson, R.J. (1993) Clinical transplantation of CD34$^+$ cells. *Experimental Hematology*, **21**, 1066.

Jones, R.J., Celano, P., Sharkis, S.J., and Sensenbrenner, L.L. (1989) Two phases of engraftment established by serial bone marrow transplantation in mice. *Blood*, **73**, 397–401.

Jones, R.J., Wagner, J.E., Celano, P., Zicha, M.S., and Sharkis, S.J. (1990) Separation of pluripotent haematopoietic stem cells from spleen colony forming cells. *Nature*, **347**, 188–9.

Kernan, N.A., Bartsch, G., Ash, R.C., et al. (1993) Analysis of 462 unrelated marrow transplants facilitated by the National Marrow Donor Program. *New England Journal of Medicine*, **328**, 593–602.

Kligman, A. (1965) Topical pharmacology and toxicology of dimethylsulfoxide – part 1. *Journal of the American Medical Association*, **193**, 151–5.

Moss, T.J., Reynolds, C.P., Reisfeld, R.A., et al. (1991) Prognostic value of immunocytologic detection of bone marrow metastases in neuroblastoma. *New England Journal of Medicine*, **324**, 219–26.

Moss, T.J., Sanders, D.G., Lasky, L.D., and Bostrom, B. (1990) Contamination of peripheral blood stem cell harvests by circulating neuroblastoma cells. *Blood*, **76**, 1879–83.

Muench, M.O., and Moore, M.A.S. (1992) Accelerated recovery of peripheral blood cell counts in mice transplanted with in vitro cytokine-expanded hematopoietic progenitors. *Experimental Hematology*, **20**, 611–18.

Noga, S.J., Cremo, C.A., Duff, S.C., et al. (1986a) Large scale separation of human bone marrow by counterflow centrifugation elutriation. *Journal of Immunological Methods*, **92**, 211–18.

Noga, S.J., Davis, J.M., Berenson, R.J., et al. (1994a) Graft engineering III: CD34$^+$ augmentation/elutriation (A/E) allows reduction in GVHD prophylaxis without affecting engraftment. *Blood*, **84**, 346a.

Noga, S.J., Davis, J., Schepers, K., Eby, L., and Berenson, R.J. (1994b) The clinical use of elutriation and positive stem cell selection columns to engineer the lymphocyte and stem cell composition of the allograft. *Progress in Clinical and Biological Research*, **398**, 317–24.

Noga, S.J., Donnenberg, A.D., Schwartz, C.L., Strauss, L.C., Civin, C.I., and Santos, G.W. (1986b) Development of a simplified counterflow centrifugation elutriation procedure for depletion of lymphocytes from human bone marrow. *Transplantation*, **41**, 220–9.

O'Donnell, J.R., Burnett, A.K., Sheehan, T., et al. (1981) Safety of dimethylsulfoxide. *Lancet*, **1**, 498.

Pinski, S.L., and Maloney, J.D. (1990) Adenosine: a new drug for acute termination of supraventricular tachycardia. *Cleveland Clinic Journal of Medicine*, **57**, 383–8.

Porro, B., Menard, S., Tagliabue, E., et al. (1988) Monoclonal antibody detection of carcinoma cells in bone marrow biopsy specimens from breast cancer patients. *Cancer*, **61**, 2407–11.

Ross, A.A., Cooper, B.W., Lazarus, H.M., et al. (1993) Detection and viability of tumor cells in peripheral blood stem cell collections from breast cancer patients using immunocytochemical and clonogenic assay techniques. *Blood*, **82**, 2605–10.

Samoszuk, M., Reid, M., and Toy, P. (1983) Intravenous dimethylsulfoxide therapy causes severe hemolysis mimicking a hemolytic transfusion reaction. *Transfusion*, **23**, 405.

Sharp, J.G., Kessinger, A., Vaughan, W.P., et al. (1992) Detection and clinical significance of minimal tumor cell contamination of peripheral stem cell harvests. *International Journal of Cell Cloning*, **10**, 92.

Shlafer, M., Matheny, J.L., and Karow, A.M. (1976) Cardiac chronotropic mechanisms of dimethylsulfoxide: inhibition of acetylcholinesterase and antagonism of negative chronotropy by atropine. *Archives Internationales de Pharmacodynamie et de Therapie*, **221**, 21–31.

Shpall, E.J., Ball, E.D., Champlin, R.E., et al. (1993) A prospective randomized phase III study using the CEPRATE SC stem cell concentrator to isolate CD34$^+$ hematopoietic progenitors for autologous marrow transplantation after high dose chemotherapy. *Blood*, **82**(Suppl.), 83.

Shpall, E.J., Franklin, W.A., Jones, R.B., et al. (1994a) Transplantation of CD34 (+) marrow and/or peripheral blood progenitor cells (PBPCs) into breast cancer patients following high-dose chemotherapy. *Blood*, **84**, 1571a.

Shpall, E.J., Jones, R.B., Franklin, W., et al. (1992) CD34$^+$ marrow and/or peripheral blood progenitor cells (PBPCs) provide effective hematopoietic reconstitution of breast cancer patients following high-dose chemotherapy with autologous hematopoietic progenitor cell support. *Blood*, **80**(Suppl.), 24.

Shpall, E.J., Jones, R.B., Franklin, W.A., et al. (1994b) Transplantation of enriched CD34 positive autologous marrow into breast cancer patients following high-dose chemotherapy: influence of CD34$^+$ peripheral blood progenitors and growth factors on engraftment. *Journal of Clinical Oncology*, **12**, 28–36.

Smith, D.M., Weisenburger, D.D., Bierman, P., et al. (1987) Acute renal failure associated with autologous bone marrow transplantation. *Bone Marrow Transplantation*, **2**, 195–201.

Stroncek, D.F., Fautsch, S.K., Lasky, L.C., Hurd, D.D., Ramsay, N.K., and McCullough, J. (1991) Adverse reactions in patients transfused with cryopreserved marrow. *Transfusion*, **31**, 521–6.

Styler, M.J., Topolsky, D.L., Crilley, P.A., et al. (1992) Transient high grade heart block following autologous bone marrow infusion. *Bone Marrow Transplantation*, **10**, 435–8.

Sutherland, D.R., and Keating, A. (1992) The CD34 antigen: structure, biology, and potential clinical applications. *Journal of Hematotherapy*, **1**, 115–29.

12
Magnetic Approaches to Cell Separation

STEFAN MILTENYI

Magnetic cell sorting has recently developed into an increasingly powerful method for the isolation of defined cell populations from complex mixtures of cells such as peripheral blood (PB) or bone marrow (BM). With magnetic cell sorting, large numbers of cells can be processed with a rather simple technology. Its increasing selectivity and other capabilities make this technique an ideal tool for the isolation of cells for cellular therapy.

Cells do not have magnetic properties, except for very minor diamagnetism because of their water content. By coupling a magnetic label to specific cell-surface molecules, cells expressing this marker can be physically separated using magnetic forces.

■ DIFFERENT APPROACHES TO MAGNETIC CELL SEPARATION

A variety of magnetic cell-separation methods have been described (Molday, Yen, and Rembaum 1977; Antoine et al. 1978; Owen and Moore 1981; Owen and Lindsay 1983; Molday and Molday 1984; Kemshead and Ugelstad 1985; Muller-Ruchholz et al. 1987; Owen 1989; Miltenyi et al. 1990). Some of the systems are commercially available or have been used in clinical trials. The major differences between the currently described magnetic cell-separation methods are the composition and size of the magnetic particles used for labeling the cells and the concept of magnetic separation.

Magnetic cell-sorting methods separate cells according to the presence or absence of cell-surface molecules recognized by monoclonal antibodies (mAB). Since most cell types in multicellular organisms perform specialized functions, they express specific "tools" on their plasma membranes. Many of these cell-surface molecules were found by raising mAB against the cells, making it possible to identify discrete cell populations (Kohler and Milstein 1975). The specificity and affinity of antibodies (Ab) used is one of the most important variables for magnetic cell sorting.

In the first step of a magnetic cell-separation procedure, magnetic particles are coupled to the target cells by Ab that are immobilized on the beads. This process is typically driven by diffusion.

The degree and specificity of the labeling is dependent on the Ab, its conjugation, the biophysical surface properties of the particles, temperature, time, media, and other factors. For most of the commercial systems, these variables have been defined and optimized.

Large magnetic particles (diameter >0.5 μm) require more time for coupling to the target cells and offer more area for nonspecific binding on their surface compared with small ones. Temperature and media must be controlled to avoid endocytosis of the particles by phagocytic cells. Depending upon the size and density of the particles, the cell suspension must be agitated to avoid settling of the beads. After coupling, cells labeled with large particles can be easily separated from unlabeled cells by a simple permanent magnet. This can be done in a test tube or in a blood bag. By using the Dynal system, high depletion rates were demonstrated (Manyonda, Soltys, and Hay 1992). Large beads have been used clinically for the purging of neuroblastoma (Kemshead and Ugelstad 1985) and leukemia cells (Trickett et al. 1991) or for the removal of T cells (Knobloch et al. 1990) from BM for autologous and allogenic transplantation. Depletion rates of 4 to 5 logs have been described (Wang et al. 1993).

For positive cell selection using large particles, the cell-bound particles must be removed to avoid damage to the cell. Various strategies to release the magnetic particles from cells have been described and commercialized. The most elegant approach is the use of anti-F(ab)$_2$ Ab to cleave the Ab from the antigen (Ag). This approach leaves the cells unlabeled; however, a compromise between efficient binding of the particles to the cells and the efficiency of their removal must be made. An indirect system using Desthiobiotin-coupled primary Ab and anti-biotin beads that can be released using free biotin has been described.

For specific cell-surface molecules, especially the CD34 molecule on hemopoietic progenitor cells, bound particles can be released using chymopapain (Civin et al. 1990; Strauss et al. 1991) or glycoproteases (Sutherland et al. 1992a, b), which cleave parts of the CD34 molecule from the selected cells. A variety of other molecules are destroyed by the enzymatic cleavage, which limits analysis or separation for other variables.

Most small-bead approaches to magnetic cell sorting use colloidal-sized particles with a diameter between 10 and 150 nm. Only particles stabilized with protein (albumin) (Owen 1989) and polysaccharide (dextran) (Abt et al. 1989) have found practical application. The characteristics of the magnetic cell-sorting (MACS) system, using 60-nm, dextran-coated magnetic particles will be described in this chapter.

The magnetic material enclosed in most magnetic particles for magnetic cell separation is superparamagnetic iron oxide. Besides iron oxide, chromium oxide, colloidal cobalt, or other ferrites such as mixed iron manganese oxides have been suggested, but are not currently used. Superparamagnetism means that in a magnetic field the particles magnetize strongly like a ferromagnetic substance, but have no remaining magnetic moment when the magnetic field is removed. Particles with a residual magnetic moment would clump together quickly. Superparamagnetism occurs in small ferromagnetic microcrystals (<20 nm in diameter) that are too small to have a defined magnetic orientation.

In a magnetic particle, many superparamagnetic microcrystal materials are encapsulated to form one magnetic particle. Polymers, such as polystyrene, latex, polysilane, and alginate, as well as polysaccharides and proteins, have been used, whereas the organic component serves as a link between the magnetic material and the Ab.

■ THE MACS CELL-SORTING SYSTEM

The concept of polysaccharide-stabilized iron oxide and high-gradient separation was originally described by Molday and Molday (1984), then improved to a laboratory system by Miltenyi et al. (1990).

The MACS system uses colloidal-sized superparamagnetic particles made of dextran and iron oxide. Several iron oxide microcrystals are bound together to form a cluster approximately 60 nm in diameter. Ab directed against cell-surface molecules, immunoglobulin subclasses, or haptens are bound covalently to the polysaccharide matrix. The resulting particles have characteristics of "magnetic Ab" (i.e., they form a stable solution and have a fast binding reaction).

For magnetic cell labeling, the cell mixture is incubated with the particles of appropriate specificity. Alternatively, cells are first coupled to a primary Ab; unbound excess Ab is removed by washing, and the cells are labeled using indirect magnetic particles recognizing the primary Ab. Some mAB are not suitable for direct magnetic labeling because of insufficient affinity, slow binding kinetics, or steric hindrance. By using the indirect approach, the cellular epitope is transformed into a secondary one that can be recognized using a high-affinity secondary labeling system. Indirect labeling usually works well for most primary Ab.

The amount of magnetic material bound to the cells is very small because of the small volume of the particles. Therefore, high-gradient magnetic fields are needed to separate cells labeled with the small-sized MACS particles. High-gradient magnetic fields can be generated in columns filled with fine ferromagnetic wires or particles. When magnetized in an external magnetic field, the column acts as a filter for magnetic particles. Magnetically labeled cells are retained, whereas those cells that are not labeled flow through. Because of the small dimensions of the magnetic filter elements, the forces induced at the surface are several thousand times stronger compared with the magnetic forces of a macroscopic magnet. To avoid potential damage to the cells, the iron matrix is coated by a thin plastic polymer layer. The cells retained in the column are released and can be removed from the matrix by removing the external magnetic field. The matrix is designed to have an extremely low, nonspecific retention rate for unlabeled material that is important for high purity of positively isolated cells.

Depending upon the total number of cells to be processed and separated, a smaller or larger matrix may be used for separation. In a laboratory-sized unit, the sample and the washing buffers are applied manually to the separation column. In a large-scale separation device, the process is performed automatically in a closed fluid system by a computer-controlled separation unit. The processing capacity ranges from a few hundred to several 10^{10} cells. The separation process takes a few minutes for a small-scale separation, and as long as 30 minutes for a large scale separation with multiple washing cycles.

Many different cell types can be separated to high purity using the technique. Typically, the enrichment factors (500 to several 10,000) or magnetic Ab cell separation allow large populations, such as CD4, CD8, T cells, and B cells in PB, to be separated to greater than 99.9% purity. Even small cell fractions such as CD34 cells in PB can be enriched from less than 0.1% to a final purity of 80% to 95%.

Alternatively, the target cells can be isolated by depletion of the unwanted cells. A cocktail of Ab against the unwanted cells is combined with an indirect magnetic labeling system followed by a depletion. The efficiency of the depletion step is dependent on the number of antigens on the labeled cells and can be up to several 10,000-fold. The advantage of this approach is that the target cells remain unlabeled in the separation process; however, for the isolation of small cell populations from complex mixtures the purity of the isolated cells is often limited by the availability of Ab against all unwanted cells.

The recovery of the target cells in the separation process is very high (>95%) if the cells are sufficiently labeled with the magnetic material. The losses of cells accrue in the washing steps of the staining procedure, and losses can add up significantly during the process.

The use of very small magnetic particles results in several unique features of the MACS separation process. The small surface per particle minimizes unspecific binding and allows the efficient isolation of rare cells. The particles form a stable colloidal solution that can be sterile filtrated and shows a fast binding to the target cells. Particles bound to the cell do not change its optical properties, the separation process can be screened using flow cytometry. Positively selected cells with bound particles have been used in cellular assays, differentiation, and in cell transfer studies showing minimal effects to the selected cells; however, depending on the Ab and the target-surface molecule, the functional status of the cell can be influenced. Polysaccharide-stabilized iron oxide has been used since 1960 for the treatment of iron deficiencies (Groden, Whitelaw, and Will 1968; Slade and Iosefa 1968) and recently as magnetic contrast agents. The particles used for cell separation have a similar composition, but carry a magnetic crystal structure of iron oxide. Particles injected into the bloodstream have been shown to be taken up and degraded by the endorecticular system of the liver and BM.

For certain applications, removal of tumor cells or T cells is desirable. Depending upon the number of target molecules on the cell surface, the undesirable cells can be depleted by many orders of magnitude.

■ MAGNETIC MULTIPARAMETER CELL SORTING

Often, target-cell populations are defined by multiple cell-surface markers. A cocktail of magnetic Ab to different markers can be used to deplete several cell types simultaneously or a depletion step may be followed by a positive selection. Examples are the isolation of $CD5^+$ B cells using a $CD3^+$ T-cell depletion followed by a $CD5^+$ selection. If the cells of interest are defined by multiple positive markers, a positive selection can be done. We have developed a fast release system to allow the combination of positive-selection steps. An enzyme is used to cleave the magnetic particle from the cell. Because the specificity of the enzyme is unique to the magnetic particle, the cell-surface molecules are not modified by the process. Release of the beads takes approximately 2 minutes. This concept is useful for the depletion of cells after and positive-selection (e.g., tumor removal from purified CD34 cells).

■ SORTING OF CELLS ACCORDING TO SECRETED MOLECULES

To date, the magnetic separation of cells has been limited to cell-surface markers. We have developed an experimental system to label and separate cells according to molecules secreted by the cell. Usually, once a molecule is secreted by a cell, it cannot be picked up by the cell again. By coupling a product-specific catching matrix on the cell-surface and deleted from cell-surface molecules, molecules secreted by the cell can be trapped at the cell surface. A high-viscosity medium around the cells prevents the cells from taking up molecules secreted by other cells. This system is in the development stage presently.

■ SUMMARY

In the past, parallel sorting methods based on binding of cells to macroscopic immunoaffinity surfaces (i.e., panning, rosetting with erythrocytes, or affinity columns), were the main tools for cell separation. These methods have low specificity. Fluorescence-activated cell sorting (FACS), including the currently available high-speed instruments, have a capacity too low for the large cell numbers needed for cellular therapy. Furthermore, such cell sorters are difficult to handle in clinical settings. Magnetic cell sorting started its development with large magnetic particles that have similar properties as macroscopic immunoaffinity surfaces, but, nevertheless, they have been widely used for depletion of cells from clinical material. For isolation of rare cell populations, a certain level of nonspecificity due to cells interacting with large bead surfaces sets the limit. Additionally, cells can be trapped mechanically in the separation process because beads aggregate during the magnetic separation.

Magnetic separation systems based on colloidal-sized particles and high-gradient separation have additional advantages in specificity, ease of operation, and speed of use. This might be of importance when cells must be purified to very high purity (e.g., isolation of hemopoietic progenitor cells for cancer patients). Positive isolation systems based on the magnetic Ab microparticle approach are entering clinical trials in 1995.

Magnetic cell sorting can isolate or deplete target cells more than 10,000-fold. By using multiparameter magnetic cell sorting, even higher specificity and efficiency can be reached.

REFERENCES

Abt, H., Emmerich, M., Miltenyi, S., Radbruch, A., and Tesch, H. (1989) CD20 positive human B lymphocytes separated with the magnetic cell sorter (MACS) can be induced to proliferation and antibody secretion in vitro. *Journal of Immunological Methods*, **125**, 19–28.

Antoine, J.C., Ternyck, T., Rodrigot, M., and Avrameas S. (1978) Lymphoid fractionation on magnetic polyacrylamide agarose beads. *Immunochemistry*, **15**, 443.

Civin, C.I., Strauss, L.C., Fackler, M.J., Trischmann, T.M., Wiley, J.M., and Loken, M.R. (1990) Positive stem cell selection–basic science. *Progress in Clinical and Biological Research*, **333**, 387–401.

Groden, B.M., Whitelaw, J., and Will, G. (1968) The treatment of iron-deficiency anaemia by iron-dextran infusion, with special reference to the effect on blood-grouping, coagulation, sedimentation and haemolysis. *Postgraduate Medical Journal*, **44**, 433–7.

Kemshead, J.T., and Ugelstad, J. (1985) Magnetic separation techniques: their application to medicine. *Molecular and Cellular Biochemistry*, **67**, 11–8.

Knobloch, C., Spadinger, U., Rueber, E., and Friedrich, W. (1990) T cell depletion from human bone marrow using magnetic beads. *Bone Marrow Transplantation*, **6**, 21–4.

Kohler, G., and Milstein, C. (1975) Continuous cultures of fused cells secreting antibody of predefined specificity. *Nature*, **256**, 495–7.

Manyonda, I.T., Soltys, A.J., and Hay, F.C. (1992) A critical evaluation of the magnetic cell sorter and its use in the positive and negative selection of CD45RO+ cells. *Journal of Immunological Methods*, **149**, 1–10.

Miltenyi, S., Muller, W., Weichel, W., and Radbruch, A. (1990) High gradient magnetic cell separation with MACS. *Cytometry*, **11**, 231–8.

Molday, R.S., and Molday, L.L. (1984) Separation of cells labeled with immunospecific iron dextran microspheres using high gradient magnetic chromatography. *FEBS Letters*, **170**, 232–8.

Molday, R.S., Yen, S.P., and Rembaum, A. (1977) Application of magnetic microspheres in labelling and separation of cells. *Nature*, **268**, 437–40.

Muller-Ruchholtz, W., Leyhausen, G., Petersen, P., Schubert, G., and Ulrichs, K. (1987) A simple methodological principle for large scale extraction and purification of collagenase-digested islets. *Transplantation Proceedings*, **19**, 911–5.

Owen, C.S. (1989) Magnetic cell sorting using colloidal protein-magnetite. *Journal of Immunogenetics*, **16**, 117–23.

Owen, C.S., and Lindsay, J.G. (1983) Ferritin as a label for high-gradient magnetic separation. *Biophysical Journal*, **42**, 145–50.

Owen, C.S., and Moore, E. (1981) High gradient magnetic separation of rosette-forming cells. *Cell Biophysics*, **3**, 141–53.

Slade, I.H., and Iosefa, R.N. (1968) Intravenous iron-dextran (Imferon) in the treatment of iron deficiency anemia. *Journal of the Medical Association of Georgia*, **57**, 137–9.

Strauss, L.C., Trischmann, T.M., Rowley, S.D., Wiley, J.M., and Civin, C.I. (1991) Selection of normal human hematopoietic stem cells for bone marrow transplantation using immunomagnetic microspheres and CD34 antibody. *American Journal of Pediatric Hematology and Onology*, **13**, 217–21.

Sutherland, D.R., Abdullah, K.M., Cyopick, P., and Mellors, A. (1992a) Cleavage of the cell-surface O-sialoglycoproteins CD34, CD43, CD44, and

CD45 by a novel glycoprotease from *Pasteurella haemolytica*. *Journal of Immunology*, **148**, 1458–64.

Sutherland, D.R., Marsh, J.C., Davidson, J., Baker, M.A., Keating, A., and Mellors, A. (1992b) Differential sensitivity of CD34 epitopes to cleavage by *Pasteurella haemolytica* glycoprotease: implications for purification of CD34-positive progenitorcells. *Experimental Hematology*, **20**, 590–9.

Trickett, A.E., Ford, D.J., Lam Po Tang, P.R., and Vowels, M.R. (1991) Immunomagnetic bone marrow purging of common acute lymphoblastic leukemia cells: suitability of BioMag particles. *Bone Marrow Transplantation*, **7**, 199–203.

13

Growth Factors and Ex Vivo Expansion of Hemopoietic Progenitor Cells

DAVID HAYLOCK, PAUL SIMMONS, LUEN BIK TO, AND CHRISTOPHER JUTTNER

The availability of a growing number of recombinant human hemopoietic growth factors (HGF) for clinical use has encouraged the development of novel and fundamentally different approaches to the manipulation of hemopoiesis. Initial HGF studies concentrated on their direct use in patients to ameliorate neutropenia after cancer chemotherapy or high-dose therapy and hemopoietic cell transplantation, or in patients with inherent cytopenic states such as hereditary neutropenia and aplastic anemia. Subsequent studies examined the role of growth factors in mobilization of hemopoietic stem cells (HSC) and progenitor cells into the circulation, both with and without chemotherapy (Gianni et al. 1989; Sheridan et al. 1992), and have demonstrated that growth factors improve mobilization, allowing the rapid hemopoietic reconstitution seen after blood-cell transplantation (BCT) to become the norm. It is predicted that BCT will ultimately replace bone-marrow transplantation (BMT) completely (Goldman 1994).

The increasing use of optimized BCT has shown that the fastest hemopoietic rescue is associated with an obligate period of neutropenia and thrombocytopenia lasting 8 to 9 days following transplant (To et al. 1992). This period is not further shortened by using massively increased doses of mobilized blood cells or by the addition of presently available HGF following transplantation. These surprising findings stimulated us to consider why there is not further shortening of neutropenia and we concluded that an optimally mobilized blood cell graft lacked the cells capable of producing progeny within 3 to 8 days of infusion. This suggested that such cells were either not present in the BC collection or that they failed to survive cryopreservation. Preliminary anecdotal data from allogeneic transplants using mobilized blood cells that have not been cryopreserved suggest that recovery may occur earlier than 8 to 9 days, although there are not authoritative data available.

This review focuses on studies aimed at ex vivo manipulation of hemopoietic stem and progenitor cells in a stroma-free liquid culture system using combinations of HGF to produce an expanded and matured hemopoietic cell population, potentially abrogating neutropenia and thrombocytopenia and allowing high-dose therapy (HDT) and hemopoietic transplantation to become an outpatient procedure. This will increase safety and reduce costs in the same way that either the addition of mobilized blood cells to BMT or their use alone has reduced costs and increased safety of hemopoietic cell transplants; however, the morbidity and mortality of BCT is now so low that it is uncertain whether a further major impact on mortality can be achieved, at least in autologous transplantation. In allogeneic transplantation, particularly using volunteer unrelated donors where morbidity and mortality remain high, it is likely that expanded and matured cells will have a major impact. There are other important potential applications for ex vivo manipulation beyond the abrogation of cytopenias (Table 13.1).

There is little evidence that lymphocyte expansion from HSC is possible, although interleukin-2 (IL-2) can generate lymphocyte-activated killer (LAK) cells from lymphocytes, and this has been used widely in immunotherapy. A major and important question relates to the true HSC, the most primitive and pluripotent cell postulated to exist. If this cell is manipulated to enter the cell cycle, is it possible that cycling can occur without irrevocable commitment to differentiation and maturation? In other words, is the concept of expansion of true primitive pluripotent HSC valid? There are no data available to support this hypothesis. There are limited data suggesting that relatively primitive HSC such as long-term culture-initiating cell (LTC-IC) can be maintained or even expanded by currently used manipulations. The field lacks assays for these true primitive cells.

The application of ex vivo manipulation in human systems clearly carries important regulatory considerations, and the guidelines offered by the U.S. Food and Drug Administration (FDA) and the National Institutes of Health (NIH) in 1993 are important reading for anyone entering the field (Kessler et al. 1993). The use of animal protein other than autologous plasma in culture systems requires careful consideration. Our current studies suggest that defined media, excluding animal protein, can produce results equivalent to the most optimized media containing fetal calf serum and bovine serum albumin. The inclusion or exclusion of stroma and other supporting

Table 13.1. Ex Vivo Expansion: Applications

	Aim	Application
1.	Post progenitor expansion/maturation	Abrogate neutropenia/thrombocytopenia after anticancer therapy
2.	Lymphocyte expansion/maturation	Adoptive immunotherapy in cancer Immunodeficiency (e.g., AIDS, CLL) Viral infections
3.	Monocyte/macrophage expansion/maturation	Deep fungal/bacterial infections
4.	Red cell expansion/maturation	Autologous red cell transfusion
5.	Neutrophil expansion	Chronic neutropenia Support anticancer therapy
6.	Platelet expansion	Amegakaryocytic thrombocytopenia Support anticancer therapy
7.	True "stem-cell" expansion *without* maturation	Transplant with minimal harvested numbers of BM or BC After purging techniques that deplete stem cells (e.g., 4-HPC ex vivo culture) Selected normal stem cells in Aplastic anemia CML Other leukemias Myelodysplasia Cancer involving BM After gene insertion
8.	Selective growth of normal cells over abnormal cells	Purging of cancer
9.	Controlled manipulation of cycling of true stem cells	Facilitate gene insertion for gene therapy

AIDS = acquired immunodeficiency syndrome; CLL = chronic lymphocytic leukemia; CML = chronic myloid leukemia.

tissues is of vital importance. The full complexity of the normal hemopoietic microenvironment is only partly reproduced and modeled in the present systems and this deficiency will most likely limit ex vivo manipulation of hemopoiesis.

Finally, it is vital to set clear targets and objectives for each of the aims in Table 13.1. A proposal that aims to achieve a target number of promyelocytes and myelocytes, such as would be necessary for abrogation of neutropenia after anticancer therapy, may be absolutely irrelevant for stem-cell expansion after purging with 4-hydroperoxycyclophosphamide (4-HPC) or for the generation of gene-bearing hemopoietic stem cells capable of providing gene replacement for the subsequent lifetime of the organism.

The remainder of this review is confined to a discussion of the approaches and practical issues concerning aim 1 of Table 13.1 (i.e., ex vivo culture of hemopoietic progenitor cells with the purpose of generating sufficient neutrophil precursors to abrogate neutropenia).

■ HEMOPOIETIC TARGET CELLS FOR EX VIVO CULTURES

In vitro assays and in vivo transplantation studies support the hypothesis that the CD34 antigen (Ag) is a marker of multipotent HSC and progenitors in humans (Civin et al. 1984; Berenson et al. 1988; Andrews, Singer, and Bernstein 1989; Wagermaker et al. 1990; Berenson et al. 1991; Baum et al. 1992; Sutherland and Keating 1992). The CD34 glycoprotein cell-surface Ag provides a means of isolating primitive human hemopoietic progenitors. A variety of cell separation systems have been developed based on the use of anti-CD34 antibodies (Ab), which allow the isolation of $CD34^+$ cells from bone marrow (BM) and peripheral blood (PB) in numbers sufficient for both laboratory and clinical applications (Miltenyi et al. 1990; Strauss et al. 1991; Hardwick et al. 1992; Heimfeld et al. 1992; Lebkowski et al. 1992; Herikstad and Lien 1994). These various technologies are described in other chapters.

It is important to emphasize the importance of $CD34^+$ cell selection in strategies for ex vivo manipulation of hemopoiesis, given the low incidence of progenitor cells in hemopoietic tissues. If unfractionated PB or BM mononuclear cells were the starting cell populations for clinical-scale, ex vivo expansion, this would of necessity require the initiation of cultures in impractically large volumes and at prohibitively high cell densities. Moreover, it is unlikely that the true potential of the $CD34^+$ cells would be realized under these suboptimal growth conditions, either because of depletion of essential nutrients from the medium, or the accumulation of toxic metabolites, or to the inhibitory effects of CD34$^-$ accessory cells in the culture.

Apart from BM, CD34$^+$ cells can be obtained from umbilical cord blood (CB) (Broxmeyer et al. 1990; Nakahata and Ogawa 1982), fetal liver and BM (Migliaccio et al. 1986; Muench et al. 1994), and from PB of patients undergoing blood cell mobilization (Siena et al. 1989, 1991; To et al. 1994). Extensive studies in our laboratory have shown that PB CD34$^+$ cells collected after various methods of mobilization have a comparable phenotype and equivalent proliferative potential to BM, as determined by production of myeloid cells in pre–colony forming cell (CFC) assays and long-term bone marrow culture (LTBMC) (To et al. 1994). Large numbers of CD34$^+$ cells can be obtained from the PB of mobilized patients. This source of cells is preferred.

■ METHODS FOR EX VIVO CULTURE OF CD34$^+$ CELLS

Ex vivo culture of CD34$^+$ cells can be performed under perfusion or static conditions with or without supporting hemopoietic stromal cells.

Perfusion Culture

Perfusion culture simulates the hemopoietic microenvironment and both metabolites and hemopoietic regulators may be removed or added in a controlled manner (Knight 1989; Schwarz et al. 1991; Schwarz, Palsson, and Emerson 1991; Palsson et al. 1993). The perfusion bioreactor systems developed by Emerson and colleagues use an irradiated stromal layer prepared 24 hours before inoculation with CD34$^+$ cells or whole BM mononuclear cells (MNC) (Koller, Emerson, and Palsson 1993b). Growth factors such as stem-cell factor (SCF), IL-3, and IL-6 can be added to compensate for variation in the ability of different sources of stroma to support hemopoiesis and to provide factors (e.g., IL-3) that are not produced by stromal cells. Initial studies indicate that LTC-IC and granulocyte-macrophage colony-forming cells (GM-CFC) can both be expanded (Koller, et al. 1993a). Koller et al. (1993a) have suggested that sufficient progenitor cells for an autologous transplant could be generated from a BM aspirate of 30 to 50 mL; however, there is no clear evidence that long-term repopulating cells are maintained during the culture. This will only be determined if transplantation with retrovirally marked cells is performed so as to indicate what contribution these cells make to long-term hemopoietic reconstitution.

Stroma-Free Static Culture

A more common approach for ex vivo culture of CD34$^+$ cells is the use of stroma-free systems with recombinant human HGF to promote cell survival, proliferation, and differentiation. This approach was used successfully by Iscove to increase the number of hemopoietic progenitors from unfractionated, murine BM nucleated cells when cultured with IL-1 and IL-3 (Iscove, Shaw, and Keller 1989). Subsequently, many investigators have performed ex vivo culture of CD34$^+$ cells or subsets of CD34$^+$ cells in stroma-free, cytokine-dependent culture systems (Brandt et al. 1990; Smith et al. 1991; Terstappen et al. 1991; Haylock et al. 1992; Lansdorp and Dragowska 1992; Muench, Schneider, and Moore 1992; Mayani, Lansdorp, and Dragowska 1993; Muench, Firpo, and Moore 1993; Sato et al. 1993; Smith et al. 1993). This culture method offers great flexibility in that according to the particular HGF added, the system can potentially be modified to facilitate selected development of particular lineages or to maintain or expand HSC. A critical issue with all stroma-free culture systems is the choice and concentrations of HGF. In part, the choice of HGF depends on the objectives of the ex vivo manipulation.

If proliferation of primitive hemopoietic cells is an objective, then combinations of at least three or four HGF including SCF, IL-3, and IL-6 are required. As suggested by Metcalf (1993), this appears to be a clear example of the need for simultaneous signaling induced by two or more regulators before the cell can respond and enter into cycle. Primitive hemopoietic cells defined as CD34$^+$CD38$^-$rhodamine^{low,} will only clone in combinations of four or six HGF, whereas more mature progenitors (which may be irreversibly committed to myeloid differentiation) such as CD34$^+$CD38^{++}rhodamine^{hi} cells are able to respond to single-lineage-specific HGF such as G-CSF, although maximal cloning is achieved with combinations of HGF (Fig. 13.1).

Previous studies in our laboratory identified a six-HGF combination (IL-1, IL-3, IL-6, G-CSF, GM-CSF, SCF) as optimal for generation of nascent CFU-GM from PB CD34$^+$ cells when grown for 7 days in a stroma-free liquid assay using Iscove's modification of Dulbeccos medium (IMDM) supplemented with 30% fetal calf serum and 1% bovine serum albumin (BSA) (Haylock et al. 1992). This was consistent with other reports showing that primitive hemopoietic precursors require combinations of direct acting and synergistic HGF for maximal proliferation (Ikebuchi et al. 1987; Moore and Warren 1987; Ikebuchi et al. 1988; Moore et al. 1990; Zsebo et al. 1990; Lowry et al. 1991; Moore 1991). HGF combinations including SCF, IL-3, granulocyte-macrophage colony-stimulating factor (GM-CSF), granulocyte colony-

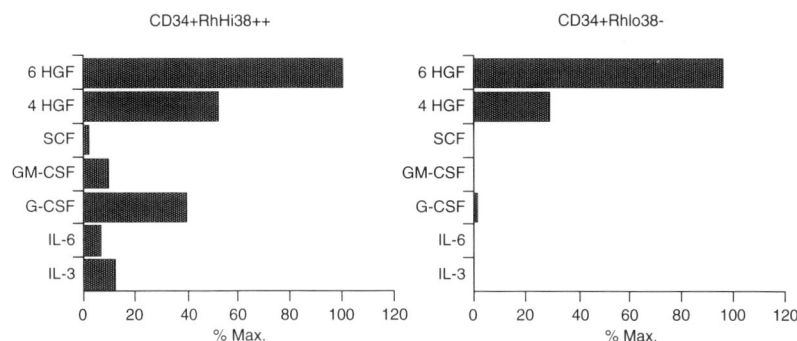

Figure 13.1 Production of myeloid progenitor cell colonies (GM-CFC) from FACS-isolated CD34$^+$rhodamine123^{bright}CD38^{++} cells (*left panel*) and CD34$^+$rhodamine123^{dull} CD38$^-$ cells (*right panel*) cultured in 0.9% methylcellulose and stimulated with either six HGF (IL-1, IL-3, IL-6, G-CSF, GM-CSF and SCF: all at 10 ng/mL) or four HGF (IL-3, IL-6, G-CSF, SCF: all at 10 ng/mL) or single HGF as indicated. Colonies were scored after 14 days' growth at 37°C and the results are shown as a proportion of the maximum number of colonies observed, which for both cell populations occurred with six-HGF stimulation.

stimulating factor (G-CSF), and erythropoietin (EPO) are also synergistic in the stimulation of human progenitor cells of the myeloid (Broxmeyer et al. 1991), erythroid (Bernstein, Andrews, and Zsebo 1991; McNiece, Langley, and Zsebo 1991; Lansdorp and Dragowska 1992; Mayani et al. 1993), and megakaryocytic lineages (Avraham et al. 1992). Another study performed by Brugger et al. (1993) investigated the effects of ten cytokines (IL-1, IL-3, IL-6, G-CSF, GM-CSF, M-CSF, SCF, EPO, leukemia-inhibiting factor [LIF], and interferon-γ [IFN-γ]) either alone or in combinations to generate nucleated cells and progenitors from CD34$^+$ cells. The combination of SCF, EPO, IL-1, IL-3, and IL-6 produced the greatest expansion of total cell numbers and clonogenic progenitors; however, it is most likely that large numbers of erythroid cells would be generated with this combination.

The concentration of individual HGF within combinations may also affect the number and type of cells generated from ex vivo culture of CD34$^+$ cells. The task of examining all the possible combinations of HGF over a restricted concentration range is certainly not practical, as there are millions of different permutations that could be tested. Our approach has been to examine the role of individual HGF within combinations so as to determine which HGF are critical for production of particular cells, and to establish which HGF can be omitted from combinations without reducing the number or type of cells generated. Where the objective for ex vivo culture is to generate large numbers of myeloid progenitors and postprogenitors from $CD34^+$ cells, IL-1 and GM-CSF can be omitted from the six-HGF combination without diminishing nucleated-cell production (Haylock et al. 1995); however, maximal production of maturing neutrophil precursors requires G-CSF, SCF, IL-6, and IL-3 at concentrations of 100, 100, 20, and 10 ng/mL, respectively. At these saturating concentrations of HGF, the growth of $CD34^+$ cells is not limited by consumption of individual growth factors, but rather by consumption of glucose and production of toxic metabolites such as lactate (unpublished observations).

Apart from the effects of single HGF or combinations of HGF on primitive and committed progenitor cells, it is also important to consider the effects of individual HGF on the later stages of myeloid maturation. We have observed that GM-CSF at doses of 0.1 ng/mL, even in the presence of 100 ng/mL G-CSF, promotes monocyte and macrophage development and suppresses the terminal stages of neutrophil maturation. Recently, Steen et al. (1994) also reported a similar effect of GM-CSF on promotion of monocytic development. Furthermore, HGF may activate mature cells generated during the culture. A consequence of this may be the production of other cytokines or regulators that inhibit the growth of hemopoietic progenitor cells still present in the culture.

Although HGF play a significant role in determining the number and type of cells generated in stroma-free static cultures, there are a number of other variables that may affect the outcome of ex vivo expansion of $CD34^+$ cells. These include the culture medium used, the purity of the $CD34^+$ cells, and the cell density during culture.

Culture Media The main consideration with culture media is whether xenogeneic serum is used to provide a source of protein and lipid. Although many investigators include fetal calf serum and BSA for laboratory studies, it is likely that regulatory authorities will insist that ex vivo culture of hemopoietic progenitors for clinical applications be performed where possible in the absence of animal protein products. In addition, we anticipate that every component of culture media will need to be defined and acceptable to the U.S. FDA before it can be used for clinical studies. Such an attitude is understandable and is of paramount importance to ensure that cells are not exposed to viruses, other infectious agents, or untested biological materials. A major advantage of completely defined, serum-free media is that cell growth may be better and more reproducible and may allow a clearer assessment of the effect of HGF in stimulation of hemopoietic cells. It is evident from studies in our laboratory that some commercially prepared complete media that contain low concentrations of pooled human serum are more effective than IMDM supplemented with high concentrations of fetal calf serum and BSA.

Purity of CD34$^+$ Cells   It is generally accepted that CD34$^+$ cells should be enriched to high purity for ex vivo culture to avoid the possible inhibitory effects of CD34$^-$ cells. There are, however, few data to substantiate this view. We have performed experiments where CD34$^-$ cells from PB apheresis collections were isolated by fluorescence-activated cell sorting (FACS), mixed and cultured with CD34$^+$ cells for 14 to 21 days with six or four HGF. Figure 13.2 shows results from three typical experiments. An excess of non-T, nonmonocytic cells (CD3$^-$,CD14$^-$) cells did not affect the production of nucleated cells from 1,000 CD34$^+$ cells after 14 days even when 10,000 CD3$^-$,CD14$^-$ cells were present in the culture. In contrast, culture of CD34$^+$ cells with an equal number of CD3$^+$ or CD14$^+$ cells (i.e., 50%

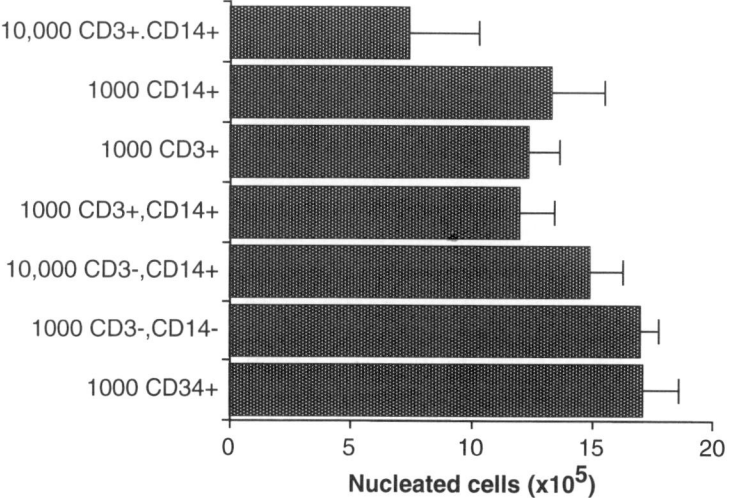

Figure 13.2   The effect of contaminating autologous CD34$^-$ cells on nucleated cell production from 1,000 PB CD34$^+$ cells after 14 days of culture in IMDM supplemented with 30% fetal calf serum and 1% bovine serum albumin and stimulated with six HGF (IL-1, IL-3, IL-6, G-CSF, GM-CSF, and SCF). The CD34$^+$, CD3$^+$, CD3$^-$CD14$^-$ and CD14$^+$ cells were obtained by FACS on a Becton Dickinson FacStar^{plus}. The results are the mean and standard error from three separate experiments.

CD34$^+$ purity) results in a 22% to 30% decrease in the number of nucleated cells after 14 days. This effect was more pronounced (57% reduction in nucleated cells) when 10,000 CD3$^+$,CD14$^+$ cells were cultured with 1,000 CD34$^+$ cells. We have previously described a similar inhibitory effect of monocytes in the GM-CFC assay of PB MNC (To et al. 1983). The mechanism for inhibition may be indirect, as a result of T-lymphocyte and/or monocyte production of soluble inhibitors such as prostaglandins or directly through cell-to-cell contact. Alternatively, HGF or other important regulators may be consumed by the CD3$^+$ or CD14$^+$ cells. These data suggest that the purity of CD34$^+$ cells is an important variable for stroma-free HGF-dependent ex vivo expansion cultures. We recommend that CD34$^+$ cells be at least 50% pure to ensure optimal myeloid cell production.

CD34$^+$ Cell Concentration   Another important variable that influences the number of cells that can be generated under static culture conditions is cell concentration. Irrespective of the initial concentration of CD34$^+$ cells, the growth rate is exponential and consistent as indicated (Fig. 13.3A) by the parallel growth curves for assays established at 300, 1,000, or 5,000 cells/mL. The other consistent feature is that above cell densities of 1.1 to 1.4 $\times$ 10^6/mL, there is increasing cell death and a reduction in the total number of viable nucleated cells. CD34$^+$ cells cultured at high density (e.g., 5,000/mL) reach a concentration of 1×10^6/mL earlier than those cultured at lower density (300/mL) (Fig. 13.3B). An extension of this observation is that 5,000 CD34$^+$ cells grown in five separate 1,000-cell/mL cultures would generate many more viable cells (possibly 15-fold more) than a single culture initiated at 5,000/mL. We have demonstrated that the growth-limiting effect of cell density can be partially overcome by daily mixing and/or media/HGF exchange (Fig. 13.4). Under these perfusion-like conditions, the system can support cell proliferation to a density of 5×10^6 /mL. Taken together, these experiments highlight the potential limitations of static culture systems and add further evidence to support the use of perfusion culture to fully capitalize on the proliferative potential of CD34$^+$ cells.

From a practical point of view, investigators need to determine the kinetics of cell growth in their systems and to be aware that cell density will influence the viability and type of cells present at any time. For example, a given number of CD34$^+$ cells could be cultured at a high initial density for 8 to 10 days to generate a target number of myeloid cells at defined stages of maturation, but 50% fewer CD34$^+$ cells could be cultured for two extra days to generate an equivalent number of the same type of myeloid cells.

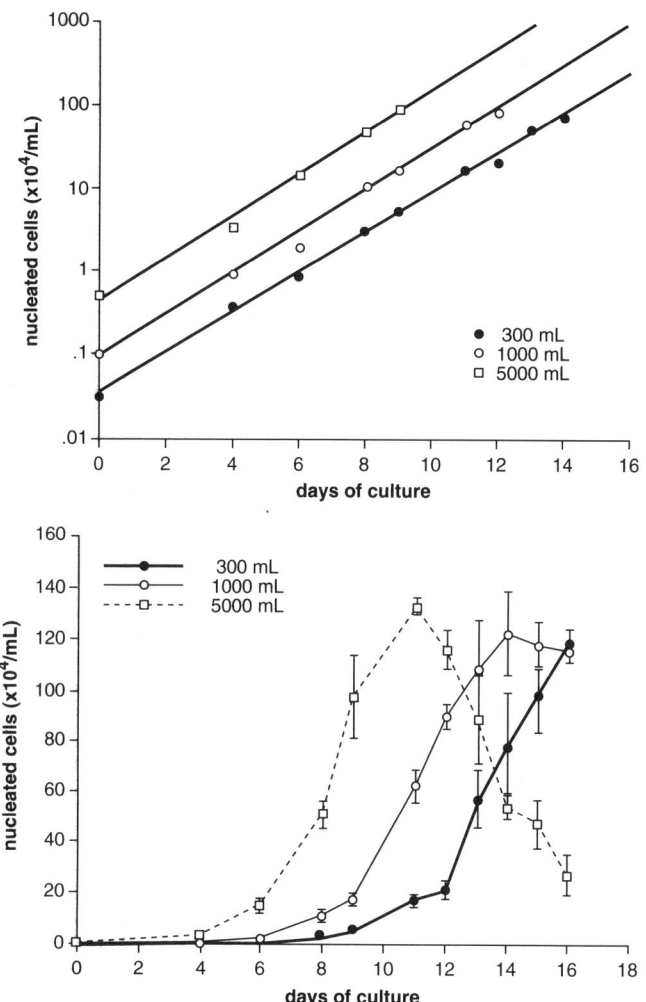

Figure 13.3 *Top panel,* Logarithmic increase in number of nucleated cells in cultures initiated with different numbers of CD34$^+$ cells obtained by FACS. Cultures were performed in IMDM, 30% fetal calf serum, 1% bovine serum albumin and IL-3 (10 ng/mL), IL-6 (20 ng/mL), G-CSF (100 ng/mL), and SCF (100 ng/mL). Each value represents the mean of three replicate wells (1 mL each) counted on the day of harvest. The data have been plotted to the day the nucleated cell counts reached approximately 1 x 10^6/mL. *Bottom panel,* Kinetics of nucleated-cell production in cultures initiated with either 300, 1,000, or 5,000 CD34$^+$ cells/mL. The CD34$^+$ cells were cultured in IMDM, 30% fetal calf serum, 1% bovine serum albumin, IL-3 (10 ng/mL), IL-6 (20 ng/mL), G-CSF (100 ng/mL), and SCF (100 ng/mL). Same experiment as given in *top panel.*

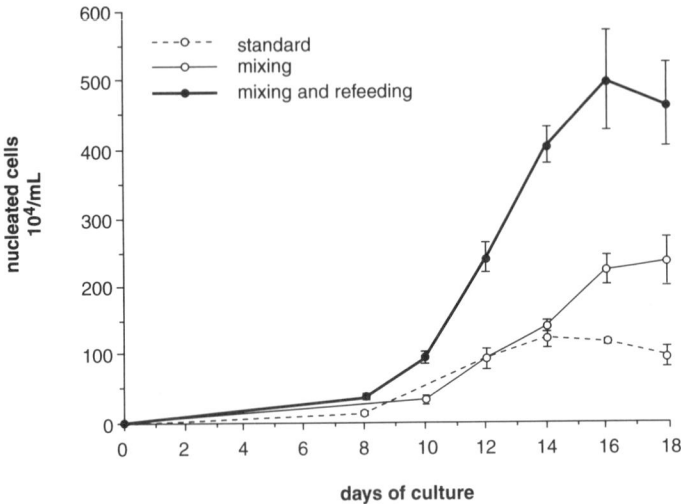

Figure 13.4   The effect of mixing cells and mixing plus refeeding of cultures on production of nucleated cells by CD34$^+$ cells. One thousand PB CD34$^+$ cells isolated by FACS were cultured in IMDM, 30% fetal calf serum, 1% bovine serum albumin, and IL-3 (10 ng/mL), IL-6 (20 ng/mL), G-CSF (100 ng/mL), and SCF (100 ng/mL). After day 7, the cells were either left undisturbed until the day of harvest (standard conditions) or a daily mixing schedule with or without removal and replacement of half the volume of the culture medium containing HGF was performed. Each data point is the mean and standard error of three experiments.

Cell growth also may be altered by the choice of culture vessel (i.e., specialized bags or tissue culture flasks) and the oxygen tension within the incubator. With the advent of new plastics and better control over gas exchange and cell adherence, there may be significant future improvements in ex vivo expansion of hemopoietic progenitor cells under both static and perfusion conditions.

■ SUMMARY

It is clear from our studies and those of other investigators that large numbers of myeloid progenitor and postprogenitor cells can be generated from CD34$^+$ cells cultured with HGF alone. Optimal ex vivo expansion of CD34$^+$ cells requires combinations of HGF including at least SCF, G-CSF, IL-3, and IL-6. Culture in stroma-free, HGF-dependent conditions allows control over the type of cells to be generated and is a more reliable and reproducible method for ex vivo expansion of CD34$^+$ cells than stromal-cell supported cultures. Culture of CD34$^+$ cells is limited under static conditions because of cell density. Despite this, sufficient neutrophil precursors can be generated for therapeutic applications and may potentially abrogate neutropenia when infused after transplant. In addition, the cell mix generated from culture of PB CD34$^+$ cells in six HGF contains 8% to 10% megakaryocytes as determined by immunocytochemical staining for P-selectin or GPIIbIIIa (Haylock et al. 1992). The recent identification and cloning of a specific thrombopoietin, the *mpl* ligand (Bartley et al. 1994; Kaushansky et al. 1994; Lok et al. 1994; Wendling et al. 1994), should facilitate the ex vivo production of sufficient megakaryocytic precursors and maturing megakaryocytes for therapeutic applications. It is envisaged that within the near future ex vivo cell "factories" will produce the necessary cell types to improve hemopoietic recovery further and possibly abrogate chemotherapy-induced cytopenia.

ACKNOWLEDGMENTS

Work in the authors' laboratory was performed with excellent technical assistance from S. Niutta, S. Trimboli, T. Dowse, and Dr. Shigeyoshi Makino, and is supported by grants from the National Health and Medical Research Council of Australia and the Anti-Cancer Foundation of the Universities of South Australia. We are also grateful for support and supply of hemopoietic growth factors from Amgen and valuable discussions with Dr. I. McNiece, Dr. W. Sheridan, and Dr. A. Gringeri.

REFERENCES

Andrews, R.G., Singer, J.W., and Bernstein, I.D. (1989) Precursors of colony-forming cells in humans can be distinguished from colony-forming cells by expression of the CD33 and CD34 antigens and their light scatter properties. *Journal of Experimental Medicine*, **169**, 1721–31.

Avraham, H., Vannier, E., Cowley, S., et al. (1992) Effects of the stem cell factor, c-kit ligand, on human megakaryocytic cells. *Blood*, **79**, 365–71.

Bartley, T.D., Bogenberger, J., Hunt, P., et al. (1994) Identification and cloning of a megakaryocyte growth and development factor that is a ligand for the cytokine receptor Mpl. *Cell*, **77**, 1117–24.

Baum, C.M., Weissman, I.L., Tsukamoto, A.S., and Buckle, A.-M. (1992) Isolation of a candidate hematopoietic stem cell population. *Proceedings of the National Academy of Sciences of the United States of America*, **89**, 2804–8.

Berenson, R.J., Andrews, R.G., Bensinger, W.I., et al. (1988) Antigen CD34-positive marrow cells engraft lethally irradiated baboons. *Journal of Clinical Investigation*, **81**, 951–5.

Berenson, R.J., Bensinger, W.I., Hill, R.S., et al. (1991) Engraftment after infusion of CD34$^+$ marrow cells in patients with breast cancer or neuroblastoma. *Blood*, **77**, 1717–22.

Bernstein, I.D., Andrews, R.G., and Zsebo, K.M. (1991) Recombinant human stem cell factor enhances the formation of colonies by CD34$^+$ and CD34$^+$lin$^-$ cells and the generation of colony-forming cell progeny from CD34$^+$lin$^-$ cells cultured with interleukin-3, granulocyte colony-stimulating factor, or granulocyte-macrophage colony-stimulating factor. *Blood*, **77**, 2316–21.

Brandt, J., Srour, E.F., Van Besien, K., Briddell, R., and Hoffman, R. (1990) Cytokine-dependent long-term culture of highly enriched precursors of hematopoietic stem cells from human bone marrow. *Journal of Clinical Investigation*, **86**, 932–41.

Broxmeyer, H.E., Cooper, S., Lu, L., et al. (1991) Effect of murine mast cell growth factor (c-kit proto-oncogene ligand) on colony formation by human hematopoietic progenitor cells. *Blood*, **77**, 2142.

Broxmeyer, H.E., Gluckman, E., Averbach, A.D., et al. (1990) Human umbilical cord blood: a clinically useful source of transplantable hematopoietic stem/progenitor cells. *International Journal of Cell Cloning*, **8**, 76–91.

Brugger, W., Mocklin, W., Heimfeld, S., Berenson, R.J., Mertelsmann, R., and Kanz, L. (1993) Ex vivo expansion of enriched PB CD34$^+$ progenitor cells by stem cell factor, interleukin-1beta (IL-1), IL-6, IL-3, interferon-gamma and erythropoietin. *Blood*, **81**, 2579–84.

Civin, C., Strauss, L.C., Brovall, C., Fackler, M.J., Schwartz, J.F., and Shaper, J.H. (1984) Antigenic analysis of hemopoiesis III: a hematopoietic progenitor cell surface antigen defined by a monoclonal antibody raised against KG1a cells. *Journal of Immunology*, **133**, 157–70.

Gianni, A.M., Siena, S., Bregni, M., et al. (1989) Granulocyte-macrophage colony stimulating factor to harvest circulating haemopoietic stem cells for autotransplantation. *Lancet*, **2**, 580–5.

Goldman, J. (1994) "Blood and marrow transplantation": a message from the editor. *Bone Marrow Transplantation*, **14**, 1.

Hardwick, A., Kulcinski, D., Mansour, V., Ishizawa, L., Law, P., and Gee A.P. (1992) Design of large-scale separation systems for positive and negative immunomagnetic selection of cells using super-paramagnetic magnetic microspheres. *Journal of Hematotherapy*, **1**, 379–86.

Haylock, D.N., To, L.B., Dowse, T.L., Juttner, C.A., and Simmons, P.J. (1992) Ex vivo expansion and maturation of peripheral blood CD34$^+$ cells into the myeloid lineage. *Blood*, **80**, 1405–12.

Haylock, D.N., To, L.B., Makino, S., Dowse, T.L., Juttner, C.A., and Simmons P.J. (1995) Ex vivo expansion of human hematopoietic progenitors with cytokines. In D.J. Levitt and R. Mertelsmann (Eds.) *Hematopoietic stem cells: biology and therapeutic applications*, pp. 49–57. New York, Marcel Dekker.

Heimfeld, S., Andrews, R., Zsebo, K., et al. (1992) Peripheral blood stem cell mobilization after stem cell factor (SCF) or G-CSF treatment: rapid enrichment for stem and progenitor cells using the CEPRATE immuno-affinity separation system. *Experimental Hematology*, **22**, 748 (abstract).

Herikstad, B.V., and Lien, E. (1994) Immunomagnetic separation of hematopoietic progenitor cells using dynabeads CD34 and DETACHaBEAD. In E. Wunder, H. Sovalat, P.R. Henon, and S. Serke (Eds.) *Hematopoietic stem cells: the Mulhouse manual*, pp. 149–60, Dayton, OH, AlphaMed Press.

Ikebuchi, K., Ihle, J.N., Hirai, Y., Wong, G.G., Clark, S.C., and Ogawa, M. (1988) Synergistic factors for stem cell proliferation: further studies of the target stem cells and the mechanism of stimulation by interleukin-1, interleukin-6 and granulocyte-colony stimulating factor. *Blood*, **72**, 2007–14.

Ikebuchi, K., Wong, G.G., Clark, S.C., Ihle, J.N., Hirai, Y., and Ogawa, M. (1987) Interleukin 6 enhancement of interleukin 3-dependent proliferation of multipotential hematopoietic progenitors. *Proceedings of the National Academy of Sciences of the United States of America*, **84**, 9035–9.

Iscove, N.N., Shaw, A.R., and Keller, G. (1989) Net increase of pluripotential hematopoietic precursors in suspension culture to IL-1 and IL-3. *Journal of Immunology*, **142**, 2332–9.

Kaushansky, K., Lok, S., Holly, R.D., et al. (1994) Promotion of megakaryocyte progenitor expansion and differentiation by the c-Mpl ligand thrombopoietin. *Nature*, **369**, 568–71.

Kessler, D.A., Siegel, J.P., Noguchi, P.D., Zoon, K.C., Feiden, K.L., and Woodcock, J. (1993) Regulation of somatic-cell therapy and gene therapy by the Food and Drug Administration. *New England Journal of Medicine*, **329**, 1169–73.

Knight, P. (1989) Hollow fibre bioreactors for mammalian cell culture. *Biotechnology*, **7**, 459–66.

Koller, M.R., Bender, J.G., Miller, W.M., and Papoutsakis, E.T. (1993a) Expansion of primitive human hematopoietic progenitors in a perfusion bioreactor system with IL-3, IL-6 and stem cell factor. *Biotechnology*, **11**, 358–63.

Koller, M.R., Emerson, S.G., and Palsson, B.O. (1993b) Large scale expansion of human stem and progenitor cells from bone marrow mononuclear cells in continous perfusion cultures. *Blood*, **82**, 378–84.

Lansdorp, P.M., and Dragowska, W. (1992) Long-term erythropoiesis from constant numbers of CD34$^+$ cells in serum-free cultures initiated with highly purified progenitor cells from human bone marrow. *Journal of Experimental Medicine*, **175**, 1501–9.

Lebkowski, J.S., Schain, L.R., Okrongly, D., Levinsky, R., Harvey, M.J., and Okarma, T.B. (1992) Rapid isolation of human CD34 hematopoietic stem cells-purging of human tumor cells. *Transplantation*, **53**, 1011–9.

Lok, S., Kaushansky, K., Holly, R.D., et al. (1994) Cloning and expression of murine thrombopoietin cDNA and stimulation of platelet production in vivo. *Nature*, **369**, 365–8.

Lowry, P.A., Zsebo, K.M., Deacon, D.H., Eichman, C.E., and Quesenberry, P.J. (1991) Effects of rrSCF on multiple cytokine responsive HPP-CFC generated from SCA$^+$Lin$^-$ murine hematopoietic progenitors. *Experimental Hematology*, **19**, 994–6.

Mayani, H., Lansdorp, P.M., and Dragowska, W. (1993) Cytokine-induced selective expansion and maturation of erythroid versus myeloid progenitors from purified cord blood precursor cells. *Blood*, **81**, 3252–8.

McNiece, I.K., Langley, K.E., and Zsebo, K.M. (1991) Recombinant human stem cell factor synergises with GM-CSF, G-CSF, IL-3 and EPO to stimulate human progenitor cells of the myeloid and erythroid lineages. *Experimental Hematology*, **19**, 226–31.

Metcalf, D. (1993) Hematopoietic regulators: redundancy or subtlety? *Blood*, **82**, 3515–23.

Migliaccio, G., Migliaccio, A.R., Petti, S., et al. (1986) Human embryonic hemopoiesis. Kinetics of progenitors and precursors underlying the yolk sac to liver transition. *Journal of Clinical Investigation*, **78**, 51–60.

Miltenyi, S., Meuller, W., Weichel, W., and Radbruch, A. (1990) High gradient magnetic cell separation with MACS. *Cytometry*, **11**, 231–8.

Moore, M.A. (1991) Clinical implications of positive and negative hematopoietic stem cell regulators. *Blood*, **78**, 1–23.

Moore, M.A., Muench, M.O., Warren, D.J., and Laver, J. (1990) Cytokine networks involved in regulation of haemopoietic stem cell proliferation and differentiation. In *Molecular control of haemopoiesis,* Ciba Symposium No. 148., p. 43. Chichester, Wiley Interscience.

Moore, M.A., and Warren, D.J. (1987) Interleukin-1 and G-CSF synergism: in vivo stimulation of stem cell recovery and hematopoietic regeneration following 5-fluorouracil treatment in mice. *Proceedings of the National Academy of Sciences of the United States of America,* **84**, 7134–8.

Muench, M.O., Cupp, J., Polakoff, J., and Roncarolo, M.G. (1994) Expression of CD33, CD38 and HLA-DR on CD34$^+$ human fetal liver progenitors with high proliferative potential. *Blood*, **83**, 3170–81.

Muench, M.O., Firpo, M.T., and Moore M.A. (1993) Bone marrow transplantation with interleukin-1 plus kit-ligand ex vivo expanded bone marrow accelerates hematopoietic reconstitution in mice without the loss of stem cell lineage and proliferative potential. *Blood*, **81**, 3463–73.

Muench, M.O., Schneider, J.G, and Moore, M.A. (1992) Interactions among colony-stimulating factors IL-1b, IL-6, and Kit-ligand in the regulation of primitive murine hematopoietic cells. *Experimental Hematology*, **20**, 339–49.

Nakahata, T., and Ogawa, M. (1982) Hematopoietic colony-forming cells in umbilical cord blood with extensive capability to generate mono- and multipotent hematopoietic progenitors. *Journal of Clinical Investigation*, **70**, 1324–8.

Palsson, B.O., Paek, S.-H., Schwartz, R.M., et al. (1993) Expansion of human bone marrow progenitor cells in a high density continous perfusion system. *Biotechnology*, **11**, 368–72.

Sato, K., Sawada, K., Koizumi, K., et al. (1993) In vitro expansion of human peripheral blood CD34$^+$ cells. *Blood*, **82**, 3600–9.

Schwarz, R.M., Emerson, S.G., Clarke, M.F., and Palsson, B.O. (1991) In vitro myelopoiesis stimulated by rapid medium exchange and supplementation with hematopoietic growth factors. *Blood*, **78**, 3155–61.

Schwarz, R.M., Palsson, B.O., and Emerson, S.G. (1991) Rapid medium perfusion rate significantly increases the productivity and longevity of human bone marrow cultures. *Proceedings of the National Academy of Sciences of the United States of America,* **88**, 6760–4.

Sheridan, W.P., Begley, C.G., Juttner, C.A., et al. (1992) Effect of peripheral blood progenitor cells mobilised by filgrastim (G-CSF) on platelet recovery after high dose chemotherapy. *Lancet*, **339**, 640–4.

Siena, S., Bregni, M., Brando, B., et al. (1991) Flow cytometry for clinical estimation of circulating hematopoietic progenitors for autologous transplantation in cancer patients. *Blood*, **77**, 400–9.

Siena, S., Bregni, M., Brando, B., Ravagnani, F., Bonadonna, G., and Gianni, A.M. (1989) Circulation of CD34$^+$ hematopoietic stem cells cells in the peripheral blood of high-dose cyclophosphamide-treated patients: enhancement by intravenous recombinant human granulocyte-marcophage colony-stimulating factor. *Blood*, **74**, 1905–14.

Smith, S.L., Bender, J.G., Maples, P.B., et al. (1993) Expansion of neutrophil precursors and progenitors in suspension cultures of CD34$^+$ cells enriched from human bone marrow. *Experimental Hematology*, **21**, 870–7.

Smith, C., Gasparetto, C., Collins, N., et al. (1991) Purification and partial characterization of a human hematopoietic precursor population. *Blood*, **77**, 2122–8.

Steen, R., Morkid, L., Tjonnfjord, G.E., and Egeland, T. (1994) c-Kit ligand combined with GM-CSF and/or IL-3 can expand CD34$^+$ hematopoietic progenitor cells for several weeks in vitro. *Stem Cells*, **12**, 214–24.

Strauss, L.C., Trischmann, T.M., Rowley, S.D., Wiley, J.M., and Civin, C.I. (1991) Selection of normal human hematopoietic stem cells for bone marrow transplantation using immunomagnetic microspheres and CD34 antibody. *American Journal of Pediatric Hematology/Oncology*, **2**, 217–81.

Sutherland, D.R., and Keating, A. (1992) The CD34 antigen: structure, biology, and potential clinical applications. *Journal of Hematotherapy*, **1**, 115–29.

Terstappen, L.W., Huang, S., Safford, M., Lansdorp, P.M., and Loken, M.R. (1991) Sequential generations of hematopoietic colonies derived from single non-lineage committed CD34$^+$CD38$^-$ progenitor cells. *Blood*, **77**, 1218–27.

To, L.B., Haylock, D.N., Dowse, T.L., Ashman, L.K., Simmons, P.J., and Juttner C.A. (1994) A comparative study of the phenotype and proliferative capacity of peripheral blood CD34$^+$ cells mobilised by 4 different protocols and those of steady state peripheral blood and bone marrow CD34$^+$ cells. *Blood*, **84**, 2930–9.

To, L.B., Haylock, D.N., Juttner, C.A., and Kimber, R.J. (1983) The effect of monocytes on the peripheral blood CFU-C assay system. *Blood*, **62**, 112–7.

To, L.B., Roberts, M.M., Haylock, D.N., et al. (1992) Comparison of hematological recovery times and supportive care requirements of autologous recovery phase peripheral blood stem cell transplants, autologous bone marrow transplants and allogeneic bone marrow transplants. *Bone Marrow Transplantation*, **9**, 277–84.

Wagermaker, G., van Gils, F.C., Bart-Baumeister, J.A., Weilenger, J.J., and Levinsky, R.J. (1990) Sustained engraftment of allogeneic CD34 positive hemopoietic stem cells in rhesus monkeys. *Experimental Hematology*, **18**, 704.

Wendling, F., Maraskovsky, E., Debili, N., et al. (1994) c-Mpl ligand is a humoral regulator of megakaryocytopoiesis. *Nature*, **369**, 571–4.

Zsebo, K.M., Wypych, J., McNiece, I.K., et al. (1990) Identification, purification and biological characterization of hematopoietic stem cell factor from buffalo rat liver–conditioned medium. *Cell*, **63**, 195–201.

—14

Bioreactors for Expansion

WILLIAM R. KIDWELL

There are two basic types of bioreactors used for cell production and/or the production of natural or recombinant products made by cells. The simplest form of bioreactor is the single batch-fed type in which cells are inoculated into a growth chamber in a fixed volume of culture medium and, over time, the cells are allowed to expand to some desired level; then the cells or cell products are harvested. With single-batch fed systems, there is no culture-medium exchange from the start-up to the termination of the culture. The single batch-fed bioreactor is usually simple to operate, and because of less manipulation steps, has a relatively low risk of contamination; however, the method often gives less than optimal cell expansion because of nutrient deprivation and the accumulation of inhibitory catabolic waste products, such as ammonium ion, lactic acid, and, as recently demonstrated, the accumulation of autocrine growth inhibitors. Not uncommonly, there is inadequate oxygenation and pH control, which adversely affects the quality and quantity of harvested cells.

A second type of bioreactor operation is one in which nutrients consumed by cells as they proliferate are replenished by the exchange of nutrient-depleted culture medium for fresh culture medium. Medium exchange may be accomplished by sequential batch exchange, or continuous exchange. For both the batch or continuous modes, medium exchange is best performed when the growing cells are confined in a small compartment of the system, with the bulk medium perfused either unidirectionally or by recirculation, from a large medium reservoir. Compartmentation substantially reduces the labor and risk of contamination during recovery of the cell mass from a large volume of nutrient-depleted medium (i.e., by centrifugation) during batch feeding or at final harvest.

The restriction of the culture to a small volume or compartmentation while allowing cells access to the total nutrients available in a large volume of perfusing culture medium in the bioreactor is achieved by the use of semipermeable membranes. Efficiency of medium exchange between the perfusion-medium compartment and the compartment containing the cell mass is highest when there is maximal membrane surface area per unit volume across which medium and components can pass by either diffusion or bulk transfer into the cell-growth compartment. Maximal membrane surface area per unit volume is achieved only with a special bioreactor configuration, the artificial capillary-perfusion culture device.

The following discussion will focus on the characteristics of an artificial capillary device that has been custom designed to accommodate the special requirements for optimal expansion of human hemopoietic cells. Each component of the system, the artificial culture module, the pump, the reservoir, and the gas-exchange mechanism, will be considered.

■ THE BIOREACTOR MODULE

There are three important requirements for optimal support of hemopoietic cell growth in the artificial capillary module: the capillary "pore" size; the ability to support attachment of anchorage-dependent feeder cells; and the biocompatibility of the capillaries, the shell, and the potting material, or adhesive, that fixes the capillaries in the shell (see the enlargement of Fig. 14.1 for the module construction and medium flow).

■ IMPORTANCE OF "PORE" SIZE

The cells are inoculated into the capillary module in a small volume of medium. The cells are separated from the medium flowing from the reservoir through the capillary lumen by the walls of the capillaries. Nutrients and oxygen are supplied from the perfusate via diffusion and/or bulk transfer across the capillary wall and products produced by the cells traverse in the opposite direction. The capillary wall material and its porosity can, therefore, greatly influence how well cells expand in the module. One might suspect that the more "open" the capillary membrane was (i.e., the higher the porosity and the larger the pore size), the better the nutrient availability would be and, therefore, the better the cells would expand. In fact, this is not always the case. Performance comparisons have been made between low-molecular-weight cutoff capillaries (ultrafiltration membranes)

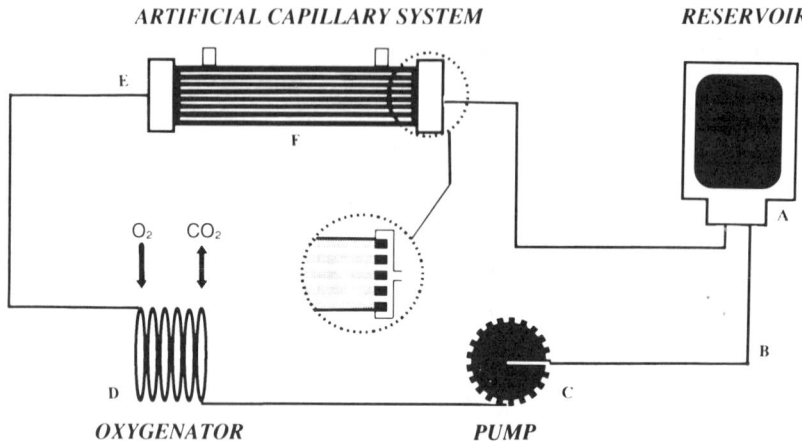

Figure 14.1 Simplified schematic demonstrating the components of the artificial capillary-perfusion system. Note that the culture medium in the reservoir recirculates from the reservoir through the capillary module, and back to the reservoir. Cells are inoculated and harvested via the side ports of the module (top of the drawing).

that limit the passage of macromolecules across the capillary wall (in both directions) and microporous membranes having capillary walls with pores in the 0.1- to 0.5-μm size. Such capillaries allow passage of molecules of many millions of daltons in and out of the capillary lumen.

Depending on the cell type, ultrafiltration-type membranes may be better or worse than microporous membranes for cell expansion. The performance difference is explained, at least in part, by whether the cells secrete macromolecular factors that stimulate or inhibit the division of the producer cells. For example, tumor-infiltrating lymphocyte (TIL) cell expansion in capillary modules made of ultrafiltration membranes with a molecular weight cutoff of 10 kDa was far superior compared with that of cultures in modules having microporous membranes (Fig. 14.2). Upon examination, the TIL cells were found to produce a growth factor that dramatically stimulated the producer TIL cells to divide (Fig. 14.3). This factor was highly purified and shown by N-terminal sequence analysis to be related to a known peptide hormone (Kidwell, Knazek, Hartman, patent pending).

In contrast, certain hybridomas were shown to produce a growth inhibitory factor, transforming growth factor-beta (TGF-β), and when these cells were cultured in modules containing ultrafiltration membranes, both proliferation and antibody (Ab) elaboration were dra-

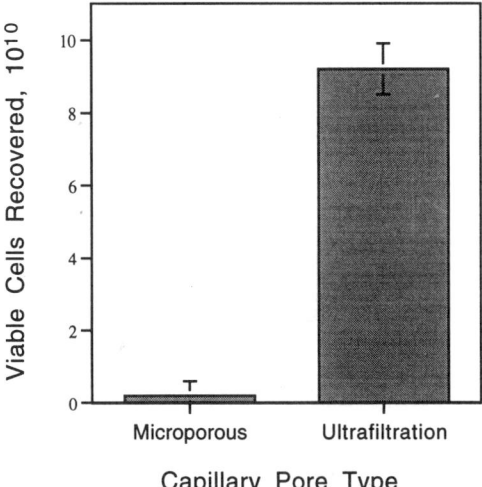

Capillary Pore Type

Figure 14.2 Effect of artificial capillary pore size on TIL proliferation. TIL were isolated from human melanoma tumors and cultured for about 5 days in plastic tissue culture flasks, then inoculated into modules having polypropylene (microporous) or cellulose (ultrafiltration) modules. After approximately 3 weeks, the cell number in the ultrafiltration modules had increased about 100-fold over the input cell number. Cultures were performed in AIM V medium (Gibco) supplemented with 1,000 IU IL-2/mL. Representative results from three separate experiments.

matically reduced (Fig. 14.4). When the same cells were cultured in microporous membrane capillary modules, cell expansion and Ab production were significantly improved. The latter modules permitted the dilution of inhibitory TGF-β by the total volume of medium in the reservoir; that is, to concentrations that were below those required for the inhibition of the hybridoma cells (Kidwell 1989).

A third cell type, the CD8$^+$ lymphocyte, exhibits a growth pattern in an artificial capillary perfusion system that is best explained by the production of both stimulatory and inhibitory factors. For example, in an artificial capillary perfusion system containing modules with ultrafiltration membranes, CD8$^+$ cells divide very poorly. They divide very well in modules containing microporous capillaries, provided the cells are inoculated at a high cell concentration (10^5 cells/mL of total medium in the flow path); however, the reservoir medium must be changed very frequently in order to sustain rapid cell expansion, indicating that the cells are producing one or more inhibitory factors. Inoculation of CD8$^+$ cells at high density does not promote cell di-

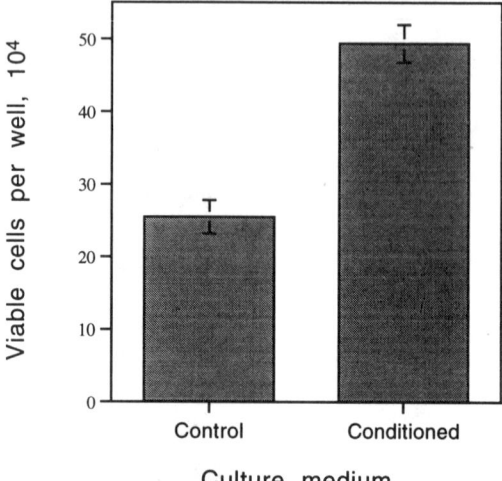

Figure 14.3 Demonstration that conditioned medium recovered from TIL cells cultured in an ultrafiltration-type membrane module contains growth-promoting factor for TIL cells. The factor has been purified to homogeneity and sequenced. The molecular weight of the factor exceeded that which would diffuse through the ultrafiltration membrane utilized (10-kDa molecular weight cutoff) and the culture conditions were 10% TIL cell-conditioned AIM V medium (Gibco) or fresh AIM V, both with 1,000 IU IL-2 (Kidwell, Knazek, and Hartman, patent pending). Representative example of more than 20 experiments.

vision when using ultrafiltration modules having a molecular weight cutoff of 10 kDa (unpublished observations).

For human hemopoietic cells, the production of inhibitory factor(s), rather than the production of growth-promoting factors, is probably a dominant limitation to successful cell expansion. It is widely known that when the inoculating $CD34^+$ cell concentration exceeds about 10^4 cells/mL, suboptimal cell expansion occurs. Furthermore, in artificial capillary systems, using human mononuclear cells (MNC), granulocyte-macrophage colony-forming cell (GM-CFC) production is markedly higher when employing microporous capillary modules that permit inhibitory molecules to escape from the cell-expansion compartment than with ultrafiltration modules that permit inhibitors to accumulate to high concentrations (Fig. 14.5). Additionally, the presence, though not the identity, of inhibitory activity has been directly demonstrated in conditioned medium recovered from MNC cultures (Fig. 14.6).

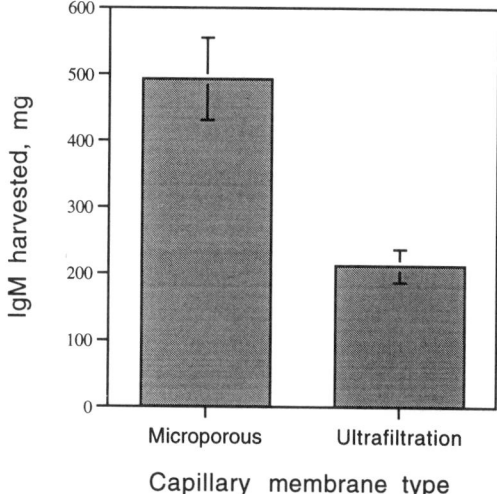

Figure 14.4 Effect of pore size on IgM yield from hybridomas cultured in the artificial capillary modules having ultrafiltration or microporous membranes. Hybridoma: END, an IgM producer. Cultures in MEM, plus 10% fetal calf serum for 21 days. The results are statistically significant at $p \geq 0.01$. Identical results have been observed with at least five hybridoma cell types.

■ SUPPORT OF ATTACHMENT-DEPENDENT CELLS

In bone marrow (BM) culture systems utilizing several cytokines, primitive stem cells are rapidly pushed toward differentiation and are rapidly depleted. This process can be slowed by co-culturing hemopoietic cells on a preformed BM stromal layer, such as that described by Dexter (Dexter, Allen, and Lajtha 1977). Quantitatively, co-cultivation with a stromal layer may retard the disappearance or even modestly increase the abundance of long-term culture-initiating cells (LTC-IC), a population of cells whose abundance correlates most positively with the long-term engrafting capabilities of harvested BM samples. Maximal long-term engraftment potential of cultured hemopoietic cells is desirable, especially for gene-therapy applications and for engrafting patients who have undergone ablative cancer therapy. Since the degree of ablation following therapy is not readily apparent, the presence of primitive stem-cell populations in BM cultures intended for patient reconstitution is probably desirable, even when the immediate objective is correction of the transient neutropenia and thrombocytopenia produced by the patient's therapy.

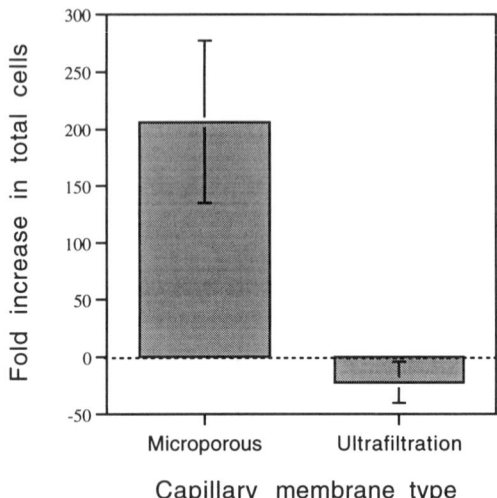

Figure 14.5 Comparison of ultrafiltration versus microporous capillary types for the culture of CD34[+] cells. Approximately 0.25×10^6/L human CD34[+] cells were isolated from a MNC BM harvest using a CellPro lab-scale device (CEPRATE LC34). These cells were inoculated into the different modules into which 10×10^6 allogeneic human BM stromal cells (irradiated with 2,000 rads) had been inoculated 2 days earlier. Cultures were performed in Iscove's medium containing 15% fetal calf serum and cytokines IL-3, IL-6, GM-CSF at 10 ng/mL, and SCF at 40 ng/mL. Cells were harvested and counted after 14 days of culture. These results have been confirmed in three separate experiments with three different BM MNC preparations.

It follows, then, that the optimal bioreactor configuration is one that would be permissive for the attachment and expansion of stromal cells that promote the survival and expansion of primitive hemopoietic cells, regardless of whether such stromal cells are endogenous to the marrow-cell preparation being cultured, or whether the stromal cells are exogenously supplied.

To this end, we have assessed the possibility that the microporous capillaries that allow passage (and dilution) of autocrine-inhibitory factors from the cell compartment might perform better if coated with a recombinant-attachment factor in support of anchorage-dependent stromal cells. That this is the case is demonstrated in Figure 14.7, wherein the CFC numbers following the culture of a MNC preparation (endogenous stromal cells) are doubled following culture in modules containing coated capillaries, compared with identical cul-

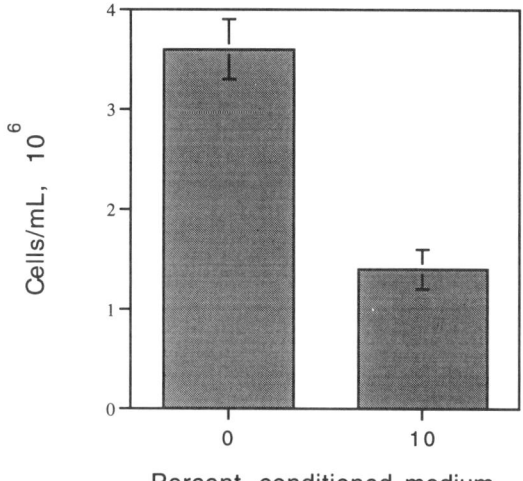

Figure 14.6 Detection of inhibitory activity in the medium recovered from human MNC cultures. Cells were cultured for 7 days (10^5 cells/mL as described in Fig. 14.5) and medium harvested, centrifuged, and sterile filtered. Fresh MNC were then cultured for 7 days in fresh Iscove's medium containing cytokines, plus or minus 10% of the above conditioned medium. These results have been reproduced with three different MNC preparations.

tures in modules without the coating (Davis, Lee, Kidwell, patent pending).

Regarding the use of exogenous stroma, our experience suggests that the abundance of stromal cells in BM MNC harvests varies considerably from patient to patient. This leads to unpredictability in cell expansion with different BM preparations. Moreover, recent experiments have indicated that only about 1% of the stromal cells recovered in BM harvests are capable of supporting primitive LTC-IC survival and expansion (Sitnicka and Wolf 1994).

For the above reasons, we and our collaborators initiated a search for a nontransformed stroma or a stroma equivalent that would support expansion of stem cells, as well as committed progenitors, while minimizing the effects of variable stromal elements. Our search led to the discovery that an endothelial cell population derived from pig brain microvessels (porcine brain microvascular endothelial cells [PMVEC] cells) supported a large expansion of blast cells, granulocyte-erythroid-macrophage-monocyte (GEMM) -CFC, GM-CFC, erythroid blast-forming cell (E-BFC), megakaryocyte (MK) -CFC, and CD34$^+$ cells (Davis, Kidwell, and Lee 1994), compared with liquid cultures in

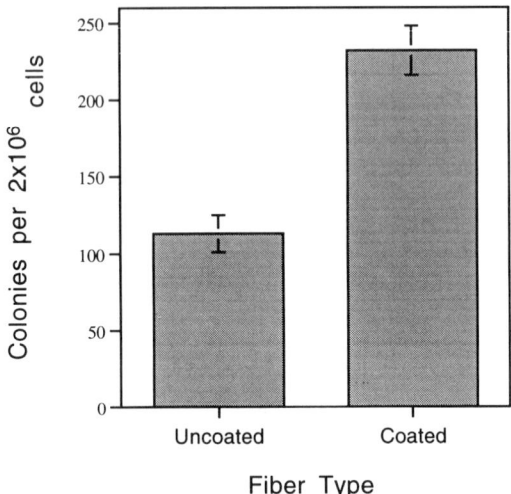

Figure 14.7 Effect of fiber coating on BM CFU-C. Human MNC were isolated and cultured in Iscove's medium plus serum and cytokines as described in the text. The modules were of the microporous fiber (polyolefin) type and were coated with recombinant attachment factor, Pronectin F (Peptide Technologies, Inc.). After 4 days, cells were harvested and CFC numbers quantitated using CFC assay test kits (Stem Cell Technologies, Inc., Vancouver, Canada, catalog #H4432). These results have also been obtained using Cellco's proprietary feeder cell line and co-cultivated isolated human CD34[+] cells (Davis, Kidwell, and Lee 1994; Davis, Lee, Kidwell, patent pending).

which these cells were omitted. These PMVEC have been shown to be sterile, mycoplasma-free, free of adventitious viruses, and nontumorigenic. Additionally, the karyotype is normal. These characteristics are the minimal requisite for use in expansion of stem cells intended for patient reinfusion. Interestingly, the use of the capillary coating results in a very tight adherence of the PMVEC to the capillaries and very few PMVEC in the harvested human hemopoietic cells following co-cultivation.

■ SURFACE-ACTIVATION PHENOMENON

In addition to the ability to support attachment of anchorage-dependent stromal cells and the ability to allow autocrine-inhibitory factors to escape from the capillary module, there is a third physical property that is important for optimal stem-cell expansion. The materials of the module with which the cell suspension come into contact must produce minimal surface activation. Surface activation is especially critical when culturing $CD34^+$ cell populations that contain macrophages and other cell types not removed during $CD34^+$ cell selection. The contaminating cells respond to such surface contact by releasing substances such as H_2O_2, NO_2, tumor necrosis factor (TNF), and interferon (IFN), which negatively affect $CD34^+$ cell expansion.

Minimal surface activation has been seen with certain materials such as polytetrafluoroethylene (PTFE), siliconized glass, and polyacrylonitrile. Materials with low surface activation potential include polyolefins, whereas unmodified cellulose has high surface activation properties. Interestingly, the use of stroma for co-cultivation does more than just provide growth factors that differentially promote primitive BM stem cell expansion and survival; it also minimizes surface activation by coating the capillaries and the shell tubing in which they are housed with a stromal cell layer, thus reducing the surface activation properties of the module-component materials with which $CD34^+$ cells (and accompanying contaminating cells) would otherwise come into direct contact.

In summary, optimal expansion of purified $CD34^+$ cells in the absence of supporting stromal cells is dependent on three major factors other than the culture-media formulation and added cytokines. These include the purity of the $CD34^+$ cells, the surface activation potential of the cell culture vessel, and the ability of the culture system to remove autocrine-growth inhibitors produced by either the $CD34^+$ cells, maturing cells derived from the $CD34^+$ cells, or contaminating cells. New materials with extremely low surface activation and low leachable properties have recently been used in simple, cost-effective manufacturing techniques to construct a new perfusion bioreactor module and system. Because of these special properties, this perfusion system appears capable of improving $CD34^+$ cell expansion, independently of the purity of the $CD34^+$ cells used for expansion.

■ THE GAS EXCHANGER

The gas exchanger used in our system is constructed of medical-grade silicone, a material of high biocompatibility that permits the equilibration of both CO_2 and O_2 in the perfusate, thus providing a means of restoring depleted O_2 levels and removing excess CO_2, which is essential for maintaining the pH. Gas exchange is simply and economically accomplished by passive diffusion across the tubing wall from the chamber of the incubator in which the cells are growing. By knowing the oxygen-consumption rate of the cells and the specific gas-transfer rate of the tubing ($0.75~\mu L~O_2/\text{min-cm}^2$ in this example), one can simply vary the length of tubing in the gas-exchange coil to provide the O_2 requirements of the cell type in question. For example, we determined that TIL cells consumed about 10 μL O_2/min/10^9 cells and that an 8-foot length of tubing was adequate to provide the O_2 needs of approximately 10^{10} TIL cells.

Empirically, it has been demonstrated that when co-cultivating with our stromal-cell line, it is the stroma, and not the CD34$^+$ cells, that determined the overall O_2 and nutrient requirements. Fortunately, the stromal line exhibits contact inhibition and in that state, low O_2 and nutrient requirements. Therefore, the stromal line is inoculated into the culture module at a concentration that produces near confluence (and near immediate contact-inhibition status) in a short time period after attachment.

■ THE PUMPING MECHANISM AND REQUIREMENTS

Oxygenation is, of course, dependent not only on the O_2 transfer rate of the gas-exchange tubing, but also on the rate at which the medium is made available to the cells. In a co-cultivation scenario or with purified CD34$^+$ cells, a pump rate of 5 to 10 mL/min is adequate for the production of a transplant quantity of CD34$^+$ cells and GM-CFC.

The pumping device, other than its output capacity, has a major requirement if it is to be operated within a closed, insulated compartment as is the case in an air:CO_2 incubator chamber. The pump must generate very low heat. We have selected a piston-driven device that minimally depresses the perfusate tubing and an in-line check valve for unidirectional flow. The piston is depressed by a rotating cam attached to the motor shaft. The tubing into which the piston is forced by the cam acts as the spring mechanism and forces the piston outward as the cam rotates. The in-line check valve provides for unidirectional flow of the medium. This mechanism is extremely efficient and generates low heat. The use of an oversized motor avoids stalling at low speed and further minimizes heat generation that would occur if the motor worked too hard in flexing the tubing during inward piston motion.

■ THE MEDIUM RESERVOIR AND TUBING

The most important consideration regarding the reservoir and tubing is that they be constructed of material that does not yield leachables into the culture medium and that they are autoclavable.

Sterilization by autoclaving is preferred over other methods, such as gas sterilization (ethylene oxide) or irradiation, both of which may produce residual or derived entities that adversely affect stem-cell viability. One additional desired property is that the tubing used to connect the reservoir to the flow path of the bioreactor be thermally weldable. Coupled with the use of a sterile connect device, this permits the reservoir to be changed at will during the culture period without opening the system and risking contamination.

■ SUMMARY

The presentation above has focused primarily on the use of artificial capillary-perfusion systems for hemopoeitic cell expansion and the maintenance of primitive stem cells by co-cultivating $CD34^+$ cells with stroma or stromal cell lines.

In the future it may be possible to simplify the expansion of primitive stem cells by replacing the stromal cells with factors that the stromal cells make. Currently, the best that is possible with stromal-cell–derived factors is to delay the rate of decline of stem cells, such as LTC-IC, during ex vivo expansion (Verfaillie 1992).

Certain cells, including $CD34^+$ cells, secrete autocrine and paracrine factors and dramatically affect how cells perform in this two-compartment, artificial capillary-perfusion system. In the construction of the system, there are important materials considerations, including the presence of leachables, appropriate sterilization procedures, and surface activation properties that dramatically impact the ability of the culture system to support optimal expansion of exquisitely sensitive hemopoietic cells.

REFERENCES

Davis, T.A., Kidwell, W.R., and Lee, K.P. (1994) Large-scale expansion of human $CD34^+$ cells on porcine endothelial cells in an artificial capillary system. *Experimental Hematology*, **22**, 802.

Dexter, T.M., Allen, T.D., and Lajtha, L.G. (1977) Conditions controlling the proliferation of hemopoietic stem cells in vitro. *Journal of Cellular Physiology*, **91**, 335–44.

Kidwell, W.R. (1989) Filtering out inhibition. *Biotechnology*, **7**, 462–63.

Sitnicka, E., and Wolf, S. (1994) Long term repopulating hemopoietic stem cells (LTRC) proliferate in vitro on only one cell type among marrow cells. *Experimental Hematology*, **22**, 770.

Verfaillie, C.M. (1992) Direct contact between human primitive hemopoietic progenitors and bone marrow stroma is not required for long-term in vitro hemopoiesis. *Blood*, **79**, 2821–6.

—15

Purging of Malignant Cells

JOHN G. GRIBBEN AND LEE M. NADLER

Despite the success of the use of combination chemotherapy for the treatment of advanced-stage malignancies, the majority of these patients die of their disease. In an attempt to overcome drug resistance, there has been increasing use of high-dose therapy with curative attempt both in patients with previously relapsed disease, and increasingly as consolidation therapy in first complete remission. The myeloablation resulting after high-dose therapy can be rescued by infusion of allogeneic or autologous bone-marrow (BM) or peripheral blood stem cells (PBSC). Autologous stem-cell support from either BM or PBSC has several potential advantages over allogeneic transplantation. It overcomes the need for an HLA-identical donor, eliminates the risk of graft-versus-host disease (GVHD), and has enabled the use of chemotherapy dose escalation for a large number of patients with a number of hematologic and solid tumors (Hurd et al. 1988; Peters, Shpall, and Jones 1988; Armitage 1989; Gribben, Goldstone, and Linch 1989a; Gribben et al. 1989b; Ball et al. 1990; Freedman et al. 1990b).

The major obstacle to the use of autologous stem cells after high-dose chemotherapy is that contaminating tumor cells infused into the patient would then contribute to subsequent relapse. To minimize this risk, most centers obtain autologous stem cells either when the patient is in complete remission or when there is no evidence by histologic examination of BM infiltration of disease. Others believe that PBSC may provide a tumor-contaminated source and use this as a rationale to move from autologous bone-marrow transplantation (BMT) to PBSC transplants. In addition, a variety of methods have been developed to "purge" malignant cells. The aim of purging is to eliminate any contaminating malignant cells and leave intact the he-

250

mopoietic stem cells (HSC) that are necessary for engraftment. The development of purging techniques has led subsequently to a number of studies of autologous BMT in patients with either a previous history of BM infiltration or even overt BM infiltration at the time of BM harvest (Takvorian et al. 1987; Hurd et al. 1988; Freedman et al. 1990a; Freedman et al. 1993). These clinical studies have demonstrated that purging can deplete malignant cells in vitro without significantly impairing hematologic engraftment. The rationale for removing tumor cells from the HSC might therefore appear compelling, yet the issue of purging remains highly controversial. To date, there have been no clinical trials testing the efficacy of purging by comparison of infusion of purged versus unpurged autologous BM. In addition, the finding that the majority of patients who relapse after autologous BM transplant do so at sites of prior disease has led to the widespread view that purging of autologous marrow could contribute little to subsequent outcome. In assessing the value of purging, we shall address three basic questions: What is the evidence that residual malignant cells are contained within autologous BM or PBSC collections? Can we purge these tumor cells using available technique? Do infused tumor cells contribute to relapse and does removal of these cells lead to improved outcome after treatment?

■ RESIDUAL DISEASE IN THE BONE MARROW

The likelihood that autologous stem cells are contaminated with neoplastic cells is determined by a number of clinical variables. BM involvement is rare in some tumors such as testicular or ovarian cancers; is more common in non-Hodgkin's lymphoma (NHL) and in solid tumors such as small-cell lung cancer (SCLC), neuroblastoma, and breast cancer; and is invariable in the leukemias. Generally, the higher the stage of the tumor, the more likely the BM is to be involved. In addition, the ability to detect malignant cells within the BM is dependent upon the sensitivity of the assay used (Fig. 15.1). Since the limit of detection of marrow infiltration by histologic examination is 5% and approximately 10^{11} cells are collected at the time of BM harvest, BM judged to be histologically normal may still contain as many as 5×10^8 malignant cells. More sensitive assays to detect the presence of malignant infiltration such as flow cytometric analysis, clonal excess of immunoglobulin light-chain expression, clonogenic assays, and molecular biologic techniques such as Southern blot analysis have greatly increased the sensitivity of detection of malignant cells. Sensitive culture techniques have demonstrated clearly that clonogenic malignant cells can be grown from marrow

DETECTION OF MARROW INFILTRATION

		Sensitivity	Disadvantage
1. Morphology	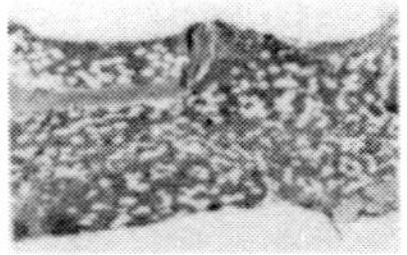	5%	• Specific, but low sensitivity
2. Flow	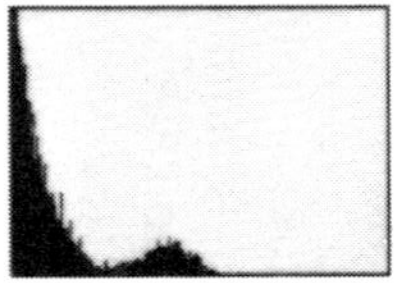	1-5%	• Lack of specificity as no lymphoma specific antigens
3. Restriction fragment analysis + Southern blotting	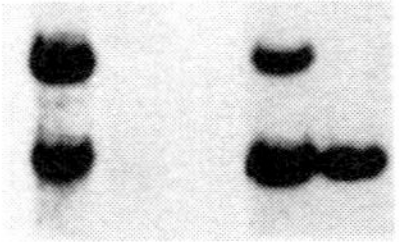	1%	• Time consuming
4. Polymerase chain reaction	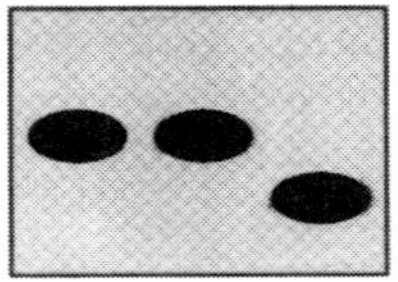	0.001%	• Requires sequence information • False positive results

Figure 15.1 Sensitivity of detection of marrow infiltration.

with no morphologic evidence of infiltration (Benjamin, et al. 1983; Estrov, Grunberger, and Dube 1986; Favrot et al. 1989). The application of the polymerase chain reaction (PCR) has greatly increased the sensitivity of detection of disease, such that one malignant cell can be detected in up to 10^6 normal cells. DNA polymerase can only add nucleotides to the 3' end of a preexisting single-stranded oligonucleotide fragment that binds to the target sequence so that sequence information is required on both sides of the gene fragments to be amplified. Nonrandom chromosomal translocations are ideal candidates for PCR amplification if the DNA sequences at the chromosomal breakpoints. For example, cloning of the t(14;18) breakpoints involving the bc1-2 protooncogene on chromosome 18 and the immunoglobulin heavy-chain locus on chromosome 14 (Bakshi et al. 1985; Cleary and Sklar 1985; Tsujimoto et al. 1985) has made it possible to use PCR amplification to detect lymphoma cells containing this translocation (Crescenzi et al. 1988; Lee et al. 1987; Ngan, Nourse, and Cleary 1989). Using this technique, residual lymphoma cells were detected in the BM at the time of initial assessment and following induction or salvage therapy of all patients with advanced stage non-Hodgkin's lymphomas containing the bc1-2 translocation (Gribben et al. l991a, b; Gribben et al. 1994).

■ PURGING OF MALIGNANT CELLS

At the same time that techniques were being developed to demonstrate the existence of minimal residual disease, attempts were being made to develop methodologies to deplete such contaminating malignant cells without impairing hematopoietic progenitors (Table 15.1). Because of their specificity, monoclonal antibodies (mAB) make ideal agents to identify and target such malignant cells. The principle for the selective depletion of contaminating residual tumor cells from hemopoietic progenitor cells is illustrated in Figure 15.2. The most likely mechanism of failure of immunologic purging is likely to be antigenic heterogeneity such that not all tumor cells express the targeted antigen.

A large number of mouse antihuman mAB have been generated with specificity for human cell-surface antigens (Ag) largely by immunizing mice with human malignant cells or malignant cell membranes. Despite the hope that unique tumor-specific cell-surface proteins would be recognized, all of the cell-surface Ag identified to date on neoplastic cells of the hemopoietic or solid tumor malignancies represent normal differentiation antigens, and true leukemia, lymphoma, or cancer-specific Ag have not been identified. The most im-

Table 15.1. Methods to "Purge" Tumor Cells from Marrow or Blood

Physical separation
  Size
  Density
  Osmotic lysis
  Lectin agglutination
  Hyperthermia
Pharmacologic
  4-hydroperoxycyclophosphamide (4-HPC)
  Asta-Z
Immunologic
  Uncoupled monoclonal antibodies
    Complement-mediated lysis
    Immunomagnetic beads
  Directly conjugated
    Chemotherapeutic agent
    Toxin
    Magnetic bead
    Radionuclide

portant factor to be determined is that the mAB target the malignant cell as specifically as possible, but have no effect on hemopoietic stem cells necessary for marrow engraftment. The ideal characteristics of mAb for purging are shown in Table 15.2. The targeted Ag should be present at high density on the cell surface to increase the efficiency of subsequent cell killing or removal. To limit antigenic heterogeneity of expression on the target cell, multiple mAB cocktails are employed targeting multiple Ag. Since mAB are not by themselves toxic, they must be used in combination with other agents to kill the targeted cell. The most widely studied methods of immunologic purging are complement-mediated lysis, immunomagnetic-bead depletion, and immunotoxins. If the mAB is used with complement, a complement-fixing isotype of antibody (Ab) must be used, the most efficient being IgM. For immunologic purging using complement-mediated lysis or immunomagnetic-bead separation, it is important that the Ag-Ab complex remains on the cell surface and is not internalized. In contrast, if immunotoxins are used, then the targeted Ag-Ab complex should be internalized to ensure intracellular delivery of the cellular toxin. Populations of cells that survive following mAB purging appear to be more resistant to subsequent treatments with the same mAB and complement treatments, associated with the emergence of subpopulations of cells with a relative decrease in the surface expression

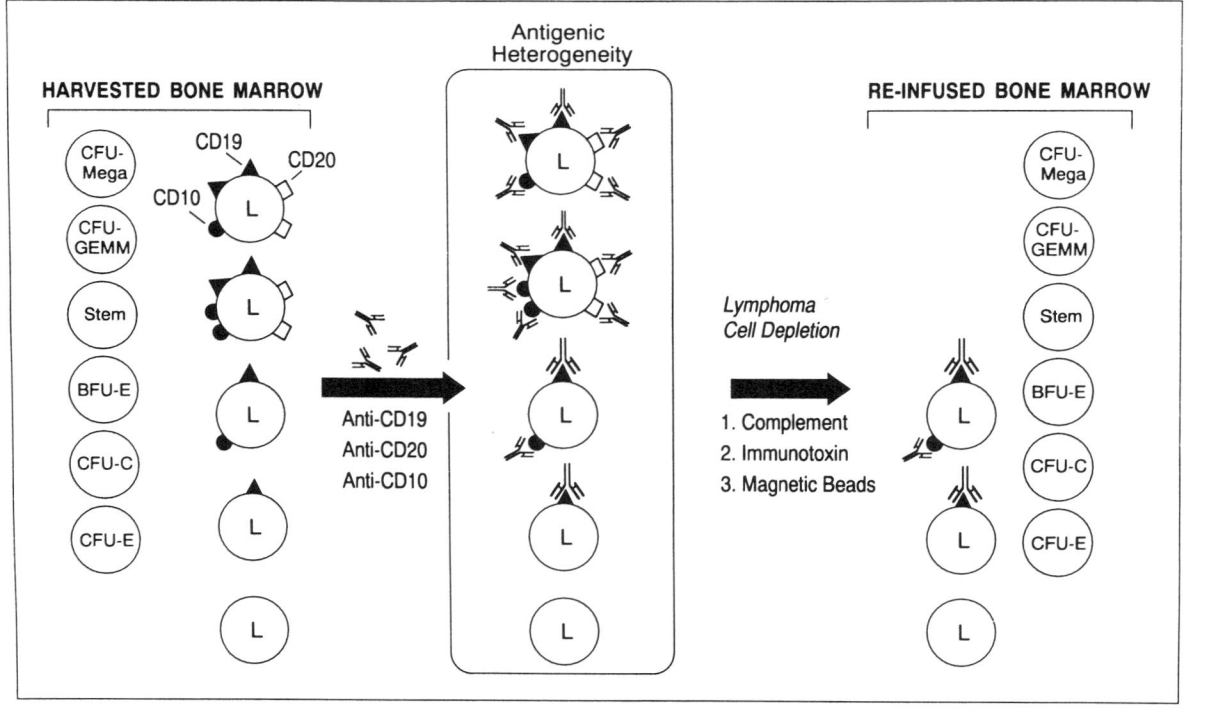

Figure 15.2 Principles of immunologic purging. Targeted antigens are present on the surface of malignant cells but are not expressed on hemopoietic progenitors. Any malignant cells escaping the purging procedure are likely to not express or express only weakly the targeted antigens.

Table 15.2. Ideal Target Antigens for Tumor Cell Purging

Not expressed on hemopoietic progenitors
Expressed on clonogenic tumor cell
High density of expression on malignant cell
Limited heterogeneity of expression on tumor cell
Lineage restriction
Depending on strategy for purging – ability to modulate

of the targeted Ag (Gee and Boyle 1988). Such changes in relative expression of Ag density also have been observed following treatment with chemotherapy. Therefore, it is important to demonstrate that the tumor to be purged should express the targeted Ag, not only at the time of diagnosis but also at the time of marrow harvest.

Purging of autologous marrow in vitro using immunotoxins is a particularly promising approach. Several exquisitely toxic candidate toxins have been identified that mediate their cytotoxic function by inhibiting cellular-protein synthesis. Because the mechanism of killing of toxins is different from that of chemotherapeutic agents, they are capable of killing cells that are resistant to chemotherapy (Fitz-Gerald et al. 1987); however, these toxins are cytotoxic to both normal and malignant cells and must be targeted to the malignant cell to demonstrate specificity. The combination of these toxins with a mAB to target delivery specifically to the neoplastic cells is, therefore, a theoretically attractive proposition (Grossbard and Nadler 1992). If native toxins were to be conjugated with mAB, the resultant immunotoxin would still be capable of binding to nonspecific targets by binding to the toxin-binding site on normal cells. This nonspecific binding is overcome by modification to the toxin moiety to delete the binding site, but leave the toxin domains intact. The most widely studied toxins have been ricin, *Pseudomonas* exotoxin, and diphtheria toxin. Most experience of in vitro marrow purging has been with ricin. Multiple, anti–T-cell, intact ricin immunotoxins have been evaluated as potential purging agents (Strong et al. 1985). The cocktail containing all four immunotoxins in equimolar concentrations eliminated greater than 4 logs of clonogenic leukemic cells at a dose that spared more than 70% of the pluripotent hemopoietic progenitors.

The combination of immunologic and pharmacologic purging is more efficient than either agent alone in eliminating clonogenic Burkitt's cell lines from human BM (De Fabritiis et al. 1985). The effectiveness of purging SCLC cell lines also was significantly increased when mAB and complement-mediated lysis was used in combination with the cyclophosphamide-derivative Asta-Z 7557, although there was significant reduction in myeloid-colony growth (Humblet et al. 1989). In a novel study, a combined approach was taken to attempt to eliminate multidrug-resistant leukemic cell lines from BM using a mAB directed against the cell-surface product of the multidrug-resistance gene (Aihara et al. 1991).

Most studies performed to date have utilized immunologic maneuvers to remove malignant cells from the autologous marrow by a process of negative selection. An alternative, and highly attractive strategy, would be to select the hemopoietic stem cell positively. There are a number of mAB that recognize the human hemopoietic progenitor-cell Ag CD34, and these Ab may be used to positively select $CD34^+$ cells. The $CD34^+$ population represents less than 2% of the low-density human mononuclear marrow cells. Precursors of all human hemopoietic lineages including B and T lymphocytes express CD34, and studies in nonhuman primates and in small number of humans have shown that isolated $CD34^+$ cells are capable of reestablishing hemopoietic engraftment (Berenson, Andrews, and Bensinger 1988; Berenson, Bensinger, and Hill 1991). Endothelial cells appear to be the only other normal cell type that expresses CD34. Although a minority of acute myeloblastic leukemia blasts express CD34 and the malignant stem cell in chronic myelogenous leukemia (CML) may also represent CD34, the clonogenic stem cells for the remaining hemopoietic malignancies and for solid tumors do not express CD34. The positive selection of $CD34^+$ cells from autologous marrow with or without negative selection to purge any more mature contaminating neoplastic cells is likely to have broad applicability in clinical autologous BMT.

Finally, increasing interest is now being placed on the use of PBSC, rather than BM as a source of hemopoietic progenitors. Further studies will be required to determine whether PBSC are indeed contaminated with fewer clonogenic tumor cells than BM, and the results of these studies will be awaited with great interest.

■ ASSESSMENT OF THE EFFICACY OF PURGING

Culture systems have been used to examine the efficacy of different complement sources (Roy et al. 1990) and to demonstrate synergy between chemotherapeutic agents and mAB-mediated purging (De Fabritiis et al. 1985). Clonogenic assays have been used to demonstrate the increased efficacy of multiple mAB and complement-mediated lysis in cell-line models (Bast et al. 1985). Multiple treatments were more efficient than single treatments and the combination of two or more Ab was more efficient than a single mAB to eliminate tumor cells (LeBien et al. 1985). PCR has been used to assess the efficacy of immunologic purging both in models using cell lines (Negrin et al. 1991) and in patient samples (Gribben et al. 1991a). The efficacy of mAB and immunomagnetic beads in removing Burkitt's lymphoma cells from normal marrow has been demonstrated in a number of studies. Clonogenic lymphoma cell assays have demonstrated that different anti–B-cell mAB differ in their efficiency of depleting lymphoma cells (Kvalheim et al. 1988). When three mAB were used in a cocktail, the efficiency of purging increased significantly. A cocktail of two mAB was used to assess the relative efficiency of purging of two different immunomagnetic particles (Trickett et al. 1991). Log-tumor-cell kill was significantly better using BioMag particles (3.1 logs) versus Dynabeads (1.8 logs) following a single cycle of treatment; however, there was no significant difference in the efficiency of purging after two treatment cycles, and greater than 4.5 logs of tumor cell depletion was obtained using either immunomagnetic bead. Treatment of harvested BM samples from lymphoma patients with either a three- or a four-mAB cocktail followed by immunomagnetic-bead depletion resulted in the loss of all PCR-detectable cells after three cycles of treatment in all patients studied (Gribben et al. 1992). This study suggests that immunomagnetic-bead depletion is significantly more efficient than complement-mediated lysis in depleting lymphoma cells, but that multiple cycles of immunomagnetic-bead depletion may still be required to remove PCR-detectable lymphoma cells. Using a single cycle of treatment with multiple mAB and beads, approximately 2.5 logs of SCLC lines could be depleted, although there was variability in the efficiency of purging different cell lines (Elias, Pap, and Bernal 1990). In parallel studies, there was no significant toxicity noted to myeloid progenitors. Anti-CD15 mAB, expressed on a variety of human cancer cell lines, was capable of depleting up to 3 logs of breast cancer cells from normal marrow using immunomagnetic-bead depletion, but minimally affected normal hemopoietic progenitors (Vrendenburgh et al. 1991). Using two SCLC lines, immunomagnetic-bead depletion was shown to result in a 4- to 5-log reduction of cancer cells and did not adversely affect BM colony growth (Vrendenburgh and Ball 1990). The combination of 4-hydroperoxycyclophosphamide (4-HPC) and immunomagnetic-bead depletion removed 4 to 5 logs of clonogenic breast cancer cells (Shpall et al. 1991). Evaluation of the purging efficiency of an immunotoxin prepared by conjugating anti-CD7 with pokeweed antiviral protein revealed that approximately 3 logs of clonogenic T cells could be eliminated, but that the addition of 2'-deoxycoformycin and deoxyadenosine to the immunotoxin resulted in the elimination of up to 6 logs of the T-cell line, but also resulted in decreased myeloid progenitor colony assay growth (Montgomery et al. 1990).

■ CLINICAL STUDIES OF IMMUNOLOGIC PURGING

Immunologic purging was first performed in NHL and has been most widely studied in this disease (Takvorian et al. 1987; Hurd et al. 1988; Freedman et al. 1990a; Freedman et al. 1993), but has also been studied in myeloma (Anderson et al. 1993), acute lymphoblastic leukemia (ALL) (Simonsson et al. 1989; Billett et al. 1993), acute myeloid leukemia (AML) (De Fabritiis et al. 1989; Ball et al. 1990; Robertson et al. 1992), breast cancer (Shpall et al. 1991), SCLC (Humblet et al. 1989; Elias et al. 1990), neuroblastoma (Kemshead et al. 1986; Combaret et al. 1989), and retinoblastoma (Saleh et al. 1988), among others. The results obtained in the larger reported trials using immunologic purging are shown in Table 15.3. These studies have confirmed that immunologic purging can be performed safely and that subsequent hemopoietic engraftment is not significantly delayed. Evaluating the efficacy of purging from these clinical trials is fraught with difficulties. No randomized or prospective study has been performed that could demonstrate whether the removal of occult or overt neoplastic cells resulted in improved disease-free survival. In addition, it is clear that in most malignancies there is a need for a more effective ablative regimen to eradicate endogenous disease. Until these regimens are developed, the relative contribution, if any, of reinfused disease may be difficult to determine.

■ CONTRIBUTION OF INFUSED TUMOR CELLS TO RELAPSE

Although no direct study has been made comparing the infusion of purged versus unpurged marrow, indirect approaches can be made to assess the clinical significance of immunologic purging. In studies at the Dana-Farber Cancer Institute, PCR amplification of the t(14;18) was used to detect residual lymphoma cells in the BM before and after purging to assess whether efficient purging had any impact on disease-free survival (Gribben et al. 1991a). In this study, 114 patients with B-cell NHL and the bcl-2 translocation were studied. Residual lymphoma cells were detected in all patients in the harvested autologous BM. Following three cycles of immunologic purging using the

Table 15.3. Results Obtained in the Larger Reported Trials Using Immunologic Purging

Disease	No. of Patients	Antigen/mAB	Days to Neutrophils >0.5×10⁹/L	Days to Platelets >20×10⁹/L	Reference
Complement					
AML	30	CD14, CD15	27 (1st CR)	38	Ball et al. 1990
AML	12	CD33	30	45	Robertson et al. 1992
ALL	54	CD10, CD19, CD7	24	40	Simonson et al. 1989
NHL	100	CD10, CD20, B5	27	29	Freedman et al. 1990b
Immunomagnetic beads					
Neuroblastoma	91	UJ13A, Thy-1, UJ127.11, UJ181.4	28	42	Combaret et al. 1989
ALL	8	CD10, CD9	15	27	Kemshead et al. 1987
Immunotoxins					
ALL	13	CD7	17	40	Preijers et al. 1989
ALL	14	CD5, CD7	27	NS	Uckun et al. 1990

AML = acute myeloid leukemia; ALL = acute lymphocytic leukemia; NHL = non-Hodgkin's lymphoma; CR = complete remission; NS = not significant.

anti–B-cell mAB J5 (anti-CD 10), B1 (anti-CD20), and B5 and complement-mediated lysis, PCR amplification detected residual lymphoma cells in 57 of these patients. The incidence of relapse was significantly increased in patients who had residual detectable lymphoma cells compared with those in whom no lymphoma cells were detectable after purging as shown in Figure 15.3. This finding was independent of the histology of the lymphoma, the degree of BM infiltration at the time of BM harvest, or remission status at the time of autologous BMT. These findings suggest that the infusion of detectable lymphoma cells is indeed associated with subsequent relapse. A major objection to this finding is that the majority of patients who relapse do so at sites of previous disease, suggesting that the major contribution to subsequent relapse came from endogenous disease; however, in 60 consecutive patients with a PCR-detectable bcl-2 translocation who had undergone immunologic purging and autologous BMT, there was also an association between the presence of residual lymphoma cells after purging and the presence of circulating lymphoma cells that could be detected as little as 2 hours after infusion of bone marrow. It is possible that these circulating lymphoma cells are capable of homing back to the sites of previous disease, and it is these sites that provide the microenvironmental conditions conducive for cell growth.

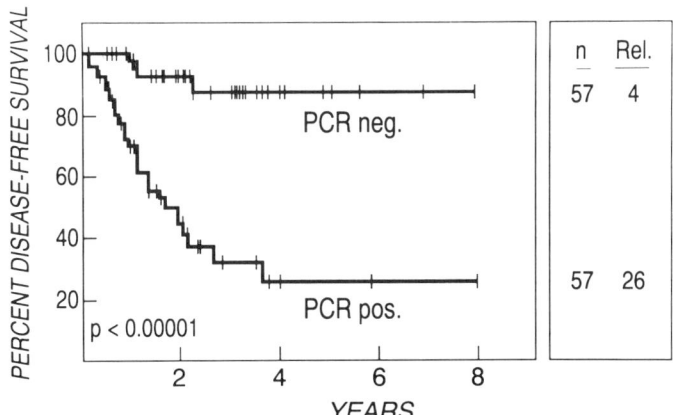

Figure 15.3 The disease free survival of lymphoma patients who were infused with autologous bone marrow with no PCR-detectable lymphoma cells (PCR neg) was significantly improved compared with those infused with a bone marrow containing residual PCR-detectable lymphoma (PCR pos). All patients had PCR-detectable lymphoma cells in the bone marrow before immunologic purging.

Second, if a marker gene were to be transfected into clonogenic malignant cells and the majority of cells at the site of relapse expressed the marker gene, this would provide compelling evidence that infused malignant cells contribute to relapse. Since the efficiency of transfection is low using existing technology, a negative result would still not be definitive; however, results published to date have demonstrated that when relapse occurs, there is evidence of malignant cells with the marker gene suggesting strongly that the infused malignant cells contributed to relapse (Brenner et al. 1993).

Finally, a randomized trial using purged versus unpurged autologous marrow would likely provide a definitive answer. This would require a multicenter study of several hundred patients; however, several ethical questions would have to be addressed in the design of such of a study. Although purging appears to have no significant toxicity, it is expensive and there are no definitive data that unpurged marrow contributes to relapse. Although data do not prove that purging is essential, they are consistent with the interpretation that minimal residual disease in the marrow may contribute to relapse. If patients with 5% marrow infiltration were randomized to receive unpurged marrows, then malignant cells would be infused. We would not wish to exclude patients with minimal marrow involvement from receiving autologous BMT, since those patients with histologic marrow involvement whose marrows purged to PCR negativity had excellent disease-free survival.

REFERENCES

Aihara, M., Aihara, Y., Schmidt-Wolf, G., et al. (1991) A combined approach for purging multidrug-resistant leukemic cell lines in bone marrow using a monoclonal antibody and chemotherapy. *Blood*, **77**, 2079–84.

Anderson, K.C., Andersen, J., Soiffer, R., et al. (1993) Monoclonal antibody-purged bone marrow transplantation therapy for multiple myeloma. *Blood*, **82**, 2568–76.

Armitage, J.O. (1989) Bone-marrow transplantation in the treatment of patients with lymphoma. *Blood*, **73**, 1749–58.

Bakshi, A., Jensen, J.P., Goldman, P., et al. (1985) Cloning the chromosomal breakpoint of t(14;18) human lymphomas: clustering around J_H on chromosome 14 and near a transcriptional unit on 18. *Cell*, **41**, 899–906.

Ball, E.D., Mills, L.E., Cornwell, G.G., et al. (1990) Autologous bone marrow transplantation for acute myeloid leukemia using monoclonal antibody-purged bone marrow. *Blood*, **75**, 1199–206.

Bast, R.C., De Fabritiis, P., Lipton, J., et al. (1985) Elimination of malignant clonogenic cells from human bone marrows using multiple monoclonal antibodies and complement. *Cancer Research*, **45**, 499–503.

Benjamin, D., Magrath, I.T., Douglass, E.C., and Corash, L.M. (1983) Derivation of lymphoma cell lines from microscopically normal bone marrow in patients with undifferentiated lymphoma: evidence of occult bone marrow involvement. *Blood*, **61**, 1017–19.

Berenson, R.J., Andrews, R.G., and Bensinger, W.I. (1988) Antigen CD34+ marrow cells engraft lethally irradiated baboons. *Journal of Clinical Investigation*, **81**, 951–5.

Berenson, R.J., Bensinger, W.I., and Hill, R.S. (1991) Engraftment after infusion of CD34+ marrow cells in patients with breast cancer or neuroblastoma. *Blood*, **77**, 1717–22.

Billett, A.L., Kornmehl, E., Tarbell, N.J., et al. (1993) Autologous bone marrow transplantation after a long first remission for children with recurrent acute lymphoblastic leukemia. *Blood*, **81**, 1651–7.

Brenner, M.K., Rill, D.R., Moen, R.C., et al. (1993) Gene-marking to trace origin of relapse after autologous bone-marrow transplantation. *Lancet*, **341**, 85–6.

Cleary, M.L., and Sklar, J. (1985) Nucleotide sequence of a t(14;18) chromosomal breakpoint in follicular lymphoma and demonstration of a breakpoint cluster region near a transcriptionally active locus on chromosome 18. *Proceedings of the National Academy of Sciences of the United States of America*, **81**, 593–7.

Combaret, V., Favrot, M.C., Chauvin, F., Bouffet, E., Philip, I., and Philip, T. (1989) Immunomagnetic depletion of malignant cells from autologous bone marrow graft: from experimental models to clinical trials. *Journal of Immunogenetics*, **16**, 125–36.

Crescenzi, M., Seto, M., Herzig, G.P., Weiss, P.D., Griffith, R.C., and Korsmeyer, S.J. (1988) Thermostable DNA polymerase chain amplification of t(14;18) chromosome breakpoints and detection of minimal residual disease. *Proceedings of the National Academy of Sciences of the United States of America*, **85**, 4869–73.

De Fabritiis, P., Bregni, M., Lipton, J., et al. (1985) Elimination of clonogenic Burkitt's lymphoma cells from human bone marrow using 4-hydroperoxy-cyclophosphamide in combination with monoclonal antibodies and complement. *Blood*, **65**, 1064–70.

De Fabritiis, P., Ferrero, D., Sandrelli, A., et al. (1989) Monoclonal antibody purging and autologous bone marrow transplantation in acute myelogenous leukemia in complete remission. *Bone Marrow Transplantation*, **4**, 669–74.

Elias, A.D., Pap, S.A., and Bernal, S.D. (1990) Purging of small cell lung cancer-contaminated bone marrow by monoclonal antibodies and magnetic beads. *Progress in Clinical and Biological Research*, **333**, 263–75.

Estrov, Z., Grunberger, T., and Dube, I.D. (1986) Detection of residual acute lymphoblastic leukemia cells in cultures of bone marrow obtained during remission. *New England Journal of Medicine*, **315**, 538–42.

Favrot, M., Philip, I., Combaret, V., et al. (1989) Monoclonal antibodies and complement purged autograft in Burkitt lymphoma and lymphoblastic leukemia. *Bone Marrow Transplantation*, **4**, 202–4.

FitzGerald, D.J., Willingham, M.C., Cardarelli, C.O., et al. (1987) A monoclonal antibody-*Pseudomonas* toxin conjugate that specifically kills multidrug-resistant cells. *Proceedings of the National Academy of Sciences of the United States of America*, **84**, 4288–92.

Freedman, A.S., Takvorian, T., Anderson, K.C., et al. (1990a) Autologous bone marrow transplantation in poor-prognosis intermediate-grade and high-grade B-cell non-Hodgkin's lymphoma in first remission: a pilot study. *Journal of Clinical Oncology*, **8**, 784–91.

Freedman, A.S., Takvorian, T., Anderson, K.C., et al. (1990b) Autologous bone marrow transplantation in B-cell non-Hodgkin's lymphoma: very low treatment-related mortality in 100 patients in sensitive relapse. *Journal of Clinical Oncology*, **8**, 1–8.

Freedman, A.S., Takvorian, T., Neuberg, D., et al. (1993) Autologous bone marrow transplantation in poor-prognosis intermediate-grade and high-grade B-cell non-Hodgkin's lymphoma in first remission: a pilot study. *Journal of Clinical Oncology*, **11**, 931–6.

Gee, A.P., and Boyle, M.D.P. (1988) Purging tumor cells from bone marrows by use of antibody and complement: a critical appraisal. *Journal of the National Cancer Institute*, **80**, 154–9.

Gribben, J.G., Freedman, A.S., Neuberg, D., et al. (1991a) Immunologic purging of marrow assessed by PCR before autologous bone marrow transplantation for B-cell lymphoma. *New England Journal of Medicine*, **325**, 1525–33.

Gribben, J.G., Freedman, A.S., Woo, S.D., et al. (1991b) All advanced stage non-Hodgkin's lymphomas with a polymerase chain reaction amplifiable breakpoint of bcl-2 have residual cells containing the bcl-2 rearrangement at evaluation and after treatment. *Blood*, **78**, 3275–80.

Gribben, J.G., Goldstone, A.H., and Linch, D.C. (1989a) Effectiveness of high-dose combination chemotherapy and autologous bone marrow transplantation for patients with non-Hodgkin's lymphomas who are still responsive to conventional dose therapy. *Journal of Clinical Oncology*, **7**, 1621–9.

Gribben, J.G., Linch, D.C., Singer, C.R.J., McMillan, A., Jarrett, K.M., and Goldstone, A.H. (1989b) Successful treatment of refractory Hodgkin's disease by high dose chemotherapy and autologous bone marrow transplantation. *Blood*, **73**, 340–4.

Gribben, J.G., Neuberg, D.N., Barber, M., et al. (1994) Detection of residual lymphoma cells by polymerase chain reaction in peripheral blood is significantly less predictive for relapse than detection in bone marrow. *Blood*, **83**, 3800–7.

Gribben, J.G., Saporito, L., Barber, M., et al. (1992) Bone marrows of non-Hodgkin's lymphoma patients with a bcl-2 translocation can be purged of polymerase chain reaction-detectable lymphoma cells using monoclonal antibodies and immunomagnetic bead depletion. *Blood*, **80**, 1083–9.

Grossbard, M.L., and Nadler, L.M. (1992) Immunotoxin therapy of malignancy. In V.T. DeVita, S. Hellman, and S.A. Rosenberg (Eds.) *Important advances in oncology*, pp. 111–35. Philadelphia, J.B. Lippincott Company.

Humblet, Y., Feyens, A.M., Sekhavat, M., Agaliotis, D., Canon, J.L., and Symann, M.L. (1989) Immunological and pharmacological removal of small cell lung cancer cells from bone marrow autografts. *Cancer Research*, **49**, 5058–61.

Hurd, D.D., LeBien, T.W., Lasky, L.C., et al. (1988) Autologous bone marrow transplantation in non-Hodgkin's lymphoma: monoclonal antibodies plus complement for ex vivo marrow treatment. *American Journal of Medicine*, **85**, 829–34.

Kemshead, J.T., Heath, L., Gibson, F.M., et al. (1986) Magnetic microspheres and monoclonal antibodies for the depletion of neuroblastoma cells from bone marrow: experiences, improvements and observations. *British Journal of Cancer*, **54**, 771–8.

Kemshead, J.T., Treleaven, J., Heath, L., Meara, A.O., Gee, A., and Ugelstad, J. (1987) Monoclonal antibodies and magnetic microspheres for the depletion of leukemic cells from bone marrow harvested for autologous transplantation. *Bone Marrow Transplantation*, **2**, 133–9.

Kvalheim, G., Sorenson, O., Fodstad, O., et al. (1988) Immunomagnetic removal of B-lymphoma cells from human bone marrow: a procedure for clinical use. *Bone Marrow Transplantation*, **3**, 31–41.

LeBien, T.W., Stepan, D.E., Bartholomew, R.M., Strong, R.C., and Anderson, J.M. (1985) Utilization of a colony assay to assess the variables influencing elimination of leukemic cells from human bone marrow with monoclonal antibodies and complement. *Blood*, **65**, 945–50.

Lee, M.S., Chang, K.S., Cabanillas, F., Freireich, E.J., Trujillo, J.M., and Stass, S.A. (1987) Detection of minimal residual disease carrying the t(l4;18) by DNA sequence amplification. *Science*, **237**, 175–8.

Montgomery, R.B., Kurtzberg, J., Rhinehardt-Clark, A., et al. (1990) Elimination of malignant clonogenic T cells from human bone marrow using chemoimmunoseparation with 2'-deoxycoformycin, deoxyadenosine and an immunotoxin. *Bone Marrow Transplantation*, **5**, 395–402.

Negrin, R.S., Kiem, H.P., Schmidt, W.I., Blume, K.G., and Cleary, M.L. (1991) Use of the polymerase chain reaction to monitor the effectiveness of ex vivo tumor cell purging. *Blood*, **77**, 654–60.

Ngan, B.Y., Nourse, J., and Cleary, M.L. (1989) Detection of chromosomal translocation t(14;18) within the minor cluster region of bcl-2 by polymerase chain reaction and direct genomic sequencing of the enzymatically amplified DNA in follicular lymphomas. *Blood*, **73**, 1759–62.

Peters, W.P., Shpall, E.J., and Jones, R.B. (1988) High dose combination alkylating agents with bone marrow support as initial treatment for metastatic breast cancer. *Journal of Clinical Oncology*, **6**, 1501–15.

Preijers, F.W.M.B., De Witte, T., Wessels, J.M.C., et al. (1989) Autologous transplantation of bone marrow purged in vitro with anti-CD7-(WT1-) ricin A immunotoxin in T-cell lymphoblastic leukemia and lymphoma. *Blood*, **74**, 1152–8.

Robertson, M.J., Soiffer, R.J., Freedman, A.S., et al. (1992) Human bone marrow depleted of CD33-positive cells mediates delayed but durable reconstitution of hematopoiesis: clinical trial of My9 monoclonal antibody-purged autografts for the treatment of acute myeloid leukemia. *Blood*, **79**, 2229–36.

Roy, D.C., Felix, M., Cannady, W.G., Cannistra, S., and Ritz, J. (1990) Comparative activities of rabbit complements of different ages using an invitro marrow purging model. *Leukemia Research*, **14**, 407–16.

Saleh, R.A., Gross, S., Cassano, W., and Gee, A. (1988) Metastatic retinoblastoma successfully treated with immunomagnetic purged autologous bone marrow transplantation. *Cancer*, **62**, 2301–3.

Shpall, E.J., Bast, R.C., Joines, W.T., et al. (1991) Immunomagnetic purging of breast cancer from bone marrow for autologous transplantation. *Bone Marrow Transplantation*, **7**, 145–51.

Simonsson, B., Burnett, A.K., Prentice, H.G., et al. (1989) Autologous bone marrow transplantation with monoclonal antibody purged marrow for high risk acute lymphoblastic leukemia. *Leukemia*, **3**, 631–6.

Strong, R.C., Uckun, F., Youle, R.J., Kersey, J., and Vallera, D.A. (1985) Use of multiple T cell-directed intact ricin immunotoxins for autologous bone marrow transplantation. *Blood*, **66**, 627–35.

Takvorian, T., Canellos, G.P., Ritz, J., et al. (1987) Prolonged disease-free survival after autologous bone marrow transplantation in patients with non-Hodgkin's lymphoma with a poor prognosis. *New England Journal of Medicine*, **316**, 1499–505.

Trickett, A.E., Ford, D.J., Lam-Po-Tang, P.R.L., and Vowels, M.R. (1991) Immuno-magnetic bone marrow purging of common acute lymphoblastic leukemia cells: suitability of BioMag particles. *Bone Marrow Transplantation*, **7**, 199–203.

Tsujimoto, Y., Gorman, J., Jaffe, E., and Croce, C.M. (1985) The t(14;18) chromosome translocations involved in B-cell neoplasms result from mistakes in VDJ joining. *Science*, **22**, 1390–3.

Uckun, F., Kersey, J H., Vallera, D.A., et al. (1990) Autologous bone marrow transplantation in high risk remission T-lineage acute lymphoblastic leukemia using immunotoxins plus 4-hydroperoxycyclophosphamide for marrow purging. *Blood*, **76**, 1723–33.

Vrendenburgh, J.J., and Ball, E.D. (1990) Elimination of small cell carcinoma of the lung from human bone marrow by monoclonal antibodies and immunomagnetic beads. *Cancer Research*, **50**, 7216–20.

Vrendenburgh, J., Simpson, J.W., Memoli, V.A., and Ball, E.D. (1991) Reactivity of anti-CD15 monoclonal antibody PM-81 with breast cancer and elimination of breast cancer cell lines from human bone marrow by PM-81 and immunomagnetic beads. *Cancer Research*, **51**, 2451–5.

Current Clinical Approaches

-16

Dose-Intensive Chemotherapy Without Hemopoietic Cell Support

RUSSELL L. BASSER AND RICHARD M. FOX

A major reason for failure to cure cancer is the lack of effective means to overcome the resistance of tumor cells to cytotoxic drugs. According to the Goldie-Coldman hypothesis, it is highly likely that chemotherapy-resistant tumor cells are present at the time of clinical presentation, or evolve during subsequent treatment (Goldie and Coldman 1979). One method used to try and overcome drug resistance is the delivery of regimens incorporating multiple, non–cross-resistant drugs to avoid selection of double-resistant clones. Another is the administration of cytotoxic agents at their maximum-tolerated doses as frequently as possible; however, substantial improvements in clinical outcome have been difficult to achieve. This has been due to both the lack of effective new agents, and the steep dose-toxicity curve of standard cancer chemotherapy. This latter phenomenon has limited the ability to test whether a dose-response relationship exists for chemosensitive tumors. The availability of recombinant hemopoietic growth factors (rHGF) (Lieschke and Burgess 1992a, b), and the development of cellular support of high-dose chemotherapy (bone marrow [BM] or peripheral blood progenitor cells [PBPC]), mean that it is now possible to investigate whether escalation of doses of cytotoxic drugs does indeed overcome tumor-cell drug resistance and produce a meaningful clinical benefit to patients; however, a number of questions remain unanswered regarding the relative merits of dose-intensive chemotherapy supported with HGF alone versus in combination with BM or PBPC. Is the in vivo dose-response curve of cytotoxic agents linear, so that ever-increasing doses result in a greater chance of response? Or does it reach a plateau, above which only greater toxicity is observed? Is the best chance of cure achieved with a single myeloablative course of chemotherapy, or multiple, nonablative cycles? What is the clinical importance of tumor cell contamination of hemopoietic cell collections (Moss et al. 1990; Cote et al. 1991; Lindemann et al. 1992; Skov, Hirsch, and Bobrow 1992; Brugger et al. 1994), and should their presence influence the method of support used? These issues are important because the use of PBPC for hemopoietic support is associated with greater demands on resources and potentially greater toxicity (Table 16.1). The major focus of this chapter will be on the degree to which dose escalation of cytotoxic chemotherapy is possible without PBPC support, with or without HGF.

■ DOSE-RESPONSE IN CANCER THERAPY

The initial evidence for a cytotoxic drug dose-response relationship came from laboratory animal studies, in which steep dose-response curves were shown for a variety of agents (Bruce, Meeker, and Valeriote 1966; Skipper 1967). Skipper recently reported a retrospec-

Table 16.1. Comparison of Chemotherapy Dose-Escalation with HGF Versus Hemopoietic Cell Support[a]

	HGF Alone	Cellular Support (PBPC or ABM) ± HGF
Maximum dose escalation	Intensive, nonablative Multiple cycles	Myeloablative Single or multiple cycles
Most common dose-limiting toxicity	Thrombocytopenia	Nonhematological (especially mucositis)
Reinfusion of tumor cells	No	Yes – reduce by purging or positive (CD34[+]) selection
Resources	Drugs and patient care facilities	Collection and storage facilities, drugs and patient care facilities
Improved response rates and duration of response[b]	Yes	Yes
Improved survival	Unknown	Unknown
Cost benefit	Unknown	Unknown

[a]HGF = hemopoietic growth factors, PBPC = peripheral blood progenitor cells, ABM = autologous bone marrow.
[b]In selected malignancies (see text).

tive analysis of a large number of animal experiments, and showed the ability to cure an experimental tumor was most closely related to the dose intensity of drug delivered (Skipper 1990). Dose intensity refers to the dose of drug and the time over which it is administered, and is expressed as milligrams per square meter per week (Hrynuik and Bush 1984). In contrast, the duration of response correlated better with the total dose of drug given in animals in which the cancer eventually relapsed. The conclusions of this study were that high dose intensity for a short duration was the best choice when the aim of treatment was cure, but that chemotherapy administration at a lower dose intensity over longer periods of time may be a superior option if the treatment intent was palliative (Skipper 1990).

Clinical data uphold the concept of dose response in a variety of malignancies. Some studies have shown that a certain critical dose of chemotherapy must be delivered to cure chemosensitive cancers, and any significant reduction from that dose results in a compromise of cure rate or shortening of survival (Fig. 16.1) (Frei and Canellos 1980; Bonadonna and Valagussa 1981; Carmo-Pereira et al. 1987; Kaye et al. 1992; Arriagada et al. 1993; Murphy et al. 1993; Wood et al. 1994). Retrospective analyses describe a relationship between dose intensity and tumor response in solid tumors and lymphomas (Hryniuk and Bush 1984; Hryniuk and Levine 1986; Levin and Hryniuk 1987; Murray 1987; Van Rijswijk et al. 1989; Meyer, Hryniuk, and Goodyear 1991; Pinedo 1993). These observations have been confirmed prospectively in studies in many cancers, in which doses of cytotoxics above previously defined "standard doses" (without the aid of HGF), have produced higher response rates than the "standard doses" (Fig. 16.2) (Ozols et al. 1988; Tannock et al. 1988; Focan et al. 1993; Neri et al. 1993; Marchner et al. 1994). Results of single-arm studies of high-dose chemotherapy with autologous hemopoietic cell rescue provide a hint that further gains might be attainable with greater escalation in cytotoxic drug dose. Response rates, and in some instances survival rates, also appear to be superior following a single cycle of myeloablative chemotherapy with BM or PBPC support when compared with low-dose regimens in a variety of malignancies (Bosly et al. 1992; Eddy 1992; Herzig 1992; Gisselbrecht et al. 1993; Gorin, Dicke, and Lowenberg 1993); however, the true benefit of such an approach is yet to be established due to the lack of randomized clinical trials.

The biological properties of solid tumors and some hematological malignancies (such as relatively slow doubling times, low growth fraction, and a microenvironment that inhibits drug access) suggest that maximum cell kill in these cancers requires delivery of multiple cycles

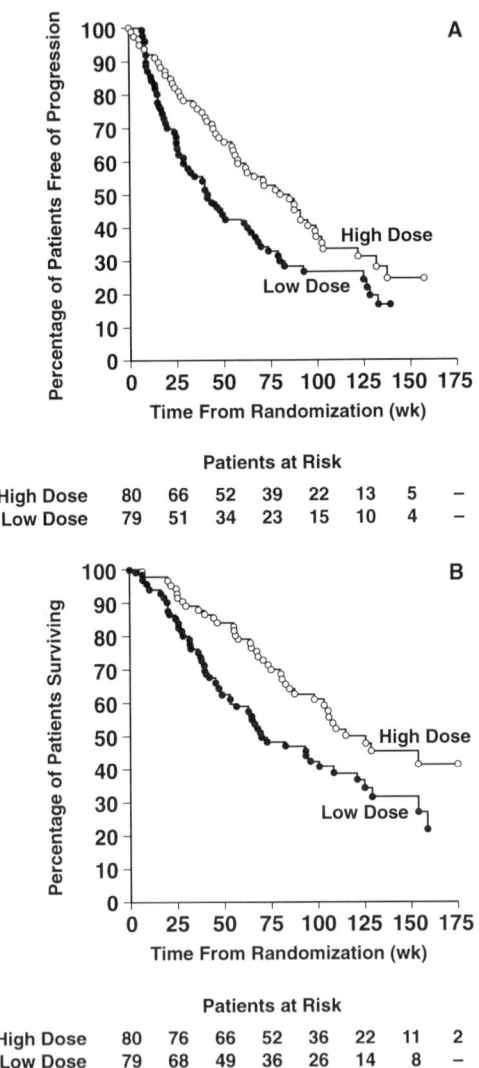

Figure 16.1 Progression-free and overall survival in women with ovarian cancer treated with cyclophosphamide and cisplatin 100 mg/m^2 (O) versus cyclophosphamide and cisplatin 50 mg/m^2 (■). Patients receiving the higher cisplatin dose had significantly improved relative progression rate ($p = 0.003$) and overall survival ($p = 0.0008$). (From Kaye et al. 1992.)

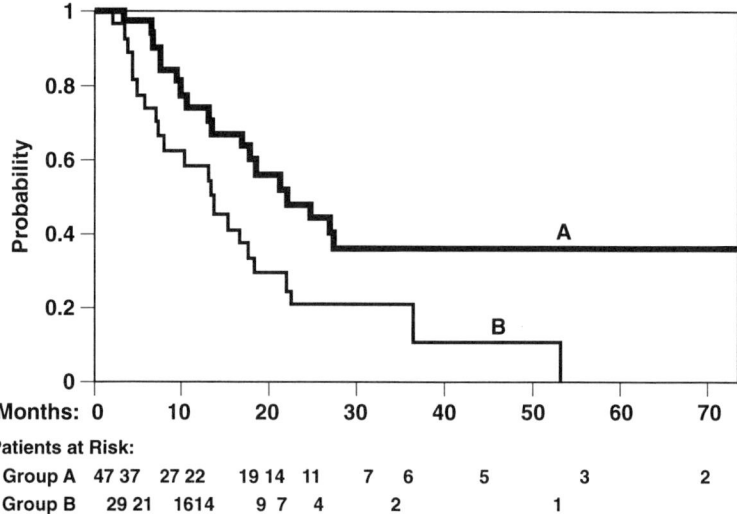

Figure 16.2 Duration of response (actuarial) in patients with metastatic breast cancer receiving either high-dose-intensity (*A*, 50 mg/m^2 on days 1 and 8) or low-dose-intensity (*B*, 50 mg/m^2 on day 1) epirubicin. Both groups were also given 5-FU and cyclophosphamide on day 1 of each cycle. Median time responding was 22 months versus 14 months, respectively; $p < 0.01$. The response rates were 69% (13% CR) versus 41% (CR 7%); $p < 0.001$. (From Focan et al. 1993.)

of chemotherapy at the "optimum" dose intensity (DeVita 1993). This "optimum" depends upon the balance between improvement in tumor outcome and the toxicity and financial costs of the technology used. Support with PBPC enables larger increases in dose intensity over multiple cycles of chemotherapy than HGF alone (Basser et al. 1995; Crown et al. 1993; Shea et al. 1993; Ayash et al. 1994), but at a greater cost. Analysis of quality of life and cost-benefit in studies using HGF- or PBPC-supported dose-intensive regimens is therefore essential for a full understanding of the impact on the treatment of a disease.

■ REDUCTION OF CHEMOTHERAPY-INDUCED MYELOSUPPRESSION WITH GROWTH FACTORS

Early studies with recombinant human granulocyte colony-stimulating factor (rHuG-CSF) or rHu granulocyte-macrophage (GM)-CSF were designed to determine whether these cytokines could abrogate episodes of neutropenia and febrile neutropenia following chemotherapy at standard doses.

Morstyn and colleagues demonstrated that filgrastim (nonglycosylated rHuG-CSF) reduced the period of neutropenia following melphalan administration in a phase I study in 15 patients with advanced malignancy (Morstyn et al. 1988, 1989). The degree of protection was related to the dose of filgrastim. Gabrilove et al. (1988) treated 27 patients with urothelial carcinoma with MVAC (methotrexate, vinblastine, doxorubicin, and cisplatin) and filgrastim. Chemotherapy was delivered as scheduled to all 18 patients receiving filgrastim, compared with 5 of 17 of the same patients treated without filgrastim. These studies showed that the period of neutropenia, but not the depth, could be reduced by the administration of filgrastim after chemotherapy.

The ability of filgrastim to prevent delays in the delivery of chemotherapy and maintenance of planned dose intensity has been substantiated in three phase III trials. Crawford et al. (1991) and Trillet-Lenoir et al. (1993), in separate trials, treated patients with small-cell lung cancer with cyclophosphamide, doxorubicin, and etoposide, and randomized them to receive filgrastim or placebo after chemotherapy. The duration of neutropenia and the incidence of febrile neutropenia and hospital admission were reduced in both studies (Fig. 16.3). In

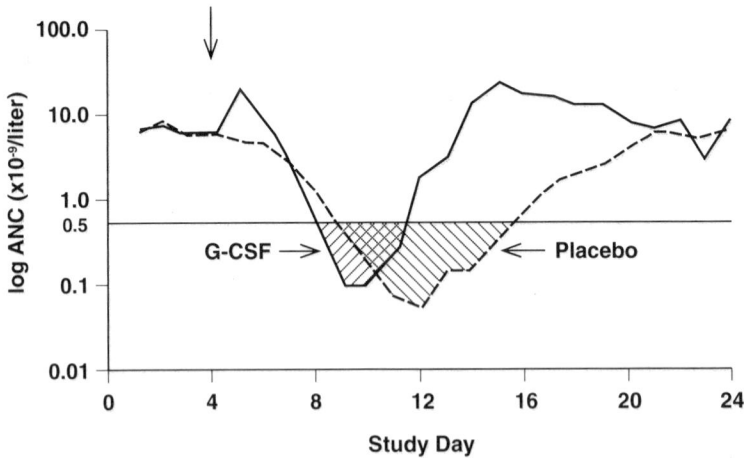

Figure 16.3 Neutrophil counts as a function of time after myelosuppressive chemotherapy. This demonstrates the effect of rHuG-CSF in patients receiving myelosuppressive chemotherapy. The arrow on the left indicates the day treatment with rHuG-CSF or placebo began. (From Crawford et al. 1991.)

the European report (Trillet-Lenoir et al. 1993), 69% of patients in the placebo group versus 29% in the filgrastim group had at least one dose reduction greater than 15%. The average relative dose intensity (taking 100% as the planned dose) was 96% in the filgrastim group and 87% in the placebo group. No difference in response or survival was detected in either study. Pettengell et al. (1992) demonstrated similar results with patients with high-grade non-Hodgkin's lymphoma (NHL) receiving VAPEC-B (vincristine, Adriamycin, prednisolone, etoposide, cyclophosphamide, and bleomycin) chemotherapy. Forty-one patients received filgrastim after chemotherapy and 39 were given placebo. There were fewer treatment delays, with shorter duration ($p = 0.01$), and a lower incidence of dose reductions in patients receiving filgrastim. The relative dose intensity of the filgrastim group was greater than 95% in 59% of patients versus 25% in the control group. Again, response was not influenced by the use of filgrastim.

Recombinant HuGM-CSF also has a favorable effect on neutropenia in uncontrolled studies (Heinrich, Gross, and Goebel 1989; Negrin et al. 1989). A large randomized study was recently reported by Gerhartz et al. (1993) in which patients with high- and intermediate-grade NHL treated with COP-BLAM (cyclophosphamide, vincristine, prednisone, bleomycin, doxorubicin, and procarbazine) chemotherapy were assigned to receive rHuGM-CSF ($n = 87$) or placebo ($n = 85$). Recombinant HuGM-CSF significantly reduced the period of neutropenia ($p = 0.01$), the days with fever ($p = 0.04$), and the days of hospitalization ($p = 0.01$). Subgroup analysis detected superior complete response (CR) rate (48% versus 28%; $p = 0.03$) and overall response rate (69% versus 48%, $p = 0.04$) in the rHuGM-CSF group for patients with "high-risk" NHL (defined as lactic dehydrogenase (LDH) above normal, and nodes ≥ 5 cm in diameter); however, the relative dose intensity of the two groups was identical, and the authors concluded that the enhanced response might have been related to immunological mechanisms enhanced by rHuGM-CSF. Toxicity required cessation of rHuGM-CSF in 11% of patients prior to the first restaging. This is consistent with results of phase I studies, in which the toxicity of rHuGM-CSF appeared to be considerably greater than rHuG-CSF (Lieschke, Cebon, and Morstyn 1989; Lieschke et al. 1989, 1990).

■ DOSE ESCALATION WITHOUT CELLULAR SUPPORT

The ability of HGF to allow dose escalation of chemotherapeutic agents has now been tested in a variety of settings, including single-agent studies and in the intensification of disease-specific regimens.

Much of the data describe the feasibility of this approach and give only hints of the efficacy.

Advanced Breast Cancer

One of the first reports of cytotoxic dose escalation of chemotherapy when given with HGF was from Bronchud et al. (1989), who treated 17 patients with advanced breast and ovarian cancer, using doxorubicin up to 150 mg/m^2 every 2 weeks for a maximum of three cycles. Patients received filgrastim on days 1 to 12. Hematological recovery occurred within 10 to 14 days of chemotherapy; however, prophylactic platelet transfusions were required in 50% of patients receiving doxorubicin doses of 125 mg/m^2 and 150 mg/m^2. In addition, nonhematological toxicities were intolerable at the highest dose, in particular mucositis and severe hand-foot desquamation. Ferguson et al. (1993) treated 18 patients with advanced breast cancer with doxorubicin 100 mg/m^2 and cyclophosphamide 500 mg/m^2 followed by 10 days of filgrastim, for a maximum of three cycles given every 2 weeks. Hematological and epithelial toxicities were also quite marked, and responses were of short duration. The strategy of decreasing the interval between doses of doxorubicin while maintaining or increasing the dose did not take into account the extremely long terminal half-life of anthracyclines in plasma and tissues. A theoretically more appropriate strategy would be to escalate doses at fixed intervals of 3 or 4 weeks. Demetri et al. (1991) did this by delivering increased doses of cyclophosphamide and doxorubicin with a fixed dose of 5-fluorouracil (5-FU) (the cyclophosphamide, doxorubicin, and fluorouracil [CAF] regimen) to women with advanced breast cancer. A maximum of four cycles were given at 28-day intervals, each supported by filgrastim for 7 to 18 days. They observed that doxorubicin 90 mg/m^2 and cyclophosphamide 2,000 mg/m^2 could be delivered safely without dose reduction and on time, with only infrequent nonhematological toxicity. Thrombocytopenia was the major hematological toxicity, and at the highest dose level the median platelet nadir was 18×10^9/L. Objective responses were noted in 13 of 15 evaluable patients. The doses of these agents were increased even further by Morgan et al. (1993), who administered two cycles of cyclophosphamide 4.2 mg/m^2 plus doxorubicin 50 mg/m^2 to 150 mg/m^2 supported by filgrastim, every 5 weeks. Patients with high-risk stage II and III breast cancer or metastatic disease responding to standard dose chemotherapy were treated. At 150 mg/m^2 of doxorubicin, severe neutropenia (absolute neutrophil count [ANC] $<0.5 \times 10^9$/L) lasted for less than 13 days; however, severe thrombocytopenia (platelets $<20 \times$

10^9/L) was more prolonged. In addition, grade 3 and 4 mucositis was almost universal and many patients required parenteral nutrition (G. Somlo, personal communication).

In an attempt to reduce the severity of epithelial toxicity, several investigators have substituted epirubicin for doxorubicin. Epirubicin is an analogue of doxorubicin that undergoes glucouronidation and more rapid elimination (Launchbury and Habboubi 1993). Compared with doxorubicin, epirubicin has reduced nonhematological and epithelial side effects and equal activity in breast cancer (Jain et al. 1985; French Epirubicin Study Group 1988; Italian Multicentre Breast Study with Epirubicin 1988; Perez et al. 1991). The maximum tolerated dose of epirubicin as a single agent has been reported as 165 to 180 mg/m^2 every 3 weeks for untreated patients, and 150 mg/m^2 every 3 weeks for previously treated patients (Case 1987; Blackstein et al. 1988; Feld et al. 1989; Holdener et al. 1988; Martoni and Pannuti 1989). Epirubicin can be administered at doses up to 120 mg/m^2 when given in conjunction with cyclophosphamide 600 mg/m^2 every 3 weeks without enhancing nonhematological toxicities (Marchner et al. 1994). Hemopoietic growth factors have been used in several studies to investigate the safety of increasing the doses of epirubicin and reducing the interval between cycles. As expected, rHuG-CSF and rHuGM-CSF have shortened intercycle intervals to 10 days. This has been achieved without debilitating mucositis or hand-foot desquamation (Piccart et al. 1995; Lalisang et al. 1994; Ardizzoni et al. 1994). In one study, support with filgrastim enabled administration of epirubicin and cyclophosphamide at 40% higher dose intensity using interval reduction compared with dose escalation at a fixed interval of 3 weeks (Lalisang et al. 1994). Overall response rates in the phase II studies using higher than standard doses of epirubicin and cyclophosphamide in metastatic breast cancer have been 70% to 100% (Ardizzoni et al. 1994; Cognetti et al. 1994), well above the 25% to 35% OR rates obtained using conventional doses (Rozencweig et al. 1984; Jain et al. 1985; Van Oosterrom et al. 1987); however, whether the degree of dose intensification possible with HGF support provides any real benefit over currently used standard doses in breast cancer will only be determined by randomized studies, and none have been published yet.

Mitoxantrone is an anthracenedione associated with less nonhematological toxicity than the anthracyclines, but also less activity in breast cancer at the standard dose (Bennett et al. 1988; Henderson et al. 1989; Cowan et al. 1991), which is 10 to 14 mg/m^2 given every 3 weeks as a single agent (Meyers and Chabner 1990). Nevertheless, mitoxantrone is an active drug in breast cancer, with a steep dose-response curve in vitro (Meyers and Chabner 1990). The lower toxicity profile theoretically allows greater dose escalation than anthracyclines. There are two preliminary reports of administration with HGF support to women with advanced breast cancer at doses of up to 32 mg/m^2 every 3 weeks. Neutropenia was reported to be the main toxicity, with little or no mucositis (ten Bokkel Huinink et al. 1990; Demetri et al. 1992). Insufficient numbers of patients had been treated to gauge the response rates at this time.

Paclitaxel (Taxol) is a promising new anticancer drug with a wide spectrum of antitumor activity. The current standard dose intensity is 175 mg/m^2 as a 3-hour infusion every 3 weeks (Thigpen et al. 1990). Although paclitaxel has a broad range of toxic effects, the predominant one is myelosuppression (McGuire et al. 1989); however, the toxicity profile alters as the dose of paclitaxel is increased. Two phase I studies of paclitaxel with filgrastim have reported that administration of doses above the maximum tolerated dose (MTD) of 250 mg/m^2 every 3 weeks was limited by peripheral neuropathy (Sarosy et al. 1992; Schiller et al. 1994). Two groups have reported that the single-agent activity of paclitaxel at this dose intensity given as first-line therapy for metastatic breast cancer is 56% to 63% (Holmes et al. 1991; Reichman et al. 1993). Although rHuG-CSF was used in one study to reduce neutropenia (Reichman et al. 1993), myelosuppression was dose limiting in both reports. Peripheral neuropathy was usually mild, and only occasionally moderate to severe.

Advanced Epithelial Ovarian Cancer

Retrospective analyses have suggested that the effectiveness of chemotherapy in ovarian cancer is directly related to the administered dose intensity of platinum compounds. As in the case of breast cancer, it is now apparent that delivery of less-than-adequate doses of chemotherapy to women with ovarian cancer compromises clinical outcome (Levin and Hryniuk 1987; Kaye et al. 1992; Murphy et al. 1993). Studies evaluating the potential for improvement with above-standard doses of platinum compounds have been reported recently. Dose escalation of carboplatin, rather than cisplatin, has been pursued due to its predominantly hematological toxicity profile. As a single agent, the MTD of carboplatin is 400 mg/m^2 every 4 weeks and 300 mg/m^2 when given with cyclophosphamide 600 mg/m^2 every 4 weeks (Alberts et al. 1985). In previously untreated patients, support with rHuGM-CSF allowed carboplatin to be given safely at doses of up to 600 mg/m^2 every 3 weeks, or 500 mg/m^2 when in combination with cyclophosphamide (Rusthoven et al. 1991). Doses of carboplatin up to 750 mg/m^2 plus cyclophosphamide up to 1,500 mg/m^2 were given with rHuG-CSF every 4 weeks to untreated patients with advanced malignancy; however, platelet transfusions for severe thrombocytopenia were commonly required at these higher doses (Toner et al. 1993). In previously treated patients, the MTD with rHuGM-CSF was 670 mg/m^2 every 5 weeks (Reed et al. 1993). These results have been disappointing in that more substantial increases in dose intensity of carboplatin have not been possible. Thrombocytopenia and cumulative toxicity were the limiting factors, and could not be overcome with HGF. A much greater increase in dose intensity is possible when cellular support is used (Shea et al. 1992).

Paclitaxel has substantial activity in advanced epithelial ovarian cancer. Response rates of approximately 40% to 50% have been observed in cisplatin-sensitive ovarian cancer, and 22% to 30% in cisplatin-resistant disease with doses of 110 to 220 mg/m^2 paclitaxel every 3 weeks (McGuire et al. 1989; Thigpen et al. 1990; Trimble et al. 1993). Sarosy et al. (1992) treated 44 women with cisplatin-resistant ovarian carcinoma using paclitaxel 250 mg/m^2 every 3 weeks. Dose delays were permitted only in extreme circumstances, and dose intensity was maintained for up to 14 cycles. A response rate of 48% (14% CR) was observed, higher than in similar groups of patients treated with paclitaxel without filgrastim (Kohn et al. 1994). Peripheral neuropathy was mild (grade 1 or 2) in 77% of patients and moderate to severe (grade 3 or 4) in 6%.

Other approaches to the treatment of women with platinum-resistant ovarian cancer have not been as successful. Doxorubicin has been particularly disappointing in this group of patients, with reported response rates of less than 10% (Stanhope, Smith, and Rudledge 1977; Hubbard, Barkes, and Young 1978). Dose-intensive therapy with doxorubicin or epirubicin and cisplatin with rHuGM-CSF support has resulted only in unacceptable toxicity, without improved rate of response (Vermorken et al. 1994).

Advanced Urothelial Cancers

The regimens of MVAC (Sternberg et al. 1988) and CMV (cisplatin, methotrexate, and vinblastine) chemotherapy (Harker et al. 1985) are currently considered the most effective combinations in advanced urothelial carcinoma. MVAC is superior to single-agent cisplatin (Loehrer et al. 1992) and other combinations (Logothetis et al. 1990a), and is likely to be similar in activity to CMV. Use of either rHuG-CSF or rHuGM-CSF reduces the myelosuppression and resultant delays in treatment with MVAC (Gabrilove et al. 1988; Moore et al. 1992).

Retrospective assessment of response rates of patients receiving MVAC suggested a dose-response relationship might exist in urothelial cancer (Scher et al. 1993), although these conclusions have been criticized on the contention of flawed methodology (Levine and Raghaven 1993). Even so, attempts have been made to improve survival and response with MVAC with the aid of HGF.

Seidman et al. (1993) increased the doses of all the agents in MVAC and reduced the intercycle interval from 21 to 14 days in 23 patients with advanced urothelial carcinoma. Each cycle was supported with rHuG-CSF. The delivered relative dose intensity was 33% higher than previously reported for MVAC without HGF support. Thrombocytopenia and leukopenia prevented maintenance of dose intensity beyond the third cycle of therapy. The results of a study by Logothetis et al. (1990b) suggested that a 20% escalated dosage of MVAC with rHuGM-CSF could be useful in the treatment of patients with refractory disease. A response was observed in 12 of 30 heavily pretreated patients (40%). Subsequently, Logothetis et al. (1992) presented a randomized study in which two groups of previously treated patients received escalated MVAC, but only half were randomized to receive rHuGM-CSF. The response rates were 83% without rHuGM-CSF versus 89% with rHuGM-CSF. The study was too small (37 patients overall) at the time of reporting to permit definitive conclusions. Loehrer et al. (1994) treated 35 patients with escalated doses of MVAC supported by filgrastim, with disappointing results. The 60% response rate was no better than with standard-dose MVAC, 14 of 35 (40%) experienced febrile neutropenia, and there were 8 (23%) early deaths. The median duration of response was 4.6 months (range 0.5 to 235+). Furthermore, only 50% of patients could be given greater than 80% of the planned dose intensity in the second cycle of therapy because of first-cycle toxicities. Such severe toxicity was not seen in patients in whom MVAC was intensified by increasing the doses of only doxorubicin and cisplatin in conjunction with rHuGM-CSF administration (Sternberg et al. 1993). A response occurred in 11 of 13 patients (85%) treated at the MTD. Toxicity was mainly hematological, and thrombocytopenia was the dose-limiting factor.

It is therefore unclear whether the use of HGF with the currently available regimens is of any benefit in urothelial cancer. This does not argue that there is no dose-response effect in this disease, simply that the use of HGF alone is ineffective in testing this question.

Non-Hodgkin's Lymphoma

Both meta-analysis (Gisselbrecht et al. 1993) and retrospective assessment of received dose intensity (Coiffier et al. 1989; Kwak et al. 1990; Lepage et al. 1993) suggest the presence of a dose-response and a dose-survival relationship in intermediate- and high-grade NHL; however, proving this prospectively has been difficult. Second- and third-generation multidrug regimens were thought to be superior to CHOP (cyclophosphamide, doxorubicin, vincristine, and prednisone) because of their higher relative dose intensity (Longo et al. 1993). Prospective trials have consistently demonstrated the lack of superior efficacy of these more complex regimens (and their greater toxicity) (Gordon et al. 1992; Fisher et al. 1993; Cooper et al. 1994), but have also shown that the received dose intensity was either equal (Cooper et al. 1994) or greater (Gordon et al. 1992) in patients given CHOP (Table 16.2). While myeloablative chemotherapy with autologous progenitor cell support appears to result in prolonged survival in patients with refractory or relapsed NHL (Bosly et al. 1992), the issue of dose intensity below this extreme is still largely unresolved.

Recent efforts to increase the dose intensity of NHL therapy have involved the escalation of individual agents, with or without HGF. In one report, a modest increase in doxorubicin dose from 50 mg/m^2 to 80 mg/m^2 in the BACOP (bleomycin, Adriamycin, cyclophosphamide, vincristine, and prednisone) regimen failed to improve rates or response or survival in patients with untreated, advanced intermediate- or high-grade NHL (Meyer et al. 1993). A preliminary report from Santoro et al. (1994) demonstrated the feasibility of intensified CHOP, incorporating cyclophosphamide up to 1,750 mg/m^2 without HGF. Recombinant HuG-CSF was administered at higher doses of cyclophosphamide and failed to impact on toxicity in this study.

Zuckerman et al. (1990) performed a series of studies in untreated patients with (mostly) high-risk intermediate-grade NHL. They delivered high-dose doxorubicin (120 mg/m^2) (Dabich et al. 1985) or epirubicin (180 mg/m^2) (Zuckerman et al. 1993) with vincristine and dexamethasone for three cycles, followed by cyclophosphamide and cytarabine for three cycles, without HGF. Complete response rates of 72% to 85% were achieved, but severe neutropenia was almost universal and treatment-related mortality was 5%. In another innovative approach, the DICEP regimen (dose-intensive cyclophosphamide 5 gm/m^2, etoposide 1,500 mg/m^2, and cisplatin 150 mg/m^2) had been developed as a way of delivering a synergistic combination that spares the BM stem cells (Neidhart et al. 1989, 1990). It is active in patients with relapsed and refractory intermediate- or high-grade NHL (Neid-

Table 16.2. Randomized Trials of Standard-Dose CHOP Versus Third-Generation Regimens for Intermediate-Grade NHL[a]

	n	% Response (CR)[b]	% Disease-Free Survival	% Overall Survival	% Treatment-Related Deaths
Gordon et al. 1992				5 years	
CHOP	199	82 (51)		48	4
mBACOD	193	86 (56)		49	5
Fisher et al. 1993			3 years	3 years	
CHOP	225	80 (44)	41	54	1
mBACOD	223	82 (48)	46	52	5
ProMACE-CytaBOM	233	87 (56)	46	50	3
MACOP-B	218	83 (51)	41	50	6
Cooper et al. 1994			4 years	4 years	
CHOP	111	92 (59)	32	51	4
MACOP-B	125	95 (51)	44	56	5

[a]No significant differences in response or survival were observed. The third-generation regimens attempted to dose intensify chemotherapy without the aid of HGF, but resulted in equal or inferior dose intensity compared with CHOP.
[b]CR = complete response.

hart et al. 1994), but has yet to be evaluated prospectively. While repeated cycles have been given without HGF (Neidhart et al. 1990), support with rHuG-CSF (Neidhart et al. 1989) or rHuGM-CSF (Neidhart et al. 1992) alone or in combination (Neidhart et al. 1993), markedly reduced the severity of myelosuppression.

Small-Cell Lung Cancer

Despite response rates to first-line, conventional chemotherapy of 50% to 90% (15% to 30% CR for extensive-stage disease, and >50% CR for limited-stage disease), almost all patients with small-cell lung cancer (SCLC) will be dead within 5 years of diagnosis (Ihde, Pass, and Glatstein 1993). After relapse, standard chemotherapy provides little or no benefit to the majority of patients. Studies investigating the use of more intensive chemotherapy have generally been small, not randomized, and produced either conflicting results or only very small survival benefits (Souhami and Ruiz De Elvira 1994). Recently, Arriagada et al. (1993) found that patients with limited disease treated with high initial doses of cyclophosphamide and cisplatin had a significantly improved 2-year survival (55% versus 43%) compared with those treated initially with low doses (Fig. 16.4). This report has strengthened the rationale for testing dose-intensification strategies in SCLC. In a phase II study, Ardizzoni et al. (1993) showed that the CDE (cyclophosphamide, doxorubicin, and etoposide) regimen could be intensified by 44% when supported with rHuGM-CSF by reducing the intercycle interval from 21 days to 15 days. Progressive anemia and thrombocytopenia prevented most patients from receiving more than four of the planned six cycles. Favaretto et al. (1992) also found that rHuGM-CSF permitted increased dose intensity of cisplatin, etoposide, and epirubicin given every 21 days. They treated two sequential cohorts of 20 patients each, the first without and the second with rHuGM-CSF. Epirubicin dose was escalated in both groups, to a maximum of 70 mg/m^2 with rHuGM-CSF. Interestingly, patients treated with rHuGM-CSF had a significantly higher response rate (94% versus 77%). In contrast, rHuGM-CSF appeared to permit no increase in the dose intensity of epirubicin above 100 mg/m^2 per cycle given every 21 days when combined with cisplatin 100 mg/m^2 in patients with untreated SCLC (Rosell et al. 1994). The results of this study should be interpreted with caution, as the dose-reduction and delay criteria were not clearly stated.

Two randomized trials have investigated the ability of HGF to allow chemotherapy for SCLC to be given with greater intensity, with different results. Fukuoka et al. (1994) showed that previously un-

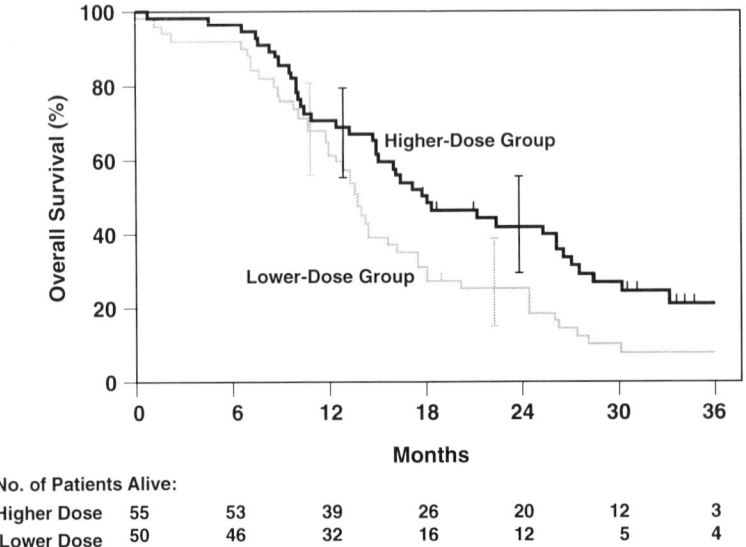

No. of Patients Alive:						
Higher Dose	55	53	39	26	20	12	3
Lower Dose	50	46	32	16	12	5	4

Figure 16.4 Overall survival of patients receiving initial high-dose cisplatin (100 mg/m^2) and cyclophosphamide (300 mg/m^2 for 4 days) compared with low-dose cisplatin and cyclophosphamide (80 mg/m^2 and 225 mg/m^2 for 4 days, respectively) for small-cell lung cancer. The 2-year survival rate was 43% in the higher dose group versus 26% in the lower dose group. The corresponding figures at 30 months were 28% and 11% (p = 0.02). Survival rates are given with 95% confidence intervals (From Arriagada et al. 1993.)

treated patients with SCLC could receive significantly more intensive CODE (cisplatin, vincristine, doxorubicin, and etoposide) chemotherapy with filgrastim than without. This did not translate into an improved response rate; however, the addition of filgrastim to a weekly chemotherapy regimen did not allow more intensive therapy to be delivered (Miles et al. 1994). These conflicting results might be in part explained by the greater ability of filgrastim to reduce the duration of neutrophil nadir than to prevent it.

The combination of carboplatin and etoposide is highly effective in SCLC, and the use of both agents is limited by myelosuppression (Bishop et al. 1987). The maximum tolerated dose of the agents when given together every 28 days is carboplatin 375 mg/m^2 and etoposide 600 mg/m^2 (Luikart et al. 1993). The addition of rHuGM-CSF has allowed etoposide to be safely escalated to 750 mg/m^2 at a reduced intercycle interval of 21 days (Luikart et al. 1991). Carboplatin has been increased to at least 650 mg/m^2 with a fixed dose of etoposide of 300 mg/m^2 with rHuG-CSF support (Fujita et al. 1993); however, the delivery of multiple cycles of higher doses has proven to be quite difficult. Bishop et al. (1991) could only administer three cycles of carboplatin 300 mg/m^2 and etoposide 360 mg/m^2 every 28 days with rHuGM-CSF to patients with untreated SCLC. Further therapy was prevented by prolonged neutropenia.

Soft-Tissue Sarcoma

Substantial progress has been made in the overall management of soft-tissue sarcomas with the use of sophisticated surgical techniques and adjuvant radiotherapy. This has led to considerable reduction in local recurrence rates in extremity lesions and prolonged disease-free survival in selected patients with metastatic disease (i.e., resection of pulmonary metastases); however, soft-tissue sarcomas tend to metastasize via hematogenous routes early on, resulting in a considerable number of patients presenting with disseminated disease or relapsing at distant sites (Lawrence et al. 1987).

Chemotherapy is for many of these patients the only available treatment modality. The most active drugs are ifosfamide, doxorubicin, epirubicin, dacarbazine, and docetaxel, which achieve response rates of 17% to 30% when used alone, and 25% to 51% when used in various combinations (Patel and Benjamin 1992; Liem and Verweij 1994). There appears to be a dose response for the anthracyclines and ifosfamide (Liem and Verweij 1994), and this has led to the use of HGF to further explore this relationship.

Escalation of single-agent ifosfamide from the maximum tolerated dose of 5 to 12 gm/m^2 has been possible with rHuG-CSF (Christman, Crapes, and Schwartz 1993) or rHuGM-CSF (Cerny et al. 1992). The dose-limiting toxicity was thrombocytopenia. In one study, a partial response was observed in four of eight patients refractory to standard-dose ifosfamide (Cerny et al. 1992). Doxorubicin has been escalated with rHuGM-CSF support from 90 to 110 mg/m^2 without any apparent improvement in response (Hoekman et al. 1994).

When given in combination without HGF, myelosuppression limits doxorubicin and ifosfamide to doses of 60 mg/m^2 and 5 gm/m^2, respectively, every 3 weeks (Loehrer et al. 1989; Schutte et al. 1990). Steward et al. (1993) used rHuGM-CSF to administer doxorubicin at 75 mg/m^2 with ifosfamide 5 gm/m^2 to 111 patients with soft-tissue sarcoma. They reported a 45% response rate (10% complete response), and the median duration of response was 9 months. Febrile neutropenia occurred in only 15 of 293 cycles, and there were two treatment-related deaths. Others have used rHuG-CSF to support the combination of epirubicin 90 mg/m^2, ifosfamide 7.5 gm/m^2, and dacarbazine 900 mg/m^2, given in divided doses over 3 days (Giannessi et al. 1994). The median intercycle interval was 20 days (range 13 to 35). Episodes of grade 3 or 4 neutropenia occurred in 60% of cycles (n = 53), but were generally of short duration (median 3 days). The dose intensity delivered was 40% above that of the regimen without rHuG-CSF, but response rate was not reported.

■ HIGH-DOSE SEQUENTIAL CHEMOTHERAPY

A novel method of administering very intensive chemotherapy, high-dose sequential (HDS) chemotherapy, has been developed by Gianni and co-workers. They initially investigated the feasibility of delivering high-dose cyclophosphamide, up to 7 gm/m^2 (Gianni et al. 1990), and etoposide, up to 2.4 gm/m^2 (Gianni et al. 1992a), when given with rHuGM-CSF. They then administered these and other agents at high doses sequentially rather than in combination, supported by HGF (rHuGM-CSF or rHuG-CSF), and followed by a single myeloablative treatment with autologous progenitor cell support. Only limited interpretation can be made of their reported phase II experiences in poor prognosis breast cancer (Gianni et al. 1992b) and multiple myeloma (MM) (Gianni et al. 1994). More interestingly, a randomized study of HDS therapy versus MACOP-B (methotrexate, doxorubicin, cyclophosphamide, vincristine, prednisone, bleomycin, and cotrimoxazole) in 75 patients with intermediate-grade NHL showed a significant improvement in complete response rate (94% versus 61%) and relapse-free survival (93% versus 68%) favoring the HDS group at 43-month follow-up. Overall survival was not different (73% versus 62%). Broader experience with HDS chemotherapy is necessary to determine whether this approach is generally feasible.

■ CONCLUSIONS

Substantial increases in the doses of chemotherapy that can safely be administered are achievable with the aid of HGF, but more data are required to understand the impact of growth factors on tumor outcome. One area where HGF have almost certainly been underinvestigated is in the maintenance of dose intensity in the elderly. There is evidence that poorer treatment outcome in elderly patients with NHL may in part be explained by less intensive chemotherapy (Goss 1993). In view of the comparable hemopoietic response to HGF between older and younger patients (Shank and Balducci 1992), investigations into the benefits of HGF-supported standard-dose chemotherapy would seem worthwhile.

One concern regarding the use of HGF to support repeated cycles of chemotherapy is the potential for "exhausting" stem cells (Moore 1992). Evidence in mice suggests that this is indeed the case (Hornung and Longo 1992). If this becomes a clinical problem, hemopoietic protection strategies, such as pretreatment with interleukin-1 (IL-1) (Hornung and Longo 1992), might need to be developed.

The major limiting factor to dose-intensive therapy with cytokines alone remains the lack of effective means to stimulate thrombopoiesis. A number of agents reduce chemotherapy-induced thrombocytopenia to a modest extent when given alone (Smith et al. 1993; Gordon et al. 1994; van Gemeren et al. 1994) or in combination (Brugger et al. 1992; Vadhan Raj et al. 1994); however, the recent cloning of the thrombopoietin c-*mpl* ligand has opened up the possibility of a markedly more effective method of overcoming this problem (Bartley et al. 1994; de Sauvage et al. 1994; Lok et al. 1994; Wendling et al. 1994). Thrombopoietin might augment PBPC in hastening platelet recovery after high-dose chemotherapy, or enable higher doses of drug to be delivered without the need for cellular support.

REFERENCES

Alberts, D., Mason, N., Surwit, E., Weiner, S., Hammond, N., and Deppe, G. (1985) Phase I trials of carboplatin-cyclophosphamide and iproplatin-cyclophosphamide in advanced ovarian cancer: a Southwest Oncology Group study. *Cancer Treatment Reviews*, **12**(Suppl. A), 83–92.

Ardizzoni, A., Venturini, M., Crino, L., et al. (1993) High dose-intensity chemotherapy, with accelerated cyclophosphamide-doxorubicin-etoposide and granulocyte-macrophage colony-stimulating factor, in the treatment of small cell lung cancer. *European Journal of Cancer*, **29A**, 687–92.

Ardizzoni, A., Venturini, M., Sertoli, M.R., et al. (1994) Granulocyte-macrophage colony-stimulating factor (GM-CSF) allows acceleration and dose intensity increase of CEF chemotherapy: a randomised study in patients with advanced breast cancer. *British Journal of Cancer*, **69**, 385–91.

Arriagada, R., Le Chevalier, T., Pignon, J.P., et al. (1993) Initial chemotherapeutic doses and survival in patients with limited small-cell lung cancer. *New England Journal of Medicine*, **329**, 1848–52.

Ayash, L.J., Elias, A., Wheeler, C., et al. (1994) Double dose-intensive chemotherapy with autologous marrow and peripheral-blood progenitor-cell support for metastatic breast cancer: a feasibility study. *Journal of Clinical Oncology*, **12**, 37–44.

Bartley, T.D., Bogenberger, J., Hunt, P., et al. (1994) Identification and cloning of a megakaryocyte growth and development factor that is a ligand for the cytokine receptor mpl. *Cell*, **77**, 1117–24.

Basser, R., To, B., Begley, G., et al. (1995) Adjuvant treatment of high-risk breast cancer using multi-cycle high-dose chemotherapy and filgrastim-mobilized peripheral blood progenitor cells. *Clinics in Cancer Research*, **1**, 715–21.

Bennett, J.M., Muss, H.B., Doroshow, J.H., et al. (1988) A randomized multicenter trial comparing mitoxantrone, cyclophosphamide, and fluorouracil with doxorubicin, cyclophosphamide, and fluorouracil in the therapy of metastatic breast carcinoma. *Journal of Clinical Oncology*, **6**, 1611–20.

Bishop, J.F., Morstyn, G., Stuart-Harris, R., et al. (1991) Dose and schedule of granulocyte macrophage colony stimulating factor (GM-CSF) carboplatin and etoposide in small cell lung cancer (small-cell lung cancer). *Proceedings of the American Society of Clinical Oncology*, **10**, 240.

Bishop, J.F., Raghavan, D., Stuart-Harris, R., et al. (1987) Carboplatin (CBDCA, JM-8) and VP-16-213 in previously untreated patients with small-cell lung cancer. *Journal of Clinical Oncology*, **5**, 1574–8.

Blackstein, M., Wilson, K., Meharchand, J., Shepherd, F., Fontaine, B., and Lassus, M. (1988) Phase I study of epirubicin in metastatic breast cancer. *Proceedings of the American Society of Clinical Oncology*, **7**, 23.

Bonadonna, G. and Valagussa, P. (1981) Dose-response effect of adjuvant chemotherapy in breast cancer. *New England Journal of Medicine*, **304**, 10–15.

Bosly, A., Coiffier, B., Gisselbrecht, C., et al. (1992) Bone marrow transplantation prolongs survival after relapse in aggressive lymphoma patients treated with the LNH-84 regimen. *Journal of Clinical Oncology*, **10**, 1615–23.

Bronchud, M.H., Howell, A., Crowther, D., Hopwood, P., Souza, L., and Dexter, T.M. (1989) The use of granulocyte colony-stimulating factor to increase the intensity of treatment with doxorubicin in patients with advanced breast and ovarian cancer. *British Journal of Cancer*, **60**, 121–5.

Bruce, W.R., Meeker, B.E., and Valeriote, F.A. (1966) Comparison of the sensitivity of normal haemopoietic and transplanted lymphoma colony-forming cells to chemotherapeutic agents. *Journal of the National Cancer Institute*, **37**, 233–45.

Brugger, W., Bross, K.J., Glatt, M., Weber, F., Mertelsmann, R., and Kanz, L. (1994) Mobilization of tumor cells and hematopoietic progenitor cells into peripheral blood of patients with solid tumors. *Blood*, **83**, 636–40.

Brugger, W., Frisch, J., Schulz, G., Pressler, K., Mertelsmann, R., and Kanz, L. (1992) Sequential administration of interleukin-3 and granulocyte-macrophage colony-stimulating factor following standard-dose combination chemotherapy with etoposide, ifosfamide, and carboplatin. *Journal of Clinical Oncology*, **10**, 1452–9.

Carmo-Pereira, J., Costa, F.O., Henriques, E., et al. (1987) A comparison of two doses of Adriamycin in the primary chemotherapy of disseminated breast cancer. *British Journal of Cancer*, **56**, 471–3.

Case, D.C. J., Gams, R., Ervin, T.J., Boyd, M.A., and Oldham, F.B. (1987) Phase I-II trial of high dose epirubicin in patients with lymphomas. *Cancer Research*, **47**, 6393–6.

Cerny, T., Leyvraz, S., Daggi, H., Varini, M., Kroner, T., and Marti, C. (1992) Phase II trials of ifosfamide and mesna in advanced soft tissue sarcomas (STS) patients: a definite dose-response relationship. *Proceedings of the American Society of Clinical Oncology*, **11**, 416.

Christman, K.L., Crapes, E.S., and Schwartz, E.K. (1993) High intensity scheduling of ifosfamide in adult patients with soft tissue sarcoma. *Proceedings of the American Society of Clinical Oncology*, **12**, 470.

Cognetti, F., Scinto, A.F., Cercato, M.C., et al. (1994) Phase II trial of high dose epirubicin and cyclophosphamide every two weeks + r-met-HuG-CSF in locally advanced and metastatic breast cancer. *Proceedings of the American Society of Clinical Oncology*, **13**, 88.

Coiffier, B., Gisselbrecht, C., Herbrecht, R., Tilly, H., Bosly, A., and Brousse, N. (1989) LNH-84 regimen: a multicenter study of intensive chemotherapy in 737 patients with aggressive malignant lymphoma. *Journal of Clinical Oncology*, **7**, 1018–26.

Cooper, I.A., Wolf, M.M., Robertson, T.I., et al. (1994) Randomized comparison of MACOP-B with CHOP in patients with intermediate grade non-Hodgkin's lymphoma. *Journal of Clinical Oncology*, **12**, 769–78.

Cote, R.J., Rosen, P.P., Lesser, M.L., Old, L.J., and Osborne, M.P. (1991) Prediction of early relapse in patients with operable breast cancer by detection of occult bone marrow micrometastases. *Journal of Clinical Oncology*, **9**, 1749–56.

Cowan, J.D., Neidhart, J., McClure, S., et al. (1991) Randomized trial of doxorubicin, bisantrene, and mitoxantrone in advanced breast cancer: a Southwest Oncology Group study. *Journal of the National Cancer Institute*, **83**, 1077–84.

Crawford, J., Ozer, H., Stoller, R., et al. (1991) Reduction by granulocyte colony-stimulating factor of fever and neutropenia induced by chemotherapy in patients with small-cell lung cancer. *New England Journal of Medicine*, **325**, 164–70.

Crown, J., Kritz, A., Vahdat, L., et al. (1993) Rapid administration of multiple cycles of high-dose myelosuppressive chemotherapy in patients with metastatic breast cancer. *Journal of Clinical Oncology*, **11**, 1144–9.

Dabich, L., Ensingeer, W.D., Zuckerman, K.S., et al. (1985) High-dose Adriamyin combination chemotherapy for intermediate and high-grade non-Hodgkin's lymphoma. *Seminars in Oncology*, **12**(Suppl. 3), 212–17.

de Sauvage, F.I., Hass, P.E., Spencer, S.D., et al. (1994) Stimulation of megakaryopoiesis and thrombopoiesis by the c-mpl ligand. *Nature*, **369**, 533–8.

Demetri, G.D., Horowitz, J., McGuire, B., Merica, E.A., Howard, G., and Henderson, I.C. (1992) Dose-intensification of mitoxantrone with adjunctive G-CSF (r-metHuG-CSF) in patients with advanced breast cancer: a phase I trial. *Proceedings of the American Society of Clinical Oncology*, **11**, 137a.

Demetri, G.D., Younger, J., McGuire, B.W., et al. (1991) Recombinant methionyl granulocyte-CSF (r-metG-CSF) allows an increase in the dose intensity of cyclophosphamide/doxorubicin/5-fluorouracil (CAF) in patients with advanced breast cancer. *Proceedings of the American Society of Clinical Oncology*, **10**, 70.

DeVita, V.T., Jr. (1993) Principles of chemotherapy. In V.T. DeVita, S. Hellamn, and S.A. Rosenberg (Eds.) *Cancer: principles and practice of oncology*, pp. 276–92. Philadelphia, J.B. Lippincott Company.

Eddy, D.M. (1992) High-dose chemotherapy with autologous bone marrow transplantation for the treatment of metastatic breast cancer. *Journal of Clinical Oncology*, **10**, 657–70.

Favaretto, A., Paccagnella, A., Sileni, V.C., et al. (1992) Correlation between GM-CSF administration and dose intensity (DI) in small-cell lung cancer. *Proceedings of the American Society of Clinical Oncology*, **11**, 304.

Feld, R., Wierzbicki, R., Walde, D., et al. (1989) High dose epirubicin given as a daily x 3 schedule in patients with untreated extensive non-small cell lung cancer. A phase I-II study. *Proceedings of the American Association for Cancer Research*, **29**, 208.

Ferguson, J.E., Dodwell, D.J., Seymour, A.M., Richards, M.A., and Howell, A. (1993) High dose, dose-intensive chemotherapy with doxorubicin and cyclophosphamide for the treatment of advanced breast cancer. *British Journal of Cancer*, **67**, 825–9.

Fisher, R.I., Gaynor, E.R., Dahlberg, S., et al. (1993) Comparison of a standard regimen (CHOP) with three intensive chemotherapy regimens for advanced non-Hodgkin's lymphoma. *New England Journal of Medicine*, **328**, 1002–6.

Focan, C., Andrien, J.M., Closon, M.T., et al. (1993) Dose-response relationship of epirubicin-based first-line chemotherapy for advanced breast cancer: a prospective randomized trial. *Journal of Clinical Oncology*, **11**, 1253–63.

Frei, E., III and Canellos, G.P. (1980) Dose: a critical factor in cancer chemotherapy. *American Journal of Medicine*, **69**, 585–94.

French Epirubicin Study Group. (1988) A prospective randomized phase III trial comparing combination chemotherapy with cyclophosphamide, fluorouracil, and either doxorubicin or epirubicin. *Journal of Clinical Oncology*, **6**, 679–88.

Fujita, J., Kamel, T., Ariyoshi, Y., Ikegami, H., Furuse, K., and Fukuoka, M. (1993) Dose intensification study of carboplatin (CBDCA) and etoposide (VP-16) with G-CSF in small cell lung cancer (small-cell lung cancer). *Proceedings of the American Society of Clinical Oncology*, **12**, 331.

Fukuoka, M., Masuda, N., Takada, M., Kodama, N., Kawahara, M., and Furuse, K. (1994) Dose-intensive chemotherapy in extensive-stage small cell lung cancer. *Seminars in Oncology*, **21**(Suppl. 1), 43–7.

Gabrilove, J.L., Jakubowski, A., Scher, H., et al. (1988) Effect of granulocyte colony-stimulating factor on neutropenia and associated morbidity due to chemotherapy for transitional-cell carcinoma of the urothelium. *New England Journal of Medicine*, **318**, 1414–22.

Gerhartz, H.H., Engelhard, M., Meusers, P., et al. (1993) Randomized, double-blind, placebo-controlled, phase III study of recombinant human granulocyte-macrophage colony-stimulating factor as adjunct to induction treatment of high-grade malignant, non-Hodgkin's lymphomas. *Blood*, **823**, 2329–39.

Giannessi, P.G., Romanini, A., Surbone, A., Michelotti, A., Bengala, C., and Conte, P.F. (1994) Treatment of metastatic soft-tissue sarcoma (MSTS) with intensified epidoxorubicin, ifosfamide, and dacarbazine + G-CSF. *Proceedings of the American Association for Cancer Research*, **35**, 238.

Gianni, A.M., Bregni, M., Siena, S., et al. (1990) Recombinant human granulocyte-macrophage colony-stimulating factor reduces hematologic toxicity and widens clinical applicability of high-dose cyclophosphamide treatment in breast cancer and non-Hodgkin's lymphoma. *Journal of Clinical Oncology*, **8**, 768–78.

Gianni, A.M., Bregni, M., Siena, S., et al. (1992a) Granulocyte-macrophage colony-stimulating factor or granulocyte colony-stimulating factor infusion makes high-dose etoposide a safe outpatient regimen that is effective in lymphoma and myeloma patients. *Journal of Clinical Oncology*, **10**, 1955–62.

Gianni, A.M., Siena, S., Bregni, M., et al. (1992b) Growth factor-supported high-dose sequential (HDS) adjuvant chemotherapy in breast cancer with

≥10 positive nodes. *Proceedings of the American Society of Clinical Oncology*, **11**, 60.

Gianni, A.M., Tarella, C., Bregni, M., et al. (1994) High-dose sequential chemoradiotherapy, a widely applicable regimen, confers survival benefit to patients with high-risk multiple myeloma. *Journal of Clinical Oncology*, **12**, 503–9.

Gisselbrecht, C., Bosly, A., Lepage, E., et al. (1993) Autologous hematopoietic stem cell transplantation in intermediate and high grade non-Hodgkin's lymphoma: a review. *Annals of Oncology*, **4**(Suppl. 1), S7–S13.

Goldie, J.H. and Coldman, A.J. (1979) A mathematical model for relating the drug sensitivity of tumors to their spontaneous mutation rate. *Cancer Treatment Reports*, **63**, 1727–33.

Gordon, L.I., Harrington, D., Andersen, J., et al. (1992) Comparison of a second-generation combination chemotherapeutic regimen (m-BACOD) with a standard regimen (CHOP) for advanced diffuse non-Hodgkin's lymphoma. *New England Journal of Medicine*, **327**, 1342–9.

Gordon, M.S., Hoffman, R., Baffisto, L., et al. (1994) Recombinant human interleukin eleven (Neumega, rhIL-11 growth factor, rhIL-11) prevents severe thrombocytopenia in breast cancer patients receiving multiple cycles of cyclophosphamide and doxorubicin chemotherapy. *Proceedings of the American Society of Clinical Oncology*, **13**, 133.

Gorin, N.C., Dicke, K., and Lowenberg, B. (1993) High dose therapy for acute myelocytic leukemia treatment strategy: what is the choice? *Annals of Oncology*, **4**(Suppl. 1), S59–S80.

Goss, P.E. (1993) Non-Hodgkin's lymphoma in elderly patients. *Leukemia and Lymphoma*, **10**, 147–56.

Harker, W.G., Meyers, F.J., Freiha, F.S., et al. (1985) Cisplatin, methotrexate, and vinblastine (CMV): an effective regimen for metastatic transitional cell carcinoma of the urinary tract: Northern California Oncology Group study. *Journal of Clinical Oncology*, **3**, 1463–70.

Heinrich, B., Gross, M., and Goebel, F.D. (1989) Methimazole-induced agranulocytosis and granulocyte-colony stimulating factor: letter. *Annals of Internal Medicine*, **111**, 621–2.

Henderson, I.C., Allegra, J., Woodcock, T., et al. (1989) Randomized clinical trial comparing mitoxantrone with doxorubicin in previously treated patients with metastatic breast cancer. *Journal of Clinical Oncology*, **7**, 560–71.

Herzig, R.H. (1992) The role of autologous bone marrow transplantation in the treatment of solid tumors. *Seminars in Oncology*, **19**(Suppl. 7), 7–12.

Hoekman, K., Wagstaff, J., Van Groenwegen, C.J., Vermorken, J.B., Meyer, S., and Pinendo, H.M. (1994) The treatment of advanced soft tissue sarcoma with high dose doxorubicin plus granulocyte-macrophage colony stimulating factor. *Annals of Oncology*.

Holdener, E.E., Jungi, W.J., Fiebig, H.H., et al. (1988) Phase I study of high-dose epirubicin in non-small cell lung cancer (Nsmall-cell lung cancer). *Proceedings of the American Society of Clinical Oncology*, **7**, 208.

Holmes, F.A., Walters, R.S., Theriault, R.L., et al. (1991) Phase II trial of Taxol, an active drug in the treatment of metastatic breast cancer. *Journal of the National Cancer Institute*, **83**, 1797–805.

Hornung, R.L. and Longo, D.L. (1992) Hematopoietic stem cell depletion by restorative growth factor regimens during repeated high-dose cyclophosphamide therapy. *Blood*, **80**, 77–83.

Hryniuk, W. and Bush, H. (1984) The importance of dose intensity in chemotherapy of metastatic breast cancer. *Journal of Clinical Oncology*, **2**, 1281–8.

Hryniuk, W. and Levine, M.N. (1986) Analysis of dose intensity for adjuvant chemotherapy trials in stage II breast cancer. *Journal of Clinical Oncology*, **4**, 1162–70.

Hubbard, S.M., Barkes, P., and Young, R.C. (1978) Adriamycin therapy for advanced ovarian carcinoma recurrent after chemotherapy. *Cancer Treatment Reports*, **62**, 1375–7.

Ihde, D.C., Pass, H.I., and Glatstein, E.J. (1993) Lung cancer: small cell lung cancer. In V.T. DeVita, Jr., S. Hellman, and S.A. Rosenberg (Eds.) *Cancer: principles and practice of oncology*, 4th edition, pp. 723–58. Philadelphia, J.B. Lippincott Company.

Italian Multicentre Breast Study with Epirubicin. (1988) Phase III randomized study of fluorouracil, epirubicin, and cyclophosphamide vs fluorouracil, doxorubicin, and cyclophosphamide in advanced breast cancer: an Italian multicentre trial. *Journal of Clinical Oncology*, **6**, 976–82.

Jain, K.K., Casper, E.S., Geller, N.L., et al. (1985) A prospective randomized comparison of doxorubicin and epirubicin in patients with advanced breast cancer. *Journal of Clinical Oncology*, **3**, 818–26.

Kaye, S.B., Lewis, C.R., Paul, J., et al. (1992) Randomised study of two doses of cisplatin with cyclophosphamide in epithelial ovarian cancer. *Lancet*, **340**, 329–33.

Kohn, E.C., Sarosy, G., Bicher, A., et al. (1994) Dose-intense Taxol: high response rate in patients with platinum-resistant recurrent ovarian cancer. *Journal of the National Cancer Institute*, **86**, 18–24.

Kwak, L.W., Halpern, J., Olshen, R.A., and Horning, S.J. (1990) Prognostic significance of actual dose intensity in diffuse large-cell lymphoma: results of a tree-structured survival analysis. *Journal of Clinical Oncology*, **8**, 963–77.

Lalisang, R., Wils, J., Nortier, J., et al. (1994) A comparative study of dose escalation versus interval reduction to obtain dose intensification of epirubicin and cyclophosphamide with G-CSF for patients with metastatic breast cancer. *Proceedings of the American Society of Clinical Oncology*, **13**, 60.

Launchbury, A.P. and Habboubi, N. (1993) Epirubicin and doxorubicin: a comparison of their characteristics, therapeutic activity, and toxicity. *Cancer Treatment Reviews*, **19**, 197–228.

Lawrence, W., Jr., Donegan, W.L., Nachimuth, N., et al. (1987) Adult soft tissue sarcomas: a pattern of care survey by the American College of Surgeons. *Annals of Surgery*, **205**, 349–59.

Lepage, E., Gisselbrecht, C., Haioun, C., et al. (1993) Prognostic significance of received dose intensity in non-Hodgkin's lymphoma patients: application to LNH-87 protocol. *Annals of Oncology*, **4**, 651–6.

Levin, L. and Hryniuk, W.M. (1987) Dose intensity analysis of chemotherapy regimens in ovarian carcinoma. *Journal of Clinical Oncology*, **5**, 756–67.

Levine, E.G. and Raghaven, D. (1993) MVAC for bladder cancer: time to move forward again. *Journal of Clinical Oncology*, **11**, 387–9.

Liem, G.S. and Verweij, J. (1994) The use of hematological growth factors to enable dose intensification in chemotherapy for soft tissue sarcomas. *Stem Cells*, **12**, 402–8.

Lieschke, G.J. and Burgess, A.W. (1992a) Granulocyte colony-stimulating factor and granulocyte-macrophage colony-stimulating factor (1). *New England Journal of Medicine*, **327**, 28–35.

Lieschke, G.J. and Burgess, A.W. (1992b) Granulocyte colony-stimulating factor and granulocyte-macrophage colony-stimulating factor (2). *New England Journal of Medicine*, **327**, 99–106.

Lieschke, G.J., Cebon, J., and Morstyn, G. (1989) Characterization of the clinical effects after the first dose of bacterially synthesized recombinant human granulocyte-macrophage colony-stimulating factor. *Blood*, **74**, 2634–43.

Lieschke, G.J., Maher, D., Cebon, J., et al. (1989) Effects of bacterially synthesized recombinant human granulocyte-macrophage colony-stimulating factor in patients with advanced malignancy. *Annals of Internal Medicine*, **110**, 357–64.

Lieschke, G.J., Maher, D., O'Connor, M., et al. (1990) Phase I study of intravenously administered bacterially synthesized granulocyte-macrophage colony-stimulating factor and comparison with subcutaneous administration. *Cancer Research*, **50**, 606–14.

Lindemann, F., Schlimok, G., Dirschedl, P., Witte, J., and Riethmuller, G. (1992) Prognostic significance of micrometastatic tumour cells in bone marrow of colorectal cancer patients. *Lancet*, **340**, 685–89.

Loehrer, P.J., Einhorn, L.H., Elson, P.J., et al. (1992) A randomized trial of cisplatin alone or in combination with methotrexate, vinblastine, and doxorubicin in patients with metastatic urothelial carcinoma: a cooperative group study. *Journal of Clinical Oncology*, **10**, 1066–73.

Loehrer, P.J., Sr., Elson, P., Dreicer, R., et al. (1994) Escalated dosages of methotrexate, vinblastine, doxorubicin, and cisplatin plus recombinant human granulocyte colony-stimulating factor in advanced urothelial carcinoma: an Eastern Cooperative Oncology Group trial. *Journal of Clinical Oncology*, **12**, 483–8.

Loehrer, P.J., Sledge, G.W., Nicaise, C., et al. (1989) Ifosfamide plus doxorubicin in metastatic adult sarcomas. *Journal of Clinical Oncology*, **7**, 1655–9.

Logothetis, C.J., Dexeus, F.H., Finn, L., et al. (1990a) A prospective randomized trial comparing MVAC and CISCA chemotherapy for patients with metastatic urothelial tumors. *Journal of Clinical Oncology*, **8**, 1050–5.

Logothetis, C.J., Dexeus, F.H., Sella, A., et al. (1990b) Escalated therapy for refractory urothelial tumors: methotrexate-vinblastine-doxorubicin-cisplatin plus unglycosylated recombinant human granulocyte-macrophage colony-stimulating factor. *Journal of the National Cancer Institute*, **82**, 667–72.

Logothetis, C.J., Finn, L., Amato, R., et al. (1992) Escalated (Esc) M-VAC +/- rhGM-CSF (Schering Plough) in metastatic transitional cell carcinoma (TCC); preliminary results of a randomized study. *Proceedings of the American Society of Clinical Oncology*, **11**, 202a.

Lok, S., Kaushansky, K., Holly, R.D., et al. (1994) Cloning and expression of murine thrombopoietin cDNA and stimulation of platelet production in vivo. *Nature*, **369**, 565–68.

Longo, D.L., DeVita, V.T., Jr., Jaffe, E.S., Mauch, P., and Urba, W.J. (1993) Lymphocytic lymphomas. In V.T. DeVita, Jr., S. Hellman, and S.A. Rosenberg (Eds.) *Cancer: principles and practice of oncology*, 4th edition, pp. 1859–927. Philadelphia, J.B. Lippincott Company.

Luikart, S.D., Goutsou, M., Mitchell, E.D., et al. (1993) Phase I/II trial of etoposide and carboplatin in extensive small-cell lung cancer. A report from the Cancer and Leukemia Group B. *American Journal of Clinical Oncology*, **16**, 127–31.

Luikart, S.D., MacDonald, M., Herzan, D., et al. (1991) Ability of daily or twice daily granulocyte-macrophage colony-stimulating factor (GM-CSF) to support dose escalation of etoposide (VP-16) and carboplatin (CBDCA) in extensive small cell lung cancer. *Proceedings of the American Society of Clinical Oncology*, **10**, 242.

Marchner, N., Kreienberg, R., Souchon, R., et al. (1994) Evaluation of the importance and relevance of dose intensity using epirubicin and cyclophosphamide in metastatic breast cancer: interim analysis of a prospective randomized trial. *Seminars in Oncology*, **21**(Suppl. 1), 10–16.

Martoni, A. and Pannuti, F. (1989) Phase I study of high dose epirubicin. *6th NCI-EORTC Symposium*, 174.

McGuire, W.P., Rowinsky, E.K., Rosenshein, N.B., et al. (1989) Taxol: a unique antineoplastic agent with significant activity in advanced ovarian epithelial neoplasms. *Annals of Internal Medicine*, **111**, 273–9.

Meyer, R.M., Hryniuk, W.M., and Goodyear, M.D.E. (1991) The role of dose intensity in determining outcome in intermediate-grade non-Hodgkin's lymphoma. *Journal of Clinical Oncology*, **9**, 339–47.

Meyer, R.M., Quirt, I.C., Skillings, J.R., et al. (1993) Escalated as compared with standard doses of doxorubicin in BACOP therapy for patients with non-Hodgkin's lymphoma. *New England Journal of Medicine*, **329**, 1770–6.

Meyers, C.E. and Chabner, B.A. (1990) Anthracyclines. In B.A. Chabner and J.M. Collins (Eds.) *Cancer chemotherapy: principles and practice*, pp. 356–81. Philadelphia, J.B. Lippincott Company.

Miles, D.W., Fogarty, O., Ash, C.M., et al. (1994) Received dose-intensity: a randomized trial of weekly chemotherapy with and without granulocyte colony-stimulating factor in small-cell lung cancer. *Journal of Clinical Oncology*, **12**, 77–82.

Moore, M.A.S. (1992) Does stem cell exhaustion result from combining hematopoietic growth factors with chemotherapy? If so, how do we prevent it? *Blood*, **80**, 3–7.

Moore, M.J., Tannock, I.F., Iscoe, N., and Brittain, M. (1992) A phase II study of methotrexate, vinblastine, doxorubicin, and cisplatin (M-VAC) + GM-CSF in patients (pts) with advanced transitional cell carcinoma. *Proceedings of the American Society of Clinical Oncology*, **11**, 199a.

Morgan, R., Jr., Doroshow, J., Somlo, G., et al. (1993) High dose doxorubicin and cyclophosphamide without bone marrow support in breast cancer. *Proceedings of the American Society of Clinical Oncology*, **12**, 74.

Morstyn, G., Campbell, L., Lieschke, G., et al. (1989) Treatment of chemotherapy-induced neutropenia by subcutaneously administered granulocyte colony-stimulating factor with optimization of dose and duration of therapy. *Journal of Clinical Oncology*, **7**, 1554–62.

Morstyn, G., Campbell, L., Souza, L.M., et al. (1988) Effect of granulocyte colony stimulating factor on neutropenia induced by cytotoxic chemotherapy. *Lancet*, **1**, 667–72.

Moss, T.J., Sanders, D.G., Lasky, L.C., and Bostrom, B. (1990) Contamination of peripheral blood stem cell harvests by circulating neuroblastoma cells. *Blood*, **76**, 1879–83.

Murphy, D., Crowther, D., Rennison, J., et al. (1993) A randomised dose intensity study in ovarian carcinoma comparing chemotherapy given at four week intervals for six cycles with half dose chemotherapy given for twelve cycles. *Annals of Oncology*, **4**, 377–83.

Murray, N. (1987) The importance of dose and dose intensity in lung cancer chemotherapy. *Seminars in Oncology*, **14**, 20–8.

Negrin, R.S., Haeuber, D.H., Nagler, A., et al. (1989) Treatment of myelodysplastic syndromes with recombinant human granulocyte colony-stimulating factor: a phase I-II trial. *Annals of Internal Medicine*, **110**, 976–84.

Neidhart, J., Ferguson, J., Parsons, A., Herman, T., Saiki, J., and Mangalik, A. (1993) Sequential GM-CSF and G-CSF allow repeated cycles of dose-intensive cyclophosphamide, etoposide, and cisplatin (DICEP) with acceptable hematological toxicity. *Blood*, **82**(Suppl. 1), 503a.

Neidhart, J.A., Kohler, W., Stidley, C., et al. (1990) Phase I study of repeated cycles of high-dose cyclophosphamide, etoposide, and carboplatin administered without bone marrow transplantation. *Journal of Clinical Oncology*, **8**, 1728–38.

Neidhart, J.A., Kubica, R., Stidley, C., Pfile, J., Clark, D., and Rinehart, J. (1994) Multiple cycles of dose-intensive cyclophosphamide, etoposide, and cisplatinum (DICEP) produce durable responses in refractory non-Hodgkin's lymphoma. *Cancer Investigation*, **12**, 1–11.

Neidhart, J., Mangalik, A., Kohler, W., et al. (1989) Granulocyte colony-stimulating factor stimulates recovery of granulocytes in patients receiving dose-intensive chemotherapy without bone marrow transplantation. *Journal of Clinical Oncology*, **7**, 1685–92.

Neidhart, J.A., Mangalik, A., Stidley, C.A., et al. (1992) Dosing regimen of granulocyte-macrophage colony-stimulating factor to support dose-intensive chemotherapy. *Journal of Clinical Oncology*, **10**, 1460–69.

Neri, B., Pacini, P., Algeri, R., et al. (1993) Conventional versus high-dose epidoxorubicin as single agent in advanced breast cancer. *Cancer Investigation*, **11**, 106–12.

Ozols, R.F., Ihde, D.C., Linehan, W.M., Jacob, J., Ostchega, Y., and Young, R.C. (1988) A randomized trial of standard chemotherapy vs a high-dose chemotherapy regimen in the treatment of poor prognosis nonseminomatous germ-cell tumors. *Journal of Clinical Oncology*, **6**, 1031–40.

Patel, S. and Benjamin, R.S. (1992) Standard and high dose chemotherapy for advanced soft tissue sarcomas. *Annals of Oncology*, **3**(Suppl. 2), S81–3.

Perez, D.J., Harvey, V.J., Robinson, B.A., et al. (1991) A randomized comparison of single-agent doxorubicin and epirubicin as first-line cytotoxic therapy in advanced breast cancer. *Journal of Clinical Oncology*, **9**, 2148–52.

Pettengell, R., Gurney, H., Radford, J.A., et al. (1992) Granulocyte colony-stimulating factor to prevent dose limiting neutropenia in non-Hodgkin's lymphoma: a randomized controlled trial. *Blood*, **80**, 1430–6.

Piccart, M., Bruning, J., Wildiers, A., et al. (1995) An EORTC pilot study of filgrastim (recombinant human granulocyte colony stimulating factor) as support to a high-dose-intensive epiadriamycin-cyclophosphamide regimen in chemotherapy-naive patients with locally advanced or metastatic breast cancer. *Annals of Oncology*, **6**, 673–7.

Pinedo, H.M. (1993) Dose effect relationship in breast cancer. *Annals of Oncology*, **4**, 351–7.

Reed, E., Janik, J., Bookman, M.A., et al. (1993) High-dose carboplatin and recombinant granulocyte-macrophage colony-stimulating factor in advanced-stage recurrent ovarian cancer. *Journal of Clinical Oncology*, **11**, 2118–26.

Reichman, B.S., Seidman, A.D., Crown, J.P.A., et al. (1993) Paclitaxel and recombinant human granulocyte colony-stimulating factor as initial chemotherapy for metastatic breast cancer. *Journal of Clinical Oncology*, **11**, 1943–51.

Rosell, R., Gomez-Codina, J., Anton, A., Sanchez, J.J., and Vadell, C. (1994) Escalating high-dose epirubicin plus cisplatin in small cell lung cancer with granulocyte-macrophage colony-stimulating factor use when appropriate. *Seminars in Oncology*, **21**(Suppl. 21), 48–53.

Rozencweig, M., Hruinink, W.B., Cavalli, F., et al. (1984) Randomized phase II trial of carminomycin versus 4′-epidoxorubicin in advanced breast cancer. *Journal of Clinical Oncology*, **2**, 275–86.

Rusthoven, J., Levin, L., Eisenhauer, E., et al. (1991) Two phase I studies of carboplatin dose escalation in chemotherapy-naive ovarian cancer patients supported with granulocyte-macrophage colony-stimulating factor. *Journal of the National Cancer Institute*, **83**, 1748–53.

Santoro, A., Balzarotti, M., Tondini, C., and Bonadonna, G. (1994) Feasibility of intensified CHOP in patients with non-Hodgkin's lymphoma (NHL). *Proceeding of the American Society of Clinical Oncology*, **13**, 374a.

Sarosy, G., Kohn, E., Stone, D.A., et al. (1992) Phase I study of Taxol and granulocyte colony-stimulating factor in patients with refractory ovarian cancer. *Journal of Clinical Oncology*, **10**, 1165–70.

Scher, H.I., Geller, N.L., Curley, T., and Tao, Y. (1993) Effect of relative cumulative dose-intensity on survival of patients with uroepithelial cancer treated with M-VAC. *Journal of Clinical Oncology*, **11**, 400–7.

Schiller, J.H., Storer, B., Tutsch, K., et al. (1994) Phase I trial of 3-hour infusion of paclitaxel with or without granulocyte colony-stimulating factor in patients with advanced cancer. *Journal of Clinical Oncology*, **12**, 241–8.

Schutte, J., Dombernowsky, P., Mourisden, H., et al. (1990) Ifosfamide plus Adriamycin in previously untreated patients with soft tissue sarcoma: final results of a phase II trial of the EORTC Soft Tissue and Bone Sarcoma Group. *European Journal of Cancer*, **26**, 558–61.

Seidman, A.D., Scher, H.I., Gabrilove, J.L., et al. (1993) Dose-intensification of MVAC with recombinant granulocyte colony-stimulating factor as initial therapy in advanced urothelial cancer. *Journal of Clinical Oncology*, **11**, 408–14.

Shank, W.A. and Balducci, L. (1992) Recombinant hemopoietic growth factors: comparative hemopoietic response in younger and older subjects. *Journal of the American Geriatric Society*, **40**, 151–4.

Shea, T.C., Mason, J.R., Storniolo, A.M., et al. (1992) Sequential cycles of high-dose carboplatin administered with recombinant human granulocyte-macrophage colony-stimulating factor and repeated infusions of autologous peripheral blood progenitor cells: a novel and effective method for delivering multiple courses of dose-intensive therapy. *Journal of Clinical Oncology*, **10**, 464–73.

Shea, T.C., Mason, J.R., Storniolo, A.M., et al. (1993) High-dose carboplatin chemotherapy with GM-CSF and peripheral blood progenitor cell support: a model for delivering repeated cycles of dose-intensive therapy. *Cancer Treatment Reviews*, **19**(Suppl. C), 11–20.

Skipper, H.E. (1967) Criteria associated with destruction of leukemia and solid tumor cells in animals. *Cancer Research*, **27**, 2636–45.

Skipper, H.E. (1990) Dose intensity versus total dose of chemotherapy: an experimental basis. In V.T. DeVita, S. Hellman, and S.A. Rosenberg (Eds.) *Important advances in oncology*, pp. 43–64. Philadelphia, J.B. Lippincott Company.

Skov, B.G., Hirsch, F.R., and Bobrow, L. (1992) Monoclonal antibodies in the detection of bone marrow metastases in small cell lung cancer. *Britsh Journal of Cancer*, **65**, 593–6.

Smith, J.W., Longo, D.L., Alvord, W.G., et al. (1993) The effects of treatment with interleukin-1a on platelet recovery after high-dose carboplatin. *New England Journal of Medicine*, **328**, 756–61.

Souhami, R.L. and Ruiz De Elvira, M.C. (1994) Chemotherapy dose intensity in small cell lung cancer. *Lung Cancer*, **10** (Suppl. 1), S175–85.

Stanhope, C.R., Smith, J.P., and Rudledge, F. (1977) Second trial drugs in ovarian cancer. *Gynecologic Oncology*, **5**, 52–8.

Sternberg, C.N., de Mulder, P.H.M., Van Oosterom, A.T., Fossa, S.D., Giannerelli, D., and Soedirman, J.R. (1993) Escalated M-VAC chemotherapy and recombinant human granulocyte-macrophage colony stimulating factor (rhGM-CSF) in patients with advanced urothelial tumors. *Annals of Oncology*, **4**, 403–7.

Sternberg, C.N., Yagoda, A., Scher, H.I., et al. (1988) M-VAC (methotrexate, vinblastine, doxorubicin, and cisplatin) for advanced transitional cell carcinoma of the urothelium. *Journal of Urology*, **139**, 462–9.

Steward, W.P., Verweij, J., Somers, R., et al. (1993) Granulocyte-macrophage colony-stimulating factor allows safe escalation of dose-intensity of chemotherapy in metastatic adult soft tissue sarcomas: a study of the European Organization for Research and Treatment of Cancer Soft Tissue and Bone Sarcoma Group. *Journal of Clinical Oncology*, **11**, 15–21.

Tannock, I., Boyd, N.F., DeBoer, G., et al. (1988) A randomized trial of two dose levels of cyclophosphamide, methotrexate, and fluorouracil chemotherapy for patients with metastatic breast cancer. *Journal of Clinical Oncology*, **6**, 1377–87.

ten Bokkel Huinink, W.W., Clavel, M., Rodenhuis, S., Franklin, H.R., and Koier, I.J. (1990) Mitoxantrone (M) and GM-CSF, a phase I study with escalated dose of M in breast cancer. *Proceedings of the American Society of Clinical Oncology*, **9**, 40a.

Thigpen, T., Blessing, J., Ball, H., et al. (1990) Phase II trial of Taxol as second-line therapy for ovarian carcinoma. *Proceedings of the American Society of Clinical Oncology*, **9**, 156a.

Toner, G., Green, M., Bishop, J., et al. (1993) Dose escalation of carboplatin (CBDCA) and cyclophosphamide (CTX) with filgrastim (r-metHuG-CSF) in advanced solid tumors. *Proceedings of the American Society of Clinical Oncology*, **12**, 274a.

Trillet-Lenoir, V., Green, J., Manegold, C., et al. (1993) Recombinant granulocyte colony-stimulating factor reduces the infectious complications of cytotoxic chemotherapy. *European Journal of Cancer*, **29**, 319–24.

Trimble, E.L., Adams, J.D., Vena, D., et al. (1993) Paclitaxel for platinum-refractory ovarian cancer: results from the first 1,000 patients registered to National Cancer Institute Treatment Referral Center 9103. *Journal of Clinical Oncology*, **11**, 2405–10.

Vadhan Raj, S., Papadopoulos, N.E., Burgess, M.A., et al. (1994) Effects of PIXY321, a granulocyte-macrophage colony-stimulating factor/interleukin-3 fusion protein, on chemotherapy-induced multilineage myelosuppression in patients with sarcoma. *Journal of Clinical Oncology*, **12**, 715–24.

van Gemeren, M.M., Willemse, P.H.B., Mulder, N.H., et al. (1994) Effects of recombinant human interleukin-6 in cancer patients: a phase I-II study. *Blood*, **84**, 1434–41.

Van Oosterrom, A.T., Mouridsen, H.T., Wildiers, J., et al. (1987) Advanced breast cancer. A comparative evaluation of epirubicin and doxorubicin. *Clinical Trials*, **24**, 131–7.

Van Rijswijk, R.E.N., Haanen, C., Dekker, A.W., De Meijer, A.J., and Verbeek, J. (1989) Dose intensity of MOPP chemotherapy and survival in Hodgkin's disease. *Journal of Clinical Oncology*, **7**, 1776–82.

Vermorken, J.B., Bolis, G., Van Rijswijk, R.E.N., et al. (1994) High-dose intensity regimens with epirubicin in ovarian cancer. *Seminars in Oncology*, **21**(Suppl. 1), 17–22.

Wendling, F., Maraskovsky, E., Debill, N., et al. (1994) c-mpl ligand is a humoral regulator of megakaryopoiesis. *Nature*, **369**, 571–4.

Wood, W.C., Budman, D.R., Korzus, A.H., et al. (1994) Dose and dose intensity of adjuvant chemotherapy for stage II, node-positive breast carcinoma. *New England Journal of Medicine*, **330**, 1253–9.

Zuckerman, K.S., Case, D.C., Jr., Gams, R.A., and Prasthofer, E.F. (1993) Chemotherapy of intermediate- and high-grade non-Hodgkin's lymphomas with an intensive epirubicin-containing regimen. *Blood*, **82**, 3564–73.

Zuckerman, K.S., LoBuglio, A.F., and Reeves, J.A. (1990) Chemotherapy of intermediate- and high-grade non-Hodgkin's lymphomas with a high-dose doxorubicin-containing regimen. *Journal of Clinical Oncology*, **8**, 248–56.

17

Clinical Potential of Hemopoietic Growth-Factor Support for High-Dose Chemotherapy

DAVID FENNELLY, GEORGE RAPTIS, JOHN P.A. CROWN, AND LARRY NORTON

The inability of chemotherapy to eradicate tumors is, in general, related to the emergence of drug resistance. Much of this drug resistance may be relative, as it appears that by increasing the dose of drug delivered, more cancer cells are often killed. Single courses of high-dose chemotherapy, such as those rescued with autologous bone marrow (BM) infusions, have achieved high rates of response in patients whose cancers grew in spite of conventional chemotherapy. These responses, however, are frequently of short duration. The use of hemopoietic progenitor cells plus recombinant human granuolocyte colony-stimulating factor (rHuG-CSF) has enabled us to deliver repeated cycles of high-dose chemotherapy at short intertreatment intervals. On the basis of our experience with curative standard chemotherapy for Hodgkin's and other diseases, we might expect that repeated application of regimens capable of producing such high response rates would improve long-term survival.

One of the major impediments to dose escalation to a truly meaningful level has always been hematological toxicity. Prolonged severe myelosuppression produces morbidity and mortality from infection and hemorrhage, and contributes to organ toxicity by two mechanisms. First, bleeding may damage organs (e.g., pulmonary hemorrhage); and second, organ damage may ensue from multiple transfusions of erythrocytes and platelets or the protracted administration of toxic antibiotics. One of the most important developments in modern medical oncology has been in the technology of hemopoietic support. Recombinant HuG-CSF and rHu granulocyte-macrophage colony-stimulating factor (GM-CSF) accelerate leukocyte recovery following chemotherapy, resulting in the amelioration of associated morbidity (Taylor et al. 1989; Gulati and Bennett 1992). These observations have prompted extensive investigations of these agents as facilitators of dose escalation (Jones et al. 1987). A general result has been a substantial reduction in the need for attenuations of dose in conventional combination regimens; however, major dose escalations of single courses have proven more difficult to achieve.

As an example, for metastatic breast cancer, the Dana-Farber group studied the use of rHuG-CSF to increase the doses of the cyclophosphamide, doxorubicin, and fluorouracil) (CAF) regimen (Younger et al. 1992). Mucositis emerged as a major dose-limiting toxicity of CAF. In a similar study in the Netherlands, the use of rHuGM-CSF permitted the use of moderately escalated doses of cyclophosphamide and doxorubicin; however, acute hematologic toxicity was considerable, and cumulative myelosuppression was observed (Hoekman et al. 1991). In a prospective Italian study, patients with metastatic breast cancer were treated with epirubicin, cyclophosphamide, and 5-fluorouracil (5-FU), randomized to receive rHuGM-CSF or not. All patients were retreated promptly on recovery from the previous cycle (Venturini et al. 1992). Use of rHuGM-CSF facilitated dose escalation, but only to approximately 130% of the doses achieved in the control group.

For many other chemotherapy agents, hemopoietic cytokines have provided even less protection from myelosuppression. A reason is that both G-CSF and GM-CSF are active primarily in leukocyte pathways. While some accelerated platelet recovery has been reported, this has not been a consistent finding (Advani et al. 1992). An attempt to escalate the dose of thiotepa by the administration of rHuGM-CSF was not successful because of thrombocytopenia (O'Dwyer et al. 1992). Thrombocytopenia and cumulative myelosuppression have also limited dose-escalation strategies for carboplatin.

The use of CSF as the only means of hemopoietic support, however, has been reported to be successful in two studies. Neidhart and colleagues (1990) have been able to administer multiple cycles of high-dose cisplatin plus cyclophosphamide and etoposide with rHuG-CSF alone, without autologous marrow reinfusion. It is important to note, relevant to the concept of dose-density, that in this study cycles could be repeated only with prolonged intertreatment intervals greater than 4 weeks. In another study using rHuGM-CSF, the Cancer and Leukemia Group B (CALGB) demonstrated that multiple cycles of high-dose cyclophosphamide could be administered to patients with various cancers, but the intertreatment interval was short, approximately 2 weeks (Lichtman et al. 1990).

The general failure of the CSF to permit major dose escalations may be because some chemotherapy drugs influence very early hemopoietic progenitors. We, therefore, look forward to the thrombopoietic effects of growth factors that act earlier in BM maturation (Crown et al. 1991). Interleukin-1 (IL-1), for example, may shorten the duration of carboplatin-induced thrombocytopenia (Smith et al. 1992; Vadhan-Raj et al. 1992). While this field develops, investigators have turned to the use of CSF plus the infusion of hemopoietic progenitor cells as a means of promoting both dose escalation and the achievement of dose density.

High-dose chemotherapy, to the degree requiring autologous bone-marrow transplant (ABMT), can produce a very high rate of complete response (CR) in patients with a variety of tumors. The use of BM-supported high-dose chemotherapy has produced long-term disease-free survivals, which for practical purposes may be tantamount to cure, for patients with lymphomas (Gulati et al. 1992) and germ-cell cancers (Motzer et al. 1992) who have had diseases refractory to standard-dose therapy. In the treatment of metastatic breast cancer, such therapy has produced high objective response rates. Some regimens have used high doses of the single agents melphalan, cyclophosphamide, and thiotepa (Jones et al. 1990; Kennedy et al. 1991; Antman et al. 1992; Bezwoda, Seymour, and Vorobiof 1992). Because of its limited nonhematological toxicity, thiotepa has particular potential for dose escalation. A phase I study published in 1992 recommended that 75 mg/m^2 be considered the phase II dose, although the dose of 30 mg/m^2 had been in use for decades (O'Dwyer et al. 1992). Use of rHuGM-CSF alone does not provide adequate protection from cumulative thiotepa-induced myelosuppression (Neidhart et al. 1990), but the infusion of autologous marrow allows for the use of a substantially higher dose. High-dose thiotepa with autologous marrow rescue has produced response and survival data similar to those reported for combination regimens (Crown et al. 1994). Above a dose of approximately 700 mg/m^2 mucosal toxicity becomes prominent (Wolff et al. 1990), and doses above 1,200 mg/m^2 produce neurological toxicity in approximately 10% of patients.

The combination of the alkylating agents cyclophosphamide, cisplatin, and carmustine (CPB) has produced a complete response rate of approximately 25% in breast cancer patients with otherwise refractory disease (Eder et al. 1986). These responses were not durable, but the results prompted a phase II evaluation of this combination in patients with more favorable disease status. Accordingly, 22 patients without prior chemotherapy for metastatic disease, who were nevertheless regarded as having a poor prognosis because their tumors were hormone receptor-negative, or who had failed prior endocrine therapies, were treated with a single application of CPB. Toxicity was substantial, but complete responses were achieved in greater than 50% of the patients. Three of the original 22 remained in unmaintained complete remissions for 5 years or longer (Peters et al. 1988). Many other single-course combinations of chemotherapy drugs with marrow support have been studied. They differ somewhat in their spectrum of toxicities, but no one regimen has emerged as clearly superior.

Exploiting the idea of multicycle regimens, some investigators have used induction chemotherapy at conventional dose levels followed by a single course of high-dose combination chemotherapy with autologous BM rescue (Antman et al. 1992). Others have tried to use repeated cycles of high-dose chemotherapy. At the M.D. Anderson Cancer Center interesting results were achieved with double applications of such high-dose chemotherapy (Dunphy and Spitzer 1992); however, toxicity required substantial intertreatment delays averaging 6 to 8 weeks. Bezwoda and colleagues (1992) have reported preliminary findings from a prospective randomized trial in which two courses of very high doses of mitoxantrone, etoposide, and cyclophosphamide were administered with autologous BM or peripheral blood (PB) –derived hemopoietic progenitor cell support (*vide infra*). The control group was conventional chemotherapy, which yielded a 70% response rate (6% CR). The experimental group, in contrast, produced a 100% response rate including 50% CR in patients who received the treatment as first chemotherapy for stage IV disease.

The CSF are an important component of therapies using autologous marrow infusions, as they contribute to more rapid leukocyte recovery (Sheridan et al. 1989; Taylor et al. 1989; Nemunaitis and Singer 1991). Another role for the CSF is in the generation of hemopoietic progenitor cells to be obtained from PB (reviewed in Chapters 8 and 9). A major clinical benefit of cytokine or cytokine plus chemotherapy-mobilized peripheral blood progenitor cells (PBPC) is accelerated hematological, especially platelet, recovery from high-dose chemotherapy. Overall, PBPC transplantation is associated with reduced morbidity and mortality compared with BMT. An interesting approach to PBPC-supported cancer treatment was reported in Gianni et al., who used a sequence of high-dose single agents with PBPC plus CSF after the last high-dose course (Frei et al. 1985). This therapy seems promising in the treatment of lymphoma and in breast cancer. We will discuss below our use of PBPC technology to improve dose density as well as dose escalation.

In the treatment of ovarian carcinoma, the use of high-dose chemotherapy with ABM support is capable of achieving high rates of response in patients failing conventional treatment regimens. This is an area of considerable interest for a number of reasons. First, ovarian cancer is a tumor with demonstrated chemosensitivity, although clearly less sensitivity than the hematological malignancies. Second, patients failing conventional therapy have a universally poor prognosis. Additionally, there is an increasing dose-response relationship for both the platinum compounds and the alkylating agents in general (Frei et al. 1985; Ozols et al. 1987). Agents such as melphalan, cyclophosphamide, and thiotepa are active in ovarian cancer, and can be substantially dose escalated with the use of autologous BM support (Mulder et al. 1989b; Shea et al. 1989). Dauplat et al. (1989), using high-dose melphalan, obtained a 36% 2-year disease-free survival rate in patients failing induction cisplatin regimens. Preclinical studies by Lidor et al. (1991) have demonstrated synergy between cisplatin and cyclophosphamide and cisplatin plus thiotepa. Shpall et al. (1990) evaluated in a phase I setting the combination of high-dose cyclophosphamide, thiotepa, and cisplatin followed by autologous BM supporting patients with advanced ovarian cancer. Cisplatin was delivered by the intraperitoneal (IP) route in an escalating dose schedule commencing at 90 mg/m^2 divided over 3 days. The overall response rate was 75% in a group of patients who had progressive disease on platinum-based therapy.

On the basis of the demonstrated activity of doxorubicin in advanced ovarian cancer, and the limited potential of this agent for dose escalation (because of dose-limiting mucositis and cardiotoxicity), investigators have turned to mitoxantrone for incorporation into dose-escalated approaches (Wallerstein et al. 1990). Mitoxantrone is an anthracene derivative, with an intercalative and nonintercalative effect on DNA (Lown et al. 1984; Bowden et al. 1985), and is cytotoxic to proliferating and nonproliferating cells in vitro (Wallace, Citarella, and Durr 1979; Drewinko et al. 1981). Clinical congestive heart failure occurs in less than 3% of patients with conventional dosing of mitoxantrone, up to cumulative doses of 100 mg/m^2 in patients previously treated with anthracyclines, and up to 160 mg/m^2 in previously untreated patients (Shenkenberg and Von Hoff 1986). In experimental systems, mitoxantrone showed some lack of cross-resistance to anthracyclines (Hill et al. 1989). In the human tumor colony-forming assay, mitoxantrone has been demonstrated to be highly cytotoxic to ovarian cancer cells (Alberts et al. 1985). It has also demonstrated clinical activity against ovarian cancer when delivered by either the intravenous (IV) (Lawton et al. 1987) or IP (Markman et al. 1991) routes. Mitoxantrone is an unusual drug to dose escalate because it is not an alkylating agent (Markman et al. 1991). Shea et al. (1992) have evaluated escalated-dose mitoxantrone (42 mg/m^2) in addition to high-dose IP carboplatin and IV thiotepa and etoposide. The Southwest Oncology Group (SWOG) is currently evaluating mitoxantrone at a dose of 75 mg/m^2 in a phase II study of high-dose chemotherapy with BM support for patients with advanced ovarian cancer, and Mulder combined either cyclophosphamide or melphalan with high-dose mitoxantrone and obtained a 66% complete response rate (Mulder et al. 1989a).

Many other single-course, dose-escalated combinations have been tested against advanced ovarian carcinoma. Legros et al. (1992) evaluated the long-term results achieved with high-dose chemotherapy and autologous BM transplant in 31 patients. All patients had received induction therapy with a cisplatin-containing regimen followed by debulking surgery. High-dose chemotherapy with autologous BM support was given for consolidation. Patients received either high-dose melphalan (140 mg/m^2) or a combination of carboplatin (1,000 to 1,500 mg/m^2) with cyclophosphamide 6 gm/m^2. With a median follow-up of 52 months, 18 of 32 patients were alive, 11 free of disease. Overall disease-free survival at 3 years was 35%. Stiff et al. (1992) published a survey of results in ovarian cancer in 11 autologous BMT centers in the United States, which included 153 ovarian carcinoma patients of whom 95% were transplanted with relapsed or refractory disease. Twenty different transplant preparative regimens were identified. The overall response rate was 71%, with a 43% CR rate. In patients with platinum-sensitive disease, overall response rate was 87%, with a 73% clinical CR rate. In patients with platinum-resistant disease, the overall response rate was 85%, with a 34% clinical CR rate. The median time to progression was 6 months, with 14% of patients disease-free at 1 year. An ongoing randomized study by SWOG is evaluating two different high-dose chemotherapy regimens with autologous BM support in patients with ovarian cancer.

■ DOSE DENSITY

Dose escalation of many chemotherapeutic agents can kill more cancer cells than conventional doses, and multiple cycles of chemotherapy seem to be associated with better clinical results. The Goldie-Coldman hypothesis has been widely tested and lacks empirical support. To use these observations in the design of improved chemotherapy regimens, we must reexamine the pattern of growth of human cancer. There is an increasing body of evidence that many cancers grow not exponentially, but by Gompertzian kinetics (Gilewski and Norton 1995). In this pattern of growth, smaller tumors are more sensitive, in terms of the fraction of cells killed, than larger tumors, but the regrowth rate is faster as well. Therefore, the overall impact of treatment will be modest even in the face of very large tumor cell kill, unless the tumor is precluded from regrowing. The best path to the permanent prevention of regrowth is the elimination of all cancer cells. This conclusion is relevant to the practical design of treatment regimens because of the concepts of drug resistance. If a whole cancer is a collection of different sublines with different proliferation rates and different sensitivities to treatment, eradicating some sublines by chemotherapy would leave others to grow. By Gompertzian kinetics, the residual sublines would have a tendency to regrow rapidly. Hence, partially effective therapies, even those killing most of the cells present, might produce only small increases in disease-free survival.

One tumor-cell subline that may be particularly difficult to eradicate with chemotherapy is that which consists of the tumor stem cells. These cells constitute an important class of undifferentiated cells that constitute less than 1% of the cells present in a cancer. They can form colonies in soft agar (Hamburger and Salmon 1977), and are thought to be able to react to the death of adjacent cells to reproduce the entire spectrum of subtypes that make up a mature tumor (Bruce and Valeriote 1968; Till et al. 1968). Hence, they could be a major source of therapeutic failure (Look, Douglass, and Meyer 1988). An optimistic side of this consideration is that some of our current chemotherapy treatments might actually be bringing us closer to total cellular eradication than we might otherwise be led to suspect by their modest impact on disease-free and overall survival.

How do we eradicate residual sublines, particularly those that are slowly growing, slowly regressing, and, therefore, harder to kill (Norton and Simon 1986)? Slower-growing cells should constitute a minority of the cells in a cancer because by the time of diagnosis they should have been overgrown by faster growing cells. We have hypothesized that the best way to cure a population of cells heterogeneous in growth rate and drug sensitivity is to eradicate the more numerous, faster-growing cells first, then the more resistant, slower-growing cells (Norton 1985). To eradicate any population of cells, treatment should include drugs to which the cells are sensitive, with minimal time between treatments to minimize opportunities for regrowth. Conventional combination chemotherapy does not accomplish this goal, since doses are reduced to permit the construction of tolerable combinations. Also, little attention is usually directed to the speed of recycling, (i.e., making minimal the intertreatment intervals).

These concepts might explain the superiority of a treatment of four 3-week courses of adjuvant doxorubicin (A) followed by eight 3-week courses of intravenous CMF (C) (AAAACCCCCCCC) over the alternating regimen of two courses of CMF alternating with one course of doxorubicin, this grouping repeated four times for a total of twelve courses (CCACCACCACCA), in the adjuvant treatment of breast cancer as described above (Buzzoni et al. 1991). The sequential regimen gave eight cycles of CMF over 33 weeks counting from the beginning of treatment, and four cycles of doxorubicin over 9 weeks. This means that the dose density of the doxorubicin was very high compared with the alternating regimen, which gave eight cycles of CMF over a similar 30 weeks, but four cycles of Adriamycin over a much longer 33 weeks. In the sequential regimen, dose density is achieved by crossover scheduling, AAAA crossing over to CCCCCCCC. It is important to note that the concept of crossover scheduling is supported by several theoretical models. Goldie and Coldman's prediction of the superiority of alternating chemotherapy, CCACCACCACCA, was dependent on the assumption of "symmetry," which means the presence of sublines with equal numbers of cells, equal proliferation rates, and equal mutation rates (Goldie and Coldman 1986). Day (1986) reconsidered the Goldie-Coldman model, but performed computer simulations of mutation to drug resistance under asymmetrical conditions. From this he predicted that the alternating plan would be inferior (Norton and Day 1991). In the laboratory, the cure of advanced murine leukemia is best accomplished by using cytosine arabinoside plus 6-thioguanine for two or three courses, followed by one high-dose treatment with cyclophosphamide plus carmustine (BCNU) (Skipper 1986). Hence, the high-dose regimens described above that use conventional-dose induction followed by a short late intensification are supported by experimental as well as clinical evidence. As another laboratory example, the complete remission rate and the median survival time of BDF1 mice bearing the M5076 tumor may be doubled by using four doses of methyl-CCNU first, then crossing over to a single dose of L-phenylalamine mustard, as compared with the use of methyl-CCNU alone (Griswold et al. 1982). In this experimental setting, L-phenylalamine mustard by itself has very weak activity because only a small subpopulation of cells is sensitive just to this drug. Yet this is the subpopulation that leads to relapse if methyl-CCNU is used alone.

Crossover scheduling is just one way of applying these concepts. Dose intensity is the total amount of drug divided by time. In the past, dose intensity could only be increased by increasing the dose level; however, the major improvements in hemopoietic technology described in this volume now allow us to shorten the intertreatment time as well.

CONCLUSIONS

A remaining and critical issue for the application of dose-intense chemotherapy is to identify the patients who will derive maximum benefit. The true efficacy of this approach will require its testing as first-line chemotherapy, without extensive prior treatment for advanced disease. For conventionally dosed as well as dose-intense regimens, bulky disease is a negative prognostic factor, so the best test may be in patients with small-volume disease. Another important field of research concerns improved methods of hemopoietic support. Efforts to expand the population of true stem cells in PBPC collections could lead to greater efficacy in marrow reconstitution and reduced costs (Shapiro et al. 1994). Just as important will be methods of reducing toxicity to organs other than the marrow. These toxicities include interstitial pneumonitis (e.g., from melphalan and BCNU), hemorrhagic myocarditis (e.g., from cyclophosphamide), neurological damage (e.g., from cisplatin and thiotepa), and renal impairment (e.g., from cisplatin). In addition, efforts to improve chemotherapeutic cell-kill by the joint use of biological therapies are under investigation (Baselga et al. 1993, 1994).

REFERENCES

Advani, R., Chao, N.J., Horning, S.J., et al. (1992) Granulocyte-macrophage colony-stimulatlng factor (GM-CSF) as an adjunct to autologous hemopoietic stem cell transplantation for lymphoma. *Annals of Internal Medicine*, **116**, 183–9.

Alberts, D.S., Young, L., Mason, N.L., et al. (1985) In vitro evaluation of anticancer against ovarian cancer at concentrations achievable by intraperitoneal administration. *Seminars in Oncology*, **12**, 38–42.

Antman, K., Ayash, L.J., Elias, A., et al. (1992) A phase II study of high dose cyclophosphamide, thiotepa, and carboplatin with autologous bone marrow support in patients with measurable advanced breast cancer responding to standard-dose therapy. *Journal of Clinical Oncology*, **10**, 102–10.

Baselga, J., Norton, L., Masui, H., et al. (1993) Anti-tumor effects of doxorubicin in combination with anti-epidermal growth factor receptor monoclonal antibody. *Journal of the National Cancer Institute*, **85**, 1327–33.

Baselga, J., Norton, L., Shalaby, R., and Mendelsohn, J. (1994) Anti HER2 humanized monoclonal antibody alone and in combination with chemotherapy against human breast carcinoma xenografts. *Proceedings of the American Society of Clinical Oncology*, **13**, 53a.

Bezwoda, W.R., Seymour, L., and Vorobiof, D.A. (1992) High dose cyclophosphamide, mitoxantrone, and VP-16 as first line treatment for metastatic breast cancer. *Proceedings of the American Society of Clinical Oncology*, **11**, 64a.

Bowden, G.T., Roberts, R., Alberts, D.S., et al. (1985) Comparative molecular pharmacology in leukemic L1210 cells of the anthracene anticancer drugs mitoxantrone and bisanthracene. *Cancer Research*, **45**, 4915–20.

Bruce, W.R., and Valeriote, F.A. (1968) Normal and malignant stem cells and chemotherapy. In *The proliferation and spread of neoplastic cells*, 21st Annual Symposium on Fundamental Cancer Research 1967, pp. 409–22, Baltimore, Williams & Wilkins.

Buzzoni, R., Bonadonna, G., Valagussa, P., and Zambetti, M. (1991) Adjuvant chemotherapy with doxorubicin plus cyclophosphamide, methotrexate, and fluorouracil in the treatment of resectable breast cancer with more than three positive axillary nodes. *Journal of Clinical Oncology*, **9**, 2134.

Crown, J., Jakubowski, A., Kemeny, N., Gordon, M., Gasparetto, C., and Wong, G. (1991) A phase I trial of recombinant human interleukin-1B alone and in combination with myelosuppressive doses of 5-fluorouracil in patients with gastrointestinal cancer. *Blood*, **78**, 1420–7.

Crown, J., Raptis, G., Vahdat, L., et al. (1994) Sequential high-dose (HD) cyclophosphamide (C), L-PAM, and thiotepa (T) in patients (pts) with metastatic breast cancer. *Annals in Oncology*, **5**, 32.

Dauplat, J., Legros, M., Condat, P., Ferriere, J.P., Ben Ahmed, S., and Plagne, R. (1989) High-dose melphalan and autologous bone marrow support for treatment of ovarian carcinoma with positive second-look operation. *Gynecologic Oncology*, **34**, 294–8.

Day, R.S. (1986) Treatment sequencing, asymmetry, and uncertainty: protocol strategies for combination chemotherapy. *Cancer Research*, **46**, 3876.

Drewinko, B., Patchen, M., Yang, L.-Y., et al. (1981) Differential killing efficacy of twenty anti-tumor drugs on proliferating and nonproliferating human tumor cells. *Cancer Research*, **41**, 2328–33.

Dunphy, F. and Spitzer, G. (1992) Use of very high-dose chemotherapy with autologous bone marrow transplantation treatment of breast cancer. *Journal of the National Cancer Institute*, **84**, 128–9.

Eder, J.P., Antman, K., Peters, W.P., et al. (1986) High-dose combination alkylating agent chemotherapy with autologous marrow support for metastatic breast cancer. *Journal of Clinical Oncology*, **4**, 1592–7.

Frei, E., Cucchi, C.A., Rosowsky, A., et al. (1985) Alkylating agent resistance: in vivo studies with human cell lines. *Proceedings of the National Academy of Sciences of the United States of America*, **82**, 2158–62.

Gilewski, T. and Norton, L. (1995) Cytokinetics of Neoplasia. In J. Mendelsohn, P. Howley, M.A. Israel, L.A. Liotta (Eds.) *The molecular basis of cancer*, pp. 143–59. Philadelphia, W.B. Saunders Company.

Goldie, J.H. and Coldman, A.J. (1986) Application of theoretical models to chemotherapy protocol design. *Cancer Treatment Reports*, **70**, 127.

Griswold, D.P., Schabel, F.M., Jr., Corbett, T.H., and Dykes, D.J. (1982) Concepts for controlling drug-resistant tumor cells. In I.-J. Fidler and R.J. White (Eds.) *Design of models for testing cancer therapeutic agents*, pp. 215–24. New York, Van Nostrand Reinhold.

Gulati, S.C. and Bennett, C.L. (1992) Granulocyte-macrophage colony-stimulating factor as adjunct therapy in relapsed Hodgkin's disease. *Annals of Internal Medicine*, **116**, 177–82.

Gulati, S., Yahalom, Y., Acaba, L., et al. (1992) Treatment of patients with relapsed and resistant non-Hodgkin's lymphoma using total body irradiation, etoposide, cyclophosphamide, and autologous bone marrow transplantation. *Journal of Clinical Oncology*, **10**, 936–41.

Hamburger, A. and Salmon, S.E. (1977) Primary bioassay of human myeloma stem cells. *Journal of Clinical Investigation*, **60**, 846.

Hill, B.T., Hoskins, L.K., Shellard, S.A., et al. (1989) Comparative effectiveness of mitoxantrone and doxorubicin in overcoming experimentally induced drug resistance in murine and human tumor cell lines *in vitro*. *Cancer Chemotherapy and Pharmacology*, **23**, 140–4.

Hoekman, K., Wagstaff, F., van Groeningen, J., et al. (1991) Effects of recombinant human granulocyte-macrophage colony-stimulating factor on myelosuppression induced by multiple cycles of high-dose chemotherapy in patients with advanced breast cancer. *Journal of the National Cancer Institute*, **83**, 1546–53.

Jones, R.B., Holland, J.F., Bhardwal, S., Norton, L., Wilfinger, C., and Strashun, A. (1987) A phase I-II study of intensive-dose Adriamycin for advanced breast cancer. *Journal of Clinical Oncology*, **5**, 172–7.

Jones, R.B., Shpall, E.J., Ross, M., Bast, R., Affronti, M., and Peters, W.P. (1990) AFM induction chemotherapy followed by intensive alkylating agent consolidation with autologous bone marrow support for advanced breast cancer. Current results. *Proceedings of the American Society of Clinical Oncology*, **9**, 9a.

Kennedy, M.J., Beveridge, R.A., Rowley, S.D., Gordon, G.B., Abeloff, M.D., and Davidson, N.E. (1991) High-dose chemotherapy with reinfusion of purged autologous bone marrow following dose-intensive induction as initial therapy for metastatic breast cancer. *Journal of the National Cancer Institute*, **83**, 920–6.

Lawton, L., Blackledge, G., Mould, J., et al. (1987) A phase II study of mitoxantrone in epithelial ovarian cancer. *Cancer Treatment Reports*, **71**, 627–9.

Legros, M., Fleury, J., Cure, P., et al. (1992) High-dose chemotherapy and autologous bone marrow transplant in 31 advanced ovarian cancers. Long-term results. *Proceedings of the American Society of Clinical Oncology*, **11**, 222a.

Lichtman, S.M., Ratain, M.J., Van Echo, D.A., et al. (1993) Phase I trial of granulocyte-macrophage colony-stimulating factor (GM-CSF) plus high dose biweekly cyclophosphamide: a CALGB study. *Journal of the National Cancer Institute*, **85**, 1319–26.

Lidor, Y.J., Shpall, E.J., Peters, W.P., and Bast, R.C., Jr. (1991) Synergistic cytotoxicity of different alkylating agents for epithelial ovarian cancer. *International Journal of Cancer*, **49**, 704–10.

Look, A.T., Douglass, E.C., and Meyer, W.I. (1988) Clinical importance of near-diploid tumor stem lines in patients with osteosarcoma of an extremity. *New England Journal of Medicine*, **318**, 1567.

Lown, J.W., Hanstock, C.C., Bradley, R.D., et al. (1984) Interactions of the antitumor mitoxantrone and bisantrene with deoxyribonucleic acids studied by electron microscopy. *Molecular Pharmacology*, **25**, 178–84.

Markman, M., Hakes, T., Reichman, B., et al. (1991) Phase II trial of weekly or bi-weekly intraperitoneal mitoxantrone in epithelial ovarian cancer. *Journal of Clinical Oncology*, **9**, 978–82.

Motzer, R., Gulati, S., Crown, J., et al. (1992) High dose chemotherapy and autologous bone marrow rescue for patients with refractory germ cell tumors. *Cancer*, **69**, 550–6.

Mulder, P.O., Sleijfer, D.T., Willemse, P.H., et al. (1989a) High-dose cyclophosphamide or melphalan with escalating doses of mitoxantrone and autologous bone marrow transplantation for refractory solid tumors. *Cancer Research*, **49**, 4654–8.

Mulder, P.O., Willemse, P.H., Azalders, J.G., et al. (1989b) High-dose chemotherapy with autologous bone marrow transplantation in patients with refractory ovarian cancer. *European Journal of Clinical Oncology*, **25**, 645–9.

Neidhart, J.A., Kohler, W., Stidley, C., et al. (1990) Phase I study of repeated cycles of high dose cyclophosphamide, etoposide, and cisplatin administered without bone marrow transplantation. *Journal of Clinical Oncology*, **8**, 1728–38.

Nemunaitis, J. and Singer, J.W. (1991) The use of recombinant human granulocyte-macrophage colony stimulating factor in autologous bone marrow transplantation. *American Journal of Clinical Oncology*, **14**, S15–8.

Norton, L. (1985) Implications of kinetic heterogeneity in clinical oncology. *Seminars in Oncology*, **12**, 231.

Norton, L. and Day, R. (1991) Potential innovations in scheduling in cancer chemotherapy. In V.T. DeVita, Jr., S. Hellman, and S.A. Rosenberg (Eds.) *Important advances in oncology 1991*, pp. 57–72. New York, J.B. Lippincott Company.

Norton, L. and Simon, R. (1986) The Norton-Simon hypothesis revisited. *Cancer Treatment Report*, **70**, 163.

O'Dwyer, P.J., LaCreta, F., Schilder, R., et al. (1992) Phase I trial of thiotepa in combination with recombinant human granulocyte-macrophage colony-stimulating factor. *Journal of Clinical Oncology*, **10**, 1352–8.

Ozols, R.F., Ostchega, Y., Myers, C.E., et al. (1987) Cisplatin in hypertonic saline in refractory ovarian cancer. *Journal of Clinical Oncology* **5**, 1246–50.

Peters, W.P., Shpall, E.J., Jones, R.B., et al. (1988) High-dose combination alkylating agents with bone marrow support as initial treatment for metastatic breast cancer. *Journal of Clinical Oncology*, **6**, 1368–76.

Shapiro, F., Yao, T.-J., Raptis, G., Reich, L., Norton, L., and Moore, M.A. (1994) Optimization of conditions for *ex-vivo* expansion of peripheral blood progenitors from patients with breast cancer. *Blood*, **84**, 3567–74.

Shea, T.C., Flaherty, M., Elias, A.M., et al. (1989) A phase I clinical and pharmacokinetic study of carboplatin and autologous bone marrow support. *Journal of Clinical Oncology*, **7**, 651–61.

Shea, T.C., Storniolo, A.M., Mason, J.R., et al. (1992) High-dose intravenous and intraperitoneal combination chemotherapy with autologous stem cell rescue for patients with advanced ovarian cancer. *Proceedings of the American Society of Clinical Oncology*, **11**, 756a.

Shenkenberg, T.D. and Von Hoff, D.D. (1986) Mitoxantrone: a new anti-cancer drug with significant clinical activity. *Annals of Internal Medicine*, **105**, 67–81.

Sheridan, W.P., Morstyn, G., Wolf, M., et al. (1989) Granulocyte colony-stimulating factor and neutrophil recovery after high-dose chemotherapy and autologous bone marrow transplantation. *Lancet*, **2**, 891–5.

Shpall, E., Clarke-Peterson, D., Soper, J., et al. (1990) High-dose alkylating agent chemotherapy with autologous bone marrow support in patients with stage III/IV epithelial ovarian cancer. *Gynecologic Oncology*, **38**, 386–91.

Skipper, H.E. (1986) Analyses of multiarmed trials in which animals bearing different burdens of L1210 leukemia cells were treated with two, three, and four drug combinations delivered in different ways with varying dose intensities of each drug and varying average dose intensities. *Southern Research Institute Booklet*, **7**, 87.

Smith, J., II, Longo, D., Alvord, W., et al. (1992) Thrombopoietic effects of IL-1α in combination with high-dose carboplatin. *Proceedings of the American Society of Clinical Oncology*, **11**, 252a.

Stiff, P., Antman, K., Randolph Broun, E., et al. (1992) Bone marrow transplantation for ovarian carcinoma in the United States: a survey of active programs. *Proceedings of the 6th International Autologous Bone Marrow Transplant Symposium*, 1–9, 1992.

Taylor, K., Jagannath, S., Spitzer, G., et al. (1989) Recombinant human granulocyte colony-stimulating factor hastens granulocyte recovery after high-dose chemotherapy and autologous bone marrow transplantation in Hodgkin's disease. *Journal of Clinical Oncology*, **7**, 1791–9.

Till, J.E., McCullock, G.A., Phillips, R.A., and Siminovitch, L. (1968) Aspects of the regulation of stem cell function. In *The proliferation and spread of neoplastic cells*, 21st Annual Symposium on Fundamental Cancer Research 1967, pp. 235–44, Baltimore, Williams & Wilkins.

Vadhan-Raj, S., Kudelka, A., Garrison, L., et al. (1992) Interleukin-1α (IL-1α) increases circulating platelet (PLT) counts and reduces carboplatin (CBDCA)-induced thrombocytopenia. *Proceedings of the American Society of Clinical Oncology*, **11**, 224a.

Venturini, M., Sertoli, M.R., Ardizzoni, A., et al. (1992) Prospective randomized trial of accelerated FEC chemotherapy (CT) with or without GM-CSF in advanced breast cancer (ABC). *Proceedings of the American Society of Clinical Oncology*, **11**, 52a.

Wallace, R.E., Citarella, R.V., and Durr, F.E. (1979) The inhibitory effects of 1,4-dihydroxy-5,8-bis((2-(2-hydroxyenthyl)amino)ethyl)amino)9,10 anthracenedione (CL232315;NSC 301739D) on dividing and non-dividing cells in-vitro. *Proceedings of the American Society of Clinical Oncology*, **20**, 12a.

Wallerstein, R., Spitzer, G., Dunphy, F., et al. (1990) A phase II study of mitoxantrone, etoposide, and thiotepa with autologous marrow support for patients with relapsed breast cancer. *Journal of Clinical Oncology*, **8**, 1782–8.

Wolff, S.N., Herzig, R.H., Fay, J.W., et al. (1990) High-dose N, N', N''-triethylenethiophosphoramide (thiotepa) with autologous bone marrow transplantation: phase I studies. *Seminars in Oncology*, **17**, 2–6.

Younger, J., Shapiro, O., Douville, L., Colecchi, C., Armstron, S., and McGuire, B. (1992) A phase I study of dose-intensified CAF chemotherapy with adjunctive r-metHuG-CSF (GCSF) in patients with advanced breast cancer. *Proceedings of the American Society of Clinical Oncology*, **11**, 108a.

-18

Treatment of Solid Tumors with High-Dose Chemotherapy Requiring Cellular Support

LOTHAR KANZ, MARION SUBKLEWE, AND
WOLFRAM BRUGGER

High-dose chemotherapy is a treatment modality that applies maximally tolerable doses of cytotoxic drugs, while accepting destruction of the hemopoietic system and the need for stem-cell (SC) transplantation. This approach represents a potentially curative treatment concept for defined chemosensitive malignancies.

In vitro experiments, animal studies, retrospective clinical evaluations, and preliminary clinical trials using high-dose chemotherapy have shown a dose-response relationship for some cytotoxic drugs, particularly alkylating agents, in a variety of tumors.

It has become evident that dose intensity (i.e., total dose per time unit) is a major determinant of outcome. The application of high-dose chemotherapy must take into account that the steepness of the dose-response curve varies greatly from tumor to tumor and is dependent on the total tumor mass. This complexity is further increased by synergism among the cytotoxic drugs, as well as a lack of extensive pharmacokinetic data for their use in high-dose regimens.

■ TUMOR-CELL CONTAMINATION IN PREPARATIONS OF PERIPHERAL BLOOD PROGENITOR CELLS

The availability of hemopoietic progenitor cells for use after high-dose chemotherapy has made it possible to study the concept of dose intensification clinically. Most data so far have been derived from studies using autologous bone marrow (BM). This source for hemopoietic SC is now widely replaced by autologous peripheral blood progenitor cells (PBPC), which are either mobilized from the BM by hemopoietic growth factors or by the combined application of

312

myelosuppressive chemotherapy plus cytokines (see Chapters 8 and 9). When compared with autologous BMT, PBPC transplantation leads to a more rapid restoration of hemopoiesis with a shortened period of pancytopenia and, as a result, the potential for a reduced risk of infection and bleeding complications (Kessinger and Armitage 1991; Sheridan et al. 1992; Brugger et al. 1993a).

Initially, PBPC collections were thought to contain significantly lower numbers of contaminating tumor cells; however, it is now quite clear that malignant cells may contaminate leukapheresis preparations (Moss et al. 1990; Ross et al. 1993; Brugger et al. 1994a; Shpall and Jones 1995) and can contribute to relapse (Brenner et al. 1993). Moreover, it has been shown that tumor cells may be mobilized concomitant with hemopoietic progenitor cells in patients with solid tumors metastasizing to the BM (Brugger et al. 1994a). Thus, there is a substantial risk of tumor cell recruitment, particularly in patients who have tumors infiltrating their BM.

Reduction of tumor-cell contamination of PBPC collections by procedures to positively select $CD34^+$ hemopoietic progenitor cells are under investigation (Brugger et al. 1994b; Shpall et al. 1994). In a recent trial, the total volume of blood processed from patients was reduced, to minimize harvesting of tumor cells; positive selection of $CD34^+$ progenitor cells was followed by ex vivo expansion using a cocktail of hemopoietic growth factors (Brugger et al. 1993b). There was rapid hemopoietic engraftment as well as long-term hemopoietic reconstitution in the ten patients (Brugger et al. 1995b). Thus, starting from a small number of PB $CD34^+$ cells, ex vivo–expanded hemopoietic progenitor cells might offer new prospects for cellular therapy (Chapter 13), including a reduced risk for tumor-cell contamination, the circumvention of leukapheresis, and the potential for repetitive cycles of high-dose chemotherapy.

■ HIGH-DOSE CHEMOTHERAPY REQUIRING CELLULAR SUPPORT IN SELECTED SOLID TUMORS

Encouraged by successful high-dose chemotherapy trials in hematological malignancies, dose-intensive chemotherapy regimens in solid tumors requiring cellular support are increasingly being studied. Most data are derived from uncontrolled phase I/II studies. High-dose chemotherapy with stem-cell rescue has not yet been definitively established as being superior to conventional approaches for any adult solid tumor; however, promising clinical results have become evident for many tumors, suggesting the need for more randomized trials. In other malignancies, such as glioma and metastatic breast cancer, the emphasis should be on the identification of new chemotherapeutic agents and the design of innovative high-dose chemotherapy protocols, including sequential administration of high-dose regimens.

Melanoma

Systemic chemotherapy for the treatment of metastatic melanoma remains disappointing. Dacarbazine, still the cornerstone of chemotherapy in this disorder, or melphalan or carmustine (BCNU) results in response rate of 10% to 20%. High-dose chemotherapy increases response rates considerably, and some complete remissions (CR) were observed (for review of response rates of published phase I/II data of high-dose treatment using autologous BMT see Antman, Elias, and Fine 1994; Fields 1992). Time-to-disease progression and overall survival were not improved; however, Lakhani et al. (1990) did not observe survival differences in patients with metastatic melanoma in a consecutive series of studies using single agents and combination standard-dose chemotherapy, as well as high-dose melphalan and high-dose BCNU plus autologous bone-marrow transplant (ABMT). Recently, investigators at Duke University (North Carolina) (Meisenberg et al. 1993) published a randomized trial comparing high-dose cyclophosphamide, high-dose BCNU and cisplatin, and observation alone in stage-II patients after resection of lymph-node metastases. Although immediate adjuvant high-dose chemotherapy prolonged the time to disease progression, the difference was not significant. No differences in overall survival were noted.

On the basis of current data, there is no role for high-dose chemotherapy in melanoma, either in the adjuvant setting, or in metastatic disease. New agents – for example, temozolamide (O'Reilly et al. 1992), fotemustine (Avril et al. 1992), camptothecin (Pantazis et al. 1992), and paclitaxel (Kirkwood 1992) – will have to be proven to be active in primary disease before further high-dose trials using such drugs are justified.

Central Nervous System Tumors

Nitrosoureas, epipodophyllotoxins, thiotepa, and cyclophosphamide are active drugs in glioma, and have been used in studies of dose escalation. High-dose chemotherapy with BMT for experimental brain tumors in rats may achieve a greater antitumor effect compared with conventional chemotherapy (Soma, Shoin, and Yamashita 1993).

Until now, however, it was not clear whether high-dose chemotherapy had any clinical role in the management of glioma. Single-agent studies (primarily with carmustine) indicate that median survival is approximately 4 months in patients with recurrent disease (Takvorian, Parker, and Hockberg 1983; Giannone and Wolff 1987) and 12 to 17 months in an adjuvant setting (Johnson, Thompson, and Corwin 1987; Mbidde, Selby, and Perren 1988; Biron, Vial, and Cauvin 1991). Studies reported recently in pediatric malignant glioma having a high risk of failure with standard treatment did not show a significant advantage using high-dose combination chemotherapy (Heideman et al. 1993; Kedar et al. 1994). More promising data have been reported in patients with recurrent medulloblastoma and primitive neuroectodermal tumors (Finlay et al. 1994).

Considering that high-dose chemotherapy in the postoperative setting is feasible; that response rates are increased compared with standard-dose treatment; that etoposide, thiotepa, cyclophosphamide, and platinum compounds (agents that can be dose-escalated) are active in these disorders; and that overall toxicity can be reduced by the use of PBPC, new high-dose protocols should be investigated in the adjuvant setting to identify patients likely to benefit from this approach.

Small-Cell Lung Cancer

Small-cell lung cancer (SCLC) is one of the most chemosensitive tumors; however, it is only rarely cured with modern combination chemotherapy. The median survival of SCLC patients treated with standard-dose regimens ranges from 12 to 16 months for those with limited-stage disease, and 7 to 11 months for extensive-disease patients (Ihde 1992). Based on the steep dose-response relationship in this malignancy (Cohen 1977), several investigators have evaluated the use of high-dose chemotherapy. The majority of these studies revealed that only patients with limited-disease at study entry were alive and disease-free 2 years following high-dose therapy, whereas patients with extensive disease uniformly relapsed and quickly died, usually within 1 year of transplantation (Seifter and Ihde 1988; Antman and Souhami 1993; Shpall et al. 1993).

The high-dose chemotherapy trials listed in Table 18.1 were performed as late-intensification strategies in both limited- and extensive-disease SCLC after at least 9 weeks of conventional-dose induction chemotherapy. The results of these trials suggest that high-dose chemotherapy with stem-cell support is no better than standard therapy; however, these investigators used high-dose regimens that would

Table 18.1. High-Dose Chemotherapy plus Stem-Cell Support in Small-Cell Lung Cancer: Published Trials Between 1986 and 1994

Author	No. of Patients	Median Age (yr)	Stage[a]	High-Dose Regimen	Disease-Free Survival (months)	Overall Survival (mo)	% Toxic Deaths	Remarks
Spitzer et al. 1986	32	59	LD	Cy, VP16, VCR + ABMT	—	14	0	Late intensification; no survival benefit
Ihde et al. 1986	8	59	ED	Cy, VP16 + ABMT	10	11	25	Only 8 of 29 patients evaluable for late intensification; no survival benefit
Humblet et al. 1987	45 (22/23)	53	LD/ED	Cy, VP16, BCNU + ABMT	7 vs. 2.5	17 vs. 14	17	Late intensification, randomized trial; DFS and OS benefit for HD
Souhami et al. 1989	9	—	ED	Carbo, VP16, Mel/Cy + ABMT	7	12	—	Multiple agents to overcome drug resistance
Elias et al. 1993	19	49	LD	Cy, CDPP, BCNU + ABMT	12	73% (1 yr) 53% (2 yr)	5	Patients in CR before HD therapy have best prognosis
Brugger et al. 1994	13	51	LD	VP16, Ifo, Carbo, Epi + PBPC	—	85% (14 mo)	0	Early intensification; median survival not reached.

[a]ED = extensive disease, LD = limited disease, Cy = cyclophosphamide, VP16 = etoposide, VCR = vincristine sulfate, OS = overall survival, BCNU = carmustine, Carbo = carboplatin, Epi = epirubicin, mo = months, yr = year, DFS = disease-free survival, HD = high-dose, Ifo = ifosfamide.

be considered only mild to moderate dose intensity by today's standards, and autologous BM support was probably unnecessary for most of these patients (Seifter and Ihde 1988).

The study by Spitzer et al. (1986) in limited-disease SCLC has shown almost identical results to patients treated with conventional therapy. It was remarkable that all of the long-term disease-free survivors were in clinical stage III at diagnosis, and that none of the patients died during chemotherapy dose intensification. This was in sharp contrast to the study by Ihde et al. (1986) in which the toxic death rate was 25%, and only 8 of the original 29 patients were eligible for late intensification. It should be noted, however, that this study only included extensive-disease patients and the majority of the patients were less than fully ambulatory at the start of treatment. Moreover, since the median age of the patients was relatively high, comorbidity might also have contributed to the high rate of fatal toxicity.

The only reported randomized study comparing conventional chemotherapy with late-intensification therapy was performed by Humblet et al. (1987). This multicenter study included a total of 101 patients, and 45 responding patients (selected for their sensitivity to the induction chemotherapy) were randomized to standard-dose consolidation or high-dose intensification chemotherapy with BMT. This study demonstrated a statistically significant increase in relapse-free survival in favor of the high-dose group; however, since relapses occurred at the primary site and the rate of fatal toxicity was 17%, overall survival was not significantly improved, although all the 2-year disease-free survivors had received high-dose therapy.

Souhami et al. (1989) included multiple chemotherapeutic agents in their high-dose regimen, in an attempt to overcome drug resistance. Although the response rate was 100% in this trial, none of the extensive-disease patients achieved a complete remission.

A recent study by Elias et al. (1993) in patients with limited-disease SCLC yielded promising results which, however, were not directly comparable to other studies because of patient selection. Over 7 years, only 19 patients were enrolled on this protocol: only patients who responded to induction therapy received late intensification, and all patients subsequently received radiotherapy for local control and prophylaxis of central nervous system (CNS) relapse. The 2-year disease-free survival rate was 53% for those patients who were in or near complete remission at the initiation of high-dose therapy. The most important prognostic factor for survival was the degree of response to induction chemotherapy.

Our approach to the treatment of limited-disease SCLC is somewhat different. We administered high-dose chemotherapy, followed by PBPC transplantation, as part of an early intensification strategy (Fig. 18.1, Table 18.1). Patients were initially treated with two cycles of etoposide (500 mg/m^2), ifosfamide (4 gm/m^2), cisplatin (50 mg/m^2), and epirubicin (50 mg/m^2) (VIP-E) and recombinant human granulocyte colony-stimulating factor (rHuG-(CSF) to combine an effective standard-dose regimen with the simultaneous mobilization of PBPC (Brugger et al. 1993a). Patients who were in partial (PR) or CR after these two induction chemotherapy cycles subsequently received high-dose intensification with cumulative doses of 1,500 mg/m^2 etoposide, 12 gm/m^2 ifosfamide, 750 to 1000 mg/m^2 carboplatin, and 150 mg/m^2 epirubicin (the high-dose VIC-E regimen), followed by autologous PBPC transplantation and rHuG-CSF administration (Brugger et al. 1994b; Brugger et al. 1995). Thus, the complete chemotherapy program was administered within approximately 7 weeks (Fig. 18.1). All patients received chest irradiation (50 Gy) following transplant, and those in complete remission additionally received prophylactic cranial irradiation (30 Gy). At a median follow-up of 14 months after transplantation, median survival in this group of patients has not yet been reached; 11 of 13 patients (84.6%) are alive with 9 of 13 (69.2%) still in complete remission. There were no treatment-related deaths, and the only clinically relevant nonhematological organ toxicity was oral mucositis (Brugger et al. 1995). We think that up-front high-dose chemotherapy with PBPC support is a promising approach, although median follow-up data at this time are limited. Based on these results,

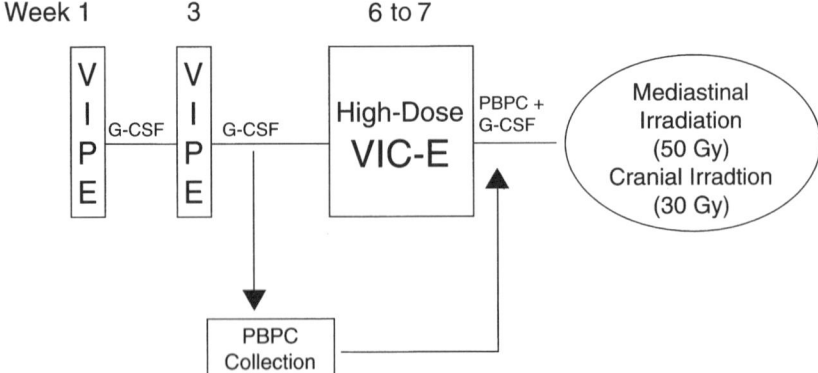

Figure 18.1 High-dose combined modality treatment in LD-SCLC (stage I-IIIB, <60 years). (From Brugger et al. 1995.)

we are planning a phase III randomized trial to provide proof of the role of this approach in the management of limited-disease SCLC.

In summary, although the initial studies (Table 18.1) (Livingston 1986; Antman and Souhami 1993) using high-dose chemotherapy with BMT in patients with SCLC did not appear to be superior to standard-dose chemotherapy, the promising approaches outlined by Elias et al. (1993) and our own experience with early high-dose intensification and PBPC support merit further testing.

Sarcoma

Ewing Sarcoma In metastatic disease, a low percentage of children and no adults are cured with conventional-dose chemotherapy. High-dose trials with SC support result in a response in approximately half of relapsing or refractory patients. These responses, however, are generally very short lasting (for review of published observations, see Antman, Elias, and Fine 1994). Preliminary data using high-dose regimens as part of the first-line treatment in high-risk patients are more promising (Marcus et al. 1988).

Other Sarcomas In metastatic disease, there are some reports on high-dose regimens in children and adults (Bader et al. 1989; Elias et al. 1991; Pinkerton 1991; Dumontet et al. 1992). Although overall response rates are clearly superior to standard approaches, there is no evidence in these phase I/II trials that long-term survival can be improved considerably.

In our own experience in ten patients with metastatic soft tissue sarcoma transplanted with PBPC after high-dose VIC-E response rate was 66% (CR 44%, PR 22%). Disappointingly, the median survival was only 8 months in these patients.

Future strategies should concentrate on the use of high-dose protocols in the adjuvant setting in patients with large volume, high-grade sarcoma after local treatment, as well as in the neoadjuvant setting for patients for whom local therapy must be marginal to preserve organ function.

Germ-Cell Tumors

Patients with relapsed and cisplatin refractory germ-cell tumors are rarely cured with conventional-dose chemotherapy. High-dose chemotherapy, supported with hemopoietic stem cells, has been shown in several series to induce a high response rate (CR rate, approximately 30%) in multiple-relapsed and mostly chemotherapy-resistant patients, and this approach is a potentially curative option in about 15% of patients (see Table 18.2).

Analysis of the heterogeneous data is complicated because the patients studied received different treatment strategies before high-dose treatment, with a varying degree of "total" chemotherapy. Additionally, some studies applied double high-dose regimens; however, it can be concluded that both the response to conventional salvage therapy before high-dose chemotherapy and the number of regimens that failed are most predictive for overall response.

It is noteworthy that patients with primary mediastinal germ-cell tumors do not seem to profit from the high-dose approach (Broun et al. 1991, 1992) although Siegert et al. (1994) did not observe a worse outcome in their five patients with this manifestation of disease.

To date, these strategies in heavily pretreated patients transplanted with BM progenitor cells have been associated with a high mortality rate (approximately 10%). Currently, most trials use PBPC as hemopoietic support, which might decrease the rate of complications.

Based on both the findings of phase I/II trials in advanced germ-cell tumors and the observation in hematological malignancies such as acute myeloid leukemia (AML) and aggressive lymphoma that early initiation of dose-intensive therapy results in a better outcome when compared with use in resistant disease, early intervention trials were performed, either in first relapse sensitive to salvage standard-dose chemotherapy or in poor-risk patients at diagnosis (Table 18.3).

At our institution (G. Dölken et al., unpublished results), we have treated five patients with primary high-risk germ-cell tumors with two cycles of PIV/rHuG-CSF (cisplatin 120 mg/m^2, ifosfamide 6 gm/m^2, etoposide 750 mg/m^2), followed by high-dose VIC with stem-cell support (VP16 1,500 mg/m^2, ifosfamide 12 gm/m^2, carboplatin 750 mg/m^2). Four patients achieved a CR, two of them following chemotherapy, and two following surgery for residual retroperitoneal masses that contained no detectable viable tumor. These patients are in continuous complete remission for 4$^+$, 6$^+$, 8$^+$, and 9$^+$ months.

Eight patients were treated for chemosensitive relapsed advanced germ cell tumors after cisplatin-based first-line chemotherapy. Salvage treatment with PIV/rHuG-CSF ($n = 5$) or VIP/rHuG-CSF ($n = 3$) was followed by high-dose chemotherapy. Four of eight patients achieved a CR (4$^+$, 6$^+$, 13$^+$, and 21$^+$ months); two patients are in CR after thoracotomy and retroperitoneal lymphadenectomy, respectively (13$^+$ and 10$^+$ months). In both groups, a total of five patients received two cycles of high-dose VIC, which was well tolerated.

Table 18.2. High-Dose Chemotherapy plus Stem-Cell Support in Germ-Cell Tumors: Advanced Malignant Disease

Author	No. of Evaluated Patients	Chemotherapy Regimen[a]	CR	CR (mo) [range]
Blijham et al. 1981	10	VP16, Cy	40%	0
Mulder et al. 1988	11	VP16, Cy	18%	1 [16]
Ghosn et al. 1988	19	VP16, Carbo, Ifo	26%	5 [6–18]
Rosti et al. 1992	32	VP16, Carbo ± Ifo	25%	4 [10–24]
Lotz et al. 1991	26	VP16, Carbo, Ifo	38%	5 [17–55]
Droz et al. 1991	15	VP16, Carbo, Cy	33%	3 [8–37]
Nichols et al. 1992	38	VP16, Carbo	24%	5 [12–20]
Broun et al. 1992	40	VP16, Carbo ± Ifo	30%	6 [24]
Motzer et al. 1993a	30	VP16, Carbo, Cy	43%	7 [6–36]
Siegert et al.[b] 1994	68	VP16, Carbo, Ifo	31%	[2–32]
Total patients	306 patients		98 patients (32%)	40 patients (16.8%)

[a]VP16 = etoposide, Cy = cyclophosphamide, Carbo = carboplatin, Ifo = ifosfamide, CR = complete response, mo = months.
[b]Relapse-free survival of patients with CR and PR with marker normalization after high-dose treatment was 67%.

Table 18.3. High-Dose Chemotherapy in Germ-Cell Tumors: Early Intervention Trials

Authors	No. of Evaluated Patients	Chemotherapy Regimen[a]	CR	cCR (mo)	Remarks
Barnett et al. 1993	21	VP16, Carbo, Ifo	71%	67% [6–78]	Poor-risk patients (15 in first relapse, 6 high-risk, first line)
Motzer et al. 1993b	22	VP16, Carbo	55%	36% [25–47]	Poor-risk first-line double high-dose chemotherapy in 14 of 22
Broun et al. 1994	18	VP16, Carbo	50%	39% [2–36]	Chemosensitive first relapse
Total patients	61 patients		36 patients (60%)	29 patients (47.6%)	

[a]VP16 = etoposide, Carbo = carboplatin, CR = complete response, mo = months, IFO = ifosfamide.

These trials indicate an excellent tolerance of early high-dose chemotherapy and the prospect of better long-term survival compared with "late-intervention" trials. Considering that poor-risk patients achieve a durable CR with conventional platinum-based chemotherapy in 30% of cases at best (Bosl et al. 1983; Vaeth et al. 1984; Birch et al. 1986; Toner et al. 1990), further high-dose trials should concentrate on this patient population.

Current strategies in germ-cell tumors do not yet provide the final answers; even with high-dose chemotherapy being part of front-line treatment in poor-risk patients, many patients still relapse. More effective approaches, particularly sequential high-dose chemotherapy using non–cross-resistant regimens, might further improve results. Finally, future trials of SC-supported high-dose chemotherapy will need to be adequately controlled by randomization to an intensified conventional-dose chemotherapy regimen, supported only by hemopoietic growth factors.

Ovarian Cancer

Ovarian cancer is very sensitive to chemotherapeutic agents, and a dose-response relationship has been shown for alkylating agents and cisplatin (Levin and Hryniuk 1987). The analysis of a potential benefit of high-dose chemotherapy in ovarian cancer must consider that conventional treatment has changed substantially in this malignancy. The introduction of paclitaxel has improved overall clinical results in suboptimally debulked stage III/IV patients, and this drug is able to induce remissions in patients who have progressed during platinum treatment (Trimble, Adams, and Vena 1993; McGuire 1994). Thus, results of high-dose chemotherapy will need to be compared with the most effective standard treatment available today.

To date, high-dose trials using stem-cell support have been reported in a limited number of patients with disease refractory to standard-dose treatment, including relapsing patients (Mulder et al. 1989; Shpall et al. 1990; Viens et al. 1990; Shea et al. 1992; Stiff et al. 1994); responsive residual disease after primary debulking surgery and front-line standard-dose chemotherapy (Daulat et al. 1989; Viens et al. 1990; Legross et al. 1992; Tepler et al. 1992); and newly diagnosed disease (after surgery) (Menichella et al. 1991; Tepler et al. 1992; Murakami et al. 1994) (For a detailed discussion of the papers cited, as well as other articles, see Schilder 1993).

It is not possible to draw firm conclusions of these phase I/II studies, as most trials included only few patients, and were heterogeneous as to stage of disease, extent of residual disease after surgery and/or initial standard-dose chemotherapy, the timing of high-dose chemotherapy, and the high-dose regimens applied. Responses are impressive (approximately 80%); however, disease-free survival rates are only increased substantially in patients with minimal residual tumor burden at the time of transplantation.

Based on these observations, high-dose chemotherapy concepts should be considered for further clinical trials in high-risk patients, such as relapsing patients with chemosensitive disease, and in patients with advanced ovarian cancer with small-volume residual disease after primary surgery and/or induction chemotherapy. An optimal conditioning regimen has not been established in ovarian cancer, although combinations including an alkylating drug and carboplatin are very active. The role of paclitaxel in high-dose regimens has not yet been defined. Moreover, whether sequential high-dose chemotherapy offers an advantage over single high-dose chemotherapy trials in these patients will need to be tested.

Breast Cancer

High-dose chemotherapy is of particular interest in breast cancer, a chemosensitive malignancy that develops in one of eight women in northern Europe and North America.

There is a threshold dose of cytotoxic drugs below which there is a significant decrease in disease-free survival in all patients and in overall survival in postmenopausal women, as studied in the adjuvant setting (Wood et al. 1994); however, it does not automatically follow that an increase in dose or dose rate of conventional chemotherapy will prove beneficial. In contrast, a modest increase in dose intensity (same dose in a 50% shorter period of time) did not improve the outcome (Wood et al. 1994).

These observations neither support nor refute the contention that more is better, but urge for adequate studies of the role of high-doses of chemotherapy.

Metastatic Disease   For advanced resistant stage IV breast cancer, phase I/II high-dose chemotherapy trials have shown that response rates were substantially higher than with standard-dose therapy (approximately 50% to 70%); however, progression occurred within a median of 6 months, and overall survival was not improved compared with that of historical controls (Henderson 1988; Antman et al. 1991; Eddy 1992).

As a consequence of the observed high response rates, high-dose chemotherapy was studied in metastatic disease responsive to induction chemotherapy (see Table 18.4). Although the trials are uncontrolled and have numerous biases, the response rate was approximately 80% with as much as 60% complete remissions. There is no doubt that this modality is the most active available treatment for induction of complete remissions in metastatic breast cancer. Importantly, in those patients achieving a complete remission, approximately 20% to 25% achieved a plateau in disease-free and overall survival beyond 2 to 3 years, which means that although the median overall survival was only in the range of 1 to 2 years, approximately 10% of all patients treated with high-dose chemotherapy might maintain durable remissions; however, median follow-up data are only in the range of 2 to 3 years, to date, and it is too early to draw firm conclusions. It is an open question whether long-term survival is confined to patients with CR after induction therapy (Antman, Ayash, and Elias 1992), or whether patients converting from PR to CR after high-dose intensification have a similar survival pattern (Dunphy et al. 1990; Kennedy, Beveridge, and Rowley 1991; Williams, Gilewski, and Mick 1992). Shorter survival after high-dose treatment in patients treated with adjuvant chemotherapy (Falkson et al. 1991) is independently predicted by disease distribution to the liver or to soft tissue (Williams, Gilewski, and Mick 1992).

Many new high-dose regimens that might be more effective, including sequential high-dose chemotherapy with non–cross-resistant drugs, or newer drugs such as paclitaxel, are currently under study. Considering the lack of established and optimized high-dose strategies, it seems premature to concentrate on randomized studies in metastatic breast cancer. Instead, it is our contention that patients with metastatic breast cancer should be included in innovative phase I/II approaches; these studies might improve results and help to define which patients are most likely to benefit.

Dose-Intensive Adjuvant Therapy in Resectable Breast Cancer Despite treatment with standard-dose, adjuvant chemotherapy in patients with extensive lymph node metastases at the time of primary therapy, relapse-free survival at 5 years is less than 30% (Tormey et al. 1983; Jones et al. 1987; Peters 1991. There is now increasing evidence that high-dose chemotherapy might be associated with superior outcome in these patients (Table 18.5). In the most advanced study, Peters et al. (1993) have reported that the actuarial projected event-free survival is 72% at 6.5 years, with a median follow-up of 3.3 years. Importantly, no patient has so far relapsed later than 28 months after transplantation. Gianni's group, using sequential high-dose che-

Table 18.4. High-Dose Chemotherapy Trials in Women with Stage IV Breast Cancer Responsive to Standard Induction Chemotherapy

Author	No. of Evaluated Patients	High-Dose Regimen Toxic Death Rate	CR	Median Disease-Free Survival	Median	Overall Survival	Remarks
Eder et al. 1986	17	Cy, Carbo, BCNU	18%	38%	4.5 mo	8 mo	Feasibility study
Vincent et al. 1988	15	L-PAM	20%	47%	7 mo	12 mo	
Peters et al. 1988	22	Cy, CDDP, BCNN	23%	54%	7 mo	10 mo	No induction chemotherapy; predominant sites of relapse in previous areas of bulk
Wallerstein et al. 1990	32	VP16, Thio, Mit	12.5%	23%	4.5 mo	9 mo	Heavily pretreated patients; 14 received double HD chemotherapy
Dunphy et al. 1990	58	Cy, CDDP	9%	55%	13 mo	23 mo	Double HD chemotherapy
Kennedy et al. 1991	24	Cy, Thio	0	46%	13 mo	22 mo	
Antman et al. 1992	29	Cy, Thio	3%	59%	6 mo	NR	17 to 31 mo from transplant
Williams et al. 1992	22	Cy, Thio	14%	56%	5.4 mo	15.1 mo	Induction with LOMAC (n = 27) (1 death)
	23	Cy, Thio, ± BCNU	30%	35%	10.5 mo	9.3 mo	Induction with FCAD (n = 32) (1 death) (12 of /59 died = 20%)
Fields et al. 1993	38	VP16, Carbo	4.5%	39.5%	6 mo	12 mo	
Crown et al. 1993	17	Sequential HD: Cy→VP16, Carbo, Cy	0	59%	9 mo	NR	

Somlo, et al. 1994	14	VP16, Cy, Dox	0	42%	9 mo	22 mo	
Ghalie et al. 1994	39	Cy, CDDP, Thio	15%	36%	8 mo	NR	HD-chemotherapy split; no induction chemotherapy in 23 of 29 patients
Ayash et al. 1994	20	Sequential HD, Melph→Cy, Carbo, Thio	0	35%	NR	NR	Feasibility study progression-free survival at 15 mo is 52 ± 15%

Carbo = carboplatin, CDDP = cisplatin, Cy = cyclophosphamide, Dox = doxorubicin, HD = high dose, Melph = melphalan, Mit = mitoxantrone, Thio = thiotepa, VP16 = etoposide, NR = not reported, mo = months.

Table 18.5. High-Dose Chemotherapy Trials in Women with High-Risk Operable Breast Cancer

Authors	No. of Evaluated Patients	High-Dose Regimen[a]	Toxic Death Rate	Recurrence-Free Survival	Median Follow-Up
Gianni et al. 1992	48	Sequential HD incl. L-PAM	2%	92%	21 mo [2–24]
Peters et al. 1993	85	Cy, CDDP, BCNU	12%[b]	72%	3.3 yr[c]
Fields et al. 1993	6	VP16, Carbo, Ifo	0	100%	14 mo [0.5–29]
Somlo et al. 1994	21	VP16, Cy, Ifo	0	90%	8 mo [4–36]
de Graaf et al. 1994	24[d]	VP16, Cy, ± Mit, ± Thio	7%	92%	36 mo [9–72]
Kanz et al., unpublished	26	VP16, Carbo, Ifo, ± Epi	0	92%	13 mo [4–27]

[a]Cy = cyclophosphamide, VP16 = etoposide, CR = complete response, Carbo = carboplatin, Ifo = ifosfamide, Thio = thiotepa, mo = months, yr = years.
[b]Primarily due to pulmonary toxicity and hemolytic-uremic syndrome.
[c]No relapses after 28 months.
[d]Includes patients ≥5 positive axillary nodes.

motherapy, observed a recurrence-free survival of 94% with a median observation of 21 months (Gianni et al. 1992).

We have studied high-dose etoposide (1,500 mg/m²), ifosfamide (12 gm/m²), and carboplatin (750 to 1,200 mg/m²) with or without epirubicin (150 mg/m²) with autologous PBPC transplant as consolidation after two cycles of standard dose VIP-E chemotherapy in 26 patients with high-risk primary breast cancer (≥10 axillary lymph nodes). PBPC were mobilized after the second cycle of VIP-E chemotherapy and rHuG-CSF administration. The total cytotoxic treatment duration, including high-dose chemotherapy, was 6 to 7 weeks only (day 1 and day 21 application of cycle 1 and cycle 2 of the standard dose VIP-E, followed 3 to 4 weeks later by high-dose VIC-E for 3 days). This approach contrasts with studies where high-dose chemotherapy is delivered as a consolidation strategy many weeks after lower dose induction therapy. Starting from week 12, patients received local radiotherapy. High-dose chemotherapy was well tolerated, with oral mucositis being the most important nonhematological toxicity. No toxic deaths were observed. At a median follow-up of 13 months (range 4 to 27) 24 of 26 patients are disease-free, and 25 patients are alive.

Current results of high-dose chemotherapy in the adjuvant setting are clearly superior to anything previously published in the high-risk adjuvant setting in breast cancer. These results provide the rationale for a series of ongoing randomized studies.

REFERENCES

Antman, K., Ayash, L., and Elias, A. (1992) A phase II study of high-dose cyclophosphamide, thiotepa, and carboplatin with autologous marrow support in women with measurable advanced breast cancer responding to standard-dose therapy. *Journal of Clinical Oncology*, **10**, 102–10.

Antman, K., Bearman, S.I., and Davidson, B. (1991) Dose intensive therapy in breast cancer: current status. In R.P. Gale and R.E. Champlin (Eds.) *New strategies in bone marrow transplantation*, pp. 423–36. New York, Alan R. Liss.

Antman, K.H., Elias, A., and Fine, H.A. (1994) Dose-intensive therapy with autologous bone marrow transplantation in solid tumors. In S.J. Forman, K.G. Blume, and E.D. Thomas (Eds.) *Bone marrow transplantation*, pp. 767–88. Boston, Blackwell Scientific Publications.

Antman, K.H. and Souhami, R.L. (1993) High-dose chemotherapy in solid tumors. *Annals of Oncology*, **4**, 29–44.

Avril, M.F., Bonneterre, J., Cupissol, D., et al. (1992) Fotemustine plus dacarbazine for malignant melanoma. *European Journal of Cancer*, **11**, 1807–11.

Ayash, L.J., Elias, A., and Wheeler, C. (1994) Double dose-intensive chemotherapy with autologous marrow and peripheral-blood progenitor-cell support for metastatic breast cancer: a feasibility study. *Journal of Clinical Oncology*, **12**, 37–44.

Bader, J.L., Horowitz, M.E., and Dewan, R. (1989) Intensive combined modality therapy of small round cell and undifferentiated sarcomas in children and young adults. *Radiotherapy and Oncology*, **16**, 187–201.

Barnett, M.J., Coppin, C.M., Murray, N., et al. (1993) High-dose chemotherapy and autologous bone marrow transplantation for patients with poor prognosis non-seminomatous germ cell tumors. *British Journal of Cancer*, **68**, 594–8.

Birch, R., Williams, S., and Cone, A. (1986) Prognostic factors for favorable outcome in disseminated germ cell tumors. *Journal of Clinical Oncology*, **4**, 400–7.

Biron, P., Vial, C., and Cauvin, F. (1991) Strategy including surgery, BCNU high dose followed by ABMT and radiotherapy in supratentorial high grade astrocytomas – a report of 98 patients. In K.A. Dicke and J. Armitage (Eds.) *Autologous bone marrow transplantation: Proceedings of the Fifth International Symposiums*, pp. 637–46. Omaha, University of Nebraska.

Blijham, G., Spitzer, G., and Litam, J. (1981) The treatment of advanced testicular carcinoma with high dose chemotherapy and autologous marrow support. *European Journal of Cancer*, **17**, 433–41.

Bosl, G., Geller, N., and Cirrincione, C. (1983) Multivariate analysis of prognostic variables in patients with metastatic testicular cancer. *Cancer Research*, **43**, 3403.

Brenner, M.K., Rill, D.R., Moen, R.C., et al. (1993) Gene-marking to trace origin of relapse after autologous bone-marrow transplantation. *Lancet*, **341**, 85.

Broun, E.R., Nichols, C.R., Einhorn, L.H., et al. (1991) Salvage therapy with high-dose chemotherapy and autologous bone marrow support in the treatment of primary non-seminomatous mediastinal germ cell tumors. *Cancer*, **68**, 1513–5.

Broun, E.R., Nichols, C.R., Kneebone, P., et al. (1992) Long-term outcome of patients with relapsed and refractory germ cell tumors treated with high-dose chemotherapy and autologous bone marrow rescue. *Annals of Internal Medicine*, **117**, 124–8.

Broun, E.R., Nichols, C.R., Turns, M., et al. (1994) Early salvage therapy for germ cell cancer using high-dose chemotherapy with autologous bone marrow support. *Cancer*, **73**, 1716–20.

Brugger, W., Birken, R., Bertz, H., et al. (1993a) Peripheral blood progenitor cells mobilized by chemotherapy + G-CSF accelerate both neutrophil and platelet recovery after high-dose VP16, ifosfamide and cisplatin. *British Journal of Haematology*, **84**, 402–7.

Brugger, W., Bross, K.J., Glatt, M., et al. (1994a) Mobilization of tumor cells and hemopoietic progenitor cells into peripheral blood of patients with solid tumors. *Blood*, **83**, 636–40.

Brugger, W., Frommhold, H., Pressler, K., et al. (1995a) Use of high-dose etoposide, ifosfamide, carboplatin, epirubicin and peripheral blood progenitor cell transplantation in limited-disease small cell lung cancer. *Seminars in Oncology*, **22**, 3–8.

Brugger, W., Henschler, R., Heimfeld, S., et al. (1994b) Positively selected autologous blood CD34 plus cell and unseparated peripheral blood progenitor cells mediate identical hemopoietic engraftment after high-dose VP16, ifosfamide, carboplatin and epirubicin. *Blood*, **84**, 1421–6.

Brugger, W., Möcklin, W., Heimfeld, S., et al. (1993b) Ex vivo expansion of enriched peripheral blood CD34 positive progenitor cells by stem cell factor, interleukin-1β, IL-6, Il-3, interferon-γ, and erythropoietin. *Blood*, **81**, 2579–83.

Brugger et al. (1995b) *New England Journal of Medicine*, **333**.

Cohen, M. (1977) Intensive chemotherapy of small cell bronchogenic carcinoma. *Cancer Treatment Report*, **61**, 344–54.

Crown, J., Kritz, A., Vahdat, L., et al. (1993) Rapid administration of multiple cycles of high-dose myelosuppressive chemotherapy in patients with metastatic breast cancer. *Journal of Clinical Oncology*, **11**, 1144–9.

Daulat, J., Legros, M., and Condat, P. (1989) High-dose melphalan and autologous bone marrow support for treatment of ovarian carcinoma with positive second-look operation. *Gynecologic Oncology*, **34**, 294–8.

deGraaf, H., Willemse, P.H., DeVries, E.G., et al. (1994) Intensive chemotherapy with autologous bone marrow transfusion as primary treatment in women with breast cancer and more than five involved axillary lymph nodes. *European Journal of Cancer*, **30A**, 150–3.

Droz, J.P., Pico, J.L., Ghosn, M., et al. (1991) Long-term survivors after salvage high dose chemotherapy with bone marrow rescue in refractory germ cell cancer. *European Journal of Cancer*, **27**, 831–5.

Dumontet, C., Biron, P., Bouffet, E., et al. (1992) High dose chemotherapy with ABMT in soft tissue sarcomas. A report of 22 cases. *Bone Marrow Transplantation*, **10**, 405–8.

Dunphy, F.R., Spitzer, G., Buzdar, A.U., et al. (1990) Treatment of estrogen receptor-negative or hormonally refractory breast cancer with double high-dose chemotherapy intensification and bone marrow support. *Journal of Clinical Oncology*, **8**, 1207–16.

Eddy, D.M. (1992) High-dose chemotherapy with autologous bone marrow transplantation for the treatment of metastatic breast cancer. *Journal of Clinical Oncology*, **10**, 657–70.

Eder, J.P., Antman, K., and Peters, W.P. (1986) High dose combination alkylating agent chemotherapy with autologous bone marrow support for metastatic breast cancer. *Journal of Clinical Oncology*, **4**, 1592–7.

Elias, A.D., Ayash, L., and Eder, J.P. (1991) A phase I study of high-dose ifosfamide and escalating doses of carboplatin with autologous bone marrow support. *Journal of Clinical Oncology*, **9**, 320–7.

Elias, A.D., Ayash, L., Frei, E., et al. (1993) Intensive combined modality therapy for limited-stage small-cell lung cancer. *Journal of the National Cancer Institute*, **85**, 559–66.

Falkson, G., Gelman, R., Falkson, C., Glick, J., and Harrison, J. (1991) Factors predicting for response, time to treatment failure, and survival in women with metastatic breast cancer treated with DAVTH: a prospective Eastern Cooperative Oncology Group study. *Journal of Clinical Oncology*, **9**, 2153–61.

Fields, K.K. (1992) Autologous bone marrow transplantation and melanoma: a focused review of the literature. *Annals of Plastic Surgery*, **28**, 70–3.

Fields, K.K., Perkins, J.P., Heimenz, J.W., et al. (1993) Intensive dose ifosfamide, carboplatin, and etoposide followed by autologous stem cell rescue: results of a Phase I/II study in breast cancer patients. *Surgical Oncology*, **2**, 87–95.

Finlay, J., Garvin, J., Allen, J., et al. (1994) High-dose chemotherapy (HDCx) with autologous bone marrow rescue (ABMR) in patients with recurrent medulloblastoma (MBO) primitive neuroectodermal tumors (PNET). *Proceedings of the American Society of Clinical Oncology*, **13**, 493A.

Ghalie, R., Richman, C.M., Adler, S.S., et al. (1994) Treatment of metastatic breast cancer with a split-course high-dose chemotherapy regimen and autologous bone marrow transplantation. *Journal of Clinical Oncology*, **10**, 342–6.

Ghosn, M., Droz, J.P., and Theodore, C. (1988) Salvage chemotherapy in refractory germ cell tumors with etoposide (VP-16) plus ifosfamide plus high-dose cisplatin. A VihP regimen. *Cancer*, **62**, 24–7.

Gianni, A.M., Siena, S., Bregni, M., et al. (1992) Growth factor-supported high-dose sequential (HDS) adjuvant chemotherapy in breast cancer with ≥10 positive nodes. *Proceedings of the American Society of Clinical Oncology*, **11**, A68.

Giannone, L. and Wolff, S. (1987) Phase II treatment of central nervous system gliomas with high dose etoposide and autologous bone marrow transplantation. *Cancer Treatment Report*, **71**, 759–61.

Heideman, R.L., Douglass, E.C., Krance, R.A., et al. (1993) High-dose chemotherapy and autologous bone marrow rescue followed by interstitial and external-beam radiotherapy in newly diagnosed pediatric malignant gliomas. *Journal of Clinical Oncology*, **11**, 1458–65.

Henderson, I.C. (1988) Chemotherapy for advanced disease. In J.R. Harris, S. Hellman, I.C. Henderson, and D.W. Kinne (Eds.) *Breast diseases*, Philadelphia, J.B. Lippincott Company.

Humblet, Y., Symann, M., Bosly, A., et al. (1987) Late intensification chemotherapy with autologous bone marrow transplantation in selected small-cell carcinoma of the lung: a randomized study. *Journal of Clinical Oncology*, **5**, 1864–73.

Ihde, D.C. (1992) Chemotherapy for lung cancer. *New England Journal of Medicine*, **327**, 1434–41.

Ihde, D.C., Deiserroth, A.B., and Lichter, A.S. (1986) Late intensification combined-modality therapy followed by autologous bone marrow infusion in extensive stage small-cell lung cancer. *Journal of Clinical Oncology*, **4**, 1443–54.

Johnson, D.B., Thompson, J.M., and Corwin, J. A. (1987) Prolongation of survival for high grade malignant gliomas with adjuvant high dose BCNU and ABMT. *Journal of Clinical Oncology*, **5**, 783–9.

Jones, S.E., Moon, T.E., and Bonadonna, G. (1987) Comparison of different trials of adjuvant chemotherapy in stage II breast cancer using a natural history data base. *American Journal of Clinical Oncology*, **10**, 387–95.

Kedar, A., Maria, B.L., Graham-Pole, J., et al. (1994) High-dose chemotherapy with marrow reinfusion and hyperfractionated irradiation for children with high-risk brain tumors. *Medical and Pediatric Oncology*, **23**, 428–36.

Kennedy, M.J., Beveridge, R.A., and Rowley, S.D. (1991) High-dose chemotherapy with reinfusion of purged autologous bone marrow following dose-intense induction as initial therapy for metastatic breast cancer. *Journal of the National Cancer Institute*, **83**, 920–6.

Kessinger, A., and Armitage, J.O. (1991) The evolving role of autologous peripheral stem cell transplantation following high-dose chemotherapy for malignancies. *Blood*, **77**, 211–14.

Kirkwood, J.M. (1992) Preclinical studies, experimental therapeutics, and clinical management of advanced melanoma. *Current Opinion in Oncology*, **4**, 368–79.

Lakhani, S., Selby, P., Bliss, J.M., et al. (1990) Chemotherapy for malignant melanoma: combinations and high doses produce more response without survival benefit. *British Journal of Cancer,* **62**, 330–4.

Legros, M., Fleury, J., Cure, X., et al. (1992) High-dose chemotherapy (HDC) and autologous bone marrow transplant (ABMT) in 31 advanced ovarian cancers: long-term results. *Proceedings of the American Society of Clinical Oncology,* **11**, 222.

Levin, L., and Hryniuk, W.M. (1987) Dose-intensity analyses of chemotherapy regimens in ovarian cancer. *Journal of Clinical Oncology,* **5**, 757–67.

Livingston, R.B. (1986) Small-cell lung cancer – whither late intensification? *Journal of Clinical Oncology,* **4**, 1437–8.

Lotz, J.P., Machover, D., and Malassagne, B. (1991) Phase I-II study of two consecutive courses of high-dose epipodophyllotoxin, ifosfamide, and carboplatin with autologous bone marrow transplantation for treatment of adult patients with solid tumors. *Journal of Clinical Oncology,* **9**, 1860–70.

Marcus, R.B., Jr., Graham-Pole, J.R., Springfield, D.S., et al. (1988) High-risk Ewing's sarcoma: end-intensification using autologous bone marrow transplantation. *International Journal of Radiation Oncology, Biology, and Physics,* **15**, 53–9.

Mbidde, E., Selby, P., and Perren, T. (1988) High dose BCNU chemotherapy with autologous bone marrow transplantation and full dose radiotherapy for grade IV astrocytomas. *British Journal of Cancer,* **58**, 779–82.

McGuire, W.P. (1994) Paclitaxel in the treatment of ovarian cancer. *Journal of Clinical Oncology,* **12**, 204–13.

Meisenberg, B.R., Ross, M., Vredenburgh, J.J., et al. (1993) Randomized trial of high-dose chemotherapy with autologous bone marrow support as adjuvant therapy for high-risk multi-node-positive malignant melanoma. *Journal of the National Cancer Institute,* **85**, 1080–5.

Menichella, G., Pierelli, L., Foddai, M.L., et al. (1991) Autologous blood stem cell harvesting and transplantation in patients with advanced ovarian cancer. *British Journal of Haematology,* **79**, 444–50.

Moss, T.J., Sanders, D.G., Lasky, L.C., and Bostrom, B. (1990) Contamination of peripheral blood stem cell harvests by circulating neuroblastoma cells. *Blood,* **76**, 1879.

Motzer, R.J., Gulati, S.C., Tong, W.P., et al. (1993a) Phase I trial with pharmacokinetic analyses of high-dose carboplatin, etoposide, and cyclophosphamide with autologous bone marrow transplantation in patients with refractory germ cell tumors. *Cancer Research,* **53**, 3730–5.

Motzer, R.J., Mazumdar, M., Subhash, C., et al. (1993b) Phase II trial of high-dose carboplatin and etoposide with autologous bone marrow transplantation in first-line therapy for patients with poor-risk germ cell tumors. *Journal of the National Cancer Institute,* **85**, 1828–35.

Mulder, P.O., DeVries, E.G., and Schrafford Koops, H. (1988) Chemotherapy with maximally tolerable doses of VP16-213 and cyclophosphamide followed by autologous bone marrow transplantation for the treatment of relapsed or refractory germ cell tumors. *European Journal of Cancer Clinical Oncology,* **24**, 675–9.

Mulder, P.O., Willemse, P.H., and Aalders, J.G. (1989) High-dose chemotherapy with autologous bone marrow transplantation in patients with refractory ovarian cancer. *European Journal of Cancer Clinical Oncology,* **25**, 645–9.

Murakami, M., Shinozuka, T., Kuroshima, Y., et al. (1994) High-dose chemotherapy with autologous bone marrow transplantation for the treatment of malignant ovarian tumors. *Seminars in Oncology*, **21**, 29–32.

Nichols, C.R., Anderson, J., and Lazarus, H.M. (1992) High-dose carboplatin and etoposide with autologous bone marrow transplantation in refractory germ cell cancer. An Eastern Cooperative Oncology Group protocol. *Journal of Clinical Oncology*, **10**, 558–63.

O'Reilly, S.M., Newlands, F.S., Stevens, M.F., et al. (1992) Temozolomide (CCRG 81045; M and B 39831; NSC 362856): a new oral cytotoxic agent with activity against melanoma, mycosis fugoides and high-grade glioma. *Proceedings of the American Association of Cancer Research*, **33**, 1267.

Pantazis, P., Hinz, H.R., Mendoza, J.T., et al. (1992) Complete inhibition of growth followed by death of human malignant melanoma cells in vitro and regression of human melanoma xenografts in immunodeficient mice induced by camptothecins. *Cancer Research*, **52**, 3980–7.

Peters, W.P. (1991) High-dose chemotherapy and autologous bone marrow support for breast cancer. In V.T. DeVita, S. Hellmann, and S.A. Rosenberg (Eds.) *Important advances in oncology*, pp. 135–50. Philadelphia, J.B. Lippincott Company.

Peters, W.P., Ross, M., Vrcndcnburgh, J.J., et al. (1993) High-dose chemotherapy and autologous bone marrow support as consolidation after standard-dose adjuvant therapy for high-risk primary breast cancer. *Journal of Clinical Oncology*, **11**, 1132–43.

Peters, W.P., Shpall, E.J., and Jones, R.B. (1988) High-dose combination alkylating agents with bone marrow support as initial treatment for metastatic breast cancer. *Journal of Clinical Oncology*, **6**, 1369–76.

Pinkerton, C.R. (1991) Megatherapy for soft tissue sarcomas. *Bone Marrow Transplantation*, **3**, 120–2.

Ross, A.A., Cooper, B.W., Lazarus, H.M., et al. (1993) Detection and viability of tumor cells in peripheral blood stem cell collections from breast cancer patients using immunocytochemical and clonogenic assay techniques. *Blood*, **82**, 2605.

Rosti, G., Albertassi, L., Salvioni, R., et al. (1992) High-dose chemotherapy supported with autologous bone marrow transplantation (ABMT) in germ cell tumors: a phase two study. *Annals of Oncology*, **3**, 809–12.

Schilder, R.J. (1993) High-dose chemotherapy with autologous hemopoietic cell support in gynecologic malignancies. In W.J. Hoskins, C.A. Perez, and R.C. Young (Eds.) *Principles and practice of gynecologic oncology updates*, pp. 1–14. Philadelphia, J.B. Lippincott Company.

Seifter, E.J. and Ihde, D.C. (1988) Therapy of small cell lung cancer: a perspective on two decades of clinical research. *Seminars in Oncology*, **15**, 278–99.

Shea, T.C., Mason, J.R., and Stornioli, A.M. (1992) Sequential cycles of high-dose carboplatin administered with recombinant human granulocyte-macrophage colony-stimulating factor and repeated infusions of autologous peripheral-blood progenitor cells: a novel and effective method for delivering multiple courses of dose-intensive therapy. *Journal of Clinical Oncology*, **10**, 464–73.

Sheridan, W.P., Begley, C.G., Juttner, C., et al. (1992) Effect of peripheral-blood progenitor cells mobilized by filgrastim (G-CSF) on platelet recovery after high-dose chemotherapy. *Lancet*, **339**, 640–4.

Shpall, E.J. and Jones, R.B. (1995) Release of tumor cells from bone marrow. *Blood*, **83**, 6232–625.

Shpall, E.J., Jones, R.B., Bearman, S.I., et al. (1994) Transplantation of enriched CD34 positive autologous marrow into breast cancer patients following high-dose chemotherapy: influence of CD34 positive peripheral blood progenitors and growth factors on engraftment. *Journal of Clinical Oncology*, **12**, 28–36.

Shpall, E.J., Pearson-Clarke, D., and Soper, J.T. (1990) High-dose alkylating agent chemotherapy with autologous bone marrow support in patients with stage III/IV epithelial ovarian cancer. *Gynecologic Oncology*, **38**, 386–91.

Shpall, E.J., Stemmer, S.M., Berarman, S.I., and Jones, R.B. (1993) Role of autotransplantation in treatment of solid tumors. *Hematology/Oncology Clinics of North America*, **7**, 674–8.

Siegert, W., Beyer, J., Strohscheer, I., et al. (1994) High-dose treatment with carboplatin, etoposide, and ifosfamide followed by autologous stem-cell transplantation in relapsed or refractory germ cell cancer: a phase I/II study. *Journal of Clinical Oncology*, **12**, 1223–31.

Soma, M., Shoin, K., and Yamashita, J. (1993) Effects of high-dose chemotherapy with syngeneic bone marrow transplantation in experimental brain tumor in rats. *Cancer*, **71**, 364–9.

Somlo, G., Doroshow, J.J., and Forman, S.J. (1994) High-dose cisplatin, etoposide, and cyclophosphamide with autologous stem cell reinfusion in patients with responsive metastatic or high-risk primary breast cancer. *Cancer*, **73**, 125–34.

Souhami, R.L., Hajichristou, H.T., Miles, D.W., et al. (1989) Intensive chemotherapy with autologous bone marrow transplantation for small-cell lung cancer. *Cancer Chemotherapy and Pharmacology*, **24**, 321–5.

Spitzer, G., Farha, P., Valdivieso, M., et al. (1986) High-dose intensification therapy with autologous bone marrow support for limited small-cell bronchogenic carcinoma. *Journal of Clinical Oncology*, **4**, 4–13.

Stiff, P.J., Scott McKenzie, R., Alberts, D.S., et al. (1994) Phase I clinical and pharmacokinetic study of high-dose mitoxantrone combined with carboplatin, cyclophosphamide, and autologous bone marrow rescue: high response rate for refractory ovarian carcinoma. *Journal of Clinical Oncology*, **12**, 176–83.

Takvorian, T., Parker, L.M., and Hockberg, F.H. (1983) Autologous bone marrow transplantation: host effects of high dose BCNU. *Journal of Clinical Oncology*, **1**, 610–20.

Tepler, I., Cannistra, S., and Anderson, K. (1992) Use of peripheral blood progenitor cells (PBPC) for support of repetitive high-dose carboplatin chemotherapy ($\times 4$) in previously untreated outpatients with cancer. *Blood*, **80**, 719.

Toner, G.C., Geller, N.L., and Tan, C. (1990) Serum tumor marker half-life during chemotherapy allows early prediction of complete response and survival in non-seminomatous germ cell tumors. *Cancer Research*, **50**, 5904–10.

Tormey, D.C., Weinberg, V.E., and Holland, J.F. (1983) A randomized trial of five and three drug chemotherapy and chemoimmunotherapy in women with operable node positive breast cancer. *Journal of Clinical Oncology*, **1**, 138–45.

Trimble, E.L., Adams, J.D., and Vena, D. (1993) Paclitaxel for platinum refractory ovarian cancer: results from the first 1,000 patients registered to the National Cancer Institute Treatment Referral Center, 9103. *Journal of Clinical Oncology*, **11**, 2405–10.

Vaeth, M., Schultz, H., von der Maase, H., et al. (1984) Prognostic factors in testicular germ cell tumors: experiences from 1058 consecutive cases. *Acta Radiologica Oncologica*, **23**, 271–85.

Viens, P., Maraninchi, D., and Legros, M. (1990) High-dose melphalan and autologous marrow rescue in advanced epithelial ovarian carcinomas: a retrospective analysis of 35 patients treated in France. *Bone Marrow Transplantation*, **5**, 227–33.

Vincent, M.D., Trevor, J., and Powles, R. (1988) Late intensification with high-dose melphalan and autologous bone marrow support in breast cancer patients responding to conventional chemotherapy. *Cancer Chemotherapy and Pharmacology*, **21**, 255–60.

Wallerstein, R.J., Spitzer, G., Dunphy, F., et al. (1990) A phase II study of mitoxantrone, etoposides, and thiotepa with autologous marrow support for patients with relapsed breast cancer. *Journal of Clinical Oncology*, **8**, 1782–8.

Williams, S.F., Gilewski, T., and Mick, R. (1992) High-dose consolidation therapy with autologous stem-cell rescue in stage IV breast cancer: follow-up report. *Journal of Clinical Oncology*, **10**, 1743–7.

Wood, W.C., Budman, D.R., Korzun, A.H., et al. (1994) Dose and dose intensity of adjuvant chemotherapy for stage II, node-positive breast carcinoma. *New England Journal of Medicine*, **330**, 1254–9.

−19

High-Dose Chemotherapy with Cellular Support for Hematological Malignancies

PHILIP J. BIERMAN, MICHAEL R. BISHOP, AND
JAMES O. ARMITAGE

High-dose therapy (HDT) followed by autologous bone-marrow transplantation (ABMT) or peripheral stem-cell transplantation (PSCT) is being used with increasing frequency for patients with various hematological malignancies. Approximately 11,000 cases have been reported to the North American Autologous Bone Marrow Transplant Registry (NAABMTR) and an estimated 25% to 30% of bone-marrow transplants (BMT) in the NAABMTR have been performed for non-Hodgkin's lymphoma (NHL); 15% to 20% for Hodgkin's disease (HD); 10% to 15% for acute myelogenous leukemia (AML); and lesser numbers for acute lymphoblastic leukemia (ALL), multiple myeloma (MM), and chronic myeloid leukemia (CML).

■ NON-HODGKIN'S LYMPHOMA

The use of ABMT for patients with recurrent and refractory intermediate- and high-grade NHL was evaluated in 100 patients from institutions in the United States and Europe (Philip et al. 1987). Prior to the HDT, relapsed patients were given a brief course of conventional salvage chemotherapy. Responders to conventional salvage chemotherapy (sensitive relapse) had a projected 3-year disease-free survival of 36%, while patients who failed to respond (resistant relapse) had a projected disease-free survival of 14%. A third group of patients who were refractory to primary therapy had a 0% projected disease-free survival. Other trials have demonstrated the prognostic significance of chemotherapy sensitivity for patients undergoing ABMT for NHL (Gribben et al. 1989; Colombat et al. 1990; Gulati et al. 1992; Lazarus et al. 1992; Rapoport et al. 1993; Vose et al. 1993). Prolonged disease-free survival is seen in 20% to 60% of patients.

Although the results of ABMT for relapsed NHL appear better than those reported for conventional salvage chemotherapy, transplanted patients may be highly selected. Increasing evidence supports the superiority of HDT for relapsed NHL, however.

Investigators in France analyzed results of 244 patients who had relapsed or achieved only a partial remission with the LNH-84 regimen (Bosly et al. 1992). Patients who received conventional salvage chemotherapy had an overall survival projected to be 7% at 4 years compared with 33% for patients who received ABMT ($p < 0.0001$). A similar study examined pediatric patients who relapsed after the LMB-84 regimen (Philip et al. 1993). Median survival after relapse was only 43 days for patients who were not transplanted, while 4 of 15 patients who received ABMT survived without relapse more than 18 months from transplantation. Another trial, the PARMA trial, is evaluating the role of ABMT for relapsed intermediate- and high-grade NHL (Philip et al. 1991). Patients who respond to conventional salvage chemotherapy with dexamethasone, cytarabine, and cisplatin (DHAP) were randomized to continue DHAP, or HDT with ABMT. Results are undergoing analysis.

Additional evidence for the utility of HDT comes from results of patients transplanted in first partial remission (PR). A trial of 17 patients with aggressive NHL in PR showed a projected survival of 75% (Philip et al. 1988). This concept has been validated in other trials (Gribben et al. 1989; Colombat et al. 1990; Gulati et al. 1992) that show disease-free survival rates of 50% to 60% for patients transplanted in first PR. The Italian Cooperative Study Group compared DHAP salvage chemotherapy with ABMT for patients with NHL who were in PR after conventional therapy (Gherlinzoni et al. 1994). Progression-free survival was estimated at 72% for transplanted patients, compared with 49% for those who received DHAP. A Dutch trial, however, failed to demonstrate improvements in outcome for patients in PR after three cycles of CHOP (cyclophosphamide, doxorubicin, vincristine, and prednisone) who were randomized between ABMT or five additional cycles of CHOP (Hagenbeek et al. 1993).

■ EARLY TRANSPLANTATION

HDT may be of greatest benefit if used as consolidation therapy for high-risk patients. A trial from Memorial Sloan-Kettering, New York, evaluated outcome in 14 poor-prognosis NHL patients who were transplanted immediately after induction chemotherapy (Gulati et al. 1988). Overall survival was 79% compared with 31% for 13 patients who continued on consolidation and maintenance phases of the protocol ($p = 0.009$).

A pilot study from the City of Hope, Los Angeles, examined the use of ABMT in 20 poor-prognosis NHL patients who had achieved complete response (CR) with conventional chemotherapy (Nademanee et al. 1992). Relapse-free survival was projected to be 84%. At the Dana-Farber Cancer Center, Boston, a similar trial of 26 poor-prognosis patients resulted in disease-free survival that was projected at 85% at 28 months (Freedman et al. 1993). Pilot trials from other institutions have demonstrated disease-free survival rates of 60% to 70% for high-risk NHL patients who undergo ABMT in first CR (Santini et al. 1989; Baro et al. 1991; Verdonck et al. 1992). A French-Belgian study randomized 464 first CR NHL patients to receive conventional consolidation therapy versus HDT with ABMT (Haioun et al. 1994). Overall survival at 3 years was projected to be 69% following ABMT, compared with 71% for patients who received sequential chemotherapy ($p = 0.60$); however, among patients with poor-prognostic features, disease-free survival was 60% following ABMT compared with 41% with conventional chemotherapy consolidation ($p = 0.07$).

■ OTHER SOURCES OF HEMOPOIETIC RESCUE

PSCT is most useful for patients with hypocellular marrow or marrow metastases. Other advantages of PSCT over ABMT include more rapid engraftment, and less malignant contamination.

A retrospective analysis at the University of Nebraska showed significantly better event-free survival for good prognosis patients with intermediate-grade NHL who received PSCT in comparison with ABMT (Vose et al. 1993), although other institutions have failed to note such differences (Liberti et al. 1993; Rapoport et al. 1993). Results of PSCT for NHL appear at least as good as ABMT.

The use of allogeneic BMT eliminates the possibility of malignant contamination and may also yield a "graft-versus-lymphoma" effect. A comparison of allogeneic and autologous BMT for 80 lymphoma patients (51 NHL, 29 HD) at Johns Hopkins (Jones et al. 1991) revealed an actuarial relapse probability of 46% following ABMT compared with 18% for allogeneic transplantation ($p = 0.02$). Although these results suggest a graft-versus-lymphoma effect, event-free survival was 47% for allograft recipients and 41% for ABMT recipients ($p = 0.8$), due to higher mortality with allogeneic transplantation. A trial from Wayne State University (Detroit, MI) also found a higher relapse rate following ABMT for NHL, in comparison with allogeneic transplantation (Ratanatharathorn et al. 1994). Procedure-related mortality was higher following allogeneic transplantation, and there were no significant differences in progression-free survival. A European case-controlled study also found no difference in progression-free survival between allogeneic and autologous transplantation for NHL (Chopra et al. 1992).

LOW-GRADE LYMPHOMA

There is relatively little experience with transplantation for low-grade lymphoma. At Dana-Farber Cancer Center, a 47% 3-year disease-free survival was projected for 51 patients with low-grade NHL following antibody (Ab) -purged ABMT (Freedman et al. 1991). Follow-up data from 142 patients shows a 51% projected disease-free survival at 4 years (Freedman et al. 1994). A continued pattern of relapse was noted and it is unclear if any patients are cured. Investigators from London reported that 35 of 64 patients receiving purged ABMT for follicular NHL remained in remission between 1 and 8 years (Rohatiner et al. 1994). Freedom from recurrence for patients transplanted in second remission was better than historical controls, although overall survival was not significantly different. At the University of Nebraska, failure-free survival at 4 years is estimated at 39% for 88 patients undergoing ABMT for follicular low-grade lymphoma. Results are not significantly different in patients receiving PSCT and those receiving unpurged BM. Similar studies of ABMT and PSCT for low-grade NHL have yielded progression-free survival rates of 35% to 84% (Colombat et al. 1994; Huebsch et al. 1994). The role of ABMT as consolidation therapy for patients with low-grade lymphoma in first remission is being investigated.

HODGKIN'S DISEASE

Several large trials have investigated the role of ABMT for HD (Reece et al. 1991; Bierman et al. 1993c; Chopra et al. 1993; Crump et al. 1993; Rapoport et al. 1993; Yahalom et al. 1993). Progression-free survival in these series is approximately 25% to 50%. Improved outcome has generally been seen in patients with good performance status and without extensive prior therapy. Other factors associated with improved survival include long initial remission duration, low serum lactate dehydrogenase (LDH), absence of systemic symptoms at relapse, and sensitivity to chemotherapy before transplant.

At Vancouver, a progression-free survival of 64% was seen for patients transplanted in first relapse (Reece et al. 1994a). Progression-free survival was 48% for patients transplanted with remission of less than 1 year and 85% for patients with longer initial remissions. At the University of Nebraska, failure-free survival was projected to be 43% for HD patients in first relapse (Bierman et al. 1993a). Patients with long initial remissions had a failure-free survival projected to be 57%, in contrast to 35% for others. Similarly, at University College Hospital (London, England), progression-free survival was 47% for HD patients transplanted in first relapse (Chopra et al. 1993).

The only reported randomized comparison of ABMT and conventional-salvage chemotherapy for HD was performed by the British National Lymphoma Investigation (Linch et al. 1993). The event-free survival was projected to be 53% following ABMT, compared with 10% for patients who received conventional salvage therapy with the same drugs. Overall survival was not significantly different, however. A retrospective analysis from Stanford University (Stanford, CA) compared transplantation results for refractory patients or those in first relapse with historical controls treated with conventional salvage therapy (Yuen et al. 1994). Freedom from progression, although not overall survival, was significantly better in transplanted patients.

HD patients who fail to enter remission with initial chemotherapy have an extremely poor prognosis. At the University of Nebraska the 3-year progression-free survival was 22% in 44 such patients following either ABMT or PSCT. Results from other institutions suggest that 20% to 40% of patients who fail to enter CR with initial chemotherapy can achieve prolonged remissions following transplantation (Chopra et al. 1993; Crump et al. 1993; Yahalom et al. 1993; Reece et al. 1994b).

As with NHL, there is evidence that transplantation of high-risk HD patients in first remission may improve outcome. In a study in Genoa, disease-free survival for 15 such patients was projected to be 87%, better than historical control patients (Carella et al. 1991).

At the University of Nebraska, no differences were observed in failure-free survival following ABMT or PSCT for HD (Bierman et al. 1993b). Similar results have been observed elsewhere (Rapoport et al. 1993). No differences in event-free survival between allogeneic and autologous transplantation for HD were noted from a study in Seattle (Anderson et al. 1993), although relapse probability was significantly higher following ABMT.

■ ACUTE MYELOGENOUS LEUKEMIA

Results of HDT and ABMT for AML have been reported in several recent trials (Körbling et al. 1989; Gorin et al. 1990; Löwenberg et al. 1990; McMillan et al. 1990; Cassileth et al. 1993; Linker et al. 1993).

Disease-free survival at 3 years averages approximately 45% to 70% for patients transplanted in first CR. These results compare favorably with allogeneic transplantation in which approximately 50% of patients achieve long-term, disease-free survival. Relapse rates following ABMT for AML in first CR are approximately 35% to 60% compared with 20% for allogeneic transplantation. Mortality following ABMT has been less than 10% in most series.

Trials of ABMT for AML patients in second and third remission have demonstrated disease-free survival rates of 35% to 50% (Körbling et al. 1989; Meloni et al. 1990; Linker et al. 1993; Selvaggi et al. 1994). Most of these trials have used purged BM. These results compare favorably with disease-free survival rates of 30% to 40% following allogeneic transplantation for AML in second or third remission.

The value of purging for AML autografting is controversial. Since relapse rates are similar to syngeneic transplantation, it is felt that most relapses result from inadequate leukemia eradication, rather than reinfusion of leukemia cells. Nevertheless, gene-marking studies indicate that at least some relapses may be due to reinfusion of clonogenic malignant cells (Brenner et al. 1993). Clinical evidence in support of purging in AML comes from the European Bone Marrow Transplant Group that retrospectively evaluated results of purging with mafosfamide for patients in first CR transplanted within 6 months of achieving CR (Gorin et al. 1990). Leukemia-free survival at 3 years was projected to be 63% for standard-risk patients transplanted with total-body irradiation and purged BM, compared with 34% for patients receiving unpurged BM ($p = 0.05$). In studies at Stanford and City of Hope, a disease-free survival of 57%, with a relapse rate of 28% was seen in AML patients in various stages of remission (Chao et al. 1993). The same regimen in 20 patients with unpurged BM resulted in a disease-free survival of 32% and relapse rate of 62%.

The optimal management for AML patients remains controversial. A Dutch study prospectively assigned first-remission AML patients to autologous or allogeneic transplantation depending on donor availability and age (Löwenberg et al. 1990). Relapse-free survival following ABMT was 35%, compared with 51% following allogeneic transplantation. Overall survival rates were 37% and 66%, respectively ($p = 0.05$). A French study randomized AML patients to allogeneic or autologous transplantation, or conventional chemotherapy following induction and consolidation (Reifers et al. 1989). The actuarial disease-free survival at 3 years was 66%, 41%, and 16%, respectively ($p < 0.004$). The Medical Research Council (London, England) randomized AML patients to allogeneic transplantation or ABMT following induction (Burnett et al. 1994). No difference in overall survival has been observed.

◼ ACUTE LYMPHOBLASTIC LEUKEMIA

Experience with ABMT for adult ALL is limited. Leukemia-free survival for patients in first CR is 20% to 60%, and 10% to 40% for patients with more advanced disease. (Doney et al. 1993; Laporte et al. 1993; Morishima et al. 1993; Soiffer et al. 1993). Most institutions have used purged BM. Factors associated with improved outcome are similar to those observed for chemotherapy treatment of adult ALL.

A prospective European study randomized ALL patients less than 50 years old to ABMT or conventional chemotherapy if they were not eligible for allogeneic transplantation (Fière et al. 1993). Disease-free survival at 3 years was 39% for patients undergoing ABMT compared with 32% for patients who received consolidation chemotherapy. Overall survival was projected to be 49% and 42%, respectively. A subsequent analysis demonstrated that results of ABMT in first CR were similar to allogeneic transplantation for standard-risk patients (Sebban et al. 1994); however, in high-risk patients, actuarial 5-year survival was 44% following allogeneic transplantation, compared with 20% for ABMT or conventional chemotherapy ($p = 0.03$).

◼ CHRONIC MYELOGENOUS LEUKEMIA

Initial attempts at ABMT for CML were performed using cells collected in chronic phase, and then transplanted after acceleration. The rationale behind these attempts was that patients might be restored to a second chronic phase. Clinical results suggest that 40% to 50% of such patients might have partial or complete elimination of the Philadelphia (Ph) chromosome (Butturini et al. 1990). Ph$^-$ hemopoiesis has been observed more than 2 years following transplantation and survival in chronic phase more than 6 years after ABMT has been seen (Reifers et al. 1993); however, most patients have clinical and cytogenetic relapses within 6 to 12 months, and it is unclear whether overall survival is prolonged.

There is considerable interest in ABMT for chronic-phase patients, who are not eligible for allogeneic transplantation. Individuals with CML may have cytogenetically normal stem cells, and the percentage of Ph$^-$ cells may increase following cytotoxic chemotherapy. Investigators from Italy reported that 60% of patients with chronic-phase CML had PBSC that were exclusively Ph$^-$ following chemotherapy (Carella et al. 1993a). Attainment of a Ph$^-$ stem-cell product was more likely in patients harvested within 2 years of diagnosis. Autologous transplantation in chronic phase might expand the population of Ph⁻ cells, which might suppress the growth of malignant clones. Furthermore, reduction of the total number of Ph⁺ cells might decrease the probability of disease acceleration and prolong survival. Several investigators have reported results of HDT followed by ABMT or PSCT for chronic-phase CML patients (Brito-Babapulle et al. 1989; Simonsson et al. 1992; Carella et al. 1993a; Carella et al. 1993b; Kantarjian et al. 1994). The Hammersmith group (London, England) has examined results of PSCT in 21 chronic-phase CML patients (Hoyle, Gray, and Goldman 1994). Survival at 5 years was 56% for autografted patients, compared with 28% for historical controls ($p = 0.003$). The Vancouver (Canada) group has shown that in vitro culture of BM from CML patients resulted in Ph⁻ hemopoiesis in 13 of 22 patients, although most patients had a cytogenetic relapse within 1 year (Barnett et al. 1994).

It is unlikely that ABMT cures patients with CML, although survival may be prolonged. Gene-marking studies have demonstrated that Ph⁺ cells in the autograft may contribute to relapse (Deisseroth et al. 1994). Efforts are underway to purge CML autografts with antisense oligonucleotides as well as pharmacologic and immunologic techniques. In addition, the use of interferon (IFN) following transplantation may be beneficial.

■ MULTIPLE MYELOMA

The steep dose-response curve for MM has led to attempts at transplantation using purged and unpurged autologous BM, and PBSC. A study in Arkansas has reported a 31% CR rate in a series of 400 patients (Vesole et al. 1994). Median event-free survival and overall survival were 24 months and 40 months, respectively. The European Bone Marrow Transplant Registry has reported a 34-month median survival for 361 patients undergoing PSCT for MM (Björkstrand et al. 1994). The use of HDT for patients with treated MM has been reported by other investigators (Jagannath et al. 1990; Jagannath et al. 1992; Fermand et al. 1993; Harousseau et al. 1992; Dimopoulos et al. 1993). Complete remission rates of 30% to 50% have been seen. Factors associated with improved outcome have been less extensive prior therapy, low β^2-microglobulin levels, non-IgA isotype, and sensitive disease. Mortality for transplantation is generally less than 5%, and transplants can be performed on patients in their seventh decade. Despite high response rates, there is a continuous pattern of relapse and it is unclear whether any patients are cured with this approach.

Transplantation is of limited value for patients with refractory disease or prolonged prior therapy (Alexanian et al. 1994).

There is now interest in intensive conventional chemotherapy followed by ABMT for newly diagnosed patients. In studies in Arkansas and Seattle, a "total therapy" program with intensive chemotherapy, double autotransplants, and IFN maintenance has been used for newly diagnosed patients (Barlogie et al. 1993). Overall survival at 3 years was projected to be 72%. The Milan group has used an intensive, high-dose, sequential regimen with autologous HSC transplantation for 13 newly diagnosed MM patients (Gianni et al. 1994). The CR rate was 77%. Although no plateau in the survival curve was seen, the median survival of 41 months was better than 14 months for a group of historical control patients ($p < 0.003$). A French pilot trial used induction chemotherapy, autologous BMT, and IFN maintenance for 31 previously untreated patients (Attal et al. 1992). The CR rate was 43%, and progression-free survival was 53% at 33 months. A subsequent prospective randomized trial has compared this approach with conventional chemotherapy for untreated patients (Attal et al. 1993). The CR rate and progression-free survival at 30 months in the transplanted patients were 25% and 67%, respectively and for chemotherapy patients, 2% and 10%, respectively, ($p < 0.01$).

HDT with BMT or PSCT has become an accepted form of therapy for some hematological malignancies. Prospective trials are underway to clarify the role and timing of this treatment in various situations. New technologies such as hemopoietic growth factors have made transplantation easier, safer, and less expensive.

It must still be noted, however, that ABMT and PSCT are relatively new procedures. Careful follow-up is necessary to identify delayed events such as late relapses and the development of second malignancies. Continued efforts are necessary to improve the results of transplantation. These efforts must include the development of better high-dose therapy regimens to increase response rates. In addition, the role of posttransplant immunotherapy to decrease relapse rates following ABMT and PSCT is under investigation.

REFERENCES

Alexanian, R., Dimopoulos, M., Smith, T., et al. (1994) Limited value of myeloablative therapy for late multiple myeloma. *Blood*, **83**, 512–16.

Anderson, J.E., Litzow, M.R., Appelbaum, F.R., et al. (1993) Allogeneic, syngeneic, and autologous marrow transplantation for Hodgkin's disease: the 21-year Seattle experience. *Journal of Clinical Oncology*, **11**, 2342–50.

Attal, M., Harousseau, J.L., Stoppa, A.M., et al. (1993) High dose therapy in multiple myeloma: a prospective randomized study of the "Intergroupe Francais Du Myelome" (IFM). *Blood*, **82**, 198a.

Attal, M., Huguet, F., Schlaifer, D., et al. (1992) Intensive combined therapy for previously untreated aggressive myeloma. *Blood,* **79**, 1130–6.

Barlogie, B., Jagannath S., Vesole, D.H., et al. (1993) Total therapy (TT) for newly diagnosed multiple myeloma (MM). *Blood,* **82**, 198a.

Barnett, M.J., Eaves, C.J., Phillips, G.L., et al. (1994) Autografting with cultured marrow in chronic myeloid leukemia: results of a pilot study. *Blood,* **84**, 724–32.

Baro, J., Richard, C., Calavia, J., et al. (1991) Autologous bone marrow transplantation as consolidation therapy for non-Hodgkin's lymphoma patients with poor prognostic features. *Bone Marrow Transplantation,* **8**, 283–9.

Bierman, P., Anderson, J., Vose, J., et al. (1993a) High-dose chemotherapy with autologous hematopoietic rescue for Hodgkin's disease (HD) following first relapse after chemotherapy. *Proceedings of the American Society of Clinical Oncology,* **12**, 366.

Bierman, P.J., Bagin, R.G., Jagannath, S., et al. (1993b) High dose chemotherapy followed by autologous hematopoietic rescue in Hodgkin's disease: long term follow-up in 128 patients. *Annals of Oncology,* **4**, 767–73.

Bierman, P., Vose, J., Anderson, J., et al. (1993c) Comparison of autologous bone marrow transplantation (ABMT) with peripheral stem cell transplantation (PSCT) for patients with Hodgkin's disease (HD). *Blood,* **82**, 445a.

Björkstrand, B., Ljungman, P., Brandt, L., et al. (1994) Autologous stem cell transplantation (ASCT) in multiple myeloma: a study of the European BMT Registry. *Blood,* **84**, 535a.

Bosly, A., Coiffier, B., Gisselbrecht, C., et al. (1992) Bone marrow transplantation prolongs survival after relapse in aggressive-lymphoma patients treated with the LNH-84 regimen. *Journal of Clinical Oncology,* **10**, 1615–23.

Brenner, M.K., Rill, D.R., Moen, R.C., et al. (1993) Gene-marking to trace origin of relapse after autologous bone-marrow transplantation. *Lancet,* **341**, 85–6.

Brito-Babapulle, F., Bowcock, S.J., Marcus, R.E., et al. (1989) Autografting for patients with chronic myeloid leukaemia in chronic phase: peripheral blood stem cells may have a finite capacity for maintaining haemopoiesis. *British Journal of Haematology,* **73**, 76–81.

Burnett, A.K., Goldstone, A.H., Stevens, R.F, et al. (1994) The role of BMT in addition to intensive chemotherapy in AML in first CR: results of the MRC AML-10 trial. *Blood,* **84**, 252a.

Butturini, A., Keating, A., Goldman, J., and Gale, R.P. (1990) Autotransplants in chronic myelogenous leukaemia: strategies and results. *Lancet,* **335**, 1255–8.

Carella, A.M., Carlier, P., Congiu, A, et al. (1991) Autologous bone marrow transplantation as adjuvant treatment for high-risk Hodgkin's disease in first compete remission after MOPP/ABVD protocol. *Bone Marrow Transplantation,* **8**, 99–103.

Carella, A.M., Podesta, M., Frassoni, F., et al. (1993a) Collection of 'normal' blood repopulating cells during early hemopoietic recovery after intensive conventional chemotherapy in chronic myelogenous leukemia. *Bone Marrow Transplantation,* **12**, 267–71.

Carella, A.M., Pollicardo, N., Pungolino, E., et al. (1993b) Mobilization of cytogenetically 'normal' blood progenitors cells by intensive conventional chemotherapy for chronic myeloid and acute lymphoblastic leukemia. *Leukemia and Lymphoma*, **9**, 477–83.

Cassileth, P.A., Andersen, J., Lazarus, H., et al. (1993) Autologous bone marrow transplantation in acute myeloid leukemia in first remission. *Journal of Clinical Oncology*, **11**, 314–19.

Chao, N.J., Stein, A.J., Long, G.D., et al. (1993) Busulfan/etoposide–initial experience with a new preparatory regimen for autologous bone marrow transplantation in patients with acute nonlymphoblastic leukemia. *Blood*, **81**, 319–23.

Chopra, R., Goldstone, A.H., Pearce, R., et al. (1992) Autologous versus allogeneic bone marrow transplantation for non-Hodgkin's lymphoma: a case-controlled analysis of the European Bone Marrow Transplant Registry data. *Journal of Clinical Oncology*, **11**, 1690–5.

Chopra, R., McMillan, A.K., Linch, D.C., et al. (1993) The place of high-dose BEAM therapy and autologous bone marrow transplantation in poor-risk Hodgkin's disease. A single-center eight-year study of 155 patients. *Blood*, **81**, 1137–46.

Colombat, P., Donadio, D., Fouillard, L., et al. (1994) Value of autologous bone marrow transplantation in follicular lymphoma: a France autogreffe retrospective study of 42 patients. *Bone Marrow Transplantation*, **13**, 157–62.

Colombat, P., Gorin, N.-C., Lemonnier, M.-P., et al. (1990) The role of autologous bone marrow transplantation in 46 adult patients with non-Hodgkin's lymphoma. *Journal of Clinical Oncology*, **8**, 630–7.

Crump, M., Smith, A.M., Brandwein, J., et al. (1993) High-dose etoposide and melphalan, and autologous bone marrow transplantation for patients with advanced Hodgkin's disease: importance of disease status at transplant. *Journal of Clinical Oncology*, **11**, 704–11.

Deisseroth, A.B., Zu, Z., Claxton, D., et al. (1994) Genetic marking shows that Ph$^+$ cells present in autologous transplants of chronic myelogenous leukemia (CML) contribute to relapse after autologous bone marrow in CML. *Blood*, **83**, 3068–76.

Dimopoulos, M.A., Alexanian, R., Przepiorka, D., et al. (1993) Thiotepa, busulfan, and cyclophosphamide: a new preparative regimen for autologous marrow or blood stem cell transplantation in high-risk multiple myeloma. *Blood*, **82**, 2324–8.

Doney, K., Buckner, C.D., Fisher, L., et al. (1993) Autologous bone marrow transplantation for acute lymphoblastic leukemia. *Bone Marrow Transplantation*, **12**, 315–21.

Fermand, J.-P., Chevret, S., Ravaud, P., et al. (1993) High-dose chemoradiotherapy and autologous blood stem cell transplantation in multiple myeloma: results of a phase II trial involving 63 patients. *Blood*, **82**, 2005–9.

Fière, D., Lepage, E., Sebban, C., et al. (1993) Adult acute lymphoblastic leukemia: a multicentric randomized trial testing bone marrow transplantation as postremission therapy. *Journal of Clinical Oncology*, **11**, 1990–2001.

Freedman, A., Neuberg, D., Gribben, J., et al. (1994) Autologous bone marrow transplantation in relapsed low grade non-Hodgkin's lymphoma. *Blood*, **84**, 203a.

Freedman, A.S., Ritz, J., Neuberg, D., et al. (1991) Autologous bone marrow transplantation in 69 patients with a history of low-grade B-cell non-Hodgkin's lymphoma. *Blood*, **77**, 2524–9.

Freedman, A.S., Takvorian, T., Neuberg, D., et al. (1993) Autologous bone marrow transplantation in poor-prognosis intermediate-grade and high-grade B-cell non-Hodgkin's lymphoma in first remission: a pilot study. *Journal of Clinical Oncology*, **11**, 931–6.

Gherlinzoni, F., Martelli, M., Mazza, P., et al. (1994) Autologous bone marrow transplantation (ABMT) vs. DHAP in aggressive non-Hodgkin's lymphoma (NHL) partially responding to first-line chemotherapy. *Blood*, **84**, 234a.

Gianni, A.M., Tarella, C., Bregni, M., et al. (1994) High-dose sequential chemoradiotherapy, a widely applicable regimen, confers survival benefit to patients with high-risk multiple myeloma. *Journal of Clinical Oncology*, **12**, 503–9.

Gorin, N.C., Aegerter, P., Auvert, B., et al. (1990) Autologous bone marrow transplantation for acute myelocytic leukemia in first remission: a European survey of the role of marrow purging. *Blood*, **75**, 1606–14.

Gribben, J.G., Goldstone, A.H., Linch, D.C., et al. (1989) Effectiveness of high-dose combination chemotherapy and autologous bone marrow transplantation for patients with non-Hodgkin's lymphomas who are still responsive to conventional-dose therapy. *Journal of Clinical Oncology*, **7**, 1621–9.

Gulati, S.C., Shank, B., Black, P., et al. (1988) Autologous bone marrow transplantation for patients with poor-prognosis lymphoma. *Journal of Clinical Oncology*, **6**, 1303–13.

Gulati, S., Yahalom, J., Acaba, L., et al. (1992) Treatment of patients with relapsed and resistant non-Hodgkin's lymphoma using total body irradiation, etoposide, and cyclophosphamide and autologous bone marrow transplantation. *Journal of Clinical Oncology*, **10**, 936–41.

Hagenbeek, A., Verdonck, L., Sonneveld, P., et al. (1993) CHOP chemotherapy versus autologous bone marrow transplantation in slowly responding patients with intermediate- and high-grade malignant non-Hodgkin's lymphoma. Results from a prospective randomized phase III clinical trial in 294 patients. *Blood*, **82**, 332a.

Haioun, C., Lepage, L., Gisselbrecht, C., et al. (1994) Comparison of autologous bone marrow transplantation with sequential chemotherapy for intermediate-grade and high-grade non-Hodgkin's lymphoma in first compete remission: a study of 464 patients. *Journal of Clinical Oncology*, **12**, 2543–51.

Harousseau, J.L., Milpied, N., Laporte, J.P., et al. (1992) Double-intensive therapy in high-risk multiple myeloma. *Blood*, **79**, 2827–33.

Hoyle, C., Gray, R., and Goldman, J. (1994) Autografting for patients with CML in chronic phase: an update. *British Journal of Haematology*, **86**, 76–81.

Huebsch, L., Leger, C., Bredeson, C., et al. (1994) High-dose chemoradiotherapy with unpurged marrow (BM) and/or blood stem cell (BC) support for follicular non-Hodgkin's lymphoma. *Blood*, **84**, 208a.

Jagannath, S., Barlogie, B., Dicke, K., et al. (1990) Autologous bone marrow transplantation in multiple myeloma: identification of prognostic factors. *Blood*, **76**, 1860–6.

Jagannath, S., Vesole, D.H., Glenn, L., et al. (1992) Low-risk intensive therapy for multiple myeloma with combined autologous bone marrow and blood stem cell support. *Blood*, **80**, 1666–72.

Jones, R.J., Ambinder, R.F., Piantadosi, S., and Santos, G.W. (1991) Evidence of a graft-versus-lymphoma effect associated with allogeneic bone marrow transplantation. *Blood*, **77**, 649–53.

Kantarjian, H.M., Talpaz, M., Andersson, B., et al. (1994) High doses of cyclophosphamide, etoposide and total body irradiation followed by autologous stem cell transplantation in the management of patients with chronic myelogenous leukemia. *Bone Marrow Transplantation*, **14**, 57–61.

Körbling, M., Hunstein, W., Fliedner, M., et al. (1989) Disease-free survival after autologous bone marrow transplantation in patients with acute myelogenous leukemia. *Blood*, **74**, 1898–1904.

Laporte, J.P., Douay, L., Lopez, M., et al. (1993) 134 patients with acute leukemia autografted (ABMT) using mafosfamide purged marrow: a ten years single institution experience. *Blood*, **82**, 82a.

Lazarus, H.M., Crilley, P., Ciobanu, N., et al. (1992) High-dose carmustine, etoposide, and cisplatin and autologous bone marrow transplantation for relapsed and refractory lymphoma. *Journal of Clinical Oncology*, **10**, 1682–9.

Liberti, G., Pearce, R., Taghipour, G., et al. (1993) Comparison of peripheral and bone marrow autologous transplantation for lymphoma patients: a case controlled analysis of the EBMT Registry data. *Fifth International Conference on Malignant Lymphoma (Lugano)*, p. 39, abstr. #37.

Linch, D.C., Winfield, D., Goldstone, A.H., et al. (1993) Dose intensification with autologous bone marrow transplantation in relapsed and resistant Hodgkin's disease: results of a BNLI randomized trial. *Lancet*, **341**, 1051.

Linker, C.A., Ries, C.A., Damon, L.E., et al. (1993) Autologous bone marrow transplantation for acute myeloid leukemia using busulfan plus etoposide as a preparative regimen. *Blood*, **81**, 311–8.

Löwenberg, B., Verdonck, L.J., Dekker, A.W., et al. (1990) Autologous bone marrow transplantation in acute myeloid leukemia in first remission: results of a Dutch prospective study. *Journal of Clinical Oncology*, **8**, 287–94.

McMillan, A.K., Goldstone, A.H., Linch, J.G., et al. (1990) High-dose chemotherapy and autologous bone marrow transplantation in acute myeloid leukemia. *Blood*, **76**, 480–8.

Meloni, G., DeFabritiis, P.D., Petti, M.C., and Mandelli, F. (1990) BAVC regimen and autologous bone marrow transplantation in patients with acute myelogenous leukemia in second remission. *Blood*, **75**, 2282–5.

Morishima, Y., Miyamura, K., Kojima, S., et al. (1993) Autologous BMT in high risk patients with CALLA-positive ALL: possible efficacy of ex vivo marrow leukemia cell purging with monoclonal antibodies and complement. *Bone Marrow Transplantation*, **11**, 255–9.

Nademanee, A., Schmidt, G.M., O'Donnell, M.R., et al. (1992) High-dose chemoradiotherapy followed by autologous bone marrow transplantation as consolidation therapy during first complete remission in adult patients with poor-risk aggressive lymphoma: a pilot study. *Blood*, **80**, 1130–4.

Philip, T., Armitage, J.O., Spitzer, G., et al. (1987) High-dose therapy and autologous bone marrow transplantation after failure of conventional chemotherapy in adults with intermediate-grade or high-grade non-Hodgkin's lymphoma. *New England Journal of Medicine*, **316**, 1493–8.

Philip, T., Chauvin, F., Armitage, J., et al. (1991) Parma international protocol: pilot study of DHAP followed by involved-field radiotherapy and BEAC with autologous bone marrow transplantation. *Blood*, **77**, 1587–92.

Philip, T., Hartmann, O., Biron, P., et al. (1988) High-dose therapy and autologous bone marrow transplantation in partial remission after first-line induction therapy for diffuse non-Hodgkin's lymphoma. *Journal of Clinical Oncology*, **6**, 1118–24.

Philip, T., Hartmann, O., Pinkerton, R., et al. (1993) Curability of relapsed childhood B-cell non-Hodgkin's lymphoma after intensive first line therapy: a report from the Société Française d'Oncolgie Pédiatrique. *Blood*, **81**, 2003–6.

Rapoport, A.P., Rowe, J.M., Kouides, P.A., et al. (1993) One hundred autotransplants for relapsed or refractory Hodgkin's disease and lymphoma: value of pretransplant disease status for predicting outcome. *Journal of Clinical Oncology*, **11**, 2351–61.

Ratanatharathorn, V., Uberti, J., Karanes, C., et al. (1994) Prospective comparative trial of autologous versus allogeneic bone marrow transplantation in patients with non-Hodgkin's lymphoma. *Blood*, **84**, 1050–5.

Reece, D.E., Barnett, M.J., Connors, J.M., et al. (1991) Intensive chemotherapy with cyclophosphamide, carmustine, and etoposide followed by autologous bone marrow transplantation for relapsed Hodgkin's disease. *Journal of Clinical Oncology*, **9**, 1871–9.

Reece, D.E., Connors, J.M., Spinelli, J.J., et al. (1994a) Intensive therapy with cyclophosphamide, carmustine, etoposide ± cisplatin, and autologous bone marrow transplantation for Hodgkin's disease in first relapse after combination chemotherapy. *Blood*, **83**, 1193–9.

Reece, D., Spinelli, J., Barnett, M., et al. (1994b) High-dose cyclophosphamide, BCNU, VP16-213 + cisplatin (CBV+P) and autologous stem cell transplantation (ASCT) for patients (pts) with Hodgkin's disease (HD) who fail to enter a complete remission (CR) after combination chemotherapy. *Blood*, **84**, 162a.

Reifers, J., Gaspard, M.H., Maraninchi, D., et al. (1989) Comparison of allogeneic or autologous bone marrow transplantation and chemotherapy in patients with acute myeloid leukaemia in first remission: a prospective controlled trial. *British Journal of Haematology*, **72**, 57–63.

Reifers, J., Montastruc, M., Cahn, J.Y., et al. (1993) Autologous blood stem-cell transplantation and recombinant interferon alfa in chronic myeloid leukemia. *Seminars in Oncology*, **30**, 51–2.

Rohatiner, A.Z., Johnson, P.W., Price, C.G., et al. (1994) Myeloablative therapy with autologous bone marrow transplantation as consolidation therapy for recurrent follicular lymphoma. *Journal of Clinical Oncology*, **12**, 1177–84.

Santini, G., Congiu, A.M., Coser, P., et al. (1991) Autologous bone marrow transplantation for adult advanced stage lymphoblastic in first CR. A study of the NHLCSG. *Leukemia*, **5**, 42–5.

Sebban, C., Lepage, E., Vernant, J.-P., et al. (1994) Allogeneic bone marrow transplantation in adult acute lymphoblastic leukemia in first complete remission: a comparative study. *Journal of Clinical Oncology*, **12**, 2580–7.

Selvaggi, K.J., Wilson, J.W., Mills, L.E., et al. (1994) Improved outcome for high-risk acute myeloid leukemia patients using autologous bone marrow transplantation and monoclonal antibody-purged bone marrow. *Blood*, **83**, 1698–705.

Simonsson, B., Öberg, G., Björeman, M., et al. (1992) Intensive treatment in order to minimize the Ph-positive clone in chronic myelogenic leukemia. *Leukemia and Lymphoma*, **7**, 55–7.

Soiffer, R.J., Roy, D.C., Gonin, R., et al. (1993) Monoclonal antibody-purged autologous bone marrow transplantation in adults with acute lymphoblastic leukemia at high risk of relapse. *Bone Marrow Transplantation,* **12**, 243–51.

Verdonck, L.F., Dekker, A.W., de Gast, G.C., et al. (1992) Autologous bone marrow transplantation for adult poor-risk lymphoblastic lymphoma in first remission. *Journal of Clinical Oncology,* **10**, 644–6.

Vesole, D., Jagganath, S., Tricot, G., et al. (1994) 400 Autotransplants (AT) for multiple myeloma (MM). *Blood,* **84**, 535a.

Vose, J.M., Anderson, J.R., Kessinger, A., et al. (1993) High-dose chemotherapy and autologous hematopoietic stem-cell transplantation for aggressive non-Hodgkin's lymphoma. *Journal of Clinical Oncology,* **11**, 1846–51.

Yahalom, J., Gulati, S.C., Toia, M., et al. (1993) Accelerated hyperfractionated total-lymphoid irradiation, high-dose chemotherapy, and autologous bone marrow transplantation for refractory and relapsing patients with Hodgkin's disease. *Journal of Clinical Oncology,* **11**, 1062–70.

Yuen, A.R., Blume, K.G., Rosenberg, S.A., et al. (1994) Comparison between autologous bone marrow transplantation (ABMT) and conventional salvage therapy for recurrent or refractory Hodgkin's disease. *Blood,* **84**, 234a.

-20

Allogeneic Marrow Transplantation as Treatment for Myeloid Malignancies: Why it Works and How it Might Be Improved

FREDERICK R. APPELBAUM

The application of allogeneic bone-marrow transplantation (BMT) to the treatment of myeloid malignancies represents a major therapeutic advance. Patients with acute myeloid leukemia (AML) who have failed chemotherapy and are incurable by other means can be cured with allogeneic BMT, and for many patients with AML in first remission, BMT is the treatment of choice. The impact of allogeneic BMT in chronic myelogenous leukemia (CML) is even greater, since this disease is incurable by any other means and transplantation can cure a large proportion of CML patients. Given the major advance represented by allogeneic BMT, it may be worthwhile to consider the mechanisms by which this technique can eradicate malignancies incapable of elimination by other methods with the hope that by understanding the reasons for success, the method can be both further improved and applied to other settings. Thus, in this chapter, the results of allogeneic BMT in the treatment of myeloid malignancies will be briefly reviewed, the mechanisms by which transplantation works will be examined, and methods to make further use of these mechanisms will be discussed.

■ ACUTE MYELOID LEUKEMIA

High-dose chemotherapy or chemoradiotherapy followed by allogeneic BMT from a matched-sibling donor can cure patients of AML who are almost certainly incurable by any other means. The clearest examples are patients who fail to enter an initial complete remission (CR) despite receiving at least two courses of induction chemotherapy. Such patients are incurable by any nontransplant means, but several studies have documented that approximately 20% of such primary induction failure patients can become long-term, disease-free survivors if treated with allogeneic BMT (Forman et al. 1991; Biggs et al. 1992). This result argues that patients with newly diagnosed AML and their families should be HLA typed as soon as possible after diagnosis so that if induction chemotherapy fails, a transplant can be done without delay.

The outcome of allogeneic BMT for patients with AML who have obtained a first remission and then relapse is somewhat better than that for primary induction failures. If patients are transplanted in second CR, approximately 25% become long-term survivors and if transplantation is carried out in first untreated relapse, 30% to 40% survival has been reported (Appelbaum et al. 1983; Clift et al. 1987; Clift et al. 1992).

The best results of allogeneic BMT in AML are seen when the procedure is performed during first remission. The initial trials of this approach, although uncontrolled and done in only a limited number of patients, demonstrated long-term, disease-free survival in 50% to 60% of transplanted patients (Thomas et al. 1979; Blume et al. 1980). Following these first reports, a number of trials were done in which patients with AML in first CR were assigned to allogeneic BMT if they had a matched-sibling donor, while those without such donors served as concurrent chemotherapy controls. Between 1984 and 1994, 14 such trials involving more than 1,000 patients were reported. In each of these studies, the disease-free survival at 3 or more years was greater in the BMT group than in the chemotherapy group, ranging from 40% to 64% for transplantation and 19% to 24% for chemotherapy (Appelbaum et al. 1984; Champlin et al. 1985; Marmont et al. 1985; Appelbaum et al. 1988; Conde et al. 1988; Zander et al. 1988; Reiffers et al. 1989; Ringden et al. 1989; Dahl et al. 1990; Cassileth et al. 1992; Schiller et al. 1992; Amadori et al. 1993; Archimbaud et al. 1994; Nesbit et al. 1994; Hewlett et al., unpublished data). While these studies demonstrate that transplantation from a matched-sibling donor in first remission offers a higher likelihood of cure than does chemotherapy, whether transplantation in first remission is superior to a combination of chemotherapy followed by transplantation as salvage therapy at first relapse remains untested.

■ CHRONIC MYELOID LEUKEMIA

The results of allogeneic BMT for CML in patients with matched siblings in many ways mirror the results obtained in AML. As in AML, if transplantation is done late, when patients are in blast crisis, the results are poor, with only 10% to 15% of patients becoming long-term survivors in most studies (Thomas et al. 1986). If transplantation is done while patients are in accelerated phase, the results improve, with cure rates averaging about 35% to 40% in most series. The accelerated phase of CML encompasses a broad range of patients, some of whom have disease essentially indistinguishable from chronic phase (CP) except for the presence of a cytogenetic abnormality in addition to the Philadelphia (Ph) chromosome, while others have more advanced disease falling just short of blast crisis. A recent analysis of Seattle results using non–T-cell–depleted marrow found that among CML patients classified as having accelerated phase on the basis of a cytogenetic abnormality only, 66% were alive 5 years after transplant, while for those with additional clinical manifestations of acceleration, the survival at 5 years was 34% (Clift et al. 1994).

The best results of transplantation for CML are obtained when the procedure is done during CP. Many centers now report 5-year disease-free survival in approximately 70% of transplanted patients (Blume and Forman 1992; Goldman et al. 1992). Patients transplanted earlier after diagnosis do better than those transplanted after longer delays, even if still in CP (Thomas and Clift 1989; Goldman et al. 1993). The improved survival seen with transplantation earlier in CP is due both to a diminished chance of disease recurrence as well as a lessened likelihood of nonrelapse mortality. Because delay increases the chances that the disease may accelerate before the transplant and has a deleterious effect on transplantation outcome even if the disease remains stable, most investigators recommend transplantation within 1 year of diagnosis for patients less than 56 years old with matched siblings. Taking this approach at Seattle, we recently reported a 90% probability of survival at 1 year after transplant and an 81% probability at 5 years after transplant (Buckner et al. 1993). We have also been using transplantation for CML patients in their sixth and seventh decades and have found that older patients with CML tolerate the procedure surprisingly well. Among 47 patients aged 50 to 65 years, 70% were alive disease-free at 3 years after allogeneic transplant for CML (Buckner et al. 1993).

■ WHY MARROW TRANSPLANTATION CURES LEUKEMIA

There are two straightforward reasons why BMT cures patients with myeloid malignancies. First, BMT allows for the administration of systemic doses of chemotherapy and radiotherapy that would be intolerable without transplantation. Second, allogeneic BMT confers a powerful graft-versus-leukemia (GVL) effect.

Dose Intensity

Evidence that the dose intensification permitted with BMT support allows for the cure of patients who are otherwise incurable comes from several observations. First, there are the results in syngeneic and autologous transplantation where, presumably, a GVL response is absent. The results of syngeneic transplantation for CML are useful examples. Without BMT, the disease is incurable, even if treated with aggressive chemotherapy. At Seattle, between May 1976 and November 1981, 14 patients with CML in CP had syngeneic BMT following a preparative regimen of dimethylbusulfan (5 mg/kg), cyclophosphamide (120 mg/kg), and 10 Gy total-body irradiation (TBI) (Fefer et al. 1994). Two patients died of interstitial pneumonia, and one patient relapsed and died. The other 11 are alive 12 to 18 years after transplantation. Of these 11, 3 have relapsed (2 of whom have undergone a second transplant and are alive in remission), and 8 are in continuous CR at a median of 16.6 years after transplantation. Bone marrow of six of these eight patients has recently been tested for *bcr/abl* transcript by polymerase chain reaction (PCR) amplification and Southern blotting and in all six patients, the assays were negative. Although one cannot absolutely dismiss the possibility that the transfer of syngeneic marrow and lymphocytes conferred an antitumor effect separate from that of the preparative regimen, evidence for any such effect is limited at best. A second argument supporting the view that dose intensification is a major reason for the cure rates seen with allogeneic BMT comes from studies demonstrating a clear relationship between the dose delivered in the preparative regimen and the chance of relapse. Two prospective randomized trials, one in AML and a second in CML, compared the outcome of allogeneic BMT from matched siblings after a preparative regimen consisting of cyclophosphamide and 12 Gy TBI with that of a regimen of cyclophosphamide and 15.75 Gy TBI (Clift et al. 1990, 1991). In the AML study, the actuarial incidence of relapse with the lower TBI dose was 34%, but with the higher TBI dose, it was only 13%. In the CML trial, the actuarial incidence of relapse after 12 Gy TBI was 30% compared with only 7% with 15.75 Gy TBI. Thus, the results of these studies argue that within the range of high-dose therapy made possible by BMT, leukemia still displays a steep dose-response curve. Unfortunately, in the above-mentioned studies, patients treated in the higher dose groups had an increased frequency of treatment-related complications including more mucositis, interstitial pneumonia, and liver disease with a final result that, despite the decreased relapse rates associated with the higher dose of radiation, there was no net gain in long-term survival.

At least three general approaches have been taken in the context of BMT to capitalize on the dose response of malignancies to chemotherapy and radiotherapy. The first, and perhaps simplest, is to try to ensure that patients receive the prescribed doses of treatment for the tumor. For some chemotherapeutic agents, there is considerable variability in pharmacokinetics among patients leading to the possibility that with any given dose, some patients may achieve only low plasma values and be undertreated, while others may develop dangerous or fatal toxicities as a consequence of excessive plasma values. The clearest example in BMT is with busulfan, where several investigators have found highly variable pharmacokinetics among patients. Of particular importance is the finding that busulfan clearance is considerably greater during the first decade of life so that children treated with a set dose of busulfan achieve much lower plasma concentrations over time than older individuals and, as a consequence, are more likely to reject grafts and perhaps to relapse (Grochow et al. 1990; Hassan et al. 1991; Slattery et al., unpublished data). In most transplant settings, busulfan is given over 4 days. This provides an opportunity for dose adjustment, and several investigators have shown that it is possible to achieve a prescribed busulfan plasma concentration by altering subsequent busulfan doses based on the metabolism of the initial busulfan dose. Data from Ayash et al. (1992) suggest that there may also be considerable variability among patients in the way cyclophosphamide is metabolized as well.

A second approach to increasing tumor dose without increased toxicity in the transplant setting has been to identify and use agents that might reduce the toxicity of the preparative regimen without diminishing its antitumor effect. Several investigators have raised the possibility that some of the toxicities of the transplant regimen are caused by inflammatory mediators such as tumor necrosis factor-alpha (TNF-α) and interleukin-1 (IL-1), and that these inflammatory mediators contribute little or no antitumor effects of their own. This hypothesis led Bianco et al. (1991) to study whether pentoxifylline, an agent which inhibits TNF mRNA transcription in vitro and suppresses the production of TNF after endotoxin exposure in vivo, might reduce the toxicities of preparative regimens allowing for delivery of higher and potentially more effective doses. Although a phase I/II trial of this approach showed some promise, when put to the test in a randomized phase III study, no positive effects of pentoxifylline were found (Clift et al. 1993). Although unsuccessful to date, exploration of this general approach continues using other agents.

A third approach to increasing the dose of therapy delivered to tumors without increasing the systemic toxicity of BMT is to target some or all of the preparative therapy specifically to sites of disease. The availability of monoclonal antibodies (mAB) reactive with distinct populations of hemopoietic cells and the ability to conjugate these antibodies (Ab) with radionuclides such as ^{131}I, which deliver the majority of their energy locally, led us and others to investigate whether targeted radiotherapy might be used as the basis for a BMT preparative regimen. Initial studies done at Seattle using murine and canine models showed that with Ab-radionuclide conjugates, it is possible to deliver at least fourfold, and as much as tenfold, more radiation to sites of leukemia or lymphoma than to normal organs (Badger et al. 1986; Appelbaum et al. 1989). These studies further demonstrated that complete remission of murine tumors could be achieved with this approach but cure was difficult because of the dose limitation imposed by marrow suppression, and also demonstrated that this limitation could be overcome with BMT, allowing for the delivery of curative doses of radioimmunotherapy. Encouraged by these preclinical results, clinical studies were initiated at Seattle adopting this approach to the treatment of leukemia and lymphoma.

Radiolabeled Anti-CD33 Antibody for the Treatment of AML

CD33 is an antigen (Ag) expressed on normal myeloid cells from the myeloblast to the metamyelocyte stage and on leukemic cells in more than 90% of cases of AML; CD33 is not found on any normal nonhemopoietic tissue. In initial studies done at Seattle, patients with recurrent AML were given an anti-CD33 Ab (p67) trace-labeled with ^{131}I to determine if more radiation could be delivered to marrow, spleen, and other sites of leukemia than to any normal organ (Appelbaum et al. 1992). If it was determined that this was the case, a situation termed "favorable biodistribution," patients were treated with a well-tolerated preparative regimen (cyclophosphamide 120 mg/kg plus 12 Gy TBI) combined with increasing doses of ^{131}I-p67. Results of the initial biodistribution studies were disappointing; only in about half of the patients was favorable biodistribution achieved and even in these cases, the ratio of radiation delivered to leukemic marrow versus normal organs was considerably less impressive than that achieved in animal models. Major limitations with the use of ^{131}I-labeled anti-CD33 Ab in our experience are the relatively few Ag sites found per cell, a feature that limited the initial uptake of the Ab-radionuclide complex, and the relatively short half-life of the radionuclide in BM, a likely result of the rapid internalization of the ^{131}I-p67 complex with subsequent deiodination of the complex and excretion of the radionuclide from the cell (van der Jagt et al. 1992). Scheinberg et al. (1991), using a different anti-CD33 Ab, found a similar limitation of initial uptake, but noted a somewhat longer retention in BM than in our study.

Two approaches to overcome these limitations have been studied. One approach is to label p67 or other internalizing Ab using methods or radiolabels that lead to intracellular retention after internalization. This has been achieved using alternative labeling techniques of ^{131}I such as tyramine cellobiose or by using other radiolabels such as [90]Y. Another approach is to target antigens that are cell surface stable.

Radiolabeled Anti-CD45 Antibody in AML and ALL The CD45 Ag is expressed on virtually all hemopoietic cells except mature red cells and platelets and is also found in 85% to 90% of all clinical specimens of AML and acute lymphocytic leukemia (ALL). The average number of antigenic sites on most acute leukemia blast cells is five- to tenfold greater than CD33 and, unlike CD33, CD45 is maintained on the cell surface after Ab binding. Based on the results of animal studies confirming our hypothesis that the increased number of antigenic sites would improve initial marrow uptake and that lack of internalization prolongs retention of the radionuclide in the marrow, Matthews et al. (1991a, b) initiated a trial of ^{131}I-labeled anti-CD45 Ab (BC8) in patients with leukemia designed similarly to the study previously described for CD33.

Biodistribution studies were done in 23 patients using 0.5 mg/kg trace-labeled ^{131}I-BC8. As recently reported, in almost all patients, we found that the radiolabeled Ab delivered more radiation to BM, spleen, and other known sites of leukemia than to any normal organ, delivering an average of 7.1 cGy per mCi injected to marrow but only 2.7 cGy per mCi to liver, 2.1 to lungs, and 0.7 to kidney (Matthews 1994). Twenty patients have been treated on the dose-escalation study to date. The study is still ongoing, but already we have found that it is possible to deliver, in addition to the usual cyclophosphamide 120 mg/kg and 12 Gy TBI, a boost dose of radiation to leukemic BM of 2,500 cGy using ^{131}I-BC8 without undue toxicity.

Anti–B-Cell Antibody-Radionuclide Conjugates for the Treatment of Lymphoma The possibility of using radiolabeled anti–B-cell Ab as the basis for a BMT preparative regimen for lymphoma has been investigated by Press et al. (1989, 1993) in a series of experiments similar to those already described for leukemia. One important difference between the lymphoma and leukemia studies is that the lymphoma studies have only been done in the autologous setting and, thus, immunosuppressive agents such as cyclophosphamide or TBI were not required to achieve engraftment, enabling us to evaluate the toxicity and efficacy of high-dose, radiolabeled, anti–B-cell Ab in the absence of other agents. In the initial experiments, 43 patients with B-cell lymphomas in relapse underwent biodistribution studies using from 0.5 to 10 mg/kg Ab trace-labeled with ^{131}I. In 24 of 43, we found that the radiolabeled Ab would deliver more radiation to all known tumor sites than to any normal organ. Favorable biodistribution was achieved more frequently in patients with low tumor burdens (<500 gm tumor) and without splenomegaly. Nineteen of the 24 were treated with escalating doses of ^{131}I, resulting in CR in 16 and a partial remission (PR) in the other 3. Nine of the 16 remain in CR from 15 to 64 months from treatment. The maximum tolerated dose of ^{131}I in this study delivered 27.75 Gy to the normal organs receiving the highest radiation dose, which were usually the lungs. A phase II study of this approach continues.

Graft-Versus-Leukemia

There is convincing evidence that the antileukemic effects of allogeneic BMT are not merely the result of the high-dose chemoradiotherapy but, instead, that alloreactivity of donor cells against leukemia provides a significant contribution. A strong correlation exists between the occurrence of acute graft-versus-host disease (GVHD) and a decreased risk of relapse, and an additional contribution has been found with the occurrence of chronic GVHD (Weiden et al. 1979; Sullivan et al. 1989a). Since T cells transferred with the donor marrow or developing from it are responsible for the development of GVHD, it seems likely that T cells are the mediators of this GVL effect, an argument supported by the substantial increase in relapse rates seen with the use of T-cell–depleted BM (Horowitz et al. 1990; Marmont et al. 1991). That does not necessarily mean, however, that the same T cells responsible for causing GVHD mediate the GVL effect. An antileukemic effect of alloreactivity can be seen even in the absence of clinically apparent GVHD, as evidenced by the increased incidence of relapse in syngeneic transplant recipients compared with allogeneic BMT recipients with no clinically evident GVHD (Fefer et al. 1987; Marmont et al. 1991). In animal models, it has also been demonstrated that the GVHD and GVL effects are not necessarily linked and that GVL can exist without GVHD (Truitt and Atasoylu 1991; Glass et al. 1992).

It is now understood that, in general, CD8$^+$ T lymphocytes recognize endogenously processed peptides presented by HLA class I molecules and that CD4$^+$ T cells react to peptides presented by HLA class II. In animal models of GVL, both CD8[+] and CD4[+] T cells contribute to the GVL effect.

The exact peptides seen by T cells and responsible for the GVL effect are unknown, but a number of categories of peptides are likely targets. After HLA-matched allogeneic transplantation, donor-derived cytotoxic T cells with specificity against minor histocompatibility (Hc) Ag can be found that are capable of recognizing and lysing a wide range of host cells including host leukemic cells (Kaminski et al. 1989; Sosman et al. 1990). T cells recognizing such broadly expressed minor Ag may be responsible for the association between GVHD and GVL, but offer little hope of achieving relative tumor specificity. Falkenburg et al. (1991) have made the important observation that allogeneic T cells can be generated with reactivity to host Ag that are relatively tissue specific (Voogt et al. 1988). This observation may explain the occurrence of GVHD involving only one organ system. Furthermore, this observation suggests that if relatively specific T cells exist with reactivity to host hemopoietic tissue, one might be able to use such cells to elicit GVL without GVHD. It is also possible that there are donor T cells reactive with true tumor-specific Ag, such as the unique protein resulting from the t(9;22) translocation in CML, the t(15;17) in APL, or the t(8;21) in AML. Chen et al. (1992) at Seattle, for example, have recently demonstrated that the p210 *bcr/abl* protein can be presented by class II molecules and recognized by T cells.

A number of relatively nonspecific attempts to capitalize on the GVL effect have been made. In several studies it has been shown that administration of less GVHD prophylaxis after transplantation can increase the incidence of GVHD (Sullivan et al. 1989b). In most circumstances, however, the increased mortality associated with GVHD has counterbalanced any observed diminution in relapse rates. Some important exceptions to this generalization exist, however, and in some circumstances, such as AML in first relapse, improved survival has been achieved by purposefully limiting the extent of GVHD prophylaxis (Clift et al. 1992). It has also been shown that complete discontinuation of GVHD prophylaxis in patients who have relapsed after allogeneic BMT can restore a complete remission that, in some cases, can be prolonged (Higano et al. 1990).

The addition of viable donor buffy coat after transplantation has also been studied in hopes of augmenting a GVL effect (Sullivan et al. 1989c). The initial study of this approach was done in patients with acute leukemia and demonstrated that buffy coat cells could result in more GVHD, but failed to show a major impact on relapse. More recently, however, the administration of viable donor buffy coat cells to patients with CML who have relapsed after an allogeneic BMT has resulted in restoration of CR (Kolb et al. 1990; Antin 1993). Other approaches to nonspecifically augment a GVL effect have included the use of interferon-α (IFN-α) after transplant in an effort to upregulate class I Ag and the administration of IL-2.

Recently, it has been convincingly demonstrated that donor-derived, Ag-specific T cells can be isolated, cloned, expanded, and infused to HLA-matched siblings following BMT without toxicity. Using cytomegalovirus infection (CMV) as a model disease, Riddell et al. (1992a) demonstrated that CMV-specific T cells from BM donors could be isolated and expanded to large numbers and infused after transplant to patients, resulting in the restoration of normal immunity to CMV. A similar finding has subsequently been made for Epstein-Barr virus (EBV), and is being studied as therapy for human immunodeficiency virus (Riddell et al. 1992b). These observations argue that it may be possible to isolate T cells with a desired tumor-specific or tissue-specific reactivity, to expand such cells to large numbers, and then use them after transplant to further augment the antileukemic effects of allogeneic BMT.

ACKNOWLEDGMENTS

This work was supported in part by grants CA-18029, CA-18221, and CA-26386 from the National Institutes of Health, DHHS.

REFERENCES

Amadori, S., Testi, A.M., Arico, M., et al. (1993) Prospective comparative study of bone marrow transplantation and postremission chemotherapy for childhood acute myelogenous leukemia. *Journal of Clinical Oncology*, **11**, 1046.

Antin, J.H. (1993) Graft-versus-leukemia: no longer an epiphenomenon. *Blood*, **82**, 2273–7.

Appelbaum, F.R., Brown, P., Sandmaier, B., et al. (1989) Antibody-radionuclide conjugates as part of a myeloblative preparative regimen for marrow transplantation. *Blood*, **73**, 2202–8.

Appelbaum, F.R., Clift, R.A., Buckner, C.D., et al. (1983) Allogeneic marrow transplantation for acute nonlymphoblastic leukemia after first relapse. *Blood*, **61**, 949–53.

Appelbaum, F.R., Dahlberg, S., Thomas, E.D., et al. (1984) Bone marrow transplantation or chemotherapy after remission induction for adults with acute nonlymphoblastic leukemia–a prospective comparison. *Annals of Internal Medicine*, **101**, 581–8.

Appelbaum, F.R., Fisher, L.D., Thomas, E.D., and the Seattle Marrow Transplant Team. (1988) Chemotherapy v marrow transplantation for adults with acute nonlymphocytic leukemia: a five-year follow-up. *Blood*, **72**, 179–84.

Appelbaum, F.R., Matthews, D.C., Eary, J.F., et al. (1992) Use of radiolabeled anti-CD33 antibody to augment marrow irradiation prior to marrow transplantation for acute myelogenous leukemia. *Transplantation*, **54**, 829–33.

Archimbaud, E., Thomas, X., Michallet, M., et al. (1994) Prospective genetically randomized comparison between intensive postinduction chemotherapy and bone marrow transplantation in adults with newly diagnosed acute myeloid leukemia. *Journal of Clinical Oncology*, **12**, 262.

Ayash, L.J., Wright, J.E., Tretyakov, O., et al. (1992) Cyclophosphamide pharmacokinetics: correlation with cardiac toxicity and tumor response. *Journal of Clinical Oncology*, **10**, 995.

Badger, C.C., Krohn, K.A., Shulman, H., Flournoy, N., and Bernstein, I.D. (1986) Experimental radioimmunotherapy of lymphoma with ^{131}I-labelled anti-T-cell antibodies. *Cancer Research*, **46**, 6223–8.

Bianco, J.A., Appelbaum, F.R., Nemunaitis, J., et al. (1991) Phase I-II trial of pentoxifylline for the prevention of transplant-related toxicities following bone marrow transplantation. *Blood*, **78**, 1205–11.

Biggs, J.C., Horowitz, M.M., Gale, R.P., et al. (1992) Bone marrow transplants may cure patients with acute leukemia never achieving remission with chemotherapy. *Blood*, **80**, 1090.

Blume, K.G., Beutler, E., Bross, K.J., et al. (1980) Bone-marrow ablation and allogeneic marrow transplantation in acute leukemia. *New England Journal of Medicine*, **302**, 1041–6.

Blume, K. and Forman, S. (1992) High dose etoposide (VP-16)-containing preparatory regimens in allogeneic and autologous bone marrow transplantation for hematologic malignancies. *Seminars in Oncology*, **19**, 63.

Buckner, C.D., Clift, R.A., Appelbaum, F.R., and Thomas, E.D. (1993) Editorial: treatment of chronic myeloid leukemia by marrow transplantation. *Blood*, **82**, 1954–6.

Cassileth, P.A., Lynch, E., Hines, J.D., et al. (1992) Varying intensity of postremission therapy in acute myeloid leukemia. *Blood*, **79**, 1924.

Champlin, R.E., Ho, W.G., Gale, R.P., et al. (1985) Treatment of acute myelogenous leukemia. A prospective controlled trial of bone marrow transplantation versus consolidation chemotherapy. *Annals of Internal Medicine*, **102**, 285–91.

Chen, W., Peace, D.J., Rovira, K., You, S.G., and Cheever, M.A. (1992) T-cell immunity to the joining region of p210bcr-abl protein. *Proceedings of the National Academy of Sciences of the United States of America*, **89**, 1468.

Clift, R.A., Bianco, J.A., Appelbaum, F.R., et al. (1993) A randomized controlled trial of pentoxifylline for the prevention of regimen-related toxicities in patients undergoing allogeneic marrow transplantation. *Blood*, **82**, 2025–30.

Clift, R.A., Buckner, C.D., Appelbaum, F.R., et al. (1990) Allogeneic marrow transplantation in patients with acute myeloid leukemia in first remission. A randomized trial of two irradiation regimens. *Blood*, **76**, 1867–71.

Clift, R.A., Buckner, C.D., Appelbaum, F.R., et al. (1991) Allogeneic marrow transplantation in patients with chronic myeloid leukemia in the chronic phase. A randomized trial of two irradiation regimens. *Blood*, **77**, 1660–5.

Clift, R.A., Buckner, C.D., Appelbaum, F.R., et al. (1992) Allogeneic marrow transplantation during untreated first relapse of acute myeloid leukemia. *Journal of Clinical Oncology*, **10**, 1723–9.

Clift, R.A., Buckner, C.D., Thomas, E.D., et al. (1987) The treatment of acute non-lymphoblastic leukemia by allogeneic marrow transplantation. *Bone Marrow Transplantation*, **2**, 243–58.

Clift, R.A., Buckner, C.D., Thomas, E.D., et al. (1994) Marrow transplantation for patients in accelerated phase of chronic myeloid leukemia. *Blood*, **84**, 4368–73.

Conde, E., Iriondo, A., Rayon, C., et al. (1988) Allogeneic bone marrow transplantation versus intensification chemotherapy for acute myelogenous leukaemia in first remission: a prospective controlled trial. *British Journal of Haematology*, **68**, 219–26.

Dahl, G.V., Kalwinsky, D.K., Mirro, J., Jr., et al. (1990) Allogeneic bone marrow transplantation in a program of intensive sequential chemotherapy for children and young adults with acute nonlymphocytic leukemia in first remission. *Journal of Clinical Oncology*, **83**, 295–303.

Falkenburg, J.H., Goselink, H.M., Van der Harst, D., et al. (1991) Growth inhibition of clonogenic leukemic precursor cells by minor histocompatibility antigen-specific cytotoxic T lymphocytes. *Journal of Experimental Medicine*, **174**, 27.

Fefer, A., Radich, J., Pavletic, Z., et al. (1994) Syngeneic bone marrow transplantation (BMT) for chronic myelogenous leukemia in chronic phase: update of the original 14 Seattle patients, including PCR results. *Blood*, **84**(Suppl. 1), 257a.

Fefer, A., Sullivan, K.M., Weiden, P., et al. (1987) Graft versus leukemia effect in man: the relapse rate of acute leukemia is lower after allogeneic than after syngeneic marrow transplantation. In R.L. Truitt, R.P. Gale, and M.M. Bortin (Eds.) *Cellular immunotherapy of cancer*, pp. 401–8. New York, Alan R. Liss.

Forman, S.J., Schmidt, G.M., Nademanee, A.P., et al. (1991) Allogeneic bone marrow transplantation as therapy for primary induction failure for patients with acute leukemia. *Journal of Clinical Oncology*, **9**, 1570.

Glass, B., Uharek, L., Gassmann, W., et al. (1992) Graft-versus-leukemia activity after bone marrow transplantation does not require graft-versus-host disease. *Annals of Hematology*, **64**, 255.

Goldman, J., McGlave, P., Szydlo, R., Gale, R.P., and Horowitz, M.M. (1992) Impact of disease duration and prior treatment on outcome of bone marrow transplantation for chronic myelogenous leukemia. *Experimental Hematology*, **62**, 830.

Goldman, J.M., Szydlo, R., Horowitz, M.M., et al. (1993) Choice of pretransplant treatment and timing of transplants for chronic myelogenous leukemia in chronic phase. *Blood*, **82**, 2235–8.

Grochow, L.B., Krivit, W., Whitley, C.B., and Blazar, B. (1990) Busulfan disposition in children. *Blood*, **75**, 1723–7.

Hassan, M., Oberg, G., Bekassy, A.M., et al. (1991) Pharmacokinetics of high-dose busulphan in relation to age and chronopharmacology. *Cancer Chemotherapy and Pharmacology*, **28**, 130–4.

Higano, C.S., Brixey, M., Bryant, E.M., et al. (1990) Durable complete remission of acute non-lymphocytic leukemia associated with discontinuation of immunosuppression following relapse after allogeneic bone marrow transplantation: a case report of a graft-versus-leukemia effect. *Transplantation*, **50**, 175–7.

Horowitz, M.M., Gale, R.P., Sondel, P.M., et al. (1990) Graft-versus-leukemia reactions after bone marrow transplantation. *Blood*, **75**, 555–62.

Kaminski, E., Hows, J., Man, S., et al. (1989) Prediction of graft versus host disease by frequency analysis of cytotoxic T cells after unrelated donor bone marrow transplantation. *Transplantation*, **48**, 608–13.

Kolb, H.J., Mittermüller, J., Clemm, C., et al. (1990) Donor leukocyte transfusions for treatment of recurrent chronic myelogenous leukemia in marrow transplant patients. *Blood*, **76**, 2462–5.

Marmont, A., Bacigalupo, A., Van Lint, M.T., Frassoni, F., and Carella, A. (1985) Bone marrow transplantation versus chemotherapy alone for acute nonlymphoblastic leukemia. *Experimental Hematology*, **13**, 40.

Marmont, A.M., Horowitz, M.M., Gale, R.P., et al. (1991) T-cell depletion of HLA-identical transplants in leukemia. *Blood*, **78**, 2120–30.

Matthews, D.C., Appelbaum, F.R., Eary, J.F., et al. (1991a) Radiolabeled anti-CD45 monoclonal antibodies target lymphohematopoietic tissue in the macaque. *Blood*, **78**, 1864–74.

Matthews, D.C., Appelbaum, F.R., Eary, J.F., et al. (1991b) Radiolabeled anti-CD45 monoclonal antibodies target lymphoid tissue in murine and macaque models. *Antibody Immunoconjugates and Radiopharmaceuticals*, **4**, 713–9.

Matthews, D.C., Appelbaum, F.R., Eary, J.F., et al. (1994) Development of a marrow transplant regimen for acute leukemia using targeted hematopoietic irradiation delivered by ^{131}I-labeled anti-CD45 antibody, combined with cyclophosphamide and total body irradiation. *Blood*, **85**, 1122–31.

Nesbit, M.E., Buckley, J.D., Feig, S.A., et al. (1994) Chemotherapy for induction of remission of childhood acute myeloid leukemia followed by marrow transplantation or multiagent chemotherapy: a report from children's cancer group. *Journal of Clinical Oncology*, **12**, 127.

Press, O.W., Eary, J.F., Badger, C.C., et al. (1989) Treatment of refractory non-Hodgkin's lymphoma with radiolabeled MB-1 (anti-CD37) antibody. *Journal of Clinical Oncology*, **7**, 1027–38.

Press, O.W., Eary, J.F., Appelbaum, F.R., et al. (1993) Radiolabeled-antibody therapy of B-cell lymphoma with autologous bone marrow support. *New England Journal of Medicine*, **329**, 1219–24.

Reiffers, J., Gaspard, M.H., Maraninchi, D., et al. (1989) Comparison of allogeneic or autologous bone marrow transplantation and chemotherapy in patients with acute myeloid leukaemia in first remission: a prospective controlled trial. *British Journal of Haematology*, **72**, 57–63.

Riddell, S.R., Greenberg, P.D., Overell, R.W., et al. (1992a) Phase I study of cellular adoptive immunotherapy using genetically modified CD8$^+$ HIV-specific T cells for HIV seropositive patients undergoing allogeneic bone marrow transplant. *Human Gene Therapy*, **3**, 319–38.

Riddell, S.R., Watanabe, K.S., Goodrich, J.M., Li, C.R., Agha, M.E., and Greenberg, P.D. (1992b) Restoration of viral immunity in immunocompromised humans by adoptive transfer of T-cell clones. *Science*, **257**, 238–41.

Ringden, O., Bolme, P., Lonnqvist, B., Gustasson, G., and Kreuger, A. (1989) Allogeneic bone marrow transplantation versus chemotherapy in children with acute leukemia in Sweden. *Pediatric Hematology and Oncology*, **6**, 137.

Scheinberg, D.A., Lovett, D., Divgi, C.R., et al. (1991) A phase I trial of monoclonal antibody M195 in acute myelogenous leukemia: specific bone marrow targeting and internalization of radionuclide. *Journal of Clinical Oncology*, **9**, 478–90.

Schiller, G.J., Nimer, S.D., Territo, M.C., Ho, W.G., Champlin, R.E., and Gajewski, J.L. (1992) Bone marrow transplantation versus high-dose cytarabine-based consolidation chemotherapy for acute myelogenous leukemia in first remission. *Journal of Clinical Oncology*, **10**, 41.

Sosman, J.A., Oettel, K.R., Smith, S.D., Hank, J.A., Fisch, P., and Sondel, P.M. (1990) Specific recognition of human leukemic cells by allogeneic T cells: II. Evidence for HLA-D restricted determinants on leukemic cells that are crossreactive with determinants present on unrelated nonleukemic cells. *Blood*, **75**, 2005.

Sullivan, K.M., Storb, R., Buckner, C.D., et al. (1989b) Graft-versus-host disease as adoptive immunotherapy in patients with advanced hematologic neoplasms. *New England Journal of Medicine*, **320**, 828–34.

Sullivan, K.M., Storb, R., Witherspoon, R.P., et al. (1989a) Deletion of immunosuppressive prophylaxis after marrow transplantation increases hyperacute graft-versus-host disease but does not influence chronic graft-versus-host disease or relapse in patients with advanced leukemia. *Clinical Transplantation*, **3**, 5–11.

Sullivan, K.M., Weiden, P.L., Storb, R., et al. (1989c) Influence of acute and chronic graft-versus-host disease on relapse and survival after bone marrow transplantation from HLA-identical siblings as treatment of acute and chronic leukemia. *Blood*, **73**, 1720–8.

Thomas, E.D., Buckner, C.D., Clift, R.A., et al. (1979) Marrow transplantation for acute nonlymphoblastic leukemia in first remission. *New England Journal of Medicine*, **301**, 597–9.

Thomas, E.D. and Clift, R.A. (1989) Indications for marrow transplantation in chronic myelogenous leukemia. *Blood*, **73**, 861–4.

Thomas, E.D., Clift, R.A., Fefer, A., et al. (1986) Marrow transplantation for the treatment of chronic myelogenous leukemia. *Annals of Internal Medicine*, **104**, 155–63.

Truitt, R.L. and Atasoylu, A.A. (1991) Impact of pretransplant conditioning and donor T cells on chimerism, graft-versus-host disease, graft-versus-leukemia reactivity, and tolerance after bone marrow transplantation. *Blood*, **77**, 2515.

van der Jagt, R.H., Badger, C.C., Appelbaum, F.R., et al. (1992) Tumor localization of radiolabeled anti-myeloid antibodies in a human acute leukemia xenograft model. *Cancer Research*, **52**, 89–94.

Voogt, P.J., Goulmy, E., Veenhof, W.F., et al. (1988) Cellularly defined minor histocompatibility antigens are differentially expressed on human hematopoietic progenitor cells. *Journal of Experimental Medicine*, **168**, 2337.

Weiden, P.L., Flournoy, N., Thomas, E.D., et al. (1979) Antileukemic effect of graft-versus-host disease in human recipients of allogeneic-marrow grafts. *New England Journal of Medicine*, **300**, 1068–73.

Zander, A.R., Keating, M., Dicke, K., et al. (1988) A comparison of marrow transplantation with chemotherapy for adults with acute leukemia of poor prognosis in first complete remission. *Journal of Clinical Oncology*, **6**, 1548–57.

PART D

Future Clinical Applications

21

Clinical Gene Therapy

CYNTHIA E. DUNBAR

Ever since the development of technology allowing the transfer of new genes into eukaryotic cells, the hemopoietic stem cell (HSC) has been an obvious and desirable target for genetic therapy. The last 5 years have witnessed an explosion of interest in this approach to treating human disease, with the initiation of multiple clinical protocols, the formation of a score of biotechnology companies hoping to market this type of technology, and the evolution of safety guidelines at regulatory agencies such as the U.S. Food and Drug Administration (FDA) and the National Institutes of Health (NIH) Recombinant DNA Advisory Committee (Karlsson 1991; Miller 1992; Kessler et al. 1993; Mulligan 1993). The major applications being pursued for hemopoietic cell-directed gene therapy fall into three major categories at present: replacement of a missing or damaged gene product in congenital deficiency disorders affecting a wide variety of cells derived from the HSC, chemoprotection during anticancer therapy by transfer of a drug-resistance gene to normal progenitor and stem cells, and "intracellular vaccination" against human immunodeficiency virus (HIV) type I infection or progression via antiviral genes transferred to stem cells or T-cell precursors.

A number of requirements for successful gene transfer to hemopoietic progenitor and HSC determine the clinical applicability of various vector systems to human disease. Chromosomal integration of the transferred gene and passage to all progeny cells is necessary in hemopoietic targets, which must continuously replenish daughter effector cells. It would be desirable for integration to occur at a specific chromosomal locus in order to avoid insertional dysregulation of growth-control genes. The gene transfer procedure must not be toxic nor disrupt the self-renewal properties of the target stem-cell pool.

Gene-transfer efficiency to true repopulating stem cells must be high enough to impact on the disease phenotype; the required efficiency varies from as low as a few percent corrected cells in some congenital enzyme deficiency disorders to much higher levels in other situations such as sickle cell anemia. A vector that integrates into the genome of a cell that is not dividing at the time of transduction could increase efficiency of gene transfer to HSC, which are likely predominately in the G^o phase of the cell cycle (Lemischka, Raulet, and Mulligan 1986; Leary et al. 1992). Gene products must be stably expressed from the vector construct at adequate levels in the correct cell lineage, requiring strong constitutive or appropriately regulated transcriptional control elements. The vector must be simple and safe enough for clinical use; care must be taken to absolutely avoid generation of replication-competent particles in any viral-based system.

Currently, retroviruses are the best understood and most widely used vectors for gene transfer to hemopoietic cells, and are the only vectors that have been used in clinical trials to date involving hemopoietic targets. The remainder of this chapter will summarize current results with retroviral gene-transfer technology in human preclinical and clinical studies directed at hemopoietic cells, and briefly mention preclinical results using the adeno-associated virus (AAV) as an alternative vector system that has recently attracted intense interest and preclinical experimentation.

■ RETROVIRUS VECTORS

Preclinical Data – Human Hemopoietic Cells

Committed human progenitor cells such as granulocyte-macrophage colony-forming cells (GM-CFC) or erythroid colony-forming cells (E-CFC) can be transduced by retroviral vectors at very high efficiencies (often >50%) in the presence of various combinations of hemopoietic growth factors. Many different combinations have been tested; the highest gene-transfer efficiencies to progenitor cells have been reported using stem-cell factor (SCF) in combination with one or two other factors active on primitive cells, such as interleukin-3 (IL-3) and IL-6 (Nolta and Kohn 1990; Cournoyer et al. 1991; Hughes et al. 1992; Cassel et al. 1993). Co-culture of the target cells on the retroviral producer line increases efficiency, but is not practical for clinical trials (Nolta and Kohn 1990). Other investigators have performed transductions in the presence of primary bone marrow (BM) stroma instead of the viral producer line, and some have reported that even without the addition of soluble hemopoietic growth factors, transduction efficiency of progenitors is very high, 40% to 50% (Cournoyer et al. 1991; Moore et al. 1992). Probably stromal cells both produce the growth factors necessary to maintain and cycle the target cells in culture, and also provide as-yet-undefined signals associated with adhesion. The use of tissue-culture plates coated with specific extracellular matrix components such as fibronectin also increases transduction efficiency (Moritz, Patel, and Williams 1994).

More primitive human long-term culture-initiating cells (LTC-IC) can be transduced at equivalent efficiencies to committed progenitors under similar transduction conditions (Hughes et al. 1989; Cournoyer et al. 1991; Hughes et al. 1992; Moore et al. 1992). Many preclinical studies on human cells use assessment of LTC-IC transduction efficiency as a marker of true "stem-cell" transduction, but there is no evidence as yet that this assay is any more predictive than standard progenitor assays of in vivo results in primates and humans.

BM has been the traditional source of hemopoietic cells for transduction, but more recent studies have suggested that peripheral blood progenitor cells (PBPC) or cord blood (CB) cells may be equally good or better targets (Bregni et al. 1992; Cassel et al. 1993). Both mobilized and nonmobilized PBPC can be transduced at efficiencies of 50% to 90% in the presence of IL-3, IL-6, and SCF (Bregni et al. 1992; Cassel et al. 1993). CB has a higher frequency of very immature $CD34^+/CD38^-$ cells, and one group has shown that colonies grown from single transduced cells from this primitive population contain the retroviral vector at very high frequencies (Lu et al. 1993). Pretransduction enrichment for progenitor and stem cells via positive selection for antigens (Ag) such as CD34 or negative selection for lineage-specific Ag has been investigated by many and does not seem to influence transduction efficiency greatly, but allows much more practical volumes for ex vivo manipulation and transduction (Berenson et al. 1988; Hughes et al. 1992; Svilvassy and Cory 1994).

Human Clinical Studies

More than 100 patients have now received retrovirally modified cells in more than 20 protocols worldwide since the first patient was infused with retrovirally marked tumor-infiltrating lymphocytes (TIL) in 1989 (Rosenberg et al. 1990). To date, no adverse events related to the gene-transfer procedures have been reported. There are at least eight protocols completed or still active that use BM, PB, or CB cells as targets for retroviral transduction. Many of the preliminary studies use nontherapeutic marker vectors to try to better define safety and feasibility. These preliminary clinical marker protocols also have been designed to try to answer important biological questions about the biology of stem-cell transplantation (SCT) and the source of tumor relapse after autologous transplantation.

It is not known whether tumor relapse following autologous transplantation originates from endogenous tumor cells surviving conditioning chemo/radiotherapy or from residual tumor cells contaminating the BM or PB graft. The value of ex vivo marrow purging has been difficult to assess because the source of relapse cannot be identified without some method of marking cells originating from the graft. Purging techniques almost invariably damage normal BM progenitor and stem cells, delaying engraftment and diminishing future hemopoietic reserve; thus, a method for assessing the utility of purging directly in a small number of patients would be very desirable. The presence of gene-marked malignant cells at relapse would be strong evidence that purging should be attempted, and could be a powerful tool for analyzing the efficacy of various purging regimens.

Studies using retroviral vectors to mark harvested autologous BM or PB cells have been undertaken in several diseases, including acute myeloid leukemia (AML), chronic myeloid leukemia (CML), neuroblastoma, breast cancer, and multiple myeloma (MM). Investigators from St. Jude Children's Research Hospital have reported on two AML patients whose blast cells at relapse contained the retrovirally transferred neomycin-resistance gene (neo R), although no tumor cells had been detectable in the harvested autologous BM used for transplantation (Brenner et al. 1993b). More recently, this group has detected the marker gene in neuroblastoma cells at relapse (Rill et al. 1994). Several patients with CML have also been shown to have the marker gene in *bcr/abl*+ colonies after autologous bone-marrow transplant (ABMT) (Deisseroth et al. 1994). No marked relapses have been detected in myeloma or breast cancer patients to date, but even if these cells were present in the graft and contributing to relapse, they may not be susceptible to gene transfer under transduction conditions that are optimized for transfer to hemopoietic cells rather than for slowly cycling tumor cells (Dunbar et al. 1995).

Studies are now in progress using two vectors to compare different purging methods in patients with AML and neuroblastoma. The marrow harvest will be split then half will be purged with one agent, such as 4HC, after marking with a retroviral vector, and the other half with a second agent such as IL-2 after marking with a second retroviral vector. This approach should give data regarding the relative efficacy of different purging methods without the necessity for large, randomized, controlled purging trials, which have been very difficult to organize and carry out.

Ongoing studies are also addressing questions about the feasibility of gene transfer to HSC in humans and the biology of hemopoietic reconstitution after autologous transplantation. Preliminary results have been quite variable depending on the patient population studied and transduction conditions utilized. The St. Jude group has reported surprisingly high percentages of marked cells and progenitors in the myeloid lineages for as long as 18 months after autologous transplantation for AML or neuroblastoma. They exposed only one-third of a nonpurified autologous marrow harvest to vector for several hours and excluded growth factors or stromal elements during transduction (Brenner et al. 1993a). Animal models, both murine and primate, and in vitro assays of gene transfer to committed progenitors would not have predicted any appreciable level of gene transfer using this transduction procedure; however, up to 20% of nonleukemic CFC present in BM for 6 to 18 months after transplantation contained the marker gene and expressed a phenotype of neo R, indicating sustained gene expression. The marker gene was much less frequent in B and T cells, and true stem-cell marking, with unique retroviral insertion site in multiple lineages, has not yet been demonstrated.

Our own group had instead chosen to use a more prolonged transduction of 72 hours in the presence of growth factors (IL-3, SCF, with or without IL-6) based on the animal studies and the preclinical human data summarized above. These studies in adults undergoing ABMT and mobilized PBPC for myeloma or breast cancer have thus far shown lower levels of gene transfer efficiency, less than 0.1% to 1% at 3 months or more after transplantation (Dunbar et al. 1993, 1994). Three patients followed for more than 2 years still have the marker gene in PB and BM in both mononuclear cells (MNC) and granulocytes (Dunbar et al. 1995). The use of two different neo R marking vectors to transduce the harvested PB and the BM has allowed discrimination of the marking source after transplantation. In patients with successful marking, all marking either originated from the PB graft or from both PB and BM grafts, and marking persisting longer than 1 year originated from the PB graft in all cases. This indicates that PBPC can engraft durably, and with further investigation will provide supportive data regarding the applicability of mobilized PB cells in allogeneic transplantation.

The differences between the results in the children at St. Jude's and adults at U.S. NIH may be based on differing cell cycle characteristics of primitive hemopoietic cells in the two groups, either because of age or because the children were harvested shortly after induction chemotherapy given for treatment of leukemia or relapsed neuroblastoma. We are currently investigating the St. Jude transduction procedure in the adult population, as well as the inclusion of primary autologous stroma during transduction, in an attempt to improve transduction efficiencies to a level useful for therapeutic applications.

A smaller number of patients have been enrolled in trials involving vectors carrying a potentially therapeutic gene directed at hemopoietic progenitor and stem cells. Two children with severe combined immunodeficiency (SCID) due to lack of functional adenosine deaminase (ADA) have received infusions of PB T cells grown in vitro with IL-2 and anti-CD3 antibody (Ab) stimulation and transduced with a retroviral vector carrying the ADA gene (Blaese et al. 1995). In the 4 years since the infusions began, both children have shown improved immune function, increased T-cell and ADA levels, and no evidence of toxicity (Blaese et al. 1995). The use of peripheral blood T cells as targets for gene correction in this disorder, however, is for several reasons not ideal: some patients with ADA-deficient SCID do not have sufficient T cells in their PB to collect and transduce; repeated collections and infusions will probably be necessary because of the limited life span of most circulating T cells; and establishment of a complete immune repertoire will be impossible unless a vast number of distinct T-cell clones are successfully transduced.

In an attempt to circumvent these problems, several groups have begun transducing marrow or recombinant human granulocyte colony-stimulating factor (rHuG-CSF) –mobilized PBSC populations instead. Fewer than five patients have been treated, and although circulating cells containing the transferred gene have been detected, it is too early to assess a clinical effect. T cells derived from corrected progenitor and stem cells should have a competitive advantage, and might efficiently repopulate the immune system even if initial transduction efficiency is very low. In another study, three newborns with prenatally diagnosed ADA-deficient SCID received autologous CB CD34$^+$ cells transduced with an ADA vector. All three have the proviral ADA gene detectable in their PB MNC, and the proportion of cells carrying the new gene is increasing over time as exogenous ADA enzyme is withdrawn, suggesting an in vivo advantage for the corrected cells (Kohn et al. 1995). CB may prove to be a particularly appropriate target for the genetic correction of disorders that can be diagnosed in utero (Lu et al. 1993).

Clinical protocols still in the process of regulatory review (December 1994) include retroviral stem and progenitor cell-directed approaches to other congenital disorders such as Gaucher's disease (GD), Fanconi's anemia (FA), and chronic granulomatous disease (CGD). FA is a particularly exciting application, because of the probable in vivo growth and proliferative advantage that corrected progenitor and stem cells would have over noncorrected cells. The Fanconi's Anemia Group C (FAGC) gene has been cloned and encodes a DNA repair protein (Strathdee et al. 1992). The defect leads to progressive BM failure and leukemia (Frickhofen, Liu, and Young 1990). Transduction of hemopoietic progenitor cells from FA patients with a retroviral vector carrying the FAGC gene normalizes colony number and size, and the cells are no longer abnormally sensitive to clastogenic agents such as mitomycin C (Walsh et al. 1994).

The application of these approaches to congenital disorders would obviously be much safer and more likely to be clinically feasible if efficient engraftment of gene-corrected progenitor and stem cells could occur without prior myeloablation. It is encouraging that several investigators have recently reported that high-level engraftment of BM in the mouse can occur without ablation (Stewart et al. 1993; Harrison 1993; Wu and Keating 1993). Very large doses of marrow cells were used in these experiments, however, and would not be practical in humans unless multiple collections of cytokine-mobilized PB could be used instead of BM. This approach will be tested in clinical protocols for GD.

Safety Issues

Retroviruses are pathogenic, in both mice and primates. The murine leukemia viruses used as vectors do not carry oncogenes, even when replication competent, but do cause lymphomas in permissive mouse strains via multiple proviral insertions in the genome of thymic T-precursor cells, eventually activating cellular growth-control genes such as *myc* and *pim* (Tsichlis 1987; Kung, Boerkoel, and Carter 1991). If a recombinant viral vector inserts only once or twice in a target cell's genome, this type of insertional activation is very unlikely to occur, given the size of the genome (Schuening et al. 1991); however, the generation of replication-competent virus via recombination in the producer cell line would make insertional mutagenesis much more likely, by allowing repetitive infections and genomic insertions in vivo after return of transduced cells to the animal or patient. It has also recently been reported that the long terminal repeat (LTR) of Moloney virus encodes a transcriptional activator for major histocompatibility complex (HC) genes and lymphocyte cell-surface Ag that might add to the potential for oncogenicity (Choi and Faller 1994).

Immunocompetent or only mildly immunosuppressed primates seem to be able to immediately clear and inactivate helper virus via complement before a productive infection is set up in vivo (Cornetta et al. 1991a); however, three rhesus monkeys transplanted after total-body irradiation (TBI) with $CD34^+$ marrow cells transduced using a helper-contaminated producer cell line never developed Ab against the helper virus, and developed fatal T-cell lymphomas 6 to 9 months after transplantation (Donahue et al. 1992). The animals were viremic; the predicted recombinant helper virus arose from recombination between the helper and the vector genomes in the producer cell line (Yoder et al. 1993; Vanin et al. 1994).

The demonstration that Moloney virus can be pathogenic in primates has been an impetus to ensure that any vector preparation used clinically is free of helper virus. All vector/producer cell line combinations used for clinical vector production have many more safeguards against the generation of replication-competent helper virus than the N2 vector produced in a co-cultured producer line used for the monkey experiments. These safeguards include removal of as much homology as possible between the vector genome and the helper genome, mutation of the ATG in the small portion of the *gag* gene remaining in the vector genome, replacement of the LTR with other promoter/enhancers in the packaging genome, and separation of the different helper genes to different locations in the packaging cell's genome (Miller and Buttimore 1986; Markowitz, Goff, and Bank 1988; Cornetta, Morgan, and Anderson 1991b).

The U.S. FDA currently requires very extensive testing for all possible types of helper virus that could arise in the producer cell line before clinical lots of vector can be made; even then up to 10% of each clinical lot must be used for helper virus screening before release. Transduced patient cells are also tested for helper virus production, and patients are followed after transplantion of transduced cells for Ab to helper virus envelope proteins, and for the presence of helper virus genomes in mononuclear cells (MNC) via polymerase chain reaction (PCR) and functional $S+L^-$ testing. The expense and effort involved in this testing is considerable, and more sensitive and specific assays for helper virus need to be developed and validated.

Another safety issue concerns the "cell therapy" aspects of these protocols. The FDA is moving towards requiring quasi-pharmaceutical regulation of all substances to which autologous or allogeneic cells are exposed ex vivo, including media, fetal calf serum, trypsin, among others (Kessler et al. 1993). It will be very difficult to comply with these requirements in the retroviral gene transfer field. Adapting producer cell lines to serum-free conditions is very difficult: an alternative approach may be the use of purified vector preparations in serum-free media (Kotani et al. 1994). Preliminary results from our group indicate that hemopoietic progenitor transductions are possible under these conditions (C. Dunbar and M. Sekhar, unpublished data).

ADENO-ASSOCIATED VIRUS – PRECLINICAL DATA

The characterization of rAAV as a gene-transfer vector is at least 5 years behind that of retroviruses. Successful gene transfer with integration and appropriately regulated gene expression in human hemopoietic cell lines has recently been reported (Walsh et al. 1992; Miller et al. 1993), with high-level, hemin-inducible expression of γ-hemoglobin genes demonstrated in K562 cells. This degree of high-level, regulated hemoglobin expression has been very difficult to achieve with retroviral vectors, because of frequent recombination events leading to low titers if enhancer elements are included in retroviral constructs.

Only recently has the potential of rAAV to deliver genes to primary hemopoietic progenitors been explored. One group used rAAV containing the neo R gene to infect murine BM and reported that variable percentages (10% to 70% over background) contained the gene and were neo R; these data, however, are clouded by the facts that rAAV is very stable in methylcellulose even in the absence of cells, is a DNA virus, and nonquantitative PCR may be positive due to residual free or cell-associated virus in the culture dish, falsely elevating estimates of gene-transfer efficiency (Miller, Edwards, and Miller 1994). Another group reported that 60% to 70% of human or rhesus CD34$^+$ cells exposed to rAAV carrying the β-galactosidase gene expressed the gene product in the nucleus (Goodman et al. 1994). Colonies grown from these cells were picked and estimated to have viral-associated DNA sequences at a copy number of one to two per cell by semiquantitative PCR, implying but not proving integration. High level γ-hemoglobin expression was shown in blast-forming unit—erythroid (BFU-E) grown from CD34$^+$ human cells exposed to rAAV carrying a marked globin gene (Miller et al. 1994).

EFFICIENCY OF GENE TRANSFER TO STEM CELLS

In order for these new technologies to have therapeutic impact, the efficiency of gene transfer to true repopulating stem cells must be increased. A number of approaches are currently addressing this problem. Ex vivo selection of successfully transduced cells has been attempted for a number of years using drug selection for neo R. This works very well in vitro with enrichment of positive CFC or LTC-IC, but seems to damage stem cells, even if they are transduced, and has not proven beneficial once these cells are given back to a recipient animal (Wong et al. 1989). More recently, several groups have designed retroviral vectors containing a gene for a constititutively expressed cell-surface protein such as CD24 or a nonfunctional truncated growth factor receptor (Mavilio et al. 1994; Pawliuk et al. 1994). Cells that are successfully transduced can be isolated nontoxically via cell sorting prior to reinfusion, or used for ex vivo expansion.

One can also select for successfully transduced cells in vivo if constructs contain the multidrug-resistance gene (p-glycoprotein). In the mouse model, three groups have shown that retroviral transfer of the multidrug resistance gene into mouse BM cells allows in vivo selection or chemoprotection after engraftment (Podda et al. 1992; Sorrentino et al. 1992; Hanania and Deisseroth 1994). After a single dose of Taxol, mice transplanted and stably engrafted with transduced cells showed dramatic and stable increases in the number of circulating cells with the transfected multidrug-resistant gene (Sorrentino et al. 1992). The persistence of this effect without further treatment with Taxol, and the transfer of these populations to secondary transplant recipients without diminution in either the proportion of cells containing the provirus or transferred chemoprotection suggests that selection has occurred in very primitive hemopoietic cells (Hanania and Deisseroth 1994). A bicistronic vector containing the multidrug-resistant gene and the GC gene has been developed and expresses both genes after drug selection (Aran, Gottesman, and Pastan 1994). Other drug-resistance genes such as dihydrofolate reductase (DHFR) and multidrug resistance–associated protein (MRP) may also be useful for in vivo selection or chemoprotection (Corey et al. 1990; Cole et al. 1992).

Several clinical protocols now in development by our own group and others will attempt to introduce the MDR1 gene into hemopoietic stem and progenitor cells of patients undergoing autologous transplantation for solid tumors such as breast and ovarian cancer. We hope that normal BM cells will be protected from posttransplantation chemotherapy, thus decreasing toxicity and allowing dose intensification. The ultimate goal of this approach is also to allow for in vivo selection of cells containing an integrated provirus that carries a second therapeutic gene such as hemoglobin that must be present in a majority of hemopoietic cells to have a clinical effect.

Transfer to stem cells may be largely unsuccessful because of insufficient cell cycling and integration, but perhaps also to insufficient viral receptor density. The amphotropic retroviral receptor was only recently identified and cloned, and the AAV receptor is as yet unknown (Miller et al. 1994). The presence, density, and functionality of these receptors on primitive human cells is unknown, and fetal liver hemopoietic cells lack functional amphotropic receptors (Richardson et al. 1994). Thus, a number of investigators have attempted to alter viral vectors to enter cells via more specific, possibly more abundant receptors. Successful alteration of the retroviral envelope protein to display single-chain Ab fragments directed against various Ag or ligands to cell-surface receptors has been reported, with conclusive evidence for functional binding of epitope by this viral-associated Ab (Russell, Hawkins, and Winter 1993). But there is little evidence for augmentation of gene-transfer efficiency to target cells bearing the epitope, nor for the ability to infect human cells with an ecotropic virus bearing an envelope carrying an Ab against an epitope on human cells (Russell et al. 1993). Simple binding of a vector particle to a cell-surface receptor may not be enough: as yet unknown internalization and uncoating machinery may not be associated with these new vector-binding moieties. In the HIV model, CD4 expression alone is not enough in every cell type to allow productive viral infection (Harrington and Geballe 1993; Brodsky et al. 1994). One group has reported some success using bispecific Ab directed against both retroviral envelope and HLA Ag on the cell surface to increase gene-transfer efficiency and allow ecotropic virus entry into human cells (Raux, Jeanteur, and Piechaczyk 1989).

■ APPROPRIATE PRECLINICAL MODELS

At least in the retroviral system, high-efficiency transduction of committed progenitor cells or even more primitive LTC-IC has not predicted equivalent success under the same conditions in transducing true repopulating stem cells in either primate models or early human clinical studies. The murine model has also not been predictive, and the use of primates or other large animals routinely for large-scale or rapid screening of vectors or transduction procedures is not feasible. The ability to engraft human HSC in various immunodeficient mouse strains is one assay that might be utilized (Dick 1991; Lapidot et al. 1992). These attempts are hampered by an inability to achieve high levels of engraftment of human cells, making quantitative determination of gene-transfer efficiency in these human cells impossible (Dick et al. 1991). The co-administration of human marrow stroma overexpressing IL-3 has allowed one group to get much higher levels of engraftment and to document high levels of transduced human BM cells and CFC for as long as 9 months after xenografting (Nolta, Handley, and Kohn 1994). Further study will determine whether the engrafted cells have characteristics of true stem cells, and whether the gene-transfer efficiencies obtained correlate with in vivo human results using the same vectors and transduction conditions. More precise phenotypic definition of human stem cells will also be useful, allowing sorting of primitive populations for analysis of transduction (Pëault et al. 1991; Terstappen et al. 1991; Baum et al. 1992).

■ CONCLUSIONS

The next 5 years will certainly be active in the gene therapy field, both because existing vector systems will be improved and, we hope, because innovative new techniques will be developed. As more clinical trials are begun, better data on safety and efficacy will become available, and the medical community and the public can make a more informed judgment on the ultimate utility of this therapeutic approach.

REFERENCES

Aran, J.M., Gottesman, M.M., and Pastan, I. (1994) Drug-selected coexpression of human glucocerebrosidase and P-glycoprotein using a bicistronic vector. *Proceedings of the National Academy of Sciences of the United States of America*, **91**, 3176–80.

Baum, C.M., Weissman, I.L., Tsukamoto, A.S., Buckle, A.-M., and Peualt, B. (1992) Isolation of a candidate human hemopoietic stem-cell population. *Proceedings of the National Academy of Sciences of the United States of America*, **89**, 2804–8.

Berenson, R.J., Andrews, R.G., Bensinger, W.I., Kalamasz, D., and Knitter, G. (1988) Antigen CD34$^+$ marrow cells engraft lethally irradiated baboons. *Journal of Clinical Investigation*, **81**, 951–5.

Blaese, R.M., Culver, K.W., Miller, A.D., Carter, C.S., Fleisher, T., Clerici, M., Shearer, G., Chang, L., Chiang, Y., Tolstoshev, P., Greenblatt, J.J., Rosenberg, S.A., Klein, H., Berger, M., Mullen, C.A., Ramsey, W.J., Muul, L., Morgan, R.A., and Anderson, W.F. (1995) T lymphocyte directed gene therapy for ADA deficiency (SCID): results of the initial trial with 4 years of observation. *Science*, **270**, 475–80.

Bregni, M., Magni, M., Siena, S., Di Nicola, M., Bonadonna, G., and Gianni, A.M. (1992) Human peripheral blood hemopoietic progenitors are optimal targets of retroviral mediated gene transfer. *Blood*, **80**, 1418–22.

Brenner, M.K., Rill, D.R., Holladay, M.S., et al. (1993a) Gene marking to determine whether autologous marrow infusion restores long-term haemopoiesis in cancer patients. *Lancet*, **342**, 1134–7.

Brenner, M.K., Rill, D.R., Moen, R.C., et al. (1993b) Gene-marking to trace origin of relapse after autologous bone marrow transplantation. *Lancet*, **341**, 85–6.

Brodsky, R.A., Jane, S.M., Vanin, E.F., et al. (1994) Purified GPI-anchored CD4DAF incorporates as a receptor for HIV-mediated gene transfer. *Human Gene Therapy*, **5**, 1231–9.

Cassel, A., Cottler-Fox, M., Doren, S., and Dunbar, C.E. (1993) Retroviral-mediated gene transfer into CD34-enriched human peripheral blood stem cells. *Experimental Hematology*, **21**, 585–91.

Choi, S.-Y. and Faller, D. (1994) The long terminal repeats of a murine retrovirus encode a trans-activator for cellular genes. *Journal of Biological Chemistry*, **269**, 19691–4.

Cole, S.P., Bhardwaj, G., Gerlach, J.H., et al. (1992) Overexpression of a transporter gene in a multidrug-resistant human lung cancer cell line. *Science*, **258**, 1650–4.

Corey, C.A., DeSilva, A.D., Holland, C.A., and Williams, D.A. (1990) Serial transplantation of methotrexate-resistant bone marrow: protection of murine recipients from drug toxicity by progeny of transduced stem cells. *Blood*, **75**, 337–43.

Cornetta, K., Moen, R.C., Culver, K., et al. (1991a) Amphotropic murine leukemia retrovirus is not an acute pathogen for primates. *Human Gene Therapy*, **1**, 12–17.

Cornetta, K., Morgan, R.A., and Anderson, W.F. (1991b) Safety issues related to retroviral-mediated gene transfer to humans. *Human Gene Therapy*, **2**, 5–14.

Cournoyer, D., Scarpa, M., Mitani, K., et al. (1991) Gene transfer of adenosine deaminase into primitive human hemopoietic progenitor cells. *Human Gene Therapy*, **2**, 203–13.

Deisseroth, A.B., Zu, Z., and Claxton, D., et al. (1994) Genetic marking shows that Ph+ cell present in autologous transplants of chronic myelogenous leukemia (CML) contribute to relapse after autologous bone marrow transplantation in CML. *Blood*, **833**, 3068–76.

Dick, J.E. (1991) Immune-deficient mice as models of normal and leukemic human hemopoiesis. *Cancer Cells*, **3**, 39–48.

Dick, J.E., Kamel-Reid, S., Murdoch, B., and Doedens, M. (1991) Gene transfer into normal human hemopoietic cells using in vitro and in vivo assays. *Blood*, **78**, 624–34.

Donahue, R.E., Kessler, S.W., Bodine, D., et al. (1992) Helper virus induced T cell lymphoma in nonhuman primates after retroviral mediated gene transfer. *Journal of Experimental Medicine*, **176**, 1125–35.

Dunbar, C.E., Nienhuis, A.W., Stewart, F.M., et al. (1993) Amendment to clinical research projects. Genetic marking with retroviral vectors to study the feasibility of stem cell gene transfer and the biology of hemopoietic reconstitution after autologous transplantation in multiple myeloma, chronic myelogenous leukemia, or metastatic breast cancer. *Human Gene Therapy*, **4**, 205–22.

Dunbar, C.E., O'Shaughnessy, J.A., Cottler-Fox, M., et al. (1994) Transplantation of retrovirally-marked CD34+ bone marrow and peripheral blood cells in patients with multiple myeloma or breast cancer. *Blood*, **82**, 854.

Dunbar, C.E., Cottler-Fox, M., O'Shaughnessy J.A., Doren, S., Carter, C.S., Berenson, R., Brown, S., Moen, R.C., Greenblatt, J., Stewart, F.M., Leitman, S.F., Wilson, W., Cowan, K.H., Young, N.S., and Nienhuis, A.W. (1995). Retrovirally-marked CD34-enriched peripheral blood and bone marrow cells contribute to long-term engraftment after autologous transplantation. *Blood*, **85**, 3048–57.

Frickhofen, N., Liu, J.M., and Young, N.S. (1990) Etiologic mechanisms of hemopoietic failure. *American Journal of Pediatric Hematology/Oncology*, **12**, 385–92.

Goodman, S., Xiao, X., Donahue, R.E., et al. (1994) Recombinant adeno-associated virus mediated gene transfer into hemopoietic progenitor cells. *Blood*, **84**, 1492–1500.

Hanania, E.G., and Deisseroth, A.B. (1994) Serial transplantation shows that early hemopoietic precursor cells are transduced by MDR-1 retroviral vector in a mouse gene therapy model. *Cancer Gene Therapy*, **1**, 21–5.

Harrington, R.D., and Geballe, A.P. (1993) Cofactor requirement for human immunodeficiency virus type 1 entry into CD4-expressing human cell line. *Journal of Virology*, **67**, 5939–47.

Harrison, D.E. (1993) Competitive repopulation in unirradiated normal recipients. *Blood*, **81**, 2473–4.

Hughes, P.F., Eaves, C.J., Hogge, D.E., and Humphries, R.K. (1989) High efficiency gene transfer to human hemopoietic cells maintained in long-term marrow culture. *Blood*, **74**, 1915–22.

Hughes, P.F., Thacker, J.D., Hogge, D., et al. (1992) Retroviral gene transfer to primitive normal and leukemic hemopoietic cells using clinically applicable procedures. *Journal of Clinical Investigation*, **89**, 1817–24.

Karlsson, S. (1991) Treatment of genetic defects in hemopoietic cell function by gene transfer. *Blood*, **78**, 2481–92.

Kessler, D.A., Siegel, J.P., Noguchi, P.D., Zoon, K.C., Feiden, K.L., and Woodcock, J. (1993) Regulation of somatic-cell therapy and gene therapy by the Food and Drug Administration. *New England Journal of Medicine*, **329**, 1169–73.

Kohn, D.B., Weinberg, K.I., Nolta, J.A., Heiss, L.N., Lenarsky, C., Crooks, G.M., Hanley, M.E., Annett, G., Brooks, J.S., El-Khoureiy, D.E., Lawrence, K., Wells, S., Moen, R.C. Bastian, J., Williams-Herman, D.E., Elder, M., Wara, D., Bowen, T., Hershfield, M.S., Mullen, C.A., Blaese, R.M., and Parkman, R. (1995) Engraftment of gene-modified umbilical cord blood cells in neonates with adenosine deaminase deficiency. *Nature Medicine*, **1**, 1017–23.

Kotani, H., Newton, P.B., Zhang, S., et al. (1994) Improved methods of retroviral vector transduction and production for gene therapy. *Human Gene Therapy*, **5**, 19–28.

Kung, H.-J., Boerkoel, C., and Carter, T. H. (1991) Retroviral mutagenesis of cellular oncogenes: a review with insights into the mechanisms of insertional activation. *Current Topics in Microbiology and Immunology*, **171**, 1–25.

Lapidot, T., Pflumio, F., Doedens, M., Murdoch, B., Williams, D.E., and Dick, J.E. (1992) Cytokine stimulation of multilineage hemopoiesis from immature human cells engrafted in SCID mice. *Science*, **255**, 1137–41.

Leary, A.G., Zeng, H.Q., Clark, S.C., and Ogawa, M. (1992) Growth factor requirements for survival in G_o and entry into the cell cycle of primitive human hemopoietic progenitors. *Proceedings of the National Academy of Sciences of the United States of America*, **89**, 4013–7.

Lemischka, I.R., Raulet, D.H., and Mulligan, R.C. (1986) Developmental potential and dynamic behavior of hemopoietic stem cells. *Cell*, **45**, 917–27.

Lu, L., Xiao, M., Clapp, D.W., Li, Z.-H., and Broxmeyer, H.E. (1993) High efficiency retroviral mediated gene transduction into single isolated immature and replatable CD34$^+$ hemopoietic stem/progenitor cells from human umbilical cord blood. *Journal of Experimental Medicine*, **178**, 2089–96.

Markowitz, D., Goff, S., and Bank, A. (1988) A safe packaging line for gene transfer: separating viral genes on two different plasmids. *Journal of Virology*, **62**, 1120–4.

Mavilio, F., Ferrari, G., Rossini, S., et al. (1994) Peripheral blood lymphocytes as target cells of retroviral vector-mediated gene transfer. *Blood*, **83**, 1988–97.

Miller, A.D. (1992) Human gene therapy comes of age. *Nature*, **357**, 455–60.

Miller, A.D. and Buttimore, C. (1986) Redesign of retrovirus packaging cell lines to avoid recombination leading to helper virus production. *Molecular and Cellular Biology*, **6**, 2895–902.

Miller, D.G., Edwards, R.H., and Miller, D. (1994) Cloning of the cellular receptor for amphotropic murine retroviruses reveals homology to that for gibbon ape leukemia virus. *Proceedings of the National Academy of Sciences of the United States of America*, **91**, 78–82.

Miller, J.L., Donahue, R.E., Sellers, S.E., Samulski, R.J., Young, N.S., and Nienhuis, A.W. (1994) Recombinant adeno-associated virus (rAAV) mediated expression of a human τ-globin gene in human progenitor derived erythroid cells. *Proceedings of the National Academy of Sciences of the United States of America*, **92**, 10183–7.

Miller, J.L., Walsh, C.E., Ney, P.A., Samulski, R.J., and Nienhuis, A.W. (1993) Single copy transduction and expression of human gamma-globin in K562 erythroleukemia cells using recombinant adeno-associated virus vectors: the effect of mutations in NFr2 and GATA-1 binding motifs within the HS2 enhancer. *Blood*, **82**, 1900–5.

Moore, K.A., Deisseroth, A.B., Reading, C.L., Williams, D.E., and Belmont, J.W. (1992) Stromal support enhances cell-free retroviral vector transduction of human bone marrow long-term culture initiating cells. *Blood*, **79**, 1393–9.

Moritz, T., Patel, V.P., and Williams, D.A. (1994) Bone marrow extracellular matrix molecules improve gene transfer into human hemopoietic cells via retroviral vectors. *Journal of Clinical Investigation*, **93**, 1451–7.

Mulligan, R.C. (1993) The basic science of gene therapy. *Science*, **260**, 926–31.

Nolta, J.A., Handley, M.B., and Kohn, D.B. (1994) Sustained human hematopoiesis in immunodeficient mice by cotransplantation of marrow stroma expressing human interleukin-3: analysis of gene transduction of long-lived progenitors. *Blood*, **83**, 3041–51.

Nolta, J.A. and Kohn, D.B. (1990) Comparison of the effects of growth factors on retroviral vector-mediated gene transfer and the proliferative status of human hemopoeitic progenitor cells. *Human Gene Therapy*, **1**, 257–68.

Pawliuk, R., Kay, R., Lansdorp, P., and Humphries, R.K. (1994) Use of a cell surface antigen, CD24, as a retroviral marker for the analysis and selection of gene transfer to long-term repopulating cells. *Blood*, **82**, 314a.

Pëault, B., Weissman, I.L., Baum, C., McCune, J.M., and Tsukamoto, A. (1991) Lymphoid reconstitution of the human fetal thymus in SCID mice with CD34$^+$ precursor cells. *Journal of Experimental Medicine*, **174**, 1283–6.

Podda, S., Ward, M., Himelstein, A., et al. (1992) Transfer and expression of the human multiple drug resistance gene into live mice. *Proceedings of the National Academy of Sciences of the United States of America*, **89**, 9676–80.

Raux, P., Jeanteur, P., and Piechaczyk, M. (1989) A versatile and potentially general approach to the targeting of specific cell types by retroviruses: application to the infection of human cells by means of major histocompatibility complex class I class II antigens by mouse ecotropic murine leukemia virus-derived viruses. *Proceedings of the National Academy of Sciences of the United States of America*, **86**, 9079–83.

Richardson, C., Ward, M., Podda, S., and Bank, A. (1994) Mouse fetal liver cells lack functional amphotropic retroviral receptors. *Blood*, **84**, 433–9.

Rill, D.R., Santana, V.M., Roberts, W.M., et al. (1994) Direct demonstration that autologous bone marrow transplantation for solid tumors can return a multiplicity of tumorigenic cells. *Blood*, **84**, 380–3.

Rosenberg, S.A., Aebersold, P., Cornetta, K., et al. (1990) Gene transfer into humans-immunotherapy of patients with advanced melanoma, using tumor-infiltrating lymphocytes modified by retroviral gene transduction. *New England Journal of Medicine*, **323**, 570–8.

Russell, S.J., Hawkins, R.E., and Winter, G. (1993) Retroviral vectors displaying functional antibody fragments. *Nucleic Acids Research*, **21**, 1081–5.

Schuening, F.G., Kawahara, K., Miller, A.D., et al. (1991) Retrovirus-mediated gene transduction into long-term repopulating marrow cells of dogs. *Blood*, **78**, 2568–76.

Sorrentino, B.P., Brandt, S.J., Bodine, D., et al. (1992) Selection of drug resistant bone marrow cells in vivo after retroviral transfer of human MDR1. *Science*, **257**, 99–103.

Stewart, F.M., Crittenden, R.B., Lowry, P.A., Pearson-White, S., and Quesenberry, P.J. (1993) Long-term engraftment of normal and post-5-fluorouracil murine marrow into normal nonmyeloablated mice. *Blood*, **81**, 2544–71.

Strathdee, C.A., Gavish, H., Shannon, W.R., and Buchwald, M. (1992) Cloning of cDNAs for Fanconi's anemia by functional complementation. *Nature*, **356**, 760–6.

Svilvassy, S., and Cory, S. (1994) Efficient retroviral gene transfer to purified long-term repopulating hemopoietic stem cells. *Blood*, **84**, 74–83.

Terstappen, L.W., Huang, S., Safford, M., Lansdorp, P.M., and Loken, M.R. (1991) Sequential generations of hemopoietic colonies derived from single nonlineage-committed $CD34^+CD38^-$ progenitor cells. *Blood*, **77**, 1218–27.

Tsichlis, P.N. (1987) Oncogenesis by Moloney murine leukemia virus. *Anticancer Research*, **7**, 171–80.

Vanin, E.F., Kaloss, M., Brocius, C., and Nienhuis, A.W. (1994) Characterization of replication-competent retrovirus from nonhuman primates with virus-induced T-cell lymphomas and observations regarding the mechanism of oncogenesis. *Journal of Virology*, (in press).

Walsh, C.E., Liu, J.M., Young, N., Xiao, X., Nienhuis, A.W., and Samulski, R.J. (1992) Regulated high level expression of a human gamma-globin gene introduced into erythroid cells by a novel adeno-associated virus (AAV) vector. *Proceedings of the National Academy of Sciences of the United States of America*, **89**, 7257–61.

Walsh, C.E., Grompe, M., Vanin, E., et al. (1994) A functionally active retrovirus vector for gene therapy in Fanconi anemia group C. *Blood*, **84**, 453–9.

Wong, P.M., Chung, S.W., Dunbar, C.E., Bodine, D.M., Ruscetti, S., and Nienhuis, A.W. (1989) Retrovirus-mediated transfer and expression of the interleukin-3 gene in mouse hemopoietic cells result in a myeloproliferative disorder. *Molecular and Cellular Biology*, **9**, 798–808.

Wu, D. and Keating, A. (1993) Hemopoietic stem cells engraft in untreated transplant recipients. *Experimental Hematology*, **21**, 251–6.

Yoder, M.C., Kang, L.Y., Zhou, S.Z., Luo, F., and Srivastava, A. (1993) In vivo gene transfer in murine hemopoietic reconstituting stem cells mediated by the adeno-associated virus 2-based vectors. *Blood*, **82**, 1373.

22

Gene Therapy of Enzyme and Immune Deficiencies in the Hemopoietic System

JEFFREY A. MEDIN, MAKOTO MIGITA, AND
STEFAN KARLSSON

Research in gene therapy has focused largely on the development of gene-transfer strategies to correct inherited single-gene disorders, in particular enzyme deficiencies or immunodeficiencies. A variety of cells including differentiated blood cells, hepatocytes, endothelial cells, muscle cells, and fibroblasts have been studied as targets for gene therapy; however, as these cells have a limited life span, it is unlikely that a permanent cure for many diseases will be established using these target cells. In contrast, hemopoietic stem cells (HSC) are capable of self-renewal and are able to differentiate into all hemopoietic lineages, lymphoid and myeloid, throughout life. Therefore, HSC are ideal target cells for corrective gene therapy. In this chapter, the current progress in gene therapy of enzyme deficiencies and immunodeficiencies in the hemopoietic system is reviewed. Progress towards corrective gene transfer in various diseases is presented followed by a discussion of new approaches and developments in the gene-therapy field.

◼ RETROVIRAL TRANSDUCTION OF HEMOPOIETIC CELLS

Retroviral-mediated gene therapy for correction of human disease has been reviewed extensively (see Miller 1992; Mulligan 1993 and references therein). In addition, considerations important in gene transfer into hemopoietic cells have been discussed in detail (Karlsson 1991) and will not be duplicated here.

Figure 22.1 provides a schematic overview of the procedures used in clinical gene-therapy protocols that have been approved by the Recombinant DNA Advisory Committee (RAC). Patient cells are col-

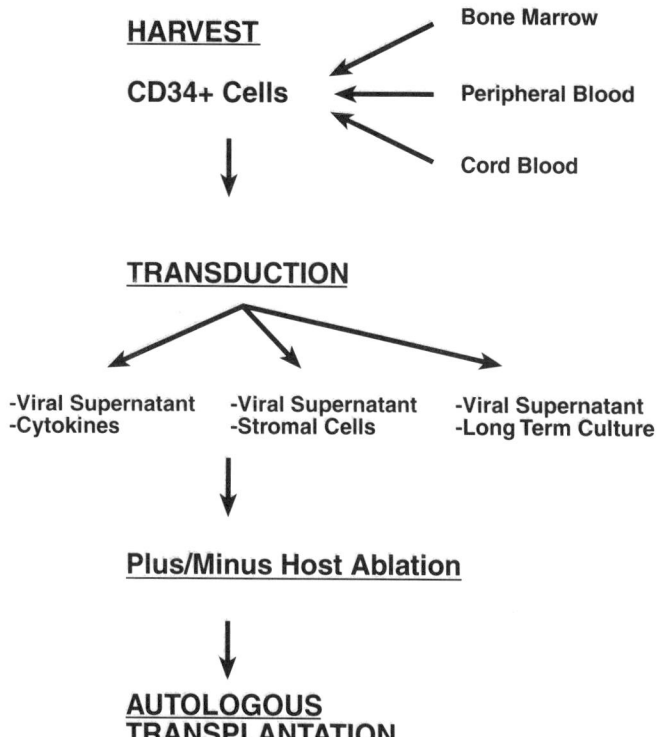

Figure 22.1 Transduction of human hemopoietic cells in various clinical protocols that have been approved by the RAC.

lected from bone marrow (BM), peripheral blood (PB), or cord blood (CB) and transduced with supernatants collected from expanded clones of high-titer amphotropic vector-producing cells. Various strategies including addition of cytokines and incubation with stromal support have been shown to enhance gene transfer into early progenitor cells and to expand the population of corrected cells. The transduced population is returned to the host that may or may not have been ablated before autologous transplantation of the cells.

Figure 22.2 diagrams the basic structures of retroviral vectors that have been found useful for transduction of murine HSC and for long-term expression in their progeny cells. The simplest vector (Fig. 22.2*A*) has the LN backbone (Miller and Rosman 1989) and uses the retroviral long terminal repeat (LTR) to drive expression of the neo R gene or a cDNA of interest (Correll et al. 1992). This vector also has internal splice donor and acceptor sites, but internal splicing of tran-

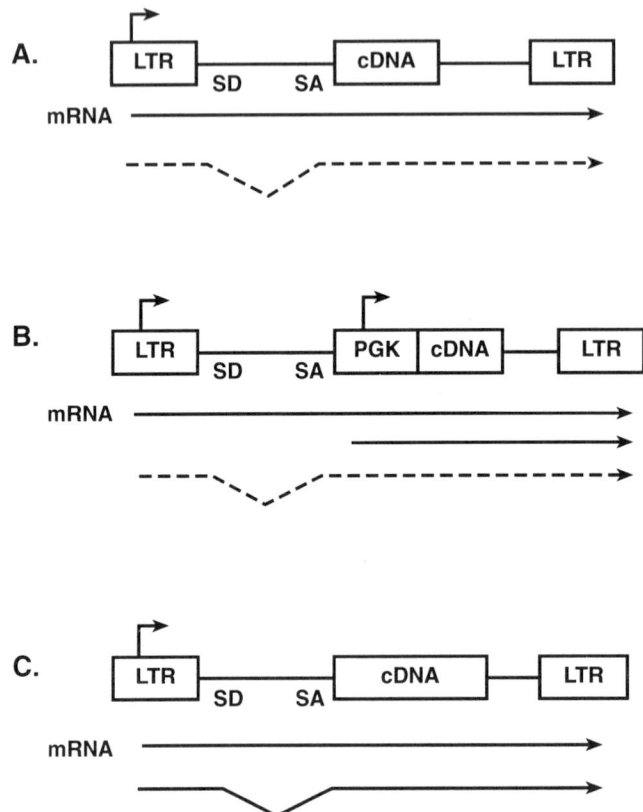

Figure 22.2 Examples of retroviral cDNA delivery vectors tested in the mouse. For details and references, see text. *A*, LN vector-derived constructs. *B*, This construct can have LN or other vector backbones. *C*, Vectors based on the MFG construct. LTR = long terminal repeat, PGK = human phosphoglycerate kinase internal promoter, SD/SA = splice donor, splice acceptor sites. The dotted lines in *A* and *B* demonstrate low levels of the spliced message.

scripts is often minimal. Many internal promoters, placed within the vector backbone to enhance expression of added cDNAs, have also been tested, but only one, the PGK promoter, has consistently given good expression levels in long-term reconstituted mice. Figure 22.2*B* shows an example of a vector with an internal promoter. These vectors can be based on the LN vector backbone (Correll, Colilla, and Karlsson 1994) or on another backbone derived in the laboratory of D.A. Williams (Lim, Williams, and Orkin 1987; Luskey et al. 1992).

The PGK promoter results in high-level expression, both by creating its own mRNA and by up-regulating the viral LTR (Correll et al. 1994). It has, however, proven to be a problem to isolate high-titer vectors containing the PGK promoter. Lastly, Figure 22.2C shows a schematic for vectors based on MFG, a vector designed in R. Mulligan's laboratory, that imitates the wild-type MMLV by adding the cDNA of interest directly at the ATG translation start site of the viral env gene (the added cDNA reading frame replaces the env sequence). This maintains the nature of wild-type splicing of the mRNA transcripts and these vectors have proven excellent for expression in long-term reconstituted mice (Ohashi et al. 1992).

■ PROGRESS TOWARDS GENE THERAPY OF HEMOPOIETIC CELLS

Many human single-gene disorders that have high associated morbidity and mortality without the availability of curative treatments have been suggested as candidates for gene therapy of hemopoietic cells. There are some fundamental requirements, however, for the application of corrective gene transfer into HSC (Karlsson 1991). The first obvious requirement is the identification and isolation of the disease-causing gene. Second, diseases should be selected that can be cured or in which symptoms can be dramatically improved by bone-marrow transplant (BMT), since gene therapy of HSC will require autologous BMT after transduction of the corrective factor. In addition, due to current shortcomings of the commonly used recombinant retroviral vector delivery systems (including low transduction efficiencies of human HSC and variable expression), candidate disorders in which low expression levels of the transgene would be expected to lead to a therapeutic effect should have preference (Karlsson 1991). For example, in adenosine deaminase deficiency (ADA), the prototype disorder for corrective gene transfer in the hemopoietic system, less than 10% of the enzyme activity of normal cells may be enough to ameliorate clinical symptoms (Blaese 1993a). In contrast, disorders like β-thalassemia or sickle cell anemia need very high levels of β-globin expression that are correctly balanced with α-globin levels. This may limit the overall effectiveness of this procedure (Karlsson 1991).

Preclinical studies for gene therapy of many disorders in the hemopoietic system have started and clinical protocols have been designed for a few conditions. Table 22.1 lists some of the current disease candidates and reports the status of each. In many diseases, correction of the defect has been shown in cells derived from patients.

Table 22.1. Gene Therapy for Hemopoietic Diseases

Disease	Target Cells	References
Diseases in which Successful Clinical Trials have Occurred		
1. ADA SCID	T-lymphocytes	Blaese 1993a
	CD34+ cells	Blaese et al. 1993b; Bordignon et al. 1994; Hoogerbrugge et al. 1994
Diseases where Gene Correction has Occurred		
In hemopoietic progenitor cells		
1. ADA SCID	Bone marrow cells	Hughes et al. 1989; Sutherland et al. 1989
2. Gaucher disease	Bone marrow cells	Fink et al. 1990, Nolta et al. 1992
	CD34+ cells	
3. LAD	Bone marrow cells	Yorifuji et al. 1993
4. CGD (p22-phox and gp91-phox)	CD34+ cells	Li et al. 1994
5. MPS type I (Hurler's syndrome)	Bone marrow and cord blood cells	Fairbairn et al. 1994[a]
In animal experiments		
1. ADA SCID	Murine	Lim et al. 1987; Kaleko et al. 1990
2. Gaucher's disease	Murine	Correll et al. 1992, 1994; Ohashi et al. 1992
3. LAD	Murine	Krauss et al. 1991
4. MLD	Murine	Learish and Barranger 1994[a]
5. β-Thalassemia	Murine	Dzierzak, Papayannopoulou, and Mulligan 1988; Karlsson et al. 1988; Bender, Gelinas, and Miller 1989
6. MPS type VI (Maroteaux-Lamy syndrome)	Feline	Fillat et al. 1994[a]

7. MPS type VII (Sly syndrome)	Murine	Wolfe et al. 1992
Patient cells in vitro		
1. ADA SCID	Lymphoid cell lines	Williams, Orkin, and Mulligan 1986
2. Gaucher's disease	Fibroblasts	Choudary et al. 1986; Fink et al. 1990
3. LAD	Lymphoid cell lines	Wilson et al. 1990
4. CGD (p22-phox, gp91-phox, and p47-phox)	Lymphoid cell lines	Cobbs et al. 1992; Li et al. 1994
5. PNP SCID	Fibroblasts	Osborne and Miller 1988
6. MLD	Fibroblasts	Rommerskirch et al. 1991; Ohashi et al. 1993
7. FA (complementation group C)	Lymphoid cell lines	Walsh et al. 1994a, b
8. Niemann-Pick disease type B	Fibroblasts	Suchi et al. 1992
9. MPS type I (Hurler's syndrome)	Fibroblasts	Anson et al. 1992a, b
10. MPS type II (Hunter's syndrome)	Lymphoid cell lines, fibroblasts	Bielicki et al. 1993; Braun et al. 1993
11. MPS type VI (Maroteaux-Lamy syndrome)	Fibroblasts	Peters et al. 1991
12. Fucosidosis	Fibroblasts	Occhiodoro et al. 1992
13. Paroxysmal nocturnal hemoglobinuria	Lymphoid cell lines	Flamm et al. 1994

[a]Presented at the September 1994 Cold Spring Harbor Meeting on Gene Therapy.
ADA SCID = adenosine deaminase severe combined immunodeficiency; LAD = leukocyte adhesion defi ciency; CGD = chronic granulomatous disease; MLD = metachromatic leukodystrophy; PND = purine nu cleoside phosphorylase; FA = Fanconi's anemia.

In some disorders, successful gene transfer has been demonstrated to cells of hemopoietic origin and, in a few cases, transfer has been demonstrated to murine HSC and human progenitor cells. Only a few clinical protocols have been initiated, most of them gene-marking studies, but many have been approved by the U.S. RAC and are being evaluated by the U.S. Food and Drug Administration (FDA).

■ ADENOSINE DEAMINASE DEFICIENCY

ADA deficiency is an autosomal recessive inherited disorder responsible for 15% to 25% of all cases of severe combined immunodeficiency (SCID) (Kredich and Hershfeld 1989). This is the first of the immunodeficiency diseases in which the disease-causing gene was identified and isolated (for review see Cournoyer and Caskey 1993; Culver and Blaese 1993). ADA catalyzes the conversion of adenosine and 2'-deoxyadenosine to inosine and 2'-deoxyinosine. The absence of functional ADA activity causes the accumulation of a toxic metabolite, deoxyadenosine triphosphate, in all cells, and this inhibits DNA synthesis and replication. The clinical effect, though, is manifested by very low numbers of T and B lymphocytes. Patients with ADA SCID present with repeated infections and usually die at an early age from a severe opportunistic infection. BMT (from a sibling source) can cure ADA SCID; however, only one-third of the patients have an HLA-identical donor (Kantoff, Freeman, and Anderson 1988). Infusions of red blood cells (RBC) (irradiated) have been used as a source of corrective ADA, but multiple infusions are necessary, with associated risks, and only limited correction has occurred (for review see Culver and Blaese 1993). Enzyme replacement therapy with bovine ADA linked to a polyethylene glycol carrier (PEG-ADA) has been successful (Polmar et al. 1976; Hershfield et al. 1987), but the replacement therapy is not a permanent cure and multiple injections are needed to maintain circulating levels of the enzyme at a high enough concentration to be clinically beneficial.

In view of the facts that replacement therapies exist to augment gene therapy, that overexpression of ADA is tolerated (Valentine et al. 1977), and that cells containing the corrective enzyme are likely to have a competitive advantage in vivo, ADA SCID was selected as the first model for the use of corrective gene therapy. In 1990, the first clinical trials of human gene therapy were started for ADA deficiency. The first protocols were attempts to transfer the recombinant ADA gene to collected PB T lymphocytes ex vivo using recombinant retroviruses as delivery vehicles. In order to harvest enough lymphocytes for gene therapy, the patients were treated with PEG-ADA to raise the number of lymphocytes and, in addition, PEG-ADA treatment has also continued following the gene transfer. Increases in enzymatic activity and overall immune function with multiple infusions of transduced T cells were seen in two patients (Blaese 1993a) for extended periods of analysis, and the patients have been able to live normal lives. Following this success, cells demonstrating high expression of the cell surface antigen (Ag) CD34 have been isolated and used as transfer target cells in an effort to enrich for more primitive progenitors and establish better long-term correction with fewer infusions (Blaese et al. 1993b). Currently, three infants diagnosed with ADA deficiency in utero were transplanted with retrovirally transduced autologous CB CD34$^+$ cells, and at least 12 months after transplantation gene expression in the progeny cells persists in multiple hemopoietic cell lineages (Blaese et al. 1994). Furthermore, two groups have recently transduced BM-derived CD34$^+$ cells with the corrective ADA enzyme cDNA (Bordignon et al. 1994; Hoogerbrugge et al. 1994).

■ GAUCHER'S DISEASE

Gaucher's disease (GD) is an autosomal recessive lysosomal storage disorder caused by a deficiency of the enzyme glucocerebrosidase (GC) (for review see Grabowski, Gatt, and Horowitz 1990; Beutler 1992). The disease is characterized by the accumulation of glucocerebroside in various tissues (Brady, Kanfer, and Shapiro 1965) due to the lack of enzyme-mediated catabolism to the products ceramide and glucose. Patients have an enlarged liver and spleen, are anemic, and some demonstrate frequent bone fractures. GD is usually classified into three types: type I (nonneuronopathic), type II (acute neuronopathic, death before the age of 2), and type III (subacute neuronopathic). The nervous system is intact in type I patients. This is the most common form and the best candidate for gene therapy of this group of disorders. BMT has been effective in correcting the systemic effects in type I GD (Hobbs et al. 1987), but matched donors are needed and complications associated with the ablation must be overcome. Genetic correction of the infantile neuronopathic type II form is not likely, since the patients are already severely affected at birth and gene transfer into neurons will be difficult to achieve. Some patients with type III GD (the Norbottnian type from Northern Sweden), who have had BMT, have also benefitted greatly both mentally and physically (Erikson et al. 1990), making this also a viable target disorder for corrective gene transfer into HSC.

The human GC gene has been transduced into murine BM stem cells and high levels of GC enzyme activity have been obtained in mouse macrophages from long-term reconstituted mice (Correll et al. 1992; Ohashi et al. 1992; Correll et al. 1994). The GC enzyme deficiency was corrected by gene transfer into GM-CFU progenitors (Fink et al. 1990) and in long-term culture-initiating cells (LTC-IC) from Gaucher patients by co-culture (Nolta et al. 1992) and by a supernatant transduction protocol (Xu et al. 1994). CD34$^+$ purified progenitor cells from PB were also transduced with high infection efficiency (Xu et al. 1994). Three clinical protocols for GD have been approved by the U.S. RAC and are currently awaiting U.S. FDA approval.

■ CHRONIC GRANULOMATOUS DISEASE

Chronic granulomatous disease (CGD) is a rare inherited disorder of blood phagocytes (for review see Gallin and Malech 1983; Curnutte 1993). Phagocytic cells from patients fail to produce superoxide and its additional microbicidal by-products hydrogen peroxide and hypochlorous acid. The oxidative agents are generated by a flavin-containing enzyme, NADPH oxidase, assembled at the cell membrane from four protein components. Patients with mutations in each component, gp91-phox, p22-phox, p67-phox, and p47-phox, have been identified. Mutations in gp91-phox are X-linked, whereas the others are autosomal recessive. Patients with CGD may show molecular heterogeneity, but the manifested clinical symptoms are similar (Clark et al. 1989). They show repeated and/or chronic life-threatening infections with granulomatous lesions in many organs. BMT has been successfully performed in this disease (Hobbs 1990) and cell lines have been established that carry each mutation. Retroviral-mediated gene transfer to these cell lines has occurred for the p47-phox, gp91-phox, and p22-phox defects (Cobbs et al. 1992; Porter et al. 1993; Li et al. 1994). In CGD the most important target cells are neutrophils whose life span is generally only hours or days (Culver and Blaese 1993), so it is necessary to transduce HSC with the therapeutic gene. Towards this goal, CD34$^+$ cells were isolated and transduced with retroviral vectors encoding p22-phox and gp91-phox (Li et al. 1994). CGD has a theoretical advantage in comparison with gene-transfer models based on other single-gene defects. Since the oxidase is a four-subunit complex, it is possible that overexpression, an issue not fully explored except in ADA SCID, of a sole component may be less detrimental to cells or organs than overexpression of a single-unit enzyme, since the functioning NADPH oxidase needs the assembly of all components to have activity. Thus, overproduction of a competent oxidase would be limited by the availability of the pool of other components and may be better tolerated.

■ FANCONI'S ANEMIA

Fanconi's anemia (FA) is an autosomal recessive disorder characterized by defective DNA repair and chromosomal instability (for review see dos Santos, Gavish, and Buchwald 1994; Liu et al. 1994). FA has been classified into four complementation groups from A to D, and the gene of the complementation group C (FACC) has recently been identified and isolated by functional complementation cloning (Strathdee, Duncan, and Shannon 1992). FACC mutations have been found to comprise about 15% of all FA patients (Whitney et al. 1993). Patients with FA clinically manifest progressive pancytopenia and physical abnormalities and have a pronounced predisposition to malignant diseases (Alter and Young 1993). At present, BMT has been thought to be the first choice for treatment if there is a histocompatible donor (Hobbs 1990), and in fact, successful BMT has been performed (Ebell, Friedrich, and Kohne 1989). FA cells show increased chromosomal breakage and have a high susceptibility to DNA cross-linking agents probably due to deficiencies in DNA repair mechanisms. Studies towards clinical gene therapy of FACC have been initiated only recently. Correction of a phenotype, in which FACC cells show hypersensitivity to a DNA cross-linking agent, has occurred in lymphoid cell lines derived from FACC patients. Both a recombinant retroviral vector (Walsh et al. 1994a) and a recombinant AAV vector have been used (Walsh et al. 1994b). The nature of the protein product and the expression pattern of the FACC gene itself has not been elucidated. Nonetheless, a clinical protocol to treat FACC patients by gene transfer with retroviral vectors has been approved by the RAC.

■ LEUKOCYTE ADHESION DEFICIENCY

Leukocyte adhesion deficiency (LAD) is an autosomal recessive disorder caused by a CD18 cell-surface marker subunit abnormality. Leukocyte adhesion molecules, LFA-1, Mac-1, and p150/95 are formed as dimers between CD18 and one of three CD11 subunits: CD11a, CD11b, and CD11c, respectively. Anomalies in these complexes result in an inability of leukocytes to migrate to sites of inflammation or infection (for review see Anderson and Springer 1987). BMT is reported to be a curative treatment (Hobbs 1990) even when the donor BM originates from HLA-nonidentical donors (three recipients were infection-free following BMT in all cases) (Le Deist et al. 1989). Cell-surface expression of CD18 and LFA-1 function itself can be restored to LAD patient lymphocytes by retroviral-mediated transfer of the CD18 molecule (Wilson et al. 1990). In addition, integration of recombinant retrovirus and expression of CD18 has been demonstrated in BM progenitor in long-term culture in cells obtained from patients with LAD (Yorifuji, Wilson, and Beaudet 1993), but to date studies have not been done using CD34$^+$ enriched cells.

■ METACHROMATIC LEUKODYSTROPHY

Metachromatic leukodystrophy (MLD) is a human autosomal recessive disorder caused by diminished ability of a lysosomal enzyme, arylsulphatase A (ASA) to catabolize galactosyl sulfatide and, to a lesser extent, lactosyl sulfatide (for review see Kolodny 1989). Patients with most forms of MLD present with abnormal lipid storage and demyelination in the central nervous system (CNS). There have been some reports that a "cross-correcting" function of BMT has improved CNS symptoms and ASA activity in PB (Hobbs 1990). BMT at early ages is recommended because after a certain degree of leukodystrophy is reached, the effects likely become irreversible (Hobbs 1990; Krivit et al. 1990). Successful transduction and expression of the ASA gene has been demonstrated in patient fibroblasts, again using retroviral vector delivery systems as a first model (Rommerskirch et al. 1991; Ohashi et al. 1993). The human ASA gene has recently been transferred into murine BM cells using a recombinant retroviral vector and high levels of human ASA enzyme activity have been demonstrated (Learish and Barranger 1994).

■ NIEMANN-PICK DISEASE

Niemann-Pick disease types A and B (sphingomyelin lipidoses) are inherited lysosomal-storage disorders caused by deficient activity of acid sphingomyelinase (ASM) (for review see Brady 1983). ASM catalyzes the breakdown of sphingomyelin to ceramide and phosphorylcholine. Patients with all types accumulate lipids, demonstrate hepatosplenomegaly, and have foam cells present in BM. Type-A patients demonstrate acute CNS symptoms and usually display a rapidly fatal course. Type-B patients have acute visceral anomalies but no CNS impairment. The differences in physiological effects between groups A and B seem to depend on the level of the enzyme activity (Graber, Salvayre, and Levade 1994). Although BMT with 100% engraftment does not correct the clinical course of type-A patients, in type-B patients BMT is known to be a curative treatment (Hobbs 1990). Retroviral-mediated gene transfer for these disorders has begun and the ASM activity of type A patient fibroblasts has been corrected with an observed concomitant decrease in lipid accumulation (Suchi et al. 1992).

■ PURINE NUCLEOSIDE PHOSPHORYLASE DEFICIENCY

Purine nucleoside phosphorylase (PNP) deficiency is an inherited autosomal recessive disorder accounting for approximately 4% of total SCID patients (for review see Markert 1991). The gene itself has been identified and isolated in 1983 (Goddard et al. 1983). PNP is involved in purine metabolism, catalyzing the conversion of inosine and guanosine into hypoxanthine and guanine. In a similar way to ADA deficiency, a toxic metabolite, deoxyguanosine triphosphate (dGTP), accumulates that likely inhibits DNA synthesis and cell division. Unlike ADA deficiency, however, B-cell function is relatively normal in most patients. Patients present with life-threatening infections, as in ADA SCID, but in PNP SCID two-thirds of the patients also have neurological disorders ranging from spasticity to mental retardation. These neurological complications may limit the overall effectiveness of PNP SCID correction by gene transfer into the hemopoietic system unless corrective measures are taken early before irreparable damage occurs. PNP SCID is also extremely rare, with 33 patients reported of whom 29 have died (Markert 1991). The success of BMT, the current treatment, has not been reported due to the limited number of patients. Efforts towards genetic correction of the deficiency had been started as early as in 1987 (McIvor et al. 1987), although limited success was seen. Patient fibroblasts have been corrected ex vivo for the enzyme defect with various retroviral constructs (Osborne and Miller 1988). A preclinical study of gene therapy using retroviral transfer into an in vitro genetic model of PNP deficiency, based on murine lymphoma cells, demonstrated a correction of the sensitivity to dGTP (Foresman, Nelson, and McIvor 1992).

■ FUTURE CANDIDATE DISEASES FOR CORRECTIVE GENE THERAPIES

Additional disorders that may be ameliorated in the future by transfer of a corrective function are listed in Table 22.2. In most cases, BMT has been shown to be beneficial, and work on isolation and characterization of the gene defect is in progress. Two major categories of common diseases in addition to the genetic diseases mentioned above are likely to become important candidates for gene therapy of hemopoietic cells. These are: (1) autoimmune diseases such as dia-

Table 22.2. Future Candidate Diseases

Disorder	Gene	BMT[a]
X-linked SCID	IL-2 receptor gamma chain (Ref: Noguchi et al. 1993)	+
X-linked hyper-IgM syndrome	CD40 ligand gene (Ref: Allen et al. 1993)	+
X-linked agammaglobulinemia	B-cell tyrosine kinase (Ref: Tsukada et al. 1993)	+
Wiscott-Aldrich syndrome	Unknown	+
Mucolipidosis II (I-cell disease)	Unknown	±
Adrenoleukodystrophy	Unknown	±
MPS IV (Morquio B)	Unknown	±
Ataxia telangiectasia	Unknown	Possibly
Mannosidosis	Unknown	Possibly

[a]+, successfully corrected; ±, partially corrected.

betes, systemic lupus erythematosus (SLE), or rheumatoid arthritis and (2) hemopoietic malignancies. Even though the molecular basis for most of these disorders is poorly understood, efforts have been initiated to develop gene therapy for these disorders, mostly by engineering immune functions to alter the state of the disease. It is beyond the scope of this chapter to discuss these approaches in detail (see review by Rosenberg 1992).

■ EFFORTS TO IMPROVE GENE TRANSFER INTO HEMOPOIETIC CELLS

Research in Hemopoiesis

The most commonly used retroviral-vector delivery systems, based on murine viruses, can introduce exogenous genes into mouse cells efficiently and stably. The efficiency, however, of delivery into human cells, especially into HSC, is relatively low. This could be due to absence or low expression of specific receptors with which the commonly used amphotropic virus constructs interact (Kavanaugh et al. 1994), but it is more likely due to the fact that these retroviral vectors need cell division for efficient integration (Miller, Adam, and Miller 1990). HSC are also rare and most are likely to be in G_0 phase and nondividing (Ogawa 1993). To overcome these disadvantages, various alternative approaches have been envisioned. One approach that is now becoming standard procedure is the enrichment of HSC before transduction by virus. A selectable surface Ag, CD34, has been described that enriches for early progenitors (for review see Silvestri et al. 1992). The selection of CD34$^+$ cells (see Chapters 11 and 12) by immunoaffinity purification allows an estimated 50-fold enrichment of HSC (Berenson et al. 1991). Enrichment of HSC for retroviral transduction of murine model HSC is less important, however, since retroviral transduction of mouse BM cells is very efficient without enrichment or purification. Nevertheless, techniques to purify and enrich murine HSC are much more advanced than those for the enrichment of human HSC. A sorting scheme (Szilvassy and Cory 1994) for low expression of Thy-1.2 Ag and high expression of H-2Kb and Ly6-A/E using a dual-laser fluorescence-activated cell sorting (FACS) device in the murine system has produced a population with both high-proliferative activity and long-term repopulation potential. Addition of this scheme to the sorting repertoire will allow more flexibility and possibly other benefits when a similar procedure is elucidated with human cells. Advances in purifying human HSC should lead to more efficient gene-transfer protocols for delivery into these cells.

Another approach to increase the efficiency of transduction is to attempt to maximize the self-renewal of hemopoietic stem cells and stimulate division of these cells using various kinds of growth factors (for review see Metcalf 1993) before and during retroviral infection. Combinations of interleukin-3 (IL-3), IL-6, and c-*kit* ligand have permitted the highest degree of gene-transfer efficiency into HSC (Bodine, Karlsson, and Nienhuis 1989; Nolta and Kohn 1990; Luskey et al. 1992; Crooks and Kohn 1993). Growth of human hemopoietic cells not only with soluble growth factors, but also with BM stroma cells (Moore et al. 1992; Nolta, Hanley, and Kohn 1994a) and extracellular matrix molecules (Moritz, Patel, and Williams 1994) enhances gene transfer into HSC. Nolta et al. (1994b) have reported increased gene-transfer efficiency of very primitive human progenitors that can repopulate BNX immunodeficient mice for 9 months or longer using stroma cell cultures.

Alternative sources to that of BM harvests of HSC exist. CD34[+] cells and HSC can also be obtained from PB (reviewed in Chapters 8 and 9) and CB. PB HSC are isolated by apheresis. From 1% to 4% of BM MNC are CD34[+], whereas only 0.02% to 0.05% of PB mononuclear cells (MNC) are CD34[+] (Serke et al. 1991). This population can be mobilized from the BM into the PB by chemotherapy or by growth factor treatment (GM-CSF, G-CSF, SCF) (Siena et al. 1991; Bodine et al. 1994; see also a review by Kessinger 1993). The great advantage of PB as a source of CD34[+] cells is the ease of the collection, that can be repeated many times if serial transduction manipulations are needed. An additional source of HSC, human CB, has been reported to contain many HSC cells (Broxmeyer et al. 1989; Abboud et al. 1992). HSC from CB are more efficiently transduced by retroviral-mediated gene transfer than adult BM cells (Moritz, Keller, and Williams 1993). In this study, introduced ADA was found to be expressed stably in progeny of LTC-IC derived from CB after 5 weeks in long-term culture. Although CB can be collected only once, it can be stored indefinitely after collection and may prove to be a promising source of cells for the correction of many genetic diseases, especially those where an in utero diagnosis has occurred or in populations where there is strong genetic predisposition to certain diseases.

A typical clinical gene transfer protocol for HSC is outlined in Figure 22.1. Cells are transduced ex vivo and then implanted into syngeneic or autologous hosts that have had marrow ablation. Marrow ablation is essential for effective engraftment, but serious complications, including fatalities from infection, can arise (for review see Armitage 1994). To avoid these risks in gene therapy, recent research has explored the feasibility of transplanting transduced hemopoietic cells into nonablated recipients. Easily detectable and unexpectedly high cell engraftment efficiencies have been reported in dogs after transfer of retrovirally marked cells (Bienzle et al. 1994). In addition, transfer of a therapeutically relevant gene (GC cDNA) into nonablated mice by repeated transplants of transduced cells has been performed and engraftment and expression of the transgene was seen in multiple tissues with no serious pathological effects observed in any recipient (Schiffmann et al. 1994).

Retroviral Vector Design Modifications

In tandem with research into general areas in hemopoiesis that directly affect gene therapy, much effort has been directed at improving transduction efficiencies and expression by improving retroviral vector-mediated gene delivery systems. One idea is to use recombinant vectors that have manifest selectability (i.e., vectors that allow transduced cells to be readily distinguished from nontransduced cells). Retroviral vectors incorporating the MDR protein allow for selective destruction of untransduced cells (Sorrentino et al. 1992) with various agents. The MDR protein is an efflux pump and selection can be done in vitro on transduced cells or in vivo after transplantation (Podda et al. 1992). CD34$^+$ cells have recently been transduced with constructs containing the MDR gene (Ward et al. 1994) and a therapeutic vector construct encoding the GC cDNA with the MDR protein has recently been made (Aran, Gottesman, and Pastan 1994), although vector transduction in that study was not demonstrated. The advantage of in vivo selection in this system is limited by the size of the MDR cloning sequence. When a second gene, in addition to the MDR cDNA, is added to the recombinant retroviral vector, the size of the derivative approaches the packaging limit and the titer of the dual system will likely be low.

Other strategies also allow selection of transduced cells. Cell-surface expression of polypeptides, built as components of recombinant retroviruses (Strair, Towle, and Smith 1988), can allow selection of transduced cell populations noninvasively by FACS, for example. Vectors have been designed that incorporate expression of small polypeptide surface Ag, human CD24 (Pawliuk et al. 1994) and the murine heat-stable antigen (HSA) (Conneally et al. 1994) to facilitate nontoxic selection of transduced hemopoietic cells. A selectable retroviral vector system for application to gene therapy for a specific disease has also been developed. High-titer, polycistronic retroviral vectors containing both the GC cDNA for the genetic correction of GD and selectable cell-surface Ag CD24 and HSA have been engineered (Medin et al. 1994; Migita et al. 1994). In these vectors, the therapeutic GC cDNA and CD24 or HSA were expressed in transduced target cells simultaneously, and, since the marker polypeptides are expressed on the cell surface and specific antibodies (Ab) exist, transduced cells could be sorted out specifically by FACS, or by other immunoselection methods. This system allows for the efficient selection of transduced cells and may be used for gene therapy for many genetic diseases by selecting transduced hemopoietic cells, and even cells of nonhemopoietic origin, prior to transplantation.

Pseudotyped vectors have recently been designed in an attempt to improve the transducibility of certain target cells or to broaden the host range (for review see Salmons and Gunzburg 1993). Pseudotyped vectors incorporate the genome of one virus into the envelope support of another. This allows the diverse properties of different viruses to be exploited. For example, pseudotyped MMLV vectors with a very broad host range have been generated using the vesicular stomatitis virus G glycoprotein (Burns et al. 1993). These vectors tolerate concentration procedures better than MMLV vectors, allowing the preparation of high-titer viral stocks. Vectors with xenotropic envelopes had been tested on human hemopoietic progenitor cells as early as 1988, but these initial efforts did not lead to higher transduction efficiencies compared with amphotropic vectors (Eglitis et al. 1988). Other pseudotyped viruses have been generated using gibbon ape leukemia virus (GALV) envelope proteins (Miller et al. 1991) and, for T-cell targeted delivery, human immunodeficiency virus (HIV) envelope proteins (Shimada et al. 1991). The GALV envelope protein is approximately twofold more efficient than the amphotropic envelope protein for targeting retroviral vectors to $CD34^+$ human hemopoietic progenitor cells because there may be more GALV receptors than amphotropic receptors on these cells. It remains to be seen whether the GALV envelope can subsequently improve transduction of HSC from humans or large out-bred animals. Investigations in which chimeric viral env proteins have been generated have recently been completed. The chimeric env proteins contain portions of the polypeptide erythropoietin (EPO) and retroviral transduction with these chimeras was increased in cells that express the EPO receptor (Kasahara, Dozy, and Kan 1994). As studies of HSC progress, it may be possible to define receptor/envelope combinations that lead to enhanced infectivity towards the earliest progenitors at transduction high efficiencies (for receptor review see Haywood 1994).

Manipulations of the proteins involved in viral assembly and integration may also lead to chimeric constructs with enhanced utility. Retroviruses of the lentivirus class (like HIV) are able to infect nondividing cells (Weinberg et al. 1991). A region in the HIV matrix protein p17 directs viral genome entry to the nucleus and allows expression in quiescent cells (Bukrinsky et al. 1993). Thus it is theoretically possible that murine leukemia viral proteins can be tailored to allow the same function. Initial studies have shown that complete exchange of HIV p17 for murine leukemia virus p15 protein allows formation of functional virus, but infectivity towards nondividing cells is not observed (Deminie and Emerman 1994). This initial attempt may be somewhat disappointing, although informative, and research into fine-tuning the amount of chimerism between these classes of retroviruses may eventually prove to be beneficial.

Future efforts in retroviral vector design will be directed towards affecting gene expression over long periods of time and only in selected cells once genomic integration of the virus has occurred. Silencing of murine retroviral LTR in progeny cells has been reported (see, e.g., Kaleko et al. 1990), with diminished expression of the transduced corrective enzyme, even though vector sequences are still present. This phenomenon has also been seen with therapeutic GC constructs and has been correlated with increased in vivo methylation of the LTR (Challita and Kohn 1994).

As retroviral integration events into host genomes become better understood, and the effects on expression of specific integration sites known, it will be possible to design vector backbones that create chromatin areas with increased or modulated transcription of the added therapeutic gene. It will also be possible to add tissue-specific elements or promoters that function only in desired cells or only in appropriate developmental milieus. Also, since retroviruses preferentially integrate into regions of DNA that are transcriptionally active or have open chromatin, there is always the potential that integration events can be deleterious to the host cell. Aberrant integration can shut down a necessary housekeeping gene, inactivate tumor-suppressing genes, or even drive overexpression of a tightly regulated protein, all with obvious and potentially drastic consequences.

Alternatives to Retroviral Gene Delivery Methods

The adeno-associated virus (AAV) system is also being explored as an alternative vehicle to recombinant retroviruses for gene transfer into hemopoietic cells (for review see Muzyczka 1992). AAV is a dependent parvovirus that is nonpathogenic and is prevalent in the human population. Advantages of AAV as a delivery vehicle include transduction of many types of human cells and the lack of any disease yet associated with infection. Wild-type AAV also preferentially integrates, by a mechanism still under study that may involve only the viral rep protein, into a specific region of 7 kb of DNA on human chromosome 19. It should be noted, however, that recombinant AAV constructs have not shown similar selectivity of integration.

Recombinant AAV virus vectors have been used to infect hemopoietic progenitor cells (Zhou et al. 1993) and marker expression has been demonstrated in murine myeloid and erythroid colonies. Expression of neomycin (as a marker) has also been demonstrated in progenitor cells derived from human CB (Zhou et al. 1994). AAV-mediated transfer into human hemopoietic progenitor cells, using β-galactosidase as a marker of infection, has also recently been demonstrated by another group (Goodman et al. 1994), thus confirming the utility of this direction of study for corrective gene transfer for human disorders.

It has been believed by some that rAAV integration into nondividing cells (Podsakoff et al. 1994b) offers a significant advantage over retroviral-mediated gene delivery, but recent studies have indicated that cell division, specifically cycling through S phase, may be necessary to get productive integration after all (Russell, Miller, and Alexander 1994). There are currently several additional shortcomings with the AAV vector system. No packaging cell lines are available to facilitate production of recombinant virus preparations totally free from possible helper virus contamination, and extremely high virus loads are necessary for the infection and genomic integration of a single cell (Russell et al. 1994). Furthermore, to date, no convincing experiments have been presented that demonstrate efficient transduction of HSC by AAV vectors. Some preliminary experiments have demonstrated marking of murine HSC by AAV vectors, but this has not been efficient (Podsakoff et al. 1994a). Future experiments will determine whether safe, high-titer AAV vectors can be developed for gene therapy of human HSC.

Corrective gene transfer based on recombinant adenovirus or herpes viruses have not been discussed, since these vectors do not normally integrate efficiently into genomic DNA and are therefore poor candidates for long-lasting therapeutic treatment of genetic disorders. These alternative gene delivery systems may be useful, though, for disorders that require temporary correction for only days or weeks such as some infectious diseases or as catalysts to boost or alter immune function of the host.

In the future, correction of enzyme-deficient stem cells may use nonviral delivery systems. For example, liposomes, encapsulating the DNA of interest in a lipid sphere, have been used in cell transfections in vitro for quite some time. Once the problem of efficient transportation of DNA from the cellular lysosome to the nucleus is solved, it may be possible to deliver the corrective gene to isolated stem cells ex vivo, supplying an integration function in *trans* (like the AAV rep protein), and direct efficient integration to a specific DNA region. This would eliminate any recombination events, however remote, that may produce helper virus or other deleterious effects.

■ CONCLUSION

Efficient gene transfer into murine HSC has been achieved and high-level expression of the transduced genes in their progeny cells has been demonstrated. Clinical gene-therapy protocols in humans have become a reality and will certainly become a more common treatment modality for inherited disorders in the future; however, the gene transfer efficiency of human HSC by retroviral-mediated transduction is still low, and expression levels of the transduced gene are variable. The accumulation of basic studies both on the biochemical mechanisms of metabolic diseases, on gene delivery systems, and on HSC will make gene therapy actually applicable to many life-threatening inherited disorders.

REFERENCES

Abboud, M., Wu, F., LaVia, M., and Laver, J. (1992) Study of early hemopoietic precursors in human cord blood. *Experimental Hematology*, **20**, 1043–7.
Allen, R.C., Armitage, R.J., Conley, M.E., et al. (1993) CD40 ligand gene defects responsible for X-linked hyper-IgM syndrome. *Science*, **259**, 990–3.
Alter, B. and Young, N.S. (1993) The bone failure syndromes. In D.G. Nathan and F.A. Oski (Eds.) *Hematology of infancy and childhood*, pp. 216–316, Philadelphia, W.B. Saunders Company.
Anderson, D.C. and Springer, T.A. (1987) Leukocyte adhesion deficiency: an inherited defect in the MAC-1, LFA-1, and p150,95 glycoproteins. *Annual Review of Medicine*, **38**, 175–94.
Anson, D.S., Bielicki, J., and Hopwood, J.J. (1992a) Correction of mucopolysaccharidosis type I fibroblasts by retroviral-mediated transfer of the human alpha-L-iduronidase gene. *Human Gene Therapy*, **3**, 371–9.
Anson, D.S., Taylor, J.A., Bielicki, J., et al. (1992b) Correction of human mucopolysaccharidosis type-VI fibroblasts with recombinant N-acetylgalactosamine-4-sulphatase. *Biochemistry Journal*, **284**, 789–94.
Aran, J.M., Gottesman, M.M., and Pastan, I. (1994) Drug-selected coexpression of human glucocerebrosidase and P-glycoprotein using a bicistronic vector. *Proceedings of the National Academy of Sciences of the United States of America*, **91**, 3176–80.
Armitage, J.O. (1994) Bone marrow transplantation. *New England Journal of Medicine*, **330**, 827–38.
Bender, M.A., Gelinas, R.E., and Miller, A.D. (1989) A majority of mice show long-term expression of a human b- globin gene after retrovirus transfer into hemopoietic cells. *Molecular and Cellular Biology*, **9**, 1426–34.

Berenson, R.J., Bensinger, W.I., Hill, R.S., et al. (1991) Engraftment after infusion of CD34⁺ marrow cells in patients with breast cancer or neuroblastoma. *Blood*, **77**, 1717–22.

Beutler, E. (1992) Gaucher disease: new molecular approaches to diagnosis and treatment. *Science*, **256**, 794–9.

Bielicki, J., Hopwood, J.J., Wilson, P.J., and Anson, D.S. (1993) Recombinant human iduronate-2-sulphatase: correction of mucopolysaccharidosis-type II fibroblasts and characterization of the purified enzyme. *Biochemistry Journal*, **289**, 241–6.

Bienzle, D., Abrams-Ogg, A.C., Kruth, S.A., et al. (1994) Gene transfer into hemopoietic stem cells: long-term maintenance of in vitro activated progenitors without marrow ablation. *Proceedings of the National Academy of Sciences of the United States of America*, **91**, 350–4.

Blaese, R.M. (1993a) Development of gene therapy for immunodeficiency: adenosine deaminase deficiency. *Pediatric Research*, **33**, S49–55.

Blaese, R.M., Culver, K.W., Chang, L., et al. (1993b) Treatment of severe combined immunodeficiency disease (SCID) due to adenosine deaminase deficiency with CD34⁺ selected autologous peripheral blood cells transduced with a human ADA gene. Amendment to clinical research project, Project 90-C-195, January 10, 1992. *Human Gene Therapy*, **4**, 521–7.

Blaese, R.M., Culver, K., Anderson, W.F., et al. (1994) Gene therapy for adenosine deaminase (ADA) deficiency: a 4 year follow-up of the original trial. (Abstract from *Cold Spring Harbor Sept. 1994 Meeting on Gene Therapy*.)

Bodine, D.M., Karlsson. S., and Nienhuis, A.W. (1989) Combination of interleukin 3 and 6 preserves stem cell function in culture and enhances retrovirus-mediated gene transfer into hemopoietic stem cells. *Proceedings of the National Academy of Sciences of the United States of America*, **86**, 8897–902.

Bodine, D.M., Seidel, N.E., Gale, M.S., Nienhuis, A.W., and Orlic, D. (1994) Efficient retrovirus transduction of mouse pluripotent hemopoietic stem cells mobilized into the peripheral blood by treatment with granulocyte colony-stimulating factor and stem cell factor. *Blood*, **84**, 1482–91.

Bordignon, C., Serrida, P., Notarangelo, L.D., et al. (1994) Long-term immune reconstitution following human somatic cell gene therapy in two patients affected by ADA deficient SCID. *Blood*, **84**, 402a.

Brady, R.O. (1983) Sphingolmyelin lipidosises; Niemann-Pick Disease. In J.B. Stanbury, J.B. Wyngarden, D.S. Fredrickson, J.L. Goldstein, and M.S. Brown (Eds.) *The metabolic basis of inherited diseases*, pp. 831–41, New York, McGraw-Hill.

Brady, R.O., Kanfer, J.N., and Shapiro, D. (1965) Metabolism of glucocerebrosides: evidence of an enzymatic deficiency in Gaucher's disease. *Biochemical and Biophysical Research Communications*, **18**, 221–5.

Braun, S.E., Aronovich, E.L., Anderson, R A., Crotty, P.L., McIvor, R.S., and Whitley, C.B. (1993) Metabolic correction and cross-correction to mucopolysaccharidosis type 2 (Hunter syndrome) by retroviral-mediated gene transfer and expression of human iduronate-2-sulfatase. *Proceedings of the National Academy of Sciences of the United States of America*, **90**, 11830–4.

Broxmeyer, H.E., Douglas, G.W., Hangoc, G., et al. (1989) Human umbilical cord blood as a potential source of transplantable hemopoietic stem/progenitor cells. *Proceedings of the National Academy of Sciences of the United States of America*, **86**, 3828–32.

Bukrinsky, M.I., Haggerty, S., Dempsey, M.P., et al. (1993) A nuclear localization signal within HIV-1 matrix protein that governs infection in non-dividing cells. *Nature*, **365**, 666–9.

Burns, J.C., Friedmann, T., Driever, W., Burrascano, M., and Yee, J.-K. (1993) Vesticular stomatitis virus G glycoprotein pseudotyped retroviral vectors: concentration to very high titer and efficient gene transfer into mammalian and nonmammalian cells. *Proceedings of the National Academy of Sciences of the United States of America*, **90**, 8033–7.

Challita, P.-M. and Kohn, D.B. (1994) Lack of expression from a retroviral vector after transduction of murine hemopoietic stem cells is associated with methylation in vivo. *Proceedings of the National Academy of Sciences of the United States of America*, **91**, 2567–71.

Choudary, P.V., Barranger, J.A., Tsuji, S., et al. (1986) Retrovirus-mediated transfer of the human glucocerebrosidase gene to Gaucher fibroblasts. *Molecular Biology and Medicine*, **3**, 293–9.

Clark, R.A., Malech, H.L., Gallin, J.I., et al. (1989) Genetic variants of chronic granulomatous disease: prevalence of deficiencies of two cytocomponents of NADPH oxidase system. *New England Journal of Medicine*, **321**, 647–52.

Cobbs, C.S., Malech, H.L., Leto, T.L., et al. (1992) Retroviral expression of recombinant p47phox protein by Epstein-Barr virus-transformed B lymphocytes from a patient with autosomal chronic granulomatous disease. *Blood*, **79**, 1829–35.

Conneally, E., Bardy, P., Chappel, S., Eaves, C.J., and Humphries, R.K. (1994) Expression of murine heat stable antigen on human hemopoietic cells as a marker of retroviral infection. *Blood*, **84**, 414a.

Correll, P.H., Colilla, S., Dave, H.P., and Karlsson, S. (1992) High levels of human glucocerebrosidase activity in macrophages of long-term reconstituted mice after retroviral infection of hemopoietic stem cells. *Blood*, **80**, 331–6.

Correll, P.H., Colilla, S., and Karlsson, S. (1994) Retroviral vector design for long-term expression in murine hemopoietic cells in vivo. *Blood*, **84**, 1812–22.

Cournoyer, D. and Caskey, C.T. (1993) Gene therapy of the immune system. *Annual Review of Immunology*, **11**, 297–329.

Crooks, G.M. and Kohn, D.B. (1993) Growth factors increase amphotropic retrovirus binding to human CD34$^+$ bone marrow progenitor cells. *Blood*, **82**, 3290–7.

Culver, C.W. and Blaese, R.M. (1993) Gene therapy for immunodeficiency disease. In S. Gupta and C. Griscelli (Eds.) *New concepts in immunodeficiency disease*, pp. 427–56, Chichester, NY, John Wiley & Sons Ltd.

Curnutte, J.T. (1993) Chronic granulomatous disease: the solving of a clinical riddle at the molecular level. *Clinical Immunology and Immunopathology*, **67**, S2.

Deminie, C.A. and Emerman, M. (1994) Functional exchange of an oncoretrovirus and a lentivirus matrix protein. *Journal of Virology*, **68**, 4442–9.

dos Santos, C.C., Gavish, H., and Buchwald, M. (1994) Fanconi anemia revisited: old ideas and new advances. *Stem Cells*, **12**, 142–53.

Dzierzak, E.A., Papayannopoulou, T., and Mulligan, R.C. (1988) Lineage-specific expression of a human beta-globin gene in murine bone marrow transplant recipients reconstituted with retrovirus-transduced stem cells. *Nature*, **331**, 35–41.

Ebell, W., Friedrich, W., and Kohne, E. (1989) Therapeutic aspects of Fanconi anaemia. In T.M. Schroeder-Kuth, A.D. Auerbach, and G. Obe (Eds.) *Fanconi anaemia: clinical, cytogenetic, and experimental aspects*, pp. 47–59. Berlin, Springer-Verlag.

Eglitis, M.A., Kohn, O.E., Moen, I.C., Blaese, R.M., and Anderson, W.F. (1988) Infection of human hemopoietic progenitor cells using a retroviral vector with a xenotropic pseudotype. *Biochemical and Biophysical Research Communications*, **151**, 201–6.

Erikson, A., Groth, C.G., Mansson, J.E., Percy, A., Ringden, O., and Svennerholm, L. (1990) Clinical and biochemical outcome of marrow transplantation for Gaucher disease of the Norrbottnian type. *Acta Paediatrica Scandinavica*, **79**, 680–5.

Fairbairn, L.J., Spooncer, E., McDermott, R.H., et al. (1994) Correction of alpha-L-iduronidase deficiency in vitro by retroviral gene transfer into hemopoietic cells from patients with Hurlers syndrome. (Abstract from *Cold Spring Harbor Sept. 1994 Meeting on Gene Therapy*.)

Fillat, C., Haskins, M.E., Yeyati, P., Abkowitz, J.L., Desnick, R.J., and Schuchman, E.H. (1994) Towards gene therapy for mucopolysaccharidosis type VI: metabolic correction of MPS VI cells by retroviral mediated gene transfer. (Abstract from *Cold Spring Harbor Sept. 1994 Meeting on Gene Therapy*.)

Fink, J.K., Correll, P.H., Perry, L.K., Brady, R.O., and Karlsson, S. (1990) Correction of glucocerebrosidase deficiency after retroviral-mediated gene transfer into hemopoietic progenitor cells from patients with Gaucher disease. *Proceedings of the National Academy of Sciences of the United States of America*, **87**, 2334–8.

Flamm, M., Richardson, C., Ward, M., and Bank, A. (1994) Retroviral gene transfer in paroxysmal nocturnal hemoglobinuria. *Blood*, **84**, 360a.

Foresman, M.D., Nelson, D.M., and McIvor, R.S. (1992) Correction of purine nucleoside phosphorylase deficiency by retroviral-mediated gene transfer in mouse S49 T cell lymphoma: a model for gene therapy of T cell immunodeficiency. *Human Gene Therapy*, **3**, 625–31.

Gallin, J.I. and Malech, H.L. (1983) Update on chronic granulomatous disease of childhood. *Journal of the American Medical Association*, **263**, 1533–7.

Goddard, J.M., Caput, D., Willlams, S.R., and Martin, D.W. (1983) Cloning of human purine nucleoside phosphorylase cDNA sequences by complement in *Escherichia coli*. *Proceedings of the National Academy of Sciences of the United States of America*, **80**, 4281–5.

Goodman, S., Xiao, X., Donahue, R.E., et al. (1994) Recombinant adeno-associated virus-mediated gene transfer into hemopoietic progenitor cells. *Blood*, **84**, 1492–500.

Graber, D., Salvayre, R., and Levade, T. (1994) Accurate differentiation of the neuronopathic and nonneuronopathic forms of Niemann-Pick disease by evaluation of the effective residual lysosomal sphingomyelinase activity in intact cells. *Journal of Neurochemistry*, **63**, 1060–8.

Grabowski, G.A., Gatt, S., and Horowitz, M. (1990) Acid β-glucosidase: enzymology and molecular biology of Gaucher disease. *Critical Reviews in Biochemistry and Molecular Biology*, **25**, 385–414.

Haywood, A.M. (1994) Virus receptors: binding, adhesion strengthening, and changes in viral structure. *Journal of Virology*, **68**, 1–5.

Hershfield, M.S., Buckley, R.H., Greenburg, M.L., et al. (1987) Treatment of adenosine deaminase deficiency with polyethylene glycol-modified adenosine deaminase. *New England Journal of Medicine*, **16**, 589–96.

Hobbs, J.R., Hugh, K., Shaw, P.J., Lindsay, I., and Hancock, M. (1987) Beneficial effect of pre-transplant splenectomy on displacement bone marrow transplantation for Gaucher's syndrome. *Lancet*, **1**, 1111–5.

Hobbs, J.R. (1990) Displacement bone marrow transplantation for some inborn errors. *Journal of Inherited Metabolic Disease*, **13**, 572–6.

Hoogerbrugge, P.M., Beusechem, V., Valerio, D., et al. (1994) Gene therapy in 3 children with adenosine deaminase deficiency. *Blood*, **84**, 402a.

Hughes, P.F., Eaves, C.J., Hogge, D.E., and Humphries, R.K. (1989) High-efficiency gene transfer to human hemopoietic cells maintained in long-term marrow culture. *Blood*, **74**, 1915–22.

Kaleko, M., Garcia, J.V., Osborne, W.R., and Miller, A.D. (1990) Expression of human adenosine deaminase in mice after transplantation of genetically-modified bone marrow. *Blood*, **75**, 1733–41.

Kantoff, P.W., Freeman, S.M., and Anderson, W.F. (1988) Prospects for gene therapy for immunodeficiency diseases. *Annual Review of Immunology*, **6**, 581–94.

Karlsson, S., Bodine, D.M., Perry, L., Papayannopoulou, T., and Nienhuis, A.W. (1988) Expression on the human β-globin gene following retroviral-mediated transfer into multipotential hemopoietic progenitors of mice. *Proceedings of the National Academy of Sciences of the United States of America*, **85**, 6062–5.

Karlsson, S. (1991) Treatment of genetic defects in hemopoietic cell function by gene transfer. *Blood*, **78**, 2481–92.

Kasahara, N., Dozy, A.M., and Kan, Y.W. (1994) Tissue-specific targeting of retroviral vectors through ligand-receptor interactions. *Science*, **266**, 1373–6.

Kavanaugh, M.P., Miller, D.P., Zhang, W., et al. (1994) Cell-surface receptors for gibbon ape leukemia virus and amphotropic murine retrovirus are inducible sodium-dependent phosphate symporters. *Proceedings of the National Academy of Sciences of the United States of America*, **91**, 7071–5.

Kessinger, A. (1993) Is blood or bone marrow better? *Stem Cells*, **11**, 290–5.

Kolodny, E.H. (1989) Metachromatic leukodystrophy and multiple sulfatase deficiency: sulfatide lipidosis. In C.R. Scriver, A.L. Beaudet, W.S. Sly, and D. Valle (Eds.) *Metabolic basis of inherited disease*, 6th ed., pp. 1721–50, New York, McGraw-Hill.

Krauss, J.C., Mayo-Bond, L.A., Rogers, C.E., Weber, K.L., Todd R.F., III, and Wilson, J.M. (1991) An in vivo animal model of gene therapy for leukocyte adhesion deficiency. *Journal of Clinical Investigation*, **88**, 1412–7.

Kredich, N.M. and Hersfield, M.S. (1989) Immunodeficiency diseases caused by adenosine deaminase deficiency and purine nucleoside phosphorylase deficiency. In C.R. Scriver, A.L. Beaudet, W.S. Sly, and D. Valle (Eds.) *Metabolic basis of inherited disease*, 6th ed., pp. 1045–75, New York, McGraw-Hill.

Krivit, W., Shapiro, E., Kennedy, W., et al. (1990) Treatment of late infantile metachromatic leukodystrophy by bone marrow transplantation. *New England Journal of Medicine*, **322**, 28–32.

Learish, R. and Barranger, J.A. (1994) Transduction by a retroviral vector containing the arylsulfatase A gene and transplantation of mouse bone marrow. (Abstract from *Cold Spring Harbor Sept. 1994 Meeting on Gene Therapy*.)

Le Deist, F., Blanche, S., Keable, H., et al. (1989) Successful HLA nonidentical bone marrow transplantation in 3 patients with the leukocyte adhesion deficiency. *Blood*, **74**, 512–6.

Li, F., Linton, G.F., Sekhsaria, S., et al. (1994) CD34$^+$ peripheral blood progenitors as a target for genetic correction of the two flavocytochrome b$_{558}$ defective forms of chronic granulomatous disease. *Blood*, **84**, 530–8.

Lim, B., Williams, D.A., and Orkin, S.H. (1987) Retrovirus-mediated gene transfer of human adenosine deaminase: expression of functional enzyme in murine hemopoietic stem cells in vivo. *Molecular and Cellular Biology*, **7**, 3459–65.

Liu, J.M., Buchwald, M., Walsh, C.E., and Young, N.S. (1994) Fanconi anemia and novel strategies for therapy. *Blood*, **84**, 3995–4007.

Luskey, B.D., Rosenblatt, M., Zsebo, K., and Williams, D.A. (1992) Stem cell factor, interleukin-3, and interleukin-6 promote retroviral mediated gene transfer into murine hemopoietic stem cells. *Blood*, **80**, 396–402.

Markert, M.L. (1991) Purine nucleoside phosphorylase deficiency. *Immunodeficiency Review*, **3**, 45–81.

McIvor, R.S., Johnson, M.J., Miller, A.D., et al. (1987) Human purine nucleoside phosphorylase and adenosine deaminase: gene transfer into cultured cells and murine hemopoietic stem cells by using recombinant amphotropic retroviruses. *Molecular and Cellular Biology*, **7**, 838–46.

Medin, J.A., Migita, M., Pawliuk, R., et al. (1994) Correction of the metabolic deficiency in Gaucher's disease using a bicistronic retroviral vector that allows selection of transduced cells. *Blood*, **84**, 356a.

Metcalf, D. (1993) Hemopoietic regulators: redundancy or subtlety? *Blood*, **82**, 3515–23.

Migita, M., Medin, J.A., Pawliuk, R., et al. (1994) The enzyme deficiency in Gaucher fibroblasts is corrected by retroviral vectors containing the genes for glucocerebrosidase gene and the selectable cell surface antigen, CD24. *Blood*, **84**, 357a.

Miller, A.D. and Rosman, G.I. (1989) Improved retroviral vectors for gene transfer and expression. *Biotechniques*, **7**, 980–90.

Miller, D.G., Adam, M.A., and Miller, A.D. (1990) Gene transfer by retrovirus vectors occurs only in cells that are actively replicating at the time of infection. *Molecular and Cellular Biology*, **10**, 4239–42.

Miller, A.D., Garcia, J.V., von Suhr, N., Lynch, C.M., Wilson, C., and Eiden, M.V. (1991) Construction and properties of retrovirus packaging cells based on gibbon ape leukemia virus. *Journal of Virology*, **65**, 2220–4.

Miller, A.D. (1992) Human gene therapy comes of age. *Nature*, **357**, 455–60.

Moore, K.A., Deisseroth, A.B., Reading, C.L., Williams, D.E., and Belmont, J.W. (1992) Stromal support enhances cell-free retroviral vector transduction of human bone marrow long term culture-initiating cells. *Blood*, **79**, 1393–9.

Moritz T., Keller D.C., and Williams, D.A. (1993) Human cord blood cells as targets for gene transfer: potential use in genetic therapies of severe combined immunodeficiency disease. *Journal of Experimental Medicine*, **178**, 529–36.

Moritz, T., Patel, V.P., and Williams, D. (1994) Bone marrow extracellular matrix molecules improve gene transfer into human hemopoietic cells via retroviral vectors. *Journal of Clinical Investigation*, **93**, 1451–7.

Mulligan, R.C. (1993) The basic science of gene therapy. *Science*, **260**, 926–32.

Muzyczka, N. (1992) Use of adeno-associated virus as a general transduction vector for mammalian cells. *Current Topics in Microbiology and Immunology*, **158**, 97–127.

Noguchi, M., Huafang, Y., Rosenblatt, H.M., et al. (1993) Interleukin-2 receptor gamma chain mutation results in X-linked severe combined immunodeficiency in humans. *Cell*, **73**, 147–57.

Nolta, J.A. and Kohn, D.B. (1990) Comparison of the effects of growth factors on retroviral vector-mediated gene transfer and the proliferative status of human hemopoietic progenitor cells. *Human Gene Therapy*, **1**, 257–63.

Nolta. J.A., Yu. X.J., Bahner, I., and Kohn, D.B. (1992) Retroviral mediated transfer of the human glucocerebrosidase gene into cultured Gaucher bone marrow. *Journal of Clinical Investigation*, **90**, 342–8.

Nolta, J.A., Hanley, M.B., and Kohn, D.B. (1994a) Sustained human hemopoiesis in immunodeficient mice by cotransplantation of marrow stroma expressing human IL-3: analysis of gene transduction of long-lived progenitors. *Blood*, **83**, 3041–51.

Nolta, J.A., Smogorzewska, E.M., and Kohn, D.B. (1994b) Late graft failure in immunodeficient mice by human CD34$^+$ progenitors transduced in the absence of stromal support. *Blood*, **84**, 343a.

Occhiodoro, T., Hopwood, J.J., Morris, C.P., and Anson, D.S. (1992) Correction of α-L-fucosidase deficiency in fucosidosis fibroblasts by retroviral vector-mediated gene transfer. *Human Gene Therapy*, **3**, 365–9.

Ogawa, M. (1993) Differentiation and proliferation of hemopoietic stem cells. *Blood*, **81**, 2844–53.

Ohashi, T., Boggs, S., Robbins, P., et al. (1992) Efficient transfer and sustained high expression of the human glucocerebrosidase gene in mice and their functional macrophages following transplantation of bone marrow transduced by a retroviral vector. *Proceedings of the National Academy of Sciences of the United States of America*, **89**, 11332–6.

Ohashi, T., Eto, Y., Learish, R., and Barranger, J.A. (1993) Correction of enzyme deficiency in metachromatic leukodystrophy fibroblasts by retroviral-mediated transfer of the human arylsulphtase A gene. *Journal of Inherited Metabolic Disease*, **16**, 881–5.

Osborne, W.R. and Miller, A.D. (1988) Design of vectors for efficient expression of human purine nucleoside phosphorylase in skin fibroblasts from enzyme-deficient humans. *Proceedings of the National Academy of Sciences of the United States of America*, **85**, 6851–5.

Pawliuk, R., Kay, R., Lansdorp, P., and Humphries, R.K. (1994) Selection of retrovirally transduced hemopoietic cells using CD24 as a marker of gene transfer. *Blood*, **84**, 2868–77.

Peters, C., Rommerskirch, W., Modaressi, S., and von Figura, K. (1991) Restoration of arylsulphatase B activity in human mucopolysaccharidosis-type-VI fibroblasts by retroviral-vector-mediated gene transfer. *Biochemistry Journal*, **276**, 499–504.

Podda, S., Ward, M., Himelstein, et al. (1992) Transfer and expression of the human multiple drug resistance gene into live mice. *Proceedings of the National Academy of Sciences of the United States of America*, **89**, 9676–80.

Podsakoff, G., Shaughnessy, E.A., Lu, D., Wong, K.K., and Chatterjee, S. (1994a) Long term in vivo reconstitution with murine marrow cells transduced with an adeno-associated virus vector. *Blood*, **84**, 256a.

Podsakoff, G., Wong, K.K., and Chatterjee, S. (1994b) Efficient gene transfer into nondividing cells by adeno-associated virus-based vectors. *Journal of Virology*, **68**, 5656–66.

Polmar, S.H., Stern, R.C., Schwartz, A.L., Wetzler, E.M., Chase, P.A., and Hirschhorn, R. (1976) Enzyme replacement therapy for adenosine deaminase deficiency and severe combined immunodeflciency. *New England Journal of Medicine*, **295**, 1337–43.

Porter, C.D., Parkar, M.H., Levinsky, R.J., Collins, M.K., and Kinnon, C. (1993) X-linked chronic granulomatous desease: correction of NAPDPH oxidase defect by retrovirus-mediated expression of gp91-phox. *Blood*, **82**, 2196–202.

Rommerskirch, W., Fluharty, A.L., Perters, C., von Figura, K., and Gieselmann, V. (1991) Restoration of arylsulphatase A activity in human-metachromatic leukodystrophy fibroblasts via retrovial-vector-mediated gene transfer. *Biochemistry Journal*, **280**, 459–61.

Rosenberg, S. (1992) The immunotherapy and gene therapy of cancer. *Journal of Clinical Oncology*, **10**, 180–99.

Russell, D.W., Miller, A.D., and Alexander, I. (1994) Adeno-associated virus vectors preferentially transduce cells in S phase. *Proceedings of the National Academy of Sciences of the United States of America*, **91**, 8915–9.

Salmons, B. and Gunzburg, W.H. (1993) Targeting of retroviral vectors for gene therapy. *Human Gene Therapy*, **4**, 129–41.

Schiffmann, R., Medin, J.A., Ward, J.M., Stahl, S., Cottler-Fox, M., and Karlsson, S. (1994) Transfer of the human glucocerebrosidase gene into hemopoietic stem cells of nonablated mice. *Blood*, **84**, 401a.

Serke, S., Sauberlich, S., Abe, Y., and Huhn, D. (1991) Analysis of CD34-positive hemopoietic progenitor cells from normal adult peripheral blood; flow cytometrical studies and in-vitro colony (CFU-GM, BFU-E) assays. *Annals of Hematology*, **62**, 45–53.

Shimada, T., Fujii, H., Mitsuga, H., and Nienhuis, A.W. (1991) Targeted and highly efficient gene transfer into CD4$^+$ cells by a recombinant human immunodeficiency virus retroviral vector. *Journal of Clinical Investigation*, **88**, 1043–7.

Siena, S., Bregni, M., Brando, B., et al. (1991) Flow cytometry for clinical estimation of circulating hemopoietic progenitors for autologous transplantation in cancer patients. *Blood*, **77**, 400–9.

Silvestri, F., Banavali, S., Baccarani, M., and Preissler, H.D. (1992) The CD34 hemopoietic progenitor cell associated antigen: biology and clinical applications. *Haematologica*, **77**, 265–72.

Sorrentino, B.P., Brandt, S.J., Bodine, D., et al. (1992) Selection of drug-resistant bone marrow cells in vivo after retroviral transfer of human MDR1. *Science*, **257**, 99–103.

Strair, R.K., Towle, M.J., and Smith, B.R. (1988) Recombinant retroviruses encoding cell surface antigens as selectable markers. *Journal of Virology*, **62**, 4756–9.

Strathdee, C.A., Duncan, A.M., and Shannon, M. (1992) Cloning of cDNA for Fanconi's anemia by functional complementation. *Nature*, **356**, 763–76.

Suchi, M., Dinur, T., Desnick, R.J., et al. (1992) Retroviral-mediated transfer of the human acid sphingomyelinase cDNA: correction of the metabolic defect in cultured Niemann-Pick disease cells. *Proceedings of the National Academy of Sciences of the United States of America*, **15**, 3227–31.

Sutherland, H.J., Eaves, C.J., Eaves, A.C., Dragowska, W., and Lansdorp, P.M. (1989) Characterization and partial purification of human marrow cells capable of initiating long-term hemopoiesis in vitro. *Blood*, **74**, 1563–70.

Szilvassy, S.J. and Cory, S. (1994) Efficient retroviral gene transfer to purified long-term repopulating hemopoietic stem cells. *Blood*, **84**, 74–83.

Tsukada, S., Saffran, D.C., Rawlings, D.J., et al. (1993) Deficient expression of a B cell cytoplasmic tyrosine kinase in human X-linked agammaglobinemia. *Cell*, **72**, 279–90.

Valentine, W.N., Paglia, D.E., Tartaglia, A.P., and Gilsanz, F. (1977) Hereditary hemolytic anemia with increased adenosine deaminase (45–70 fold) and decreased adenosine triphosphates. *Science*, **195**, 783–5.

Walsh, C.E., Grompe, M., Vanin, E., et al. (1994a) A functionally active retroviral vector for gene therapy in Fanconi anemia group C. *Blood*, **84**, 453–9.

Walsh, C.E., Nienhuis, A.W., Samulski, R.J., et al. (1994b) Phenotypical correction of Fanconi anemia in human hemopoietic cells with a recombinant adeno-associated virus vector. *Journal of Clinical Investigation*, **94**, 1440–8.

Ward, M., Richardson, C., Pioli, P., et al. (1994) Transfer and expression of the human multiple drug resistance gene in human CD34$^+$ cells. *Blood*, **84**, 1408–14.

Weinberg, J.B., Matthews, T.J., Cullen, B.R., and Malim, M.H. (1991) Productive human immunodeficiency virus type 1 (HIV-1) infection of nonproliferating human monocytes. *Journal of Experimental Medicine*, **174**, 1477–82.

Whitney, M.A., Saito, H., Jakobs, P.M., Gibson, R.A., Moses, R.E., and Grompe, M. (1993) A common mutation in the FACC gene causes Fanconi anaemia in Ashkenazi Jews. *Nature Genetics*, **4**, 202–5.

Williams, D.A., Orkin, S.H., and Mulligan, R.C. (1986) Retrovirus-mediated transfer of human adenosine deaminase gene sequences into cells in culture and into murine hemopoietic cells in vivo. *Proceedings of the National Academy of Sciences of the United States of America*, **83**, 2566–70.

Wilson, J.M., Ping, A.J., Krauss, J.C., et al. (1990) Correction of CD18-deficient lymphocytes by retrovirus-mediated gene transfer. *Science*, **248**, 1413–16.

Wolfe, J.H., Sands, M.S., Barker, J.E., et al. (1992) Reversal of pathology in murine mucopolysaccharidosis type VII by somatic cell gene transfer. *Nature*, **360**, 749–53.

Xu, L., Stahl, S.K., Dave, H.P., et al. (1994) Correction of the enzyme deficiency in hematopietic cells of Gaucher patients using a clinically acceptable retroviral supernatant transduction protocol. *Experimental Hematology*, **22**, 223–30.

Yorifuji, T., Wilson, R.W., and Beaudet, A.L. (1993) Retroviral mediated expression of CD18 in normal and deficient human bone marrow progenitor cells. *Human Molecular Genetics*, **2**, 1443–8.

Zhou, S.Z., Broxmeyer, H.E., Cooper, S., Harrington, M.A., and Srivastava, A. (1993) Adeno-associated virus 2-mediated gene transfer in murine hemopoietic progenitor cells. *Experimental Hematology*, **21**, 928–33.

Zhou, S.Z., Cooper, S., Kang, L.Y., et al. (1994) Adeno-associated virus 2-mediated high efficiency gene transfer into immature and mature subsets of hemopoietic progenitor cells in human umbilical cord blood. *Journal of Experimental Medicine*, **179**, 1867–75.

-23

Cellular Therapy Approaches to the Treatment of AIDS

RANDAL A. BYRN AND MARGO R. ROBERTS

Cellular approaches to acquired immunodeficiency syndrome (AIDS) therapy are designed to achieve diverse goals and they employ diverse strategies. This field is in its infancy and, at present, is characterized by a large number of theoretical concepts and a much smaller number of tested applications. This lack of practical feedback from the clinic leaves ample room for speculation but also provides little foundation on which to build new therapeutic modalities.

The approaches will be grouped into three categories for the purposes of this discussion: direct antiviral therapies, secretory therapies or cell-based vaccines, and therapies aimed at immune reconstitution.

◼ ANTIVIRAL THERAPIES

The rationale for cellular antiviral therapies in AIDS is derived from the natural course of the disease. Initial infection by human immunodeficiency virus (HIV) is usually followed by a period of vigorous viral replication, characterized by viremia in plasma and symptoms generally associated with acute viral syndromes. This period usually is relatively brief, 2 to 4 weeks, and is followed by a period in which the viral infection appears to be under control. Viral symptoms are diminished and the standard measures of HIV in the circulation, either infectious virions or infectious lymphocytes, are greatly reduced. At one point this period of "clinical latency" was thought to represent viral quiescence, but recent studies, using more sensitive polymerase chain reaction (PCR) methodologies, have shown that viral replication is continuing at a robust rate (Ho et al. 1995; Wei et al. 1995). After this clinically stable period lasting from months to more than 10 years, the clinical course deteriorates with the manifes-

414

tations of opportunistic infections, reduced CD4 cell levels in the blood, and the reappearance of elevated levels of virus in the circulation (Fig. 23.1).

The transition from initial vigorous virus replication to more controlled infection occurs without an effective antibody (Ab) response and is concurrent with the appearance of a cellular immune response (Koup et al. 1994b). Specific cytotoxic T lymphocytes (CTL) have been demonstrated during this early period and generally remain present during the entire period of clinical latency. Nonspecific cellular components of the immune system, such as natural killer (NK) cells, are also functional during this period. It is tempting, without a better hypothesis, to conclude that the cellular immune response has brought the infection under partial control. A steady-state model of HIV infection proposes that CD4 cell destruction by virus is balanced by CD4 cell production (Coffin 1995). It is a small additional step in theory to suggest that augmentation of the natural cellular immune response, or supplementation with additional cellular responses, could tip this balance in the favor of the host and possibly improve the outcome for the patient.

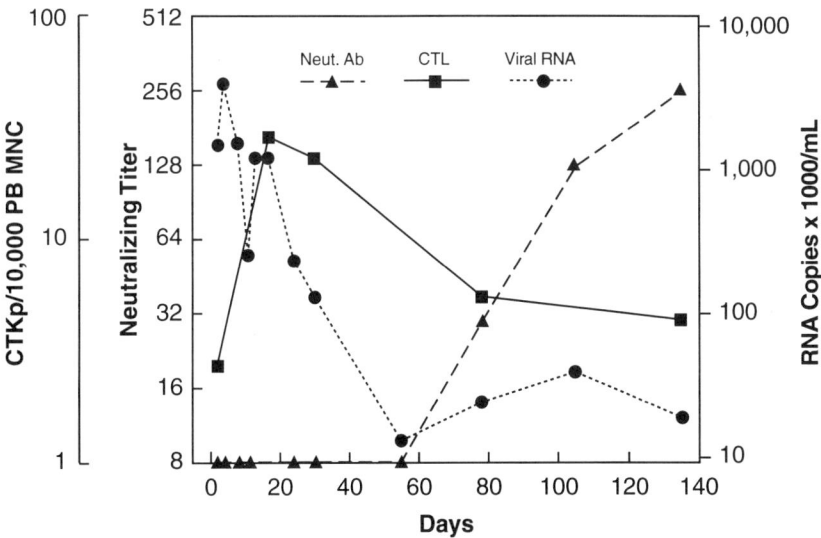

Figure 23.1 Temporal changes in viremia, frequency of HIV-1–specific CTL precursors (CTLp) per 10^4 PB MNC, and neutralizing Ab response in a patient with acute HIV-1 infection. (Adapted from Koup, R.A., and Ho, D.D. [1994a] Shutting down HIV. *Nature*, **370**, 416.)

The limitations of this conceptual approach are the lack of a clear demonstration that the cellular response is in fact controlling the virus (and not merely a concurrent phenomenon), the limited understanding of which components of the cellular response may be responsible, and little experience with therapeutic manipulation of any cellular immune responses.

The most direct cellular therapeutic approach for AIDS is to generate a broad mixture of immune effector cells from a syngeneic uninfected source and administer them to infected individuals. This approach has been taken in several forms. In a major study performed at the National Institutes of Health (NIH) (Lane et al. 1990), lymphocyte transfusions and bone-marrow transplant (BMT) was performed between identical twin pairs while the HIV-positive recipient was receiving azidothymidine (AZT) treatment. Four lymphapheresis transfusions were performed during week 10 of AZT treatment, two lymphapheresis transfusions were performed on week 12 of AZT treatment, and then BMT took place (week 12). Each lymphapheresis consisted of approximately 10×10^{10} lymphocytes and the BM administrations consisted of 2×10^{10} nucleated marrow cells. Significant temporary increases in $CD4^+$ lymphocyte levels were observed in the recipients, but the values returned to baseline after 1 month. Engraftment of the donor lymphoid cells was suggested by changes in delayed type hypersensitivity, but these changes were temporary as well. There were no conclusive benefits to the treatment regimen and it was concluded that further attempts should await the arrival of more effective antiretroviral therapies to protect the graft. One report of allogeneic BMT after cytoablative treatment was unsuccessful in spite of support of the recipient with AZT and interferon-α (IFN-α) (Contu et al. 1993).

An alternative to this approach is to administer expanded cell populations having specific anti-HIV cytolytic activity. This can take the form of either nonspecific ex vivo expansion of a broad mixture of autologous cells from an HIV-positive individual (which usually contain some anti-HIV activity), followed by reinfusion, or the form of antigen (Ag) -specific stimulation and expansion of CTL, ex vivo, followed by infusion. Infusion of the activated cells may or may not be combined with administration of immunoregulatory cytokines such as recombinant interleukin-2 (rIL-2).

In one study (Bex et al. 1994), an HIV-negative twin was vaccinated by vaccinia virus expressing the envelope gene of his HIV-infected brother. After an intramuscular (IM) booster injection with purified recombinant gp120, lymphocytes were collected by leukapheresis and transferred to the infected twin. On a second occasion lymphocytes were collected by leukapheresis, incubated in vitro for 2 hours with recombinant gp120, then administered to the infected twin. No adverse clinical events were associated with either lymphocyte transfer, but 1 week following the second transfer a temporary dramatic increase in cellular virus load was observed. This burst of virus production and the rapid disappearance of the infused CD4$^+$ lymphocytes in the recipient led the authors to caution against administering CD4$^+$ cells until adequate antiviral protection could accompany the cell infusions.

Two studies have been performed using autologous ex vivo–activated CD8 cells in patients with AIDS or AIDS-related complex. In both cases the subjects were lymphapheresed, removing up to 20% of the peripheral blood lymphocytes. The CD8 cells were purified by CELLector devices (Applied Immune Sciences), and the cells expanded by activation with phytohemagglutinin (PHA) and IL-2 over a period of several weeks (Herberman 1992; Klimas 1992; Ho et al. 1993; Whiteside et al. 1993; Klimas et al. 1994). Multiple infusions of 10^8 to 10^{10} cells were performed on each patient, with the final infusion followed by continuous infusion (CI) IL-2 treatment for 5 days. One study included tissue localization studies using ^{111}In-labeled cells; the CD8 cells were found to rapidly accumulate in the lungs, and after 24 hours cells were redistributed to the liver, spleen, and BM. These small studies demonstrated that the cellular collection, expansion, and infusion procedures were technically feasible and well tolerated. Anecdotal evidence for clinical improvement was reported for a subset of patients and both studies ended with appeals for expanded clinical trials. An independent group confirmed the safety of lymphapheresis for HIV-infected patients and observed the separated lymphocytes were replaced from extravascular stores within 1 hour (van Lunzen et al. 1994).

The most elegant demonstration of this virus-specific methodology in a non-AIDS setting is the expansion and administration of cytomegalovirus (CMV) specific CTL in the context of allogeneic BMT. In pioneering work by Greenberg and colleagues (Riddell et al. 1992), the fate of the reinfused major histocompatibility (HC) identical lymphocytes was followed and their activity was still detectable several weeks after administration. The most positive aspect of the study was the improved clinical outcome of the patients who received the cellular therapy. Recurrence of CMV infection was not detected in the patients who had received the immunotherapy. This approach is being explored in the context of AIDS and the initial studies are just entering clinical testing. The results of these studies are awaited with great interest.

A related Ag-specific approach is being explored by Dr Lieberman and colleagues (1995). Bulk ex vivo expansion of CTL is performed concurrent with peptide mapping of the major anti-HIV CTL activities in the individual. Once specific peptide epitopes are identified, they are used for several rounds of Ag-specific expansion of the bulk CTL. These anti-HIV enriched CTL are then infused into the autologous donor. Preliminary results with this approach have produced temporary elevations in Ag-specific, and nonspecific, anti-HIV CTL activity in vivo, followed by a return to baseline values.

Instead of relying on naturally occurring anti-HIV CTL activity, other groups have engineered new classes of anti-HIV effector cells. The team headed by Roberts at Cell Genesys Inc., constructed chimeric molecules termed universal-receptors (UR) that can be used to redirect $CD8^+$ cell activity against any Ag of choice (Roberts et al. 1994). In the case of AIDS, two different UR have been constructed and both have been shown to be very active in vitro.

The first type of UR was constructed by linking the extracellular portion of CD4, the cell surface molecule with high affinity for the envelope protein of HIV, with the cytoplasmic region of ζ, a nonpolymorphic component of the T-cell receptor complex. A second type of UR was constructed by linking a single-chain antibody (SAB), reactive with HIV-1 gp41, as the extracellular recognition domain to the cytoplasmic region of ζ. When the extracellular portion of either chimeric receptor is cross-linked by interaction with its cognate ligand, the cytoplasmic portion initiates a cascade of events resulting in cell activation. When UR of this type are introduced into a primitive $CD4^+$ lymphoid cell line, such as Jurkat cells, cross-linking of the receptors results in IL-2 secretion. When the UR are introduced into primary $CD8^+$ CTL, cross-linking of the receptors, as might occur upon contact of the UR cell with an Ag-expressing target cell, results in cytolysis of the target and T cell proliferation (Fig. 23.2).

Other investigators had shown chimeric receptor-ζ constructs could initiate cytolysis in transient expression systems or using cell lines selected on the basis of their ease of genetic manipulation (Romeo and Seed 1991; Eshhar et al. 1993). Roberts et al. (1994) developed a technique for the generation of stable UR-expressing primary human CD8 T cells in a manner consistent with direct clinical application.

The design of the optimum chimeric receptors was one important aspect of the approach. Both the CD4-ζ and the SAB-ζ constructs were capable of high-level expression in the cell and only required a single polypeptide chain for activity. The region of ζ chain that normally associated with the T-cell receptor (CD3) complex was omitted from

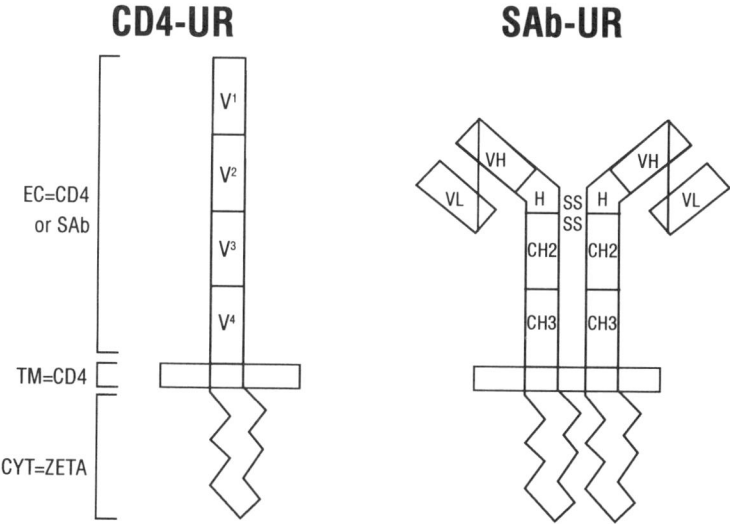

Figure 23.2 Structure of HIV-specific CD4⁻ and SAB-UR. Both UR possess the transmembrane domain of CD4 (residues 372 to 395 of the mature CD4 chain) and the cytoplasmic domain of ζ (residues 31 to 142 of the mature ζ chain) (Adapted from Roberts, M.R., Qin, L., Zhang, D., et al. [1994] Targeting of human immunodeficiency virus-infected cells by CD8+ T lymphocytes armed with universal T-cell receptors. *Blood*, **84**, 2878–89.)

the chimeric molecule so expression levels would not be limited to the level of CD3 (Fig. 23.3).

Another important requirement was the development of a method for efficient introduction of the UR gene into primary T cells (Finer et al. 1994). A murine amphotropic retrovirus system, *kat*, was developed by combining retroviral packaging plasmids and vectors encoding high levels of packagable transcripts, in the human producer cell line 293. This system allowed stable transduction efficiencies of primary CD8 cells of 10% to 40%. Expression levels of the CD4-ζ UR on CD8 lymphocytes was similar to, or higher than, expression levels of the native (endogenous) TCR/CD3 on normal lymphocytes. With high-efficiency, high-level expression, there was no need to include selectable markers in the expression vector. Large numbers of primary lymphocytes could be produced with a minimum of expansion time or selection. This allowed the development of clinical strategies in which patients could receive genetically modified therapeutic cells within several weeks of their initial donation.

Preclinical studies indicated that UR-CD8 cells could perform Ag-specific lysis of HIV-infected lymphoid target cells at exceptionally low effector/target ratios. The UR-CD8 cells also appeared to be active against cell lines expressing low levels of gp120. Lysis could occur for target cell lines in which Ag expression was undetectable by standard immunofluorescence methodology. Cytolysis experiments were performed in the presence of high concentrations of human serum or plasma from either HIV$^-$ or HIV$^+$ donors, and no interference was observed. In blocking experiments using HIV$^+$ serum and added virus, no interference was observed. Thus it appears that this method of cytolysis is operational in the presence of normal IgG levels, conditions that block standard antibody-dependent cellular cytotoxicity (ADCC) lysis, and that neither anti-HIV Ab in serum or HIV-Ag in serum block the UR-CD8 cell-target interaction.

UR-CD8 cells bearing the CD4-ζ construct appear to be CD4/CD8 $^{++}$ by fluorescence-activated cell sorting (FACS) analysis. This raises the possibility that the CD4 on the surface might serve as a receptor for HIV infection or for syncytium formation with gp120-expressing cells. We have examined this in a number of experiments, but we have never observed significant HIV-1 infection of UR-CD8$^+$ cells. When UR-CD8$^+$ and HIV-1–infected targets were prestained with fluorescent dyes and then co-incubated at 37°C, we observed destruction of target cells, but never syncytium formation. This resistance of mature CD8 cells to infection by HIV-1, even while expressing CD4 receptors, is a phenomenon worthy of further study.

Because the UR-CD8$^+$ cell approach involves genetic manipulation of the effector cells approval by the NIH Recombinant DNA Advisory Committee (RAC) was required. A clinical protocol using purified CD8 cells donated by a noninfected identical twin, genetic modification to express CD4-ζ, and infusion into the HIV-1–infected twin was approved in the autumn of 1994. Safety results should be

---

Figure 23.3 Surface expression of UR (*A*) and native TCR (*B*) in transduced human PB MNC-derived CD8$^+$ T-cell populations. Genetically modified and unmodified CD8$^+$ T-cell populations derived from identical donors were labeled with PE-conjugated anti-CD8 mAB and either FITC-conjugated anti-CD4, antihuman Fc mAB, or anti-CD3 to detect expression of CD4-UR, SAB-UR, or native TCR/CD3, respectively. Quadrants were set by labeling each T-cell population with FITC- and PE-conjugated isotype-matched control Ab. (Adapted from Roberts, M.R., Qin, L., Zhang, D., et al. [1994] Targeting of human immunodeficiency virus-infected cells by CD8+ T lymphocytes armed with universal T-cell receptors. *Blood*, **84**, 2878–89.)

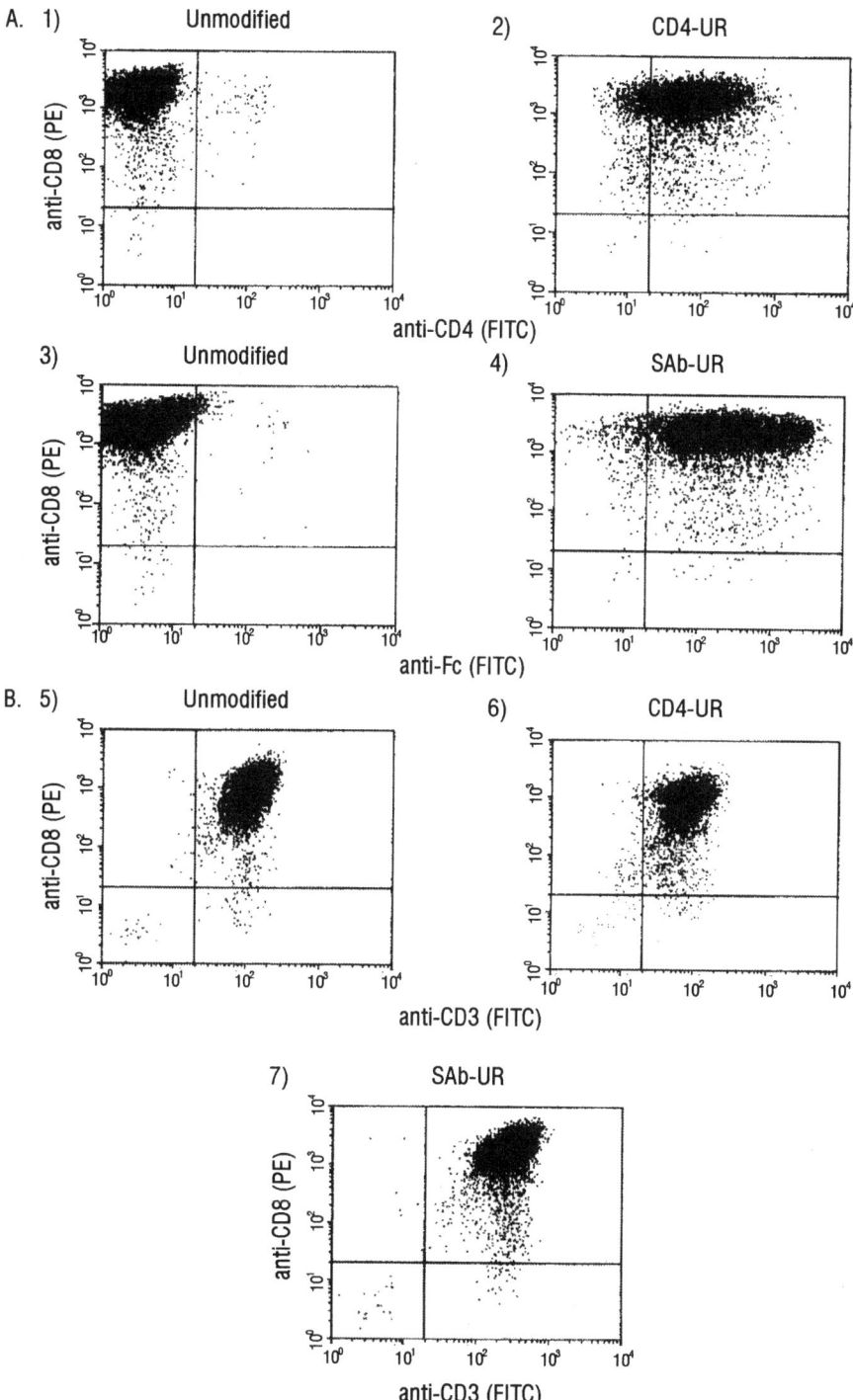

available by the end of 1995. This combination of cellular therapy and gene therapy may represent an important new methodology in AIDS treatment.

■ SECRETORY THERAPIES AND CELL-BASED VACCINES

Examples of cellular therapies for AIDS in this category can be divided into two types: cells expressing molecules that serve as vaccines, and cells that secrete proteins with some direct therapeutic effect. Both of these approaches use injected cells as "internal bioreactors" to produce therapeutic proteins. The advantages of cellular protein factories, as opposed to the standard external production-purification-injection process, may include continuous secretion of the protein over extended periods, secretion into an inaccessible anatomic site or pharmacological compartments, secretion of labile proteins that have highly localized effects, or presentation of the protein on a cell membrane for optimum immunoreactivity. Possible disadvantages of this approach include difficulties in the genetic manipulation of the secretory cells and regulation of the secretion.

Vaccination with syngeneic fibroblasts transduced with a retroviral gp120 expression vector has been proposed as a test system for direct injection of the expression vector in vivo (Galpin, Casciato, and Richards 1994). It is hoped that gp120, presented in the context of self-major HC Ag, will provide a potent stimulus for the generation of anti-HIV CTL. Initial trials of the concept are designed for HIV[+] volunteers. It is unclear how this approach will prove superior to the use of vaccinia vectors, or recombinant soluble gp120, in immunization strategies that have produced increases in Ag-specific proliferation and CTL.

Examples of cell-based secretion of therapeutic molecules include secretion of soluble CD4 or CD4-IgG (Morgan et al. 1990, 1994) and a single-chain Fab fragment reactive with HIV-1 gp120 (Chen et al. 1994). When cells induced to secrete soluble CD4 or CD4-IgG were mixed with susceptible target cells, it was shown that the overall extent of infection by HIV was significantly reduced. This inhibition, in vitro, seems of modest magnitude and must be interpreted in light of the disappointing clinical trials already completed in which much higher plasma levels of CD4-IgG were achieved in patients without any appreciable benefit. The cellular secretion of the Fab Ab fragment occurs as a by-product of its primary function as a means of intracellular protection. Intracellular expression of the Fab fragment interferes with HIV production by the cell and could serve as a means of protecting cells introduced into HIV patients while attempting immune reconstitution.

The therapeutic use of cells designed to secrete cytokines is an interesting theoretical possibility. It is already known that cytokine administration can partially correct some of the hematologic cellular deficiencies observed in AIDS. Recombinant forms of IL-2, granulocyte-macrophage colony-stimulating factor (GM-CSF), and erythropoietin (EPO) have been shown to effectively alter cell counts in HIV[+] volunteers (Groopman 1990; Miles 1991). One of the limitations to the development of cytokine administration is the modest duration of effect. Conceivably, these limitations could be partially overcome by the generation of cells transduced with the appropriate cytokine expression vectors.

■ IMMUNE RECONSTITUTION

Progress in attempts at immune reconstitution for patients with HIV infection is severely limited by our ignorance about the basic mechanisms of AIDS pathogenesis. As discussed earlier, it now appears that HIV replication is an active, continuous process. The resulting immunodeficiency is the combined result of processes that actively destroy CD4[+] cells, affect the regeneration of CD4[+] cells (and other hemopoietic lineages), and affect the regulation of the immune system. It is unclear which processes are of primary importance, under a given set of conditions, and further, it is unclear how these processes change over time.

The basic principles of hemopoietic reconstitution have been discussed in Chapters 1 and 2. It is generally believed that success in immune reconstitution will require, as a first step, development of adequate means of protection of the donor cells so they do not fall victim to HIV infection themselves. If this is accomplished, then the difficult project of reintroducing progenitor cells into a host with a severely damaged regulatory system can be started. It is unclear at this time if remaining problems such as destroyed germinal center architecture and thymic microenvironments can be circumvented by the newly introduced cells.

Gene therapy of hemopoietic progenitor cells is an exciting challenge for molecular biologists. In the field of AIDS, a large number of protective approaches have been demonstrated in vitro, on a variety of cell types, and several are proceeding through the clinical regulatory system toward clinical evaluation (Yu, Poeschla, and Wong-Staal 1994; Anderson 1994). One example of a protective approach is the expression of *trans*-dominant viral proteins, which block the function of the wild-type viral protein and prevent viral replication (Nabel et al. 1994). Targets for *trans*-dominant control include regulatory proteins rev, tat, and vpx and the structural proteins gag and env. Intracellular expression of soluble CD4, transport-redirected sCD4, or anti-gp120 SAB all have been shown to reduce virus production by controlling gp120 processing. Intracellular Ab to rev or env have been demonstrated in vitro. Several RNA decoy strategies targeting the TAR and RRE interactions with tat and rev, respectively, have been tested (Sullenger et al. 1991). An interesting body of work using antisense RNA has developed over the years. Different targets for antisense intervention have included tat, rev, gag, TAR, and the primer binding site. These molecules may arrest transcription, translation, and initiate RNAse H activity for their target sequences (Chattergee, Johnson, and Wong 1992). An alternative RNA strategy employs ribozymes, or catalytic RNA molecules. Both hammerhead-type and hairpin-type ribozymes have been developed (Sarver and Rossi 1993; Yamada et al. 1994).

The ideal gene therapy protection for a hemopoietic progenitor cell graft would block HIV infection before entry (or at least integration), would be protective in all hemopoietic lineages at all stages of development, and would be deliverable by an efficient vector system. Only limited information is available about how well any of these criteria are met by currently available technologies, but this is the challenge for molecular biologists and hematologists in the years to come. It is expected that progress in this area will be rapid and will accelerate as technical advances in gene delivery systems become available.

REFERENCES

Anderson, W.F. (1994) Gene therapy for AIDS. *Human Gene Therapy*, **5**, 149–50.

Bex, F., Hermans, P., Sprecher, S., et al. (1994) Syngeneic adoptive transfer of anti-human immunodeficiency virus-1 (HIV-1)-primed lymphocytes from a vaccinated HIV-seronegative individual to his HIV-1-infected identical twin. *Blood*, **84**, 3317–26.

Chattergee, S., Johnson, P.R., and Wong, K.K., Jr. (1992) Dual- target inhibition of HIV-1 in vitro by means of an adeno-associated virus antisense vector. *Science*, **258**, 1485–8.

Chen, S.Y., Khouri, Y., Bagley, J., and Marasco, W.A. (1994) Combined intra- and extracellular immunization against human immunodeficiency virus type 1 infection with a human anti-gp120 antibody. *Proceedings of the National Academy of Sciences of the United States of America*, **91**, 5932–6.

Coffin, J.M. (1995) HIV population dynamics in vivo: implications for genetic variation, pathogenesis and therapy. *Science*, **27**, 483–9.

Contu, L., Nasa, G.L., Arras, M., et al. (1993) Allogeneic bone marrow transplantation combined with multiple anti-HIV treatment in a case with AIDS. *Bone Marrow Transplantation,* **12,** 669–71.

Eshhar, Z., Waks, T., Gross, G., and Schindler, D.G. (1993) Specific activation and targeting of cytotoxic lymphocytes through chimeric single chains consisting of antibody-binding domains and the gamma or zeta subunits of the immunoglobulin and T-cell receptor. *Proceedings of the National Academy of Sciences of the United States of America,* **90,** 720–4.

Finer, M.H., Dull, T.J., Qin, L., Farson, D., and Roberts, M.R. (1994) *kat:* a high-efficiency retroviral transduction system for primary human T lymphocytes. *Blood,* **83,** 43–50.

Galpin, J.E., Casciato, D.A., and Richards, S.B. (1994) A phase I clinical trial to evaluate the safety and biological activity of HIV-IT (TAF) (HIV-1IIIB env-transduced, autologous fibroblasts) in asymptomatic HIV-1 infected subjects. *Human Gene Therapy,* **5,** 997–1017.

Groopman, J.E. (1990) Granulocyte-macrophage colony-stimulating factor in human immunodeficiency virus disease. *Seminars in Hematology,* **27,** 8–14.

Herberman, R.B. (1992) Adoptive therapy with purified CD8 cells in HIV infection. *Seminars in Hematology,* **29,** 35–40.

Ho, M., Armstrong, J., McMahon, D., et al. (1993) A phase 1 study of adoptive transfer of autologous CD8+ T lymphocytes in patients with acquired immunodeficiency syndrome (AIDS)-related complex or AIDS. *Blood,* **81,** 2093–101.

Ho, D.D., Neumann, A.U., Perepson, A.S., Chen W., Leonard, J.M., and Markowitz, M. (1995) Rapid turnover of plasma virions and CD4 lymphocytes in HIV infection. *Nature,* **373,** 123–6.

Klimas, N.G. (1992) Clinical impact of adoptive therapy with purified CD8 cells in HIV infection. *Seminars in Hematology,* **29,** 40–44.

Klimas, N., Patarca, R., Walling, J., et al. (1994) Clinical and immunological changes in AIDS patients following adoptive therapy with activated autologous CD8 cells and interleukin-2 infusion. *AIDS,* **8,** 1073–81.

Koup, R.A. and Ho, D.D. (1994a) Shutting down HIV. *Nature,* **370,** 416.

Koup, R.A., Safrit, J.T., Cao, Y., et al. (1994b) Temporal association of cellular immune responses with the initial control of viremia in primary human immunodeficiency virus type 1 syndrome. *Journal of Virology,* **68,** 4650–5.

Lane, H.C., Zunich, K.M., Wilson, W., et al. (1990) Syngeneic bone marrow transplantation and adoptive transfer of peripheral blood lymphocytes combined with zidovudine in human immunodeficiency virus (HIV) infection. *Annals of Internal Medicine,* **113,** 512–9.

Lieberman, J. (1995) Treatment of HIV infection with viral specific cytotoxic T-lymphocytes: a progress report. *Second National Conference on Human Retroviruses and Related Infections.* Washington, DC, Jan. 30, 1995.

Miles, S.A. (1991) The use of hematopoietic growth factors in HIV infection and AIDS-related malignancies. *Cancer Investigation,* **9,** 229–38.

Morgan, R.A., Baler-Bitterlich, G., Ragheb, J.A., Wong-Staal, F., Gallo, R.C., and Anderson, W.F. (1994) Further evaluation of soluble CD4 as an anti-HIV type 1 gene therapy: demonstration of protection of primary human peripheral blood lymphocytes from infection by HIV type 1. *AIDS Research and Human Retroviruses,* **10,** 1507–15.

Morgan, R.A., Looney, D.J., Muenchau, D.D., Wong-Staal, F., Gallo, R.C., and Anderson, W.F. (1990) Retroviral vectors expressing soluble CD4: a potential gene therapy for AIDS. *AIDS Research and Human Retroviruses*, **6**, 183–91.

Nabel, G.J., Fox, B.A., Post, L., Thompson, C.B., and Woffendin, C. (1994) Clinical protocol: a molecular genetic intervention for AIDS–effects of a transdominant negative form of *rev*. *Human Gene Therapy*, **5**, 79–92.

Riddell, S.R., Watanabe, K.S., Goodrich, J.M., Li, C.R., Agha, M.E., and Greenberg, P.D. (1992) Restoration of viral immunity in immunodeficient humans by the adoptive transfer of T cell clones. *Science*, **257**, 228–241.

Roberts, M.R., Qin, L., Zhang, D., et al. (1994) Targeting of human immunodeficiency virus-infected cells by CD8+ T lymphocytes armed with universal T-cell receptors. *Blood*, **84**, 2878–89.

Romeo, C. and Seed, B. (1991) Cellular immunity to HIV activated by CD4 fused to T cell or Fc receptor polypeptides. *Cell*, **64**, 1037–43.

Sarver, N. and Rossi, J. (1993) Gene therapy: a bold direction for HIV-1 treatment. *AIDS Research and Human Retroviruses*, **9**, 483–7.

Sullenger, B.A., Gallardo, H.F., Ungers, G.E., and Gilboa, E. (1991) Analysis of trans-acting response decoy RNA-mediated inhibition of human immunodeficiency virus type 1 transactivation. *Journal of Virology*, **65**, 6811–16.

van Lunzen, J., Schmitz, J., Dengler, K., Schmidt, L., Schmitz, H., and Dietrich, M. (1994) Recovery of T-lymphocytes for adoptive immunotherapy by lymphapheresis of HIV-infected patients without alterations of virological, immunological or clinical parameters. *British Journal of Haematology*, **88**, 46–51.

Wei, X., Ghosh, S.K., Taylor, M.E., et al. (1995) Viral dynamics in human immunodeficiency virus type 1 infection. *Nature*, **373**, 117–22.

Whiteside, T.L., Elder, E.M., Moody, D., et al. (1993) Generation and characterization of ex vivo propagated autologous CD8+ cells used for adoptive immunotherapy of patients infected with human immunodeficiency virus. *Blood*, **81**, 2085–92.

Yamada, O., Yu, M., Yee, J.K., Kraus, G., Looney, D., and Wong- Staal, F. (1994) Intracellular immunization of human T-cells with a hairpin ribozyme against human immunodeficiency virus type 1. *Gene Therapy*, **1**, 38–45.

Yu, M., Poeschla, E., and Wong-Staal, F. (1994) Progress towards gene therapy for HIV infection. *Gene Therapy*, **1**, 13–26.

Experimental and Clinical Cellular Immunotherapy

24

Adoptive Immunotherapy with T Cells

VERA MALKOVSKA AND PAUL M. SONDEL

It has long been known that T lymphocytes recognize and kill transformed cells in vitro and in animal tumor models. Although adoptively transferred tumor-specific T cells could eradicate various experimental neoplasms, it was not clear that such treatment would be feasible in human malignancy. For a long time the evidence for T-cell–mediated antitumor responses in humans was indirect and anecdotal. Spontaneous tumor regressions presumably mediated by the immune system have been observed, but the mechanism was not understood and the involvement of T cells was only hypothetical. In 1985, Rosenberg and co-workers suggested that adoptively transferred human lymphocytes exerted antitumor activity in patients with advanced cancer (Rosenberg et al. 1985). They found that in vitro interleukin-2 (IL-2) –activated autologous peripheral lymphocytes (LAK cells) plus IL-2 or IL-2 alone induce tumor regressions in about 19% of patients with "immunogenic" tumors, namely melanoma and renal cell carcinoma (Rosenberg et al. 1987). It was hypothesized that the success of the therapy was dependent on the recruitment of autologous tumor-reactive T cells which played a crucial role in tumor killing (Parmiani 1990). The low response rates observed were explained by the lack of tumor-specific T cells in the majority of cancer patients (Parmiani 1990). In agreement with this hypothesis, tumor-infiltrating lymphocytes (TIL) expanded in vitro in the presence of IL-2 appeared to have a greater antitumor activity than LAK cells with IL-2. The adoptive transfer of TIL in melanoma induced tumor regression in approximately 36% of patients (Rosenberg et al. 1988; S.A. Rosenberg, personal communication).

Strong evidence that T cells have clinically useful antitumor activity comes from studies in patients receiving allogeneic bone-marrow transplant (BMT) for leukemia. Statistical analyses of large series of patients show that the depletion of T cells from the transplanted bone marrow (BM) results in higher leukemic relapse rates (Apperley et al. 1986; Maranichi et al. 1987; Goldman et al. 1988; Horowitz et al. 1990). Thus, the allogeneic T lymphocytes in the donor marrow exert a strong antileukemic activity: the so-called graft-versus-leukemia (GVL) effect (see Chapter 31). Recent clinical studies have shown that the administration of donor lymphocytes to patients who relapsed after BMT induce remissions in certain types of leukemia (Kolb et al. 1990; Cullis et al. 1992; Drobyski et al. 1993) (see Chapter 30). Although the specificity of allogeneic T cells mediating GVL is not known, several studies suggest that the antileukemic activity is clinically separable from graft-versus-host disease (GVHD) (reviewed by Sosman and Sondel 1987; Jiang et al. 1991; Falkenburg et al. 1993).

Taken together, these observations show that adoptively transferred autologous or allogeneic lymphocytes, and specifically T cells, have therapeutic potential. Several groups of investigators have isolated T-cell lines or clones with specific reactivity against a variety of human tumors in vitro and suggested that such cells might be useful for therapy (reviewed by Anichi, Fossati, and Parmiani 1987; Parmiani 1990); however, the development of clinical protocols was hindered by the facts that both the isolation of these tumor-reactive T cells was not reproducible and the antigenic determinants were not defined.

Recent advances in several areas of tumor immunology have overcome these obstacles and opened the possibility of developing rational strategies for T-cell therapy. First, the molecular structures on the T cell and tumor cell surface involved in antigen (Ag) recognition have been better characterized, including the identification of the first tumor Ag recognized by autologous T cells. Second, the co-stimulatory signals necessary for the induction of tumor-reactive T cells are better understood. New technologies allow the reproducible generation and expansion of T cells of chosen specificity for clinical use. Moreover, both the T cells and the tumor cells can be altered by genetic manipulations designed to augment the immune response.

This chapter reviews in vitro, animal, and clinical studies relevant for the development of new strategies in T-cell immunotherapy. We discuss the challenges to therapy of human tumors with T cells and compare this approach with active immunotherapy with vaccines. The following questions are addressed: Is it possible to find tumor peptides that can serve as rejection Ag? Will these be sufficiently specific to allow tumor destruction by immune cells while preserving vital organs? What is the use for autologous versus allogeneic T cells? Finally, we discuss the role of T-cell immunotherapy in the context of traditional treatments for cancer.

■ PRINCIPLES OF TUMOR RECOGNITION BY T CELLS

In order to design effective immunotherapy with T cells, it is important to understand how T cells recognize tumors, how they become activated, and which effector mechanisms are involved in tumor killing. The molecular structures involved in recognition by T cells are well defined: Ag receptors on the T-cell surface bind to peptides positioned in the groove of major histocompatibility complex (HC) molecules. Initial studies suggested that cellular proteins processed internally are presented by class I major HC molecules to cytotoxic CD8 T cells. In contrast, class II major HC bind peptides derived from exogenous proteins that are picked up by antigen-presenting cells (APC). These are recognized by CD4 T cells. According to this paradigm, tumor-derived proteins are either processed by the tumor cell itself and presented by class I major HC molecules or taken up by various APC and bound to their class II major HC molecules (reviewed by Moudgil et al. 1993); however, several studies indicate that there are exceptions to these rules. The major HC class I can present exogenous Ag, whereas the major HC class II molecules also present a variety of endogenously derived peptides (Bevan 1976; Lanzavecchia 1985; Staerz, Karasugama, and Garner 1987). Recently, it has been shown that APC derived from murine BM present exogenous proteins in the context of class I major HC molecules and are crucial for the generation of tumor-reactive cytotoxic T cells (Huang et al. 1994). This observation might have important implications for immunotherapy with tumor-reactive class I–restricted cytotoxic T lymphocytes (CTL). Since other APC present the tumor antigens, the tumor itself does not have to be a good Ag-presenting cell. Moreover, only the APC (but not the tumor) has to be HLA-matched with the responding T cells. This would obviate the difficulties in obtaining autologous or HLA-matched tumor cells in each patient.

Most CD4 T cells recognize tumor Ag presented by professional APC; however, leukemias and lymphomas that express class II major HC molecules could also present endogenous proteins to CD4 T cells (Lanzavecchia 1985; Sosman et al. 1990). Therefore, the presentation of tumor-specific peptides can involve a variety of mechanisms depending on the system studied.

■ TUMOR-DERIVED PEPTIDES AS TARGETS FOR T-CELL IMMUNOTHERAPY

The goal of immunotherapy with T cells is to eliminate tumor cells without causing severe damage to the patient's vital organs. Therefore, the T cells should recognize Ag that are either expressed exclusively on tumor cells or expressed only on those normal cells that are not important for the patient's survival. The T cells responding to such Ag should be able to reject the tumor directly or by recruiting secondary effector cells.

From the early days of tumor immunology, investigators have been searching for tumor-specific Ag. Early studies in animal models showed that such Ag are expressed in experimental tumors and can induce immune responses resulting in tumor rejections (Baldwin 1955; Klein et al. 1960; Prehn 1962); however, many doubted the existence of therapeutically useful tumor Ag in spontaneous human neoplasms. This idea has been resurrected with the discovery of defined molecular changes in human cancer-related genes that result in the production of unique tumor-specific proteins. These genetic changes include translocations, deletions, and point mutations encoding aberrant proteins that control cell growth and differentiation. If unique peptide sequences from these proteins are processed and presented effectively to T cells they might serve as potential tumor-rejection Ag. Tumor-rejection Ag also could be derived from normal cellular genes, provided that the resulting immune response discriminates between the cancer and vital normal tissues. Such Ag include overexpressed oncogene products or differentiation Ag of restricted tissue distribution. Finally, in the minority of cancers associated with viral infections, viral peptides could be targeted. The identification of immunogenic peptides in tumor proteins has been facilitated by recently acquired knowledge about the precise length of peptides and the amino acid motifs that bind to major HC molecules (Falk et al. 1991; Hill et al. 1992; DiBirno et al. 1993).

A variety of tumor-specific proteins have now been studied as potential tumor-rejection Ag. The p21^{ras} proteins are intermediary signaling proteins that regulate cell growth and differentiation (Bourne, Sanders, and McCormick 1990). Activating-point mutations of *ras* protooncogenes are relatively common (they occur in 20% of human malignancies) and the numbers of resulting single amino acid substitutions are limited (reviewed by Cheever et al. 1993). Therefore, only a restricted set of tumor-specific determinants would need to be targeted in a relatively large patient population. In murine studies, synthetic peptides corresponding to the mutated segment elicit both class

II–restricted CD4$^+$ T cell responses and class I–restricted CD8$^+$ T-cell responses specific for mutated p21^{ras} protein (Peace et al. 1991). Moreover *ras* peptide-specific cytotoxic T cells specifically lyse a mouse fibroblast cell line transfected with a vector encoding the mutated p21^{ras} protein (Peace et al. 1994). It is not known if human tumors process and present the mutated *ras* peptides or if they are susceptible to killing by *ras*-specific T cells.

The p210*BCR/ABL* protein also has features of a target for T-cell therapy. It is coded for by the *bcr/abl* fusion gene that results from the most common translocation in chronic myelogenous leukemia (CML), the t(9;22). The *bcr/abl* translocation plays an important role in the development of CML (reviewed by Gishizky, Johnson-White, and Witte 1993). Only three potential joining region segments are commonly observed and they are easily identifiable in individual patients (Kawasaki et al. 1988). The segments are composed of unique sequences of amino acids that are potentially immunogenic. Preliminary studies suggested that *bcr/abl* peptides can be presented by both murine and human major HC molecules and elicit cytotoxic lymphocyte responses specific for the peptide (Chen et al. 1992a; Cheever et al. 1993). Unfortunately, attempts to generate *bcr/abl*-specific T cells that would selectively kill human leukemic targets have not been successful to date (Oettel et al. 1994). Disappointingly, Witte's group has recently suggested that the patients' leukemic progenitors do not express the fusion protein (Gishizky et al. 1993).

Gambacorti-Passerini et al. (1993) studied the immunogenicity of fusion peptides coded by the junction region of the chromosomal translocation t(15;17) in promyelocytic leukemia. They found that human CD4 T cells recognize both the fusion peptide and the whole protein expressed in an autologous lymphoblastoid cell line. Whether the fusion peptide is processed and presented by the leukemia cells remains uncertain.

Cheever and co-workers (1993) generated human CTL against two HLA-A2–binding peptides from the the HER-2/neu protein, a protooncogene product overexpressed in a variey of human cancers (reviewed by Disis et al. 1994). Although indirect evidence suggests that some breast cancer patients have helper T-cell immunity to the HER-2/neu protein, it is not known if human cancer cells present HER-2/neu–derived peptides recognizable by CTL (Disis et al. 1994).

Although the above studies show that selected tumor-specific proteins or peptides can be immunogenic in various experimental systems, they do not ensure that tumor cells process the same peptides and present them on the cell surface for T-cell recognition. Some investigators, therefore, used tumor-reactive CTL isolated from melanoma patients as tools for isolation of tumor Ag. Two basic strategies are applied. First, the peptides were eluted from the class I major HC molecules on tumor cells and resolved by high-performance liquid chromatography (HPLC). Peptide fractions that were capable of stimulating melanoma-specific T-cell clones were then identified (Slingluff et al. 1993; Storkus et al. 1993). The sequencing of the stimulatory peptides has been hindered by the very small amounts of material obtainable from the fractions. Recently, Cox and co-workers (1994) used mass spectrometry with a novel chromatography separation method to identify a peptide epitope recognized by five different melanoma-specific cytotoxic cell lines. The technique allowed the identification of a peptide of very low abundance in a mixture estimated to contain at least 10,000 species.

Other investigators used a genetic approach to identify tumor peptides recognized by CTL. A cDNA library was generated from the melanoma cells and transfected into COS-7 cells (together with the appropriate major HC gene) or into suitable tumor cells capable of Ag processing. The transfected cells were then screened for expression of the tumor-specific Ag by their ability to stimulate tumor-specific T-cell clones. The inserted genes were then isolated. By this approach Boon and co-workers identified a family of MAGE genes (MAGE 1, MAGE 2, and MAGE 3) and the melanocyte-specific gene for tyrosinase (Van der Bruggen et al. 1991; Brichard et al. 1993; Coulie et al. 1994; Gaugler et al. 1994). MAGE 1 and 3 are expressed in many melanomas and other tumors but not in most normal tissues except for testes. Using a similar strategy Kawakami et al. (1994a) identified the MART-1 gene that codes for a melanocyte-specific protein different from tyrosinase.

It is of considerable interest that all of the presumed tumor-specific Ag identified so far by CTL recognition of gene products from melanoma cell libraries are products of normal genes. These genes do not appear to be modified in the tumor cells and are present in all tissues. The melanoma "specificity" results from their preferential (but not exclusive) expression in melanoma cells. The successful in vitro induction of CTL responses against these self-proteins implies that autoreactive T cells have not been deleted. The experiments show that it is possible to break tolerance against these Ag presented by melanoma cells, at least in vitro. Encouraging therapeutic results with TIL suggest that these proteins can become true tumor-rejection Ag.

The melanoma Ag identified to date are presented by either HLA-A1 or HLA-A2 molecules. Studies on melanoma-specific T-cell lines from several laboratories suggest that there could be a variety of yet undiscovered peptides presented by other major HC molecules (Chen and Hersey 1992; Hom et al. 1993). It might therefore be possible to use T-cell therapy in melanoma patients of other HLA types.

Although melanoma appears to be the most immunogenic of well-studied malignancies, there is more limited experimental evidence for tumor-specific Ag expressed by other human neoplasms. Cytotoxic T-cell lines that recognized autologous tumor cells have been generated in vitro from peripheral blood (PB), TIL, or tumor-draining lymph nodes of patients with renal-cell carcinoma, lymphoma, sarcoma, breast carcinoma, and other tumors (reviewed in Yssel, Spits, and DeVries 1984; Anichi et al. 1987; Wright et al. 1989; Jerome et al. 1991; Wang et al. 1992; Yasumura et al. 1993). The immunoglobulin idiotype expressed in B-cell malignancies appears to be an ideal target for immunotherapy. T cells specific for the peptide encoded by the immunoglobulin hypervariable region prevented the outgrowth of lymphoma in a mouse model (Wilson et al. 1990). Both idiotype-specific $CD8^+$ CTL and $CD4^+$ helper cells exerted antitumor activity against B-cell malignancies in animal models (Chakrabarti and Ghosh 1992; Lauritzsen and Bogen 1993). A clinical study demonstrated that patients with B-cell lymphomas can generate both humoral and cellular anti-idiotype immune responses following immunization with idiotype proteins from their individual tumors (Kwak et al. 1992). This team is now pursuing immunization of BMT donors with the idiotypic peptides from the patients' tumors. The goal is to induce an immune response in the donor that can be subsequently transplanted to the recipient. It remains to be seen which of the anti-idiotype therapies, namely antibodies (Ab), vaccines, or adoptively transfered T cells, will be most effective in B-cell malignancies.

Finn (1993) and co-workers studied the antigenicity of epithelial cell mucin encoded by the MUC-1 gene expressed by various carcinomas. They found that CTL derived from patients with breast adenocarcinoma recognize an epitope present on the protein core of a mucin preferentially expressed on malignant cells (Jerome et al. 1991). Both peptides derived from the tandem-repeat domain as well as the whole mucin molecule have also been tested for tumor-rejection properties in mice. Thus mucin Ag are another example of a self-Ag that might be preferentially recognized on tumor cells (Finn 1993).

Human malignancies associated with viral infections represent an immunologically distinct group of tumors in which viral peptides may serve as specific targets for T cells. Although most human neoplasms are not thought to be due to viral infections, the number of viruses found to cause cancer is rising. The list of viruses and associated human tumors now includes: Epstein-Barr virus (EBV) in African Burkitt's lymphoma, Hodgkin's disease (HD) (especially in childhood), and lymphomas in immunocompromised individuals; human T-lymphotropic virus I (HTLV-1) in adult T-cell leukemia; human papilloma viruses (HPV) in genital cancers; and hepatitis-B virus in hepatocellular carcinoma (reviewed by Melief and Kast 1992). T-cell immunity against virus-induced tumors parallels in many ways antiviral immunity in general. In some cases, antiviral immune response recognizes viral peptides on the tumor cell, and creates potent antitumor T-cell immunity. The strategies for immunotherapy of tumors induced by viruses has been recently reviewed elsewhere (Melief and Kast 1992).

■ SECOND SIGNALS AND ACTIVATION OF TUMOR-REACTIVE T CELLS

The need for co-stimulatory signals is an important consideration for T-cell therapy. It has been known for many years that T cells need other signals in addition to the specific Ag to become fully activated and initiate an immune response (Jenkins et al. 1987). Recently, molecular structures (B7-1, B7-2, CD28, cytotoxic T-lymphocyte–associated Ag-4) involved in co-stimulation have been defined (reviewed in Linsley and Ledbetter 1993). It has also become clear that tumors might escape immune attack by failing to express co-stimulatory molecules. Indeed, many naturally occurring tumors lack B7-1 (CD80).

Fortunately for tumor immunotherapy, the co-stimulatory molecules are critical for the T-cell induction phase, but not necessarily for the effector phase of tumor killing. Melanomas that grow progressively in immunocompetent mice are rejected by CD8[+] T cells after transfection of the melanoma cells with the B7 gene (Chen et al. 1992b; Baskar et al. 1993; Townsend and Allison 1993). The immune response elicited by the B7[+] cells eliminated B7[−] variants of the same melanoma (Chen et al. 1992b; Baskar et al. 1993). Ramarathinam et al. (1994) showed that this may not be the case in every tumor: in a murine melanoma model the B7/BB1 functions not only as a co-stimulatory molecule at the initiation of the immune response but also plays a major role in T-cell recruitment and effector function.

For reproducible generation of T cells for therapy, it is necessary to choose APC that provide appropriate co-stimulatory signals. These could be "professional" APC such as monocytes or dendritic cells obtained from patients' PB or BM. Alternatively, tumor cells expressing co-stimulatory molecules naturally or after genetic modification can also serve as APC (Chen et al. 1992b). The induction of immune responses against tumors also can be improved by a variety of other genetic manipulations of the stimulatory tumor cells or APC (Pardoll

1993). This approach has been used not only for adoptive T-cell therapy but also for therapy with vaccines and has been reviewed elsewhere in this monograph.

■ IN VITRO EXPANSION OF T CELLS FOR ADOPTIVE THERAPY

Trials with LAK cells and TIL led to the develoment of cell-culture technology for growing large quantities of human lymphocytes for clinical use. These cultures contained polyclonal, mostly nonspecific T cells expanded in high doses of IL-2 (Rosenberg et al. 1985, 1988). Techniques for large-scale expansion of stable Ag-specific T-cell lines or clones have also been developed (Herin et al. 1987; Riddel et al. 1992). Successful techniques involved repeated stimulations of T cells with the Ag of choice in the presence of IL-2 and autologous APC. In situations where the availability of autologous APC was limiting, the T cells could be stimulated with monoclonal antibodies (mAB) against the T-cell receptor and T-cell activation molecules (Chen, Reese, and Cheever 1990; Crossland et al. 1991; Riddell, Gilbert, and Greenberg 1993). The first study in humans to evaluate the efficacy of adoptively transferred CD8[+] T-cell clones for reconstitution of specific immunity was performed in allogeneic BMT recipients at risk of developing cytomegalovirus (CMV) disease (reviewed by Riddell et al. 1993). CD8[+] T-cell clones specific for immunodominant CMV Ag were expanded to large numbers ($>10^9$ cells) and administered to the immunodeficient hosts. The transferred T cells reconstituted CMV-specific immune responses equivalent to or greater in magnitude than those observed in the immunocompetent BM donors (Riddell et al. 1992). By using polymerase chain reaction (PCR) to identify T-cell–receptor gene rearrangements in the donor clones, it was demonstrated that transferred cells persist in the recipient for more than 12 weeks after infusion (Riddell et al. 1993). These findings hold great promise both for treatment of viral infections in immunocompromised patients and for adoptive therapy of cancer.

■ EFFECTOR MECHANISMS INVOLVED IN TUMOR KILLING IN VIVO

T cells can kill tumors either through direct cell-mediated cytotoxicity or through recruitment of secondary effector cells such as natural killer (NK) cells and macrophages. The two major T-cell populations defined by phenotype are the CD4[+]CD8[−] cells that recognize Ag in the context of class II HC molecules and the CD4[−]CD8[+] cells that see peptides presented by class I molecules. Studies of T-cell functions have demonstrated that the majority of CD4$^+$ cells act as helper cells and produce cytokines that induce other immune cells to lyse tumors, while most CD8$^+$ T cells are directly cytotoxic; however, there are important exceptions to this rule. Cytolytic CD4$^+$ T cells and CD8$^+$ T cells that produce cytokines and act as helper cells have been well described (Swain 1981; Widmer and Bach 1981; Golding and Singer 1985; Mizuochi et al. 1988).

Since most tumor cells express class I HC molecules and are therefore recognizable by cytolytic CD8$^+$ T cells, many investigators focused on the CD8$^+$ T cells as the main subset to promote tumor eradication (reviewed by Greenberg 1991). The in vivo antitumor activity of cytolytic T cells derived from the CD8$^+$ subset has been demonstrated in a wide range of murine tumors, including hematological malignancies, sarcoma, glioma, melanoma, and epithelial cancers (Dailey, Pillemer, and Weissman 1982; Evans 1984; Rosenstein, Eberlein, and Rosenberg 1984; Wortzel, Urban, and Schreiber 1984; Yamasaki et al. 1984; Greenberg 1986; De Graaf, Horak, and Brookman 1988; Ward et al. 1988; Fan and Edington 1989; reviewed by Melief and Kast 1992). In many of these models the therapeutic activity of CD8$^+$ T cells depends on or is enhanced by the presence of CD4$^+$ helper cells or exogenous IL-2. Some CD8$^+$ T-cell clones produce IL-2 and can by themselves eliminate disseminated tumors after adoptive transfer into T-cell–deficient hosts (Greenberg 1991); however, the amount of IL-2 produced by CD8$^+$ cells can be limiting, and exogenously administered IL-2 enhances their antitumor activity (Rosenberg et al. 1988; Greenberg 1991).

Tumor rejection mediated by CD4$^+$ T cells without contribution of CD8$^+$ T cells has been described in several models (Fujiwara et al. 1984; Greenberg 1991). The CD4$^+$ T cells can eradicate tumors through different effector mechanisms. Cytotoxic CD4$^+$ T cells can directly lyse tumors expressing class II major HC molecules, as is the case in many leukemias or lymphomas (reviewed by Greenberg 1991). Interestingly, although such human and murine tumors can be killed effectively by the T cells, class II–expressing normal APC are resistant to lysis by cytotoxic CD4$^+$ T cells (Woods, Kitagami, and Ochi 1989). In most systems, the CD4$^+$ cells are not directly cytotoxic and kill tumors through recruitment of macrophages, NK cells, and possibly other cell types. The CD4$^+$ cells release macrophage-activating cytokines inducing tumoricidal macrophages that bind selectively to tumor cells and deliver a cytolytic signal (De Graaf et al. 1988; Paulnock 1994). The pathways of macrophage activation and mechanisms of tumor killing have been recently reviewed elsewhere (Paulnock 1994).

CD4$^+$ T cells release cytokines, particularly IL-2 and interferon-γ (IFN-γ) that are powerful inducers of NK activity. They are also synergistic in inducing tumor killing by NK cells (Brunda, Tarnowski, and Davatelis 1986). NK cells mediate most of the LAK cell activity inducible in PB mononuclear cells (MNC) by high-doses of IL-2 (Rosenberg et al. 1985). LAK cells kill a wide range of cancer cells in vitro including NK-resistant tumors, and it has therefore been suggested that they might play a role in antitumor immunity in vivo (Rosenberg et al. 1985); however, it is not clear if LAK cell activity is induced by T-cell–derived cytokines in the tumor microenvironment. Indeed NK cells are not significant effectors in many animal models of T-cell immunotherapy (Greenberg et al. 1989). On the other hand, their antitumor activity may be crucial in certain settings. For example, the susceptibility of tumor targets to NK lysis correlates with reduced expression of class I major HC molecules (Harel-Bellan et al. 1986; Karre et al. 1986; Storkus and Dawson 1991). Therefore, it is tempting to speculate that NK cells have developed to eliminate tumor cells or virus-infected cells that fail to express adequate levels of self-major HC class I gene products (Karre et al. 1986). Thus, NK cells represent a potentially important tool for the elimination of class I–deficient tumor variants that cannot be targeted directly by T cells. A detailed description of NK cell activity in cancer is beyond the scope of this chapter and has been the subject of a recent review (Klein and Mantovani 1993).

The results discussed above show that either CD8$^+$ T cells, CD4$^+$ T cells, or both can mediate tumor regressions, and their respective involvement is distinct in different models. For the design of therapeutic trials, more information is needed about the variables that determine the in vivo recognition and susceptibility of human tumors to killing by different types of T cells. Although the murine models discussed above provided valuable information about the principles of T-cell therapy, their relevance is limited because of the fundamental differences between experimental murine tumors and human cancer. The discovery that severe combined immunodeficiency (SCID) mice can be transplanted with human tumors and human T cells opened the possibility to generate preclinical models for T-cell therapy (Mosier et al. 1988; McCune et al. 1988). First studies have shown that human PB T cells injected intraperitoneally (IP) into SCID mice can respond to antigenic stimulation. Moreover, lymphoma cell line-reactive human T cells can confer specific antitumor immunity against the lymphoma after adoptive transfer into SCID mice (Malkovska et al. 1992; Malkovska, Cigel, and Storer 1994). Such xenogeneic models may provide information relevant to clinical immunotherapy with T cells.

■ GENETIC MODIFICATIONS OF EFFECTOR CELLS FOR ADOPTIVE THERAPY

The antitumor activity of T cells used for adoptive therapy can be further enhanced by in vitro transfer of genes coding for cytokines and other proteins. Rosenberg and colleagues (1990) took the first steps towards this goal by introducing a "marker" gene encoding for neomycin resistance into human TIL. The gene transfection did not impair the proliferative or cytolytic functions of the TIL, some of which survived for several weeks after transfer. More recently these investigators inserted the human tumor necrosis factor gene into human TIL.

A major limiting factor in adoptive therapy of most tumors is the inability of lymphocytes to selectively recognize tumor cells. Therefore, some investigators have used Ab to target cytotoxic lymphocytes to tumors. Several Ab can bind selectively to human tumors and induce an antibody-dependent cellular cytotoxicity (ADCC). Trials combining such Ab with lymphocyte activators (i.e., IL-2) have been successful in murine models and are now being tested clinically (Berinstein, Starnes, and Levy 1988; Hank et al. 1990). An extension of this approach is to introduce an "artificial receptor" into T cells or NK cells. Such receptors consist of the Fab fragment of the antitumor Ab, linked to a transmembrane triggering structure such as the CD3-ζ component of the Fc-γ receptor. This has been accomplished in vitro by transfection of a chimeric gene that fuses a single-chain Fab Ab gene to the FcR-γ or CD3-ζ component (Hwu et al. 1993). The transfected cells can recognize tumors via the chimeric receptor and trigger T-cell activation through the CD3 complex. As chimeric and humanized mAB with greater tumor selectivity are developed, these may become incorporated into chimeric receptors for insertion into human T or NK cells.

■ IMMUNOTHERAPY WITH ALLOGENEIC T CELLS

Allogeneic human T cells have a powerful antitumor activity as evidenced by the GVL phenomenon and the success of donor-lymphocyte transfusions for treatment of leukemic relapse after BMT. The increase in donor CTL precursor frequencies against recipient leukemia after BMT (Jiang et al. 1991) and after donor lymphocyte transfusion to treat relapse (Jiang et al. 1993) is direct evidence for an in vivo alloresponse to recipient leukemia; however, the precise specificity of the CTL was not defined in these studies. In clinical studies, the beneficial effect of GVL is often offset by the morbidity from GVHD. Considerable efforts are therefore directed towards the isolation of donor T cells that recognize the leukemic cells but not normal tissues (Sosman et al. 1990; Jiang et al. 1991; Falkenberg et al. 1993; Datta et al. 1994; Oettel et al. 1994). Currently, little is known about the specificity of the T lymphocytes involved in the clinical GVL response. For example, it is not clear whether the T cells recognize leukemia-specific Ag or normal differentiation Ag. Sosman et al. described HLA-restricted T-cell lines that strongly recognized allogeneic leukemic cells with minimal recognition of EBV-transformed lymphocytes from the same patient (Sosman et al. 1989, 1990). Falkenburg and co-workers (1993) could reproducibly generate donor-derived HLA class I– or class II–restricted CTL lines that specifically lysed the patients' leukemic cells and, in most cases, did not lyse their IL-2–stimulated lymphocytes. The actual Ag recognized by CTL in any of these studies still remain to be defined. Datta et al. (1994) developed a technique for the in vitro separation of polyclonal CML-reactive donor T cells from lymphocyte-reactive T cells. This approach could be used to deplete donor T cells recognizing certain tissue Ag while preserving leukemia-reactive T-cell populations for adoptive therapy.

In solid tumors, the therapeutic potential of allogeneic lymphocytes has not been extensively explored, although there could be theoretical advantages to this approach. Most of the tumor rejection Ag identified to date using autologous T cells appear to be normal proteins expressed preferentially but not exclusively on tumor cells; however, tumor-specific T cells have been more difficult to isolate from patients with tumors other than melanoma. It is therefore possible that in most cancer patients, T cells recognizing self-proteins expressed on tumor cells might have been deleted during the generation of tolerance. In contrast, it might be feasible to induce donor T-cell responses against differentiation alloantigens expressed preferentially on recipient tumor cells. An important caveat of this approach is the potential damage of normal tissues caused by alloreactive T cells. In hematological malignancy, the allografted BM replaces the recipient's hemopoietic system. Therefore, there is no disadvantage in using T cells directed against tissue-restricted alloantigens expressed on both malignant and normal hemopoietic cells. In solid tumors, however, the alloreactive tissue-specific donor T cells could damage the recipient's normal tissues from which the cancer originated.

■ THE POTENTIAL AND THE LIMITATIONS OF ADOPTIVE THERAPY WITH T CELLS

Recent advances in molecular tumor immunology form a basis for treatment strategies using adoptive transfer of in vitro–induced and expanded T cells. A parallel approach involves the establishment of immune response in vivo by vaccination. Both adoptive and active immunotherapy have their respective potential strengths and weaknesses, depending on the type of tumor and the clinical situation.

The use of T cells activated and grown in vitro can avoid the in vivo control mechanisms that limit antitumor T-cell expansion (Greenberg 1991). The identification of the antigenic proteins and the understanding of Ag presentation have facilitated the development of reproducible in vitro conditions for the production of tumor-specific T cells. It could be argued that such conditions can be better controlled in vitro than in patients where individual variables are difficult to predict. Since large numbers of T cells generated in vitro can be infused over short periods of time, the tumor killing can occur rapidly, decreasing the chance of tumor escape. For the same reason it could be advantageous to simultaneously infuse T-cell lines directed against multiple epitopes. The adoptive approach also allows the in vitro gene transfer and modifications of the T cells in order to augment their cytotoxic potential and other antitumor properties (Rosenberg et al. 1990; Hwu et al. 1993).

There are also several disadvantages to adoptive therapy with T cells. The induction and expansion of T cells in long-term cultures is costly and labor intensive. The optimal source of suitable APC still needs to be defined; it is often difficult to obtain sufficent numbers of a patient's PB monocytes or fresh tumor cells. Moreover, these cells are not the optimal Ag presenters and better APC, such as dendritic cells or genetically modified tumor cell lines, are being studied. Another concern is the preservation of T-cell homing and other functions during long-term in vitro culture. Although animal studies and first clinical trials with adoptively transferred T cells are encouraging, the trafficking of cultured human T cells is still poorly understood (Riddel et al. 1992).

■ ADOPTIVE IMMUNOTHERAPY: FUTURE APPLICATIONS

Just as chemotherapeutic treatments can select tumor cells that are drug resistant, studies in animal models document a number of ways whereby tumor cells can be modulated or selected to escape immune response (Melief and Kast 1992; Hank et al. 1994). The combined use of modalities directed against different Ag or using distinct antitumor mechanisms may potentially prevent such immune escape. For example, T cells reactive against MART and GP-100 as well as Ab-dependent cell killing against the GD-2 Ag could all be directed against melanoma and potentially used in combination or sequentially (Kawakami et al. 1994b; Hank et al. 1994).

Murine models of adoptive immunotherapy clearly demonstrate the power of protection that can be provided by tumor-reactive T cells. The Ag recognized on human cancer cells appear to be less immunogenic and less tumor-specific than those identified on experimental murine tumors. The in vitro activation, selection, and expansion of tumor-reactive lymphocytes is complex, and not reproducibly effective for most human tumors studied to date. Nevertheless, specific clinical examples indicate that tumor-reactive T cells can, in some cases, preferentially recognize human tumors and destroy them selectively. Progress in identifying the molecular targets of lymphocyte-tumor interactions have been possible through this research; however, if these concepts are to be clinically useful, they may need to be incorporated into a less complex clinical program that does not require individualized large-scale in vitro T-cell expansion, selection, and infusion. It is hoped that the principles learned from this approach may allow creation of treatment strategies that can induce the direct in vivo expansion of tumor-reactive lymphocytes. The different immunotherapeutic approaches, including cytokine administration, vaccination, and in vivo transfer of genes into tumors or lymphoid cells, are all focused on this goal.

ACKNOWLEDGMENTS

This work was supported by NIH grants and contracts CA-55623, CA-14520, CA-05436, CA-32685, CM-87290, CA-13539, and CM-47669.

REFERENCES

Anichi, A., Fossati, G., and Parmiani, G. (1987) Clonal analysis of the cytolytic T cell response to human tumors. *Immunology Today*, **8**, 385–9.

Apperley, J.F., Jones, L., Hale, G., et al. (1986) Bone marrow transplantation for patients with chronic myeloid leukaemia: T-cell depletion with Campath-1 reduces the incidence of graft-versus-host disease but may increase the risk of leukaemia relapse. *Bone Marrow Transplantation*, **1**, 53–7.

Baldwin, R.W. (1955) Immunity to methylcholanthrene-induced tumours in inbred rats following atrophy and regression of the implanted tumours. *British Journal of Cancer*, **9**, 652–7.

Baskar, S., Nabavi, N., Glimcher, L.H., and Ostrand-Rosenberg, S. (1993) Tumor cells expressing major HC class II and B7 activation molecules stimulate potent tumor-specific immunity. *Journal of Immunotherapy*, **14**, 209–15.

Berinstein, N., Starnes, C.O., and Levy, R. (1988) Specific enhancement of the therapeutic effect of anti-idiotype Ab on a murine B cell lymphoma by IL-2. *Journal of Immunology*, **140**, 2839–45.

Bevan, M.J. (1976) Cross-priming for a secondary cytotoxic response to minor H Ag with H2-congenic cells which do not cross-react in the cytotoxic assay. *Journal of Experimental Medicine*, **143**, 1283–8.

Bourne, H.R., Sanders, D.A., and McCormick, F. (1990) The GTPase superfamily: a conserved switch for diverse cell functions. *Nature*, **348**, 125–32.

Brichard, V., Van Pel, A., Wolfel, T., et al. (1993) The tyrosinase gene codes for an Ag recognized by autologous cytolytic T lymphocytes on HLA-A2 melanomas. *Journal of Experimental Medicine*, **178**, 489–95.

Brunda, M.J., Tarnowski, D., and Davatelis, V. (1986) Interaction of recombinant interferons with recombinant interleukin-2: differential effects on natural killer cell activity and interleukin-2-activated killer cells. *International Journal of Cancer*, **37**, 787–93.

Chakrabarti, D. and Ghosh, S.K. (1992) Induction of syngeneic cytotoxic T lymphocytes against a B cell tumor: III. MHC-class I-restricted CTL recognize the processed form(s) of idiotype. *Cellular Immunology*, **144**, 455–64.

Cheever, M.A., Chen, W., Disis, M.L., Takahashi, M., and Peace, D.J. (1993) T-cell immunity to oncogenic proteins including mutated *ras* and chimeric *bcr/abl*. *Annals of the New York Academy of Science*, **690**, 101–12.

Chen, L., Ashe, S., Brady, W.A., et al. (1992b) Costimulation of antitumor immunity by the B7 counterreceptor for the T lymphocyte molecules CD28 and CTLA-4. *Cell*, **71**, 1093–102.

Chen, Q.M. and Hersey, P. (1992) MHC-restricted responses of CD8[+] and CD4[+] T-cell clones from regional lymph nodes of melanoma patients. *International Journal of Cancer*, **51**, 218–24.

Chen, W., Peace, D.J., Rovira, D.K., You, S.G., and Cheever, M.A. (1992a) T-cell immunity to the joining region of p210*BCR/ABL* protein. *Proceedings of the National Academy of Sciences of the United States of America*. **89**, 1468–72.

Chen, W., Reese, V.A., and Cheever, M.A. (1990) Adoptively transferred Ag-specific T cells can be grown and maintained in large numbers in vivo for extended periods of time by intermittent restimulation with specific Ag plus IL-2. *Journal of Immunology*, **144**, 3659–66.

Cox, A.L., Skipper, J., Chen, Y., et al. (1994) Identification of a peptide recognized by five melanoma-specific human cytotoxic T cell lines. *Science*, **264**, 716–19.

Coulie, P.G., Brichard, V., Van Pel, A., et al. (1994) A new gene coding for a differentiation Ag recognized by autologous cytolytic T lymphocytes on HLA-A2 melanomas. *Journal of Experimental Medicine*, **180**, 35–42.

Crossland, K.D., Lee, V.K., Chen, W., Riddell, S.R., Greenberg, P.D., and Cheever, M.A. (1991) T cells from tumor-immune mice non-specifically expanded in vitro with anti-CD3 plus IL-2 retain specific function in vitro and can eradicate disseminated leukemia in vivo. *Journal of Immunology*, **146**, 4414–20.

Cullis, J.O., Jiang, Y.Z., Schwarer, A.P., Hughes, T.P., Barrett, A.J., and Goldman, J.M. (1992) Donor leukocyte infusions in the treatment of chronic myeloid leukaemia in relapse following allogeneic bone marrow transplantation. *Blood*, **79**, 1379–81.

Dailey, M.O., Pillemer, E., and Weissman, I.L. (1982) Protection against syngeneic lymphoma by a long-lived cytotoxic T cell clone. *Proceedings of the National Academy of Sciences of the United States of America*, **79**, 5384–7.

Datta A.R., Barrett A.J., Jiang Y.Z., et al. (1994) Distinct donor T-cell populations distinguish between lymphocytes and myeloid cells in marrow recipients with chronic myelogenous leukemia. *Bone Marrow Transplantation*, **14**, 517–24.

De Graaf, P.W., Horak, E., and Brookman, M.A. (1988) Adoptive immunotherapy of syngeneic murine leukemia is enhanced by the combination of IFN-gamma and a tumor-specific cytotoxic T cell clone. *Journal of Immunology*, **140**, 2853–7.

DiBirno, M., Parker, K.C., Schiloach, J., et al. (1993) Endogenous peptides bound to HLA-A3 possess a specific combination of anchor residues that permit identification of potential antigenic peptides. *Proceedings of the National Academy of Sciences of the United States of America*, **90**, 1508–12.

Disis, M.L., Smith, J.W., Murphy, A.E., Chen, W., and Cheever, M. (1994) In vitro generation of human cytolytic T-cells specific for peptides derived from the HER-2/neu protooncogene protein. *Cancer Research*, **54**, 1071–6.

Drobyski, W.R., Keever, C.A., Roth, M.S., et al. (1993) Salvage immunotherapy using donor leukocyte infusions as treatment for relapsed chronic myelogenous leukemia after allogeneic bone marrow transplantation: efficacy and toxicity of a defined T-cell dose. *Blood*, **82**, 2310–18.

Evans, R. (1984) Phenotypes associated with tumor rejection mediated by cyclophosphamide and syngeneic tumor-sensitized T lymphocytes: potential mechanisms of action. *International Journal of Cancer*, **33**, 381–8.

Falk, K., Rotzschke, O., Stevanovic, S., Jung, G., and Rammensee, H.G. (1991) Allele-specific motifs revealed by sequencing of self-peptides eluted from major HC molecules. *Nature*, **351**, 290–6.

Falkenburg, J.H.F., Faber, L.M., Van Den Elshout, M., et al. (1993) Generation of donor-derived antileukemic cytotoxic T lymphocyte responses for treatment of relapsed leukemia after allogeneic HLA-identical bone marrow transplantation. *Journal of Immunotherapy*, **14**, 305–9.

Fan, S.T. and Edgington, T.S. (1989) Sufficiency of the $CD8^+$ T cell lineage to mount an effective tumoricidal response to syngeneic tumor-bearing novel class I MHC antigen. *Journal of Immunology*, **143**, 4287–91.

Finn, O.J. (1993) Tumor-rejection Ag recognized by T lymphocytes. *Current Opinion in Immunology*, **5**, 701–8.

Fujiwara, H., Fukuzawa, M., Yoshioka, T., Nakajima, H., and Hamaoka, T. (1984) The role of tumor-specific $Lyt1^+2^-$ T cells in eradicating tumor cells in vivo. I. $Lyt1^+2^-$ T cells do not necessarily require recruitment of host's cytotoxic T cell precursors for implementation of in vivo immunity. *Journal of Immunology*, **133**, 1671–6.

Gambacorti-Passerini, C., Grignani, F., Arienti, F., Pandolfi, P.P., Pelicci, P.G., and Parmiani, G. (1993). Human CD4 lymphocytes specifically recognize a peptide representing the fusion region of the hybrid protein pml/RAR alpha present in acute promyelocytic leukemia cells. *Blood*, **81**, 1369–75.

Gaugler, B., Van den Eynde, B., van der Bruggen, P., et al. (1994) Human gene MAGE-3 codes for an Ag recognized on a melanoma by autologous cytolytic T lymphocytes. *Journal of Experimental Medicine*, **179**, 921–30.

Gishizky, M.L., Johnson-White, J., and Witte, O.N. (1993) Evaluating the effect of P210 BCR/ABL on growth of hematopoietic progenitor cells and its role in the pathogenesis of human chronic myelogenous leukemia. *Seminars in Hematology*, **30**, 6–8.

Golding, H. and Singer, A. (1985) Specificity, phenotype and precursor frequency of primary cytolytic T lymphocytes specific for class II major histocompatibility Ag. *Journal of Immunology*, **135**, 1610–15.

Goldman, J.M., Gale, R.P., Horowitz, M.M., et al. (1988) Bone marrow transplantation for chronic myelogenous leukemia in chronic phase. Increased risk of relapse associated with T-cell depletion. *Annals of Internal Medicine,* **108**, 806–14.

Greenberg, P.D. (1991) Adoptive T cell therapy of tumors: mechanisms operative in the recognition and elimination of tumor cells. *Advances in Immunology,* **49**, 281–355.

Greenberg, P.D. (1986) Therapy of murine leukemia with cyclophosphamide and immune Lyt-2$^+$ cells: cytolytic T cells can mediate eradication of disseminated leukemia. *Journal of Immunology,* **136**, 1917–22.

Greenberg, P.D., Klarnet, J.P., Kern, D.E., Okuno, K., Riddell, S., and Cheever, M.A. (1989) Specific adoptive immunotherapy. *Progress in Clinical and Biological Research,* **288**, 349–61.

Hank, J.A., Robinson, R., Surfus, J., et al. (1990) Augmentation of antibody dependent cell-mediated cytotoxicity following in vivo therapy with recombinant IL-2. *Cancer Research,* **50**, 5234–9.

Hank, J.A., Surface J., Gan J., et al. (1994) Treatment of neuroblastoma patients with anti-GD2 antibody plus interleukin 2 induces antibody dependent cellular cytotoxicity against neuroblastoma detected in vitro. *Journal of Immunotherapy,* **15**, 29–37.

Harel-Bellan, A., Quillet, A. Marchiol, C., DeMars, R., Tursz, T., and Fradelizi, D. (1986) Natural killer susceptibility of human cells may be regulated by genes in the HLA region of chromosome 6. *Proceedings of the National Academy of Sciences of the United States of America,* **83**, 5688–92.

Herin, M., Lemoine, C., Weynants, P., et al. (1987) Production of stable cytolytic T cell clones directed against autologous human melanoma. *International Journal of Cancer,* **39**, 390–6.

Hill, A.V.S., Elvin, J., Willis, A.C., et al. (1992) Molecular analysis of the association of HLA-B53 and resistence to severe malaria. *Nature,* **360**, 434–9.

Hom, S.S., Schwatzentruber, D.J., Rosenberg, S.A., and Topalian, S.L. (1993) Specific release of cytokines by lymphocytes infiltrating human melanomas in response to shared melanoma antigens. *Journal of Immunotherapy,* **13**, 18–30.

Horowitz, M.M., Gale, R.P., Sondel, P.M., et. al. (1990) Graft-versus-leukaemia reactions after bone marrow transplantation. *Blood,* **75**, 555–62.

Huang, A.Y.C., Golumbek, P., Ahmadzadeh, M., Jaffee, E., Pardoll, D., and Levitsky, H. (1994) Role of bone marrow-derived cells in presenting MHC class I-restricted tumor antigens. *Science,* **24**, 961–5.

Hwu, P., Shafer, G.E., Treisman, J., et al. (1993) Lysis of ovarian cancer cells by human lymphocytes redirected with a chimeric gene composed of an antibody variable region and the Fc receptor gamma chain. *Journal of Experimental Medicine,* **178**, 361–6.

Jenkins, M.K., Pardoll, D.M., Mizuguchi, J., Quill, H., and Schwartz, R.H. (1987) T cell responsiveness in vivo and in vitro: fine specificity of induction and molecular characterization of the unresponsive state. *Immunological Review,* **95**, 113–35.

Jerome, K.R., Barnd, D.L., Bendt, K.M., et al. (1991) Cytotoxic T-lymphocytes derived from patients with breast adenocarcinoma recognize an epitope present on the protein core of a mucin molecule preferentially expressed by malignant cells. *Cancer Research,* **51**, 2908–16.

Jiang, Y.Z., Cullis, J.O., Kanfer, E.J., Goldman, J.M., and Barrett, A.J. (1993) T-cell and NK cell mediated graft-versus-leukemia reactivity following donor buffy coat transfusion to treat relapse after bone marrow transplantation for chronic myeloid leukemia. *Bone Marrow Transplantation*, **11**, 133–8.

Jiang, Y.Z., Kanfer, E.J., Macdonald, D., Cullis, J.O., Goldman, J.M., and Barrett, A.J. (1991) Graft-versus-leukemia following allogeneic bone marrow transplantation: emergence of cytotoxic T lymphocytes reacting to host leukemia cells. *Bone Marrow Transplantation*, **8**, 253–8.

Karre, K., Ljunggren, H.G., Piontek, G., and Kiessling, R. (1986) Selective rejection of H-2 deficient lymphoma variants suggests alternative immune defence strategy. *Nature*, **319**, 675–8.

Kawakami, Y., Eliyahu, S., Delgado, C.H., et al. (1994a) Cloning of the gene coding for a shared melanoma Ag recognized by autologous T cells infiltrating into tumor. *Proceedings of the National Academy of Sciences of the United States of America*, **91**, 3515–19.

Kawakami, Y., Eliyahu, S., Delgado, C.H., et al. (1994b) Identification of a human melanoma Ag recognized by tumor infiltrating lymphocytes associated with in vivo tumor rejection. *Proceedings of the National Academy of Sciences of the United States of America*, **91**, 6459–62.

Kawasaki, E.S., Clark, S.S., Coyne, M.Y., et al. (1988). Diagnosis of chronic myeloid and acute lymphocytic leukemias by detection of leukemia-specific mRNA sequences amplified in vitro. *Proceedings of the National Academy of Sciences of the United States of America*, **85**, 5698–702.

Klein, E. and Mantovani, A. (1993) Action of natural killer cells and macrophages in cancer. *Current Opinion in Immunology*, **5**, 714–18.

Klein, G., Sjorgen, H.O., Klein, E., and Hellstrom, K.E. (1960) Demonstration of resistance against methylcholanthrene-induced sarcomas in the primary autochtonous host. *Cancer Research*, **20**, 1561–72.

Kolb, H.J., Mittermuller, J., Clemm, C.H., et al. (1990) Donor leucocyte transfusions for treatment of recurrent chronic myelogenous leukemia in marrow transplant patients. *Blood*, **76**, 2462–5.

Kwak, L.W., Campbell, M.J., Czerwinski, D.K., Hart, S., Miller, R.A., and Levy, R.L. (1992) Induction of immune responses in patients with B cell lymphoma against the surface immunoglobulin idiotype expressed by their tumor. *New England Journal of Medicine*, **327**, 1209–15.

Lanzavecchia, A. (1985) Antigen-specific interaction between T and B cells. *Nature*, **314**, 537–9.

Lauritzsen, G.F. and Bogen, B. (1993) The role of idiotype-specific, CD4$^+$ T cells in tumor resistance against major histocompatibility complex class II molecule negative plasmocytoma cells. *Cellular Immunology*, **148**, 177–88.

Linsley, P.S. and Ledbetter, J.A. (1993) The role of CD28 receptor during T cell responses to Ag. *Annual Review of Immunology*, **11**, 191–212.

Malkovska, V., Cigel, F.K., Armstrong N., Storer, B.E., and Hong, R. (1992) Antilymphoma activity of human $\gamma\delta$ T-cells in mice with severe combined immune deficiency. *Cancer Research*, **52**, 5610–16.

Malkovska, V., Cigel, F., and Storer, B.E. (1994) Human T cells in hu-PBL-SCID mice proliferate in response to Daudi lymphoma and confer anti-tumor immunity. *Clinical and Experimental Immunology*, **96**, 158–65.

Maranichi, D., Gluckman, E., Blaise, D., et al. (1987) Impact of T-cell depletion on outcome of allogeneic bone marrow transplantation for standard risk leukaemias. *Lancet*, **2**, 175–8.

McCune, J.M., Namikawa, R., Kaneshima, H., Shultz, L.D., Lieberman, M., and Weissman, I.L. (1988) The SCID-hu mouse: murine model for the analysis of human hematolymphoid differentiation and function. *Science*, **241**, 1632–9.

Melief, C.J. and Kast, W.M. (1992) Lessons from T cell responses to virus induced tumours for cancer eradication in general. *Cancer Surveys*, **13**, 81–99.

Mizuochi, T., Golding, H., Rosenberg, S.A., Glimcher, L.H., Malek, T.R., and Singer, A. (1988). Both L3T4+ and Lyt2+ helper T cells initiate cytotoxic T lymphocyte responses against allogeneic major histocompatibility Ag but not against trinitrophenyl-modified self. *Journal of Experimental Medicine*, **162**, 427–43.

Mosier, D.E., Gulizia, R.J., Baird, S.M., and Wilson, D.B. (1988) Transfer of functional human immune system to mice with severe combined immunodeficiency. *Nature*, **335**, 256–9.

Moudgil, K.D., Ametani, A., Grewal, I.S., Kumar, V., and Sercarz, E.E. (1993) Processing of self-proteins and its impact on shaping T cell repertoire, autoimmunity and immune regulation. *International Review of Immunology*, **10**, 365–77.

Oettel, K.R., Wesly, O.H., Albertini, M.R., et al. (1994) Allogeneic T cell clones able to selectively destroy Philadelphia chromosome-bearing (Ph1+) human leukemia lines can also recognize Ph1− cells from the same patients. *Blood*, **83**, 3390–402.

Pardoll, D.M. (1993). New strategies for enhancing the immunogenicity of tumors. *Current Opinion in Immunology*, **5**, 719–25.

Parmiani, G. (1990) An explanation for the variable clinical response to interleukin 2 and LAK cells. *Immunology Today*, **11**, 113–15.

Paulnock, D.M. (1994) The molecular biology of macrophage activation. *Immunology Series*, **60**, 47–62.

Peace, D.J., Chen, W., Nelson, H., and Cheever, M.A. (1991) T cell recognition of transforming proteins encoded by mutated ras proto-oncogenes. *Journal of Immunology*, **146**, 2059–65.

Peace, D.J., Smith, J.W., Chen, W., You, S.G., Blake, J., and Cheever, M.A. (1994) Lysis of ras oncogene-transformed cells by specific cytotoxic lymphocytes elicited by primary in vitro immunization with mutated ras peptide. *Journal of Experimental Medicine*, **179**, 473–9.

Prehn, R.T. (1962) Specific isoantigenicities among chemically-induced tumors. *Annals of the New York Academy of Science*, **101**, 107–13.

Ramarathinam, L., Castle, M., Wu, Y., and Liu, Y. (1994) T cell costimulation by B7/BB1 induces CD8 T cell-dependent tumor rejection: an important role of B7/BB1 in the induction, recruitment, and effector function of antitumor T cells. *Journal of Experimental Medicine*, **179**, 1205–14.

Riddell, S.R., Gilbert, M.J., and Greenberg, P.D. (1993) CD8+ cytotoxic T cell therapy of cytomegalovirus and HIV infection. *Current Opinion in Immunology*, **5**, 484–91.

Riddell, S., Watanabe, K., Goodrich, J., Li, C.R., Agha, M., and Greenberg, P. (1992) Restoration of viral immunity in immunodeficient humans by the adoptive transfer of T cell clones. *Science*, **257**, 238–41.

Rosenberg, S., Aebersold, P., and Cornetta, K., et. al. (1990) Gene transfer into humans: immunotherapy of patients with advanced melanoma using tumor infiltrating lymphocytes modified by retroviral gene transfer. *New England Journal of Medicine*, **323**, 570–8.

Rosenberg, S.A., Lotze, M.T., Muul, L.M., et al. (1987) A progress report on the 157 patients with advanced cancer using lymphokine-activated killer cells and intereukin-2 or high-dose interleukin-2 alone. *New England Journal of Medicine*, **316**, 889–97.

Rosenberg, S.A., Lotze, M.T., Muul, L.M., et al. (1985) Observations on the systemic administration of autologous lymphokine-activated killer cells and recombinant interleukin-2 to patients with metastatic cancer. *New England Journal of Medicine*, **313**, 1485–92.

Rosenberg, S.A., Packard, B.S., Aebersold, P.M., et al. (1988). Use of tumor-infiltrating lymphocytes and interleukin-2 in the immunotherapy of patients with metastatic melanoma. A preliminary report. *New England Journal of Medicine*, **319**, 1676–80.

Rosenstein, M., Eberlein, T., and Rosenberg, S.A. (1984) Adoptive immunotherapy of established syngenenic solid tumors: role of T lymphoid subpopulations. *Journal of Immunology*, **132**, 2117–22.

Slingluff, C.L., Jr., Cox, A.L., Henderson, R.A., Hunt, D.F., and Engelhard, V.H. (1993) Recognition of human melanoma cells by HLA-A2.1-restricted cytotoxic T lymphocytes is mediated by at least six shared peptide epitopes. *Journal of Immunology*, **150**, 2955–63.

Sosman, J.A., Oettel, K.R., Hank, J.A., Fisch, P., and Sondel, P.M. (1989) Specific recognition of human leukemic cells by allogeneic T cell lines. *Transplantation*, **48**, 486–95.

Sosman, J.A., Oettel, K.R., Smith, S.D., Hank, J.A., Fish, P., and Sondel, P.M. (1990) Specific recognition of human leukemic cells by allogeneic T cells: II. Evidence for HLA-D restricted determinants on leukemic cells that are crossreactive with determinants present on unrelated nonleukemic cells. *Blood*, **75**, 1–12.

Sosman, J.A. and Sondel, P.M. (1987) The graft versus leukemia (GVL) effect following bone marrow transplantation (BMT): a review of laboratory and clinical data. *Hematology Review*, **2**, 77–91.

Staerz, U.D., Karasugama, H., and Garner, A.M. (1987) Cytotoxic T lymphocytes against a soluble protein. *Nature*, **32**, 449–51.

Storkus, W.J. and Dawson, J.R. (1991) Target structures involved in natural killing (NK): characteristics, distribution and candidate molecules. *Critical Reviews in Immunology*, **10**, 393–416.

Storkus, W.J., Zeh, H.J., III, Maeurer, M.J., Salter, R.D., and Lotze, M.T. (1993) Identification of human melanoma peptides recognized by class I restricted tumor infiltrating T lymphocytes. *Journal of Immunology*, **151**, 3719–27.

Swain, S.L. (1981) Significance of Lyt phenotypes: Lyt2 Ab block activities of T cells that recognize class I major histocompatibility complex Ag regardless of their function. *Proceedings of the National Academy of Sciences of the United States of America*, **78**, 7101–5.

Townsend, S.E. and Allison, J.P. (1993) Tumor rejection after direct costimulation of CD8$^+$ T cells by B7-transfected melanoma cells. *Science*, **259**, 368–70.

Van der Bruggen, P., Traversari, C., Chomez, P., et al. (1991) A gene encoding an Ag recognized by cytolytic T lymphocytes on a human melanoma. *Science*, **254**, 1643–7.

Wang, P., Vegh, Z., Vanky, F., and Klein, E. (1992) HLA-B5-restricted auto-tumor-specific cytotoxic T cells generated in mixed lymphocyte-tumor-cell culture. *International Journal of Cancer*, **52**, 517–22.

Ward, B.A., Shu, S., Chou, T., Perry-Lalley, D., and Chang, A.E. (1988) Cellular basis of immunologic interactions in adoptive T cell therapy of established metastases from a syngeneic murine sarcoma. *Journal of Immunology*, **141**, 1047–53.

Widmer, M.B. and Bach, F.H. (1981) Antigen-driven helper cell-independent cytolytic T lymphocytes. *Nature*, **294**, 750–2.

Wilson, A., George, A.J., King, C.A., et al. (1990) Recognition of a B cell lymphoma by antiidiotypic T cells. *Journal of Immunology*, **145**, 3937–43.

Woods, G., Kitagami, K., and Ochi, A. (1989). Evidence for an involvement of T4+ cytotoxic T cells in tumor immunity. *Cellular Immunology*, **118**, 126–35.

Wortzel, R.D., Urban, J.L., and Schreiber, H. (1984) Malignant growth in the normal host after variant selection in vitro with cytolytic T cell lines. *Proceedings of the National Academy of Sciences of the United States of America*, **81**, 2186–90.

Wright, A., Lee, J.E., Link, M.P., et al. (1989) Cytotoxic T lymphocytes specific for self tumor immunoglobulin express T cell receptor gamma chain. *Journal of Experimental Medicine*, **169**, 1557–64.

Yamasaki, T., Handa, H., Yamashita, J., Watanabe, Y., Namba, Y., and Hanaoka, M. (1984) Specific adoptive immunotherapy with tumor-specific cytotoxic T-lymphocyte clone for murine malignant gliomas. *Cancer Research*, **44**, 1776–83.

Yasumura, S., Hirabayashi, H., and Schwartz, D.R., et al. (1993) Human cytotoxic T cell lines with restricted specificity for squamous cell carcinoma of the head and neck. *Cancer Research*, **53**, 1461–8.

Yssel, H., Spits, H., and DeVries, J.E. (1984) A cloned human T cell line cytotoxic for autologous and allogeneic B lymphoma cells. *Journal of Experimental Medicine*, **160**, 239–54.

25

Cellular Adoptive Immunotherapy with Natural Killer Cells

WILLIAM E. CARSON AND MICHAEL A. CALIGIURI

Natural killer (NK) cells are bone marrow (BM)–derived large granular lymphocytes (LGL) that neither express CD3 T-cell surface antigens (Ag) nor display functional rearrangements of the T-cell receptor or B-cell immunoglobulin genes (Robertson and Ritz 1990). These cells comprise approximately 10% to 20% of human peripheral blood mononuclear cells (PBMC) and are an important component of the innate system of immunity that also consists of monocyte/macrophages, granulocytes, and eosinophils (Brown, Atkinson, and Fearon 1994). Resting or unstimulated NK cells express abundant cytolytic granules and cellular adhesion molecules in comparison to T cells and engage in non–major histocompatibility complex–restricted cytotoxicity against virally infected cells and tumor-target cells without prior sensitization (Trinchieri 1989). The surface expression of a low-affinity receptor for the Fc portion of immunoglobulin (FcRγIII or CD16) also enables NK cells to interact with antibody (Ab) -coated target cells and mediate Ab-dependent cellular cytotoxicity (ADCC) (Trinchieri et al. 1984).

All human NK cell express the CD56 surface Ag, an isoform of the neural cell-adhesion molecule whose function on LGL remains unknown (Robertson and Ritz 1990). CD56 is also expressed on a small subset of CD3[+] and CD8[+] T cells. Approximately 10% of NK cells have high-density cell-surface expression of CD56 (CD56[bright]). These CD56[bright] NK cells are unique in their constitutive expression of a high-affinity heterotrimeric interleukin-2 receptor (IL-2R), composed of α, β, and γ transmembrane protein subunits, which binds IL-2 at very low concentrations (Kd, 10 pm or approximately 2.3 U/mL) (Caligiuri et al. 1990; Nagler, Lanier, and Phillips 1990). This cell population also expresses an intermediate-affinity IL-2R composed of β

451

and γ subunits that noncovalently associate as a heterodimer (Kd, 1 nM or approximately 230 U/mL). The more abundant CD56^{dim} NK cells (the remaining 90% of NK cells) constitutively express only the intermediate-affinity heterodimeric IL-2R (Siegel et al. 1987; Tsudo et al. 1987; Kehrl et al. 1988; Voss, Sondel, and Robb 1992). It has been shown that the binding of IL-2 to the high-affinity IL-2R expressed on CD56^{bright} NK cells results in a strong proliferative signal, while complete saturation of the intermediate-affinity IL-2R on either CD56^{bright} or CD56^{dim} NK cells results in enhanced cytotoxic activity with little or no effect on proliferation (Caligiuri et al. 1990). Thus, the high- and intermediate-affinity IL-2R appear to mediate relatively distinct functional responses following the binding of IL-2. Importantly, the NK cell is the only lymphocyte to constitutively express functional isoforms of the IL-2 receptor in the resting or unactivated state and is, therefore, poised to respond to the exogenous administration of this cytokine in the absence of antigenic stimulation (Smith 1993).

The role of the NK cell in the normal immune response continues to be the focus of intense research. The availability of purified monoclonal antibodies (mAB) and recombinant cytokines, as well as recent advances in the field of flow cytometry, have greatly aided this effort. The activity of NK cells against tumor targets in vitro has provided the impetus for investigators to test the efficacy of this cell population as an antitumor effector in animal models as well as in humans with malignancy. Initial trials conducted in the early 1980s involved the infusion of high-dose IL-2 in combination with IL-2–activated PB lymphocytes subsequently found to have many characteristics of human NK cells (Robertson and Ritz 1990). More recently, attempts have been made to expand pure populations of NK cells in vitro with IL-2 for use in adoptive cellular immunotherapy. In a refinement of this concept, several investigators have succeeded in expanding the CD56$^+$ NK cell population in vivo through the prolonged administration of low doses of IL-2. In this chapter, a chronological review of these studies will be presented to provide a broad overview of the history and possible future applications of cellular therapy with human NK cells.

■ LYMPHOKINE-ACTIVATED KILLER CELL THERAPY

Culture of PBMC with IL-2 produces a population of cytotoxic lymphocytes with the ability to lyse fresh tumor cells without prior sensitization and without major histocompatibility complex (HC) restriction. These effector cells have been defined as lymphokine-activated killer (LAK) cells and have been used to treat human malignancies in many clinical trials (Robertson and Ritz 1990; Grimm et al. 1982). The available evidence indicates that the majority of functional LAK cells are $CD56^+$ LGL whose phenotype is similar, if not identical, to that of the human NK cell (Phillips and Lanier 1986; Phillips et al. 1987; McMannis et al. 1988; Kolitz and Mertelsmann 1991; Hiserodt 1993). We will review the evidence that implicates the NK cell as the primary effector cell in LAK cultures and summarize the important clinical trials that have used LAK cells in adoptive immunotherapy.

Cell suspensions derived from fresh autologous tumor are essentially resistant to lysis by unstimulated NK cells; however, these preparations can be readily lysed by LAK cells generated from the culture of PBMC in crude or recombinant IL-2 for 3 to 5 days. LAK-cell activity is routinely measured in short-term ^{51}Cr release assays that do not allow prolonged contact between effector cell and the tumor target. This brief interaction excludes significant contributions to the lysis of target cells by activated macrophages or granulocytes, both of which require much longer periods of time to exert their cytolytic effects (Hiserodt 1993). The mechanisms used by LAK cells to recognize and lyse tumor cell targets have not been adequately defined, but are not directed by the major HC complex and may, therefore, be referred to as major HC-unrestricted. In this sense, LAK-cell activity appears to be operationally identical to the cytotoxic effector mechanisms used by the NK cell (Kolitz and Mertelsmann 1991; Hiserodt 1993). LAK-cell activity can be generated from the PBMC of normal individuals as well as patients with malignancy. The resulting effector cells are active against a wide array of targets including fresh autologous and allogeneic tumor cells, tumor cell lines, and cells derived from xenogeneic sources (Rosenberg and Lotze 1986). LAK cells, however, do not appear to have cytolytic efficacy against freshly isolated normal tissues (Hiserodt 1993).

Numerous studies have dealt with the characterization of the LAK-cell phenotype since the original description of the phenomenon by Grimm et al. (1982). LAK cells are derived from PBMC cultures of a mixture of cell types. This has made it difficult to correctly identify the cell population(s) responsible for mediating LAK-cell activity. Early studies were hampered also by limitations in mAB technology and flow cytometry (Hiserodt 1993). Consequently, investigators could not precisely determine whether LAK-cell effectors arose from NK cell and/or T-cell precursors, or whether LAK cells constituted a novel lineage. There is now good evidence indicating that LAK-cell precursors are contained primarily within the LGL population, express the NK-surface markers CD56 and CD16, and lack the T-cell marker CD5 (Ortaldo, Mason, and Overton 1986; Phillips and Lanier 1986; Herberman et al. 1987; Phillips et al. 1987; McMannis et al. 1988; Kolitz and Mertelsmann 1991; Hiserodt 1993).

Separation of IL-2–cultured PBMC by flow cytometric cell sorting reveals that nearly all LAK activity is contained within the $CD56^+$ lymphocyte population; CD3 and CD5 populations are largely devoid of LAK activity (Ortaldo et al. 1986; Phillips and Lanier 1986). Additional proof comes from experiments in which LAK-cell activity can be abrogated by depleting PBMC of $CD56^+$ LGL before culture with IL-2 (Hiserodt 1993). As mentioned, NK cells are the only resting lymphocyte to constitutively express a functional IL-2R. The majority of NK cells express an intermediate-affinity IL-2R, thus explaining the relatively high concentrations of IL-2 that are required to generate LAK cells (Rosenberg and Lotze 1986; Kolitz and Mertelsmann 1991; Hiserodt 1993). The majority of T cells do not express a functional IL-2R before Ag-specific stimulation, and as such, are not IL-2 responsive. A notable exception is a small and highly variable population of T cells that express CD56 and CD3 and comprise less than 5% of all T cells. This cell population exhibits NK-like cytolytic activity and develops LAK activity in response to high concentrations of IL-2 without antigenic activation. The total contribution of these cells, however, to the cytotoxic activity of standard LAK-cell cultures is probably less than 10%. Other investigators have suggested that $CD11b^+$ T cells and $\gamma\delta$ T-cell populations can function as LAK precursors and mediate major HC-unrestricted cytotoxicity in response to IL-2. These cell types, however, appear to contribute little to the cytotoxic activity of LAK-cell cultures (Dianzani et al. 1989; Fox and Rosenberg 1989). Consequently, the cytolytic effector cell containing the majority of LAK activity in the adoptive transfer of IL-2–activated PBMC appears to be the NK cell (Robertson and Ritz 1990; Kolitz and Mertelsmann 1991; Hiserodt 1993).

IL-2 must be available in concentrations approximating 1,000 U/mL for significant LAK-cell activity to be generated. In the original experiments, IL-2 was provided as crude supernatants from cultures of Jurkat cells, but with the development of rIL-2 in 1984, it has since been shown that LAK cells can be grown in medium containing rIL-2 without loss of activity (Lotze et al. 1985a, b). Several investigators have reported the generation of LAK cells by culture of PBMC in cytokines other than IL-2. For instance, IL-7 can stimulate the development of LAK activity from cultures of fresh lymphocytes; however, very little clinical experience has been gained with these preparations and it is not apparent that they exhibit any advantage over standard

IL-2–generated LAK preparations (Alderson, Sassenfeld, and Widmer 1990). Importantly, as LAK-cell cultures are a heterologous collection of cell types, "bystander" cells, such as monocytes and macrophages, can be activated by the cytokines produced by IL-2–activated NK cells. These cells can, in turn, secrete factors that further contribute to the generation or suppression of LAK cells (Kolitz and Mertelsmann 1991; Hiserodt 1993).

The clinical use of LAK cells for the treatment of cancer through adoptive immunotherapy followed reports of success with IL-2/LAK therapy in animal models, where a number of studies showed that IL-2 in combination with LAK infusions resulted in superior antitumor effects in comparison to therapy with either modality alone (Lafreniere and Rosenberg 1985; Mule et al. 1986; Papa, Mule, and Rosenberg 1986; Charak and Mazumder 1993). From these initial observations, hundreds of trials have been conducted in humans. The most impressive results have been seen in patients with metastatic or unresectable malignant melanoma or renal cell carcinoma (RCCA). We will, therefore, focus on trials involving these two cancers and review the progress that has been made over the past 10 years.

Rosenberg et al. (1985) reported the first use of LAK and rIL-2 in the treatment of human malignancy. Remarkable regressions of metastatic disease were achieved with this regimen and considerable interest was generated in the field of immunotherapy. Objective responses were noted in 11 of 25 patients with metastatic cancer, but these were most common in patients with metastatic malignant melanoma or RCCA. In this phase I trial, one of seven patients with advanced malignant melanoma achieved a complete response (CR) and three others achieved partial responses (PR). Furthermore, all three patients with RCCA who were treated with this regimen went on to exhibit PR. In the high-dose regimen used in this study, 6×10^5 U/kg rIL-2 was administered as an intravenous (IV) bolus every 8 hours on days 1 to 5 and again on days 12 to 16. Administration of rIL-2 at these doses resulted in a profound lymphopenia beginning 24 to 48 hours after the initiation of IV rIL-2 that was not reversed until day 5 or 6 when the rIL-2 infusion finished and a rebound lymphocytosis was seen. Patients had leukapheresis on days 8 to 12 and PBMC were cultured for 4 days in 6×10^3 U rIL-2. These cells were harvested for infusion on days 12, 13, and 15 to coincide with the second cycle of IV IL-2. Of note, this protocol and subsequent modifications all resulted in significant systemic toxicities including hypotension, fluid retention, oliguria, and hepatic dysfunction, and close observation in an intensive care unit setting was required for all patients (Lafreniere and Rosenberg 1985; Lanier et al. 1985; Lotze et al. 1985a, b; Rosenberg et al. 1985; Mule et al. 1986; Ortaldo et al. 1986; Papa et al. 1986; Rosenberg and Lotze 1986; Schmidt et al. 1986; Herberman et al. 1987; Dianzani et al. 1989; Fox and Rosenberg 1989; Alderson et al. 1990; Charak and Mazumder 1993). As experience was gained, however, it was found that specific support measures could be instituted to anticipate and minimize the more serious side effects. If there were life-threatening toxicities, the discontinuation of rIL-2 resulted in a prompt reversal of symptoms, indicating that these toxicities arose primarily from the infusion of high-dose rIL-2 and were not related to the administration of LAK cells.

Rosenberg et al. (1987) updated the National Cancer Institute (NCI) experience and reported an objective response in 6 of 23 patients with malignant melanoma, 2 of which were CR. A subsequent report from the NCI reviewed the results of a similarly designed trial that had a total of 652 participating patients, 48 of whom received LAK and rIL-2 for malignant melanoma. A CR was noted in 4 of 48 patients (18%) and another 6 patients (13%) achieved a PR. Unfortunately, these responses were of relatively short duration and permanent regressions of disease were not obtained (Rosenberg et al. 1989). Two subsequent studies conducted by the NCI extramural IL-2 working group (ILWG) focused specifically on the treatment of patients with malignant melanoma using rIL-2/LAK therapy (Dutcher et al. 1989; Bar et al. 1990). In the first study, 3% CR and 14% PR were achieved in 36 patients with metastatic or unresectable malignant melanoma. Sites of disease responding to therapy included skin, lymph nodes, and lung as well as visceral metastases, which are generally resistant to traditional chemotherapeutic regimens. In the second study, rIL-2 was given as a continuous infusion (CI) during the administration of LAK cells in an attempt to maximize the exposure of cells to a high concentration of cytokine. The sites of response were similar to the previous study, as were the overall results: one patient experienced a CR (2%) and six had PR (12%). In both of these trials, it was found that patients with lower tumor burdens were more likely to respond to therapy.

Evidence suggests that CI of IL-2 might result in greater LAK-cell activation with less clinical toxicity (Sondel et al. 1988; Waleski et al. 1989; Sparano and Dutcher 1993). Also, West et al. had reported a 50% PR in a group of ten patients with malignant melanoma given rIL-2 as a CI (West et al. 1987). Therefore, several studies were initiated in which rIL-2 was given as a CI to patients with malignant melanomas (Gaynor et al. 1990; Richards et al. 1990; Dillman et al. 1991; Dutcher et al. 1991). Disease burdens were similar to those of patients in previous trials, yet overall response rates were consistently less than 10% and no CR were observed.

More recently, there has been an attempt to define the role of adoptively transferred LAK cells in the immunotherapy of malignant melanoma. In contrast to animal models, clinical studies using high-dose IL-2 alone in a bolus schedule showed results comparable with those in which IL-2 was used in combinations with the infusion of ex vivo–expanded LAK cells (Whitehead et al. 1989; Parkinson et al. 1990a). A recent report from the NCI reviewed the progress of 181 patients who had been randomized between rIL-2 alone and rIL-2 plus LAK cells (Rosenberg et al. 1993). Of the 26 patients with melanoma, 3 CR and 3 PR were noted in patients receiving infusions of both rIL-2 and LAK cells, whereas no CR were noted in patients receiving rIL-2 alone. More importantly, a trend towards improved survival at 2 years was seen for patients receiving LAK cells and rIL-2 compared with those who received rIL-2 alone (32% versus 15%; $p = 0.064$). To date, however, there is no conclusive evidence that the administration of LAK cells to patients with advanced malignant melanoma results in improved survival. This form of cellular therapy may deliver superior results with further refinement.

Therapy with LAK cells in combination with high-dose IV rIL-2 has also been used successfully in the treatment of advanced RCCA. Rosenberg's initial report included three patients with RCCA, all of whom exhibited partial regression of pulmonary metastases (Rosenberg et al. 1985). Subsequent reports confirmed the effectiveness of this therapy for patients with advanced cancers, and in the 1989 review of the NCI experience, Rosenberg documented an overall response rate of 35% in 72 patients with RCCA. Of particular interest was the observation that 8 of 25 patients who experienced objective responses went on to achieve a CR. In a confirmatory study by the ILWG, 2 PR and 3 CR were observed in 32 patients receiving the standard rIL-2/LAK-cell regimen (Fisher et al. 1988). This translated into an overall response rate of 16%, again lower than that observed in the NCI trials. Nonetheless, this activity was noteworthy, given the general resistance of this tumor type to chemotherapeutic-based treatments. Further analysis revealed that patients who had had nephrectomy or pulmonary and soft tissue sites of disease were more likely to respond to rIL-2/LAK-cell therapy. A subsequent phase II trial by ILWG used a hybrid regimen in which the delivery of rIL-2 during the period of LAK-cell treatment was changed to a 144-hour CI (Parkinson et al. 1990b). Again, the rationale was to reduce rIL-2 toxicity as well as increase the exposure of adoptively transferred LAK cells to rIL-2. This modified schedule, however, resulted in only a 9% response rate without significant improvement in toxicity. In another phase II trial, 94 patients were randomized between LAK therapy in conjunction with either bolus or CI rIL-2. Despite a CI schedule that delivered only 25% of the total dose of rIL-2 received by patients in the bolus group, the incidence of grade III and IV toxicities was equal in both groups (Weiss et al. 1992). Moreover, response rates for the CI and bolus regimens were similar (15% and 20%, respectively) and it was concluded that CI rIL-2 held no inherent advantage. Several additional studies by the National Biotherapy and the European Multicenter study groups have confirmed the efficacy of CI rIL-2 given in conjunction with LAK cells and have reported response rates for RCCA between 22% and 28% (West et al. 1987; West 1989; Weiss et al. 1992).

At this point in the development of rIL-2/LAK-cell therapy for RCCA, several lines of evidence indicated that LAK cells were an important component of this treatment. In 1989, Rosenberg had reviewed the NIH experience with rIL-2–based protocols, and had reported a slightly improved response rate when rIL-2 was used in conjunction with LAK-cell therapy (24% versus 33%) (Hawkins 1988; Rosenberg et al. 1989). These two patient groups, however, were not part of a randomized trial and could not be compared statistically. Additionally, a small phase II trial of high-dose rIL-2 alone conducted by the ILWG had produced no objective responses among 16 patients with RCCA (Abrams et al. 1990), indicating that LAK cells were important in the immunotherapy of this human malignancy. On the other hand, it was known that LAK cells do not preferentially accumulate at tumor sites in humans. Histologic studies had established that lymphocytes that do invade the tumor stroma had the phenotype of T-cytotoxic/suppressor cells and lacked detectable NK cell-surface markers (Lotze et al. 1980; Finke et al. 1990). Collectively, these data provided the impetus for additional trials in which patients were randomized between treatments consisting of rIL-2 alone or rIL-2 with the adoptive transfer of LAK cells (Marincola 1994).

In a study of 49 patients with RCCA, Bajorin and co-workers examined the effects of LAK-cell treatments in combination with CI rIL-2 (Bajorin et al. 1990). Patients received 3×10^6 U/m^2/d on days 1 to 5, 13 to 17, 21 to 24, and 28 to 31 and were randomized to receive either rIL-2 alone or rIL-2 plus LAK cells. The LAK cells were given on days 13 to 15 and the median number of LAK cells administered was 73×10^9. The number of CR and PR in each group were not statistically different and it was concluded that in RCCA the response rates for CI rIL-2 were similar regardless of LAK-cell administration. In a phase III trial in which 69 patients were randomized between rIL-2 and rIL-2 with LAK, McCabe et al. reported that LAK cells did not significantly improve patient outcome (McCabe, Stablein, and Hawkins 1991). In this study, patients received rIL-2 every 8 hours at a dose of 100,000 U/kg on days 1 to 5 and days 11 to 15. Patients randomized to LAK-cell therapy received infusions of LAK cells on days 11, 12, and 17. One CR and two PR were seen in RCCA patients treated with rIL-2 alone, whereas patients in the group receiving rIL-2 plus LAK cells had no CR and four PR. This study included 98 patients with malignant melanoma who were randomized between rIL-2 or rIL-2 and LAK and again the addition of LAK cells to the regimen did not lead to significant improvement in the response rate to rIL-2. Furthermore, a subsequent report from the surgery branch of the NCI found no statistically significant difference in overall survival among 97 patients with RCCA who were randomized between high-dose rIL-2 alone or in combination with LAK-cell therapy (Rosenberg et al. 1993). Based on these studies and the results of similar trials from Europe (Palmer et al. 1992), it appears that rIL-2 alone is capable of mediating the antitumor effect seen in this disease.

The seeming requirements for LAK-cell administration in conjunction with rIL-2 in animal models is a distinct contrast to the results obtained in humans, where rIL-2 alone can mediate the regression of established tumors in 10% to 20% of cases, and the addition of adoptively transferred LAK cells does not add significantly to these results (Lafreniere and Rosenberg 1985; Mule et al. 1986; Papa et al. 1986). Thus, the true potential of LAK-cell therapy in the treatment of human malignancy remains unproven. It is possible that the therapeutic benefit of LAK-cell therapy is restricted to a specific patient subgroup or is most efficacious in the setting of minimal disease. Alternatively, given the evidence that points to the NK cell as the primary cytolytic cell of the LAK preparations (Ortaldo et al. 1986; Phillips and Lanier 1986; Herberman et al. 1987), better results might be obtained with purified populations of activated NK effectors or with techniques that maximize the intensity and duration of the interaction between the effector and target cell (discussed later). Based on the preceding studies, several investigators have attempted to delineate the efficacy of purified NK cells in the treatment of experimental tumors in animals as well as in the setting of advanced malignant disease in humans.

■ ADOPTIVE CELLULAR THERAPY WITH NATURAL KILLER CELLS

Previous animal studies have implicated the NK cell as the primary mediator of antitumor activity within LAK-cell preparations

(Charak and Mazumder 1993). Based on these data, investigators at the University of Pittsburgh have developed a method for generating large numbers of adherent LAK (A-LAK) cells highly enriched for CD56$^+$ NK cells (Melder et al. 1988; Vujanovic et al. 1993). The PBMC cells are cultured for 24 hours in medium containing 1,000 U/mL rIL-2. Under these conditions, approximately 1% to 4% of cells become adherent to plastic. Analysis of the adherent cell population reveals a CD3$^-$ CD56$^+$ cell type that possesses cytolytic activity against NK-sensitive and NK-resistant targets. Adherent cells are then collected and expanded for 7 to 12 additional days in medium supplemented with rIL-2. Over the course of this culture period, there is a 130- to 1,100-fold increase in cell number and a steady increase in expression of the CD56 surface Ag such that 60% to 95% of A-LAK are CD56$^+$ when tested on day 12. In these studies, A-LAK exhibit superior cytolytic capacity against a variety of targets compared with unfractionated LAK cells and can mediate ADCC against Ab-coated targets. Interestingly, A-LAK can be generated from the PBMC of cancer patients, but not at the same efficiency as with normal donors (Melder et al. 1988; Vujanovic et al. 1993).

Animal Studies with Adherent Lymphokine-Activated Killer Cells

Basse et al. studied the tissue distribution of IV murine A-LAK in C57BL/6 mice bearing lung and liver metastases of the B16 melanoma, MCA 102 sarcoma, and Lewis lung carcinoma (Basse et al. 1991). A dose-dependent specific infiltration of lung metastases (as compared with surrounding normal tissues) was found after IV injection of fluorescently labeled A-LAK cells, whereas substantial infiltration of liver metastases was seen only after intraportal injection of A-LAK cells. IL-2 activation was critical to the development of this infiltrative capacity, since fresh murine NK cells failed to accumulate in metastatic sites of disease with any degree of specificity. In a similar experiment, Kuppen et al. found that the number of adoptively transferred A-LAK cells localizing within established colon carcinoma lung metastases in WAG rats increased over time compared with normal tissues (Kuppen et al. 1994). At 24 hours, 10% of the injected A-LAK cells had localized to these metastases and the estimated effector cell/tumor cell ratio was 1:3. In contrast, very low numbers of A-LAK cells were found within the liver, spleen, or lung. These data suggest that IL-2–activated A-LAK cells possess specific properties that permit their infiltration into regions of metastatic tumor growth in preference to normal tissues.

Schwarz et al. examined the antimetastatic activity of adoptively transferred murine A-LAK cells in Fischer 344 rats bearing experimentally induced pulmonary or hepatic metastases of the NK-resistant mammary adenocarcinoma cell line MAD B106 (Schwarz, Vujanovic, and Hiserodt 1989b). The A-LAK cells were administered IV and IL-2 (5×10^4 U twice daily for 5 days) was given intraperitoneally (IP). Treatment groups received either control, IL-2 alone, A-LAK cells plus IL-2, or unfractionated LAK cells plus IL-2. Unfractionated LAK cells in combination with IL-2 were able to mediate significant regression of pulmonary and hepatic metastases that resulted in improved survival compared with control animals receiving either no treatment or IL-2 alone. Adoptive transfer of A-LAK, however, in combination with IL-2 was superior against metastatic disease at both sites and improved survival time ($p < 0.03$). The authors concluded that adoptive immunotherapy with purified populations of A-LAK cells plus IL-2 led to improved outcome compared with standard LAK-cell therapies.

More recently, Whiteside et al. have devised an elegant animal model of liver metastases using a human gastric carcinoma cell line to test the efficacy of adoptive immunotherapy with A-LAK cells (Yasumura et al. 1994). Intrasplenic injection of 1×10^7 carcinoma cells into nude mice depleted of endogenous NK-cell activity by pretreatment with cyclophosphamide and anti-asialo G_M1 led to the development of numerous micrometastases (groups of 10 to 20 cells) by day 4 and macrometastases by day 7. Animals developed ascites and died within 30 to 40 days of injection. Animals bearing 3-day micrometastases received an intrasplenic injection of 1×10^7 A-LAK cells with IP IL-2 (6×10^4 U twice daily for 5 days) or IL-2 alone. Histologic examination of the mouse livers at various times revealed the elimination of the vast majority of microscopic disease within 24 hours of A-LAK-cell treatment, whereas IL-2 alone had no significant effect on the extent of liver disease. Similarly, A-LAK-cell treatment to mice bearing 7-day macrometastases significantly decreased the number of liver lesions as well as improved survival compared with mice receiving IL-2 alone ($p < 0.0001$). Interestingly, two mice in the A-LAK–treatment group exhibited no evidence of tumor on gross or histologic examination at 60 days.

Other investigators have examined the efficacy of human A-LAK-cell treatments in immunosuppressed mice xenografted with human tumors to create a workable animal model of localized disease. Sacchi et al. investigated the effects of A-LAK cells on xenografted squamous-cell carcinoma of the head and neck (SCCHN) in a nude mouse model (Sacchi et al. 1990). To ensure tumor-cell growth, nude mice were spelenectomized at least 2 weeks before treatment and received cyclophosphamide the day before the injection of SCCHN tumor cells. Mice with established tumors were treated beginning on day 3 or day 7 with 1×10^7 LAK or A-LAK cells administered as a peritumoral injection. A total of six treatments was administered in combination with daily local injections of rIL-2 (1,000 CU). Despite similar in vitro cytolytic profiles, A-LAK cells mediated complete regression of all day-3 and day-7 tumors, whereas LAK cells did not. Furthermore, labeled A-LAK cells could be localized to the tumor stroma within 24 hours of injection and their presence coincided with the initiation of an inflammatory response that was followed by accelerated tumor differentiation and involution.

Additional work by this group of investigators showed that adoptively transferred A-LAK cells that had infiltrated the stroma of SCCHN tumors in nude mice expressed increased levels of IL-2Rα, IL-2Rβ, and IFN-γ at both the mRNA and protein levels. Functionally, it was shown that irradiated tumor cells enhanced the proliferative and cytotoxic capacities of A-LAK cells cultured in IL-2. Also, supernatants from cultures containing A-LAK and irradiated tumor cells were able to inhibit tumor-cell proliferation in vitro, an activity that could be partially blocked by neutralizing Ab to IFN-γ and tumor necrosis factor-α (TNF-α). Interestingly, perilesional injection of supernatants from IL-2–activated A-LAK cells led to regression of tumors in nude mice, and this activity could be duplicated using IFN-γ alone (1×10^5 U, three times a week for 2 weeks). These findings imply that tumor cells may stimulate adoptively transferred A-LAK cells to release immunomodulatory cytokines that may mediate the regression of the malignant lesion.

Human Studies with Adherent Lymphokine-Activated Killer Cells

The success of future studies will depend, in large part, on our ability to efficiently expand NK cell effectors in vitro and deliver them in a safe and timely manner to the patient with malignancy. It is also apparent from animal studies that a physical interaction between the NK cell and the tumor target might be an essential step in this process. Whether this interaction provides for the optimal release of cytokines by the NK cell or reflects the importance of direct NK cytolytic mechanisms is still unresolved. It was previously assumed that the effector functions of the NK cell were centered around its cytotoxic capacities. It is now known, however, that the secretion of cytokines (such as IFN-γ) by the NK cell is critical to host defense against pathogenic organisms, and it is possible that similar cytokine networks will be important in the function of adoptively transferred NK cells (Rabinowich et al. 1992; Bancroft 1993). Thus, strategies to direct NK cells to sites of disease and augmentation of NK activity through the administration of exogenous cytokines may prove critical to the success of NK cell–based therapies.

Rabinowich et al. (1991) described the use of mitogen-activated feeder cells to enhance the proliferation, cytolytic activity, and purity of human A-LAK cells. The A-LAK cells were obtained by adherence to plastic during a 24-hour culture with rIL-2 (1,000 CU/mL) and then cultured with IL-2 for 14 days in the presence of either Con A-stimulated peripheral blood lymphocytes (PBL) or an Epstein-Barr virus (EBV) –transformed lymphoblastoid cell line. Under these conditions, there was a five- to tenfold increase in A-LAK cells numbers compared with cultures without feeder cells, and a 30% increase in the number of $CD3^-$ $CD56^+$ cells. Also, the presence of feeder cells led to higher A-LAK cells cytotoxic activity as measured against NK-cell–resistant and –sensitive tumor-target cells. This technique was used to generate A-LAK cells from patients with metastatic melanoma, RCCA, and other solid malignancies. Although feeder cells permitted greater expansion of the $CD3^-$ $CD56^+$ cell population, sufficient numbers of A-LAK cells for adoptive therapy could be generated in only 21 of 54 (39%) of the patients in this study. Nonetheless, such studies are very useful in the development of strategies to maximize effector-cell production. The role of the feeder-cell population in providing specific cytokines enhancing NK cell number and function will need to be further investigated.

Other researchers have attempted to generate A-LAK cells from the PBMC of patients with either early or advanced chronic myeloid leukemia (CML). In this study, A-LAK cells generated from patients with advanced CML were significantly worse cytolytic effectors than those obtained from patients with earlier stage disease (Verfaille et al. 1990). The A-LAK cells were generated from the PBMC of seven early chronic phase (CP) patients and ten advanced-disease (AD) patients by culture in rIL-2 for 14 days. At the end of this period, cells from both patient populations were greater than 80% $CD3^-$ $CD56^+$ with the morphology of large granular lymphocytes. When these effectors were tested against the NK-sensitive cell line K562, it was found that A-LAK cells from CP patients were able to mediate $80\pm7\%$ cytotoxicity as compared with $31\pm3\%$ for the AD patients. The authors concluded that the ability to generate cytotoxic A-LAK cells from the PBMC of patients with CML varied according to their disease staging.

In an attempt to generate greater numbers of pure A-LAK, patients had leukapheresis using counterflow centrifugal elutriation that resulted in a twofold enrichment of cells bearing the CD56 surface Ag (Melder et al. 1989). The A-LAK cells were then isolated by rIL-2–induced adherence to plastic for 24 hours and cultured for 8 to 14 days in 1,000 U/mL rIL-2. Using this technique, sufficient numbers of A-LAK cells (about 1×10^8) could be generated from the PBMC of patients with advanced cancer for adoptive immunotherapy (Melder et al. 1989). Other researchers have had some success using other cytokines in combination with IL-2 to enhance the outgrowth of NK effectors, such as IL-1 and TNF-α (Owen-Schaub, Gutterman, and Grimm 1988; Crump, Owen-Schaub, and Grimm 1989). Schwartz et al. have shown that A-LAK cells can be efficiently generated from the PB of patients with primary or metastatic liver malignancy if PBMC are obtained before the initiation of chemotherapy or radiation therapy (Schwarz et al. 1989a).

Early work by French investigators showed that NK cells could be isolated from the PB of patients with metastatic RCCA and better expanded in vitro in the presence of IL-2 and 1% leukocyte-conditioned medium as opposed to medium supplemented with IL-2 alone (Hercend et al. 1990). The NK cells were cultured in microtiter plates on an irradiated feeder consisting of allogeneic PBMC and EBV$^+$ lymphoblastoid cell line (LAZ 388). After 4 to 5 weeks of culture, the remaining lymphokine-activated NK cells (LANAK) were greater than 80% CD3$^-$ CD56$^+$ and showed significantly enhanced cytotoxicity (average 100-fold increase) against an NK-sensitive target cell compared with autologous LAK cells generated in the standard fashion. Nine of 12 patients completed the planned course of therapy and received an average of 45.1×10^9 cells that were administered twice at 3-week intervals. Recombinant IL-2 (3×10^6 U/m^2/d) was given as a 24-hour CI both immediately before and during the transfusion of LANAK. Administration of LANAK cells did not induce significant toxicity and there were only five episodes of chills during 38 transfusions. In contrast to animal models, labeled LANAK cells did not preferentially localize to tumor sites. Three patients showed partial responses to this combination of rIL-2 and LANAK, but there was no group given rIL-2 with standard LAK cells or rIL-2 alone with which to compare these results.

Purified NK cells have been used to treat the surgical bed of resected malignant gliomas. Kawamoto et al. isolated NK cells from the PB of patients using fluorescence-activated cell sorting (FACS) (Kawamoto et al. 1991). In vitro studies with NK cells from six patients showed significant cytolytic activity against four separate glioma cell lines and six different cultured surgical specimens. Subsequently, NK cells were administered through an Ommaya reservoir to the bed of the resected glioma without any ill effects. The use of adoptive immunotherapy in the treatment of malignant glioma is an attractive concept, not only because of the dismal prognosis for patients with current therapies, but also because of the ability to directly access the tumor site after surgical debulking. Through the use of an implanted Ommaya reservoir, multiple cell treatments can be administered along with cytokines. Similar studies have been conducted by Munari et al. (1990) demonstrating that this technique may be useful for the delivery of NK cells to the postsurgical bed of intracranial malignancies with acceptable toxicity.

The adoptive immunotherapy of these intracranial tumors is not solely dependent on the balance between numbers of cytotoxic effector cells and residual tumor. The cytokine milieu present in the brain cavity may explain some of the negative results that have been obtained in previous trials with unfractionated LAK cells. Ruffini et al. generated A-LAK cells from patients with recurrent glioblastoma multiforme and tested whether there were immunosuppressive factors present in the fluid that collects in the cavity left after subtotal resection of tumor (Ruffini et al. 1993). They found that every sample of glioblastoma cavity fluid tested exerted a dose-dependent inhibitory effect upon the proliferation and antitumor cytotoxicity of A-LAK cells tested after 7 days of culture in rIL-2. The identity of the suppressive factor was confirmed when the neutralizing Ab against TNF-β was found to abrogate the inhibitory effects of the cavity fluid.

The in vitro generation of LAK and A-LAK cells for adoptive transfer to patients requires specialized technical expertise and dedicated laboratory space. The high cost of these resources, the difficulty in generating effector cells in patients with advanced malignancy, and the failure to show clear improvements in survival with NK-cell therapy has led investigators to develop other methods of delivering large numbers of activated NK cells to patients with cancer. Specifically, it has now been shown that prolonged continuous IV infusion of low-dose rIL-2 can result in a selective expansion of CD56$^+$ cells in patients without any significant clinical toxicity in the outpatient setting (Caligiuri 1993).

■ MODULATION OF HUMAN NATURAL KILLER CELLS WITH LOW-DOSE rIL-2

It has been shown that the CD56^{bright} NK cell is the only resting PBMC to constitutively express a functional high-affinity IL-2R (Caligiuri et al. 1990; Nagler et al. 1990). While monocytes and CD56^{dim} NK cells also constitutively express an IL-2R, it is of the intermediate-affinity class and is activated at 100-fold higher concentrations of IL-2 than is the high-affinity IL-2R (Taniguchi and Minami 1993). In addition, resting T and B cells do not express a functional form of the IL-2R and, therefore, would not be expected to respond to exogenously administered IL-2. Initial studies using very-low-dose IL-2 were first reported by Caligiuri et al. (1991). The hypothesis was that prolonged continuous in vivo administration of low-dose IL-2 would result in serum IL-2 concentrations that selectively saturate the high-affinity IL-2R expressed on the CD56[bright] NK cell subset, leading to a selective expansion of this cell type in vivo.

In the initial trial, 21 patients with advanced cancer received prolonged CI rIL-2 at doses that ranged from 50,000 U/m²/d (3.3 $\mu g/m^2/$d) to 600,000 U/m²/d (40 $\mu g/m^2/$d) (Caligiuri et al. 1991, 1993). Serum levels of IL-2 were measured during therapy in 11 patients. These data revealed that the three lowest doses (3.3, 10, and 30 $\mu g/m^2/$d) gave serum IL-2 levels that selectively saturated the high-affinity IL-2R. Even at the highest prolonged IL-2 infusion of 40 $\mu g/m^2/$d, the resultant serum IL-2 concentrations were estimated to saturate only 26% of the intermediate-affinity receptors. As predicted, a gradual, progressive expansion of NK cells was seen in the PB of patients receiving rIL-2 and no plateau effect was encountered during the 3 months of therapy. In contrast, the absolute number of T cells, B cells, and monocytes remained essentially unchanged. At IL-2 doses of 40 $\mu g/m^2/$d, the absolute number of total NK cells went from a pretherapy mean of 165/μL to 2,425/μL at week 12 (approximate 15-fold increase). Although the CD56[bright] NK cell subset normally represents less than 10% of NK cells, this cell population accounted for the majority of CD56[+] cells after 12 weeks of low-dose rIL-2. In fact, some patients experienced a 100-fold or greater increase in the absolute number of CD56[bright] cells, with this cell type representing 50% to 80% of all PBL near the completion of therapy. Following discontinuation of therapy, however, the numbers of CD56[bright] NK cells steadily declined until pretherapy levels had been reached. Flow cytometric analysis of IL-2R on expanded NK cells revealed a significant increase in the IL-2Rβ subunit during infusion of IL-2, but little increase in the IL-2Rα subunit (Caligiuri et al. 1993).

Unsorted PBMC from patients receiving rIL-2 infusions exhibited a significant increase in the lysis of NK-sensitive targets in vitro when compared with PBMC obtained pretherapy, largely due to the selective expansion of the CD3[−] CD56[+] lymphocyte subset (Caligiuri et al. 1991, 1993). When cells were further incubated with higher concentrations of rIL-2 that saturate the intermediate-affinity IL-2R (i.e., 1 nM or approximately 230 U/mL), a significant increase in cytotoxicity in vitro against NK-cell–sensitive and –resistant, and in ADCC was seen. Hence, one plausible scenario for adoptive immunotherapy with purified NK-cell populations would be to expand NK cells in vivo using low-dose rIL-2, followed by apheresis, in vitro activation, and reinfusion of the IL-2–activated NK cell.

Alternatively, the prolonged in vivo expansion of NK cells achieved with low-dose rIL-2 could be followed by an incremental increase in the dose of rIL-2 infused in order to activate the cytolytic mechanisms of the expanded effector cell population. The latter approach is currently being investigated in patients with acute myeloid leukemia (AML) in first remission (Frankel et al. 1994).

Interestingly, the selective expansion of $CD56^+$ NK cells in patients being treated with low-dose IL-2 does not appear to result from the proliferation of this PB NK population in response to IL-2, as might have been predicted by earlier in vitro investigations (Caligiuri et al. 1990). Our preliminary investigation reveals that the fraction of $CD56^{bright}$ NK cells in the G_2/M phases of the cell cycle in patients who are receiving rIL-2 does not increase compared with similar patients not receiving rIL-2. The expanded population of NK cells, however, does have very high levels of the antiapoptotic gene product, Bcl-2 (Bluman et al. 1994). Thus, exogenous IL-2 may be expanding the $CD56^{bright}$ NK cell population in vivo by the prevention of cell death rather than increasing cell numbers through enhanced replication. Further investigation of this observation, including the effect of low-dose rIL-2 on BM NK precursor cells is underway.

The in vivo expansion of human NK cells in patients undergoing outpatient administration of rIL-2 in a nontoxic fashion may prove to be a feasible form of immune therapy for cancer and/or chronic infections. Trials are presently underway to identify SC dose of rIL-2 that will allow in vivo NK cell expansion comparable to that seen with the outpatient CI therapy (Bernstein et al. 1994; Meropol et al. 1994). Outpatient low-dose IL-2 therapy, while more time consuming than the LAK-cell trials described earlier, is significantly less toxic, requires less commitment of laboratory resources, and can be performed with little interruption of a patient's daily activities. Such qualities may make low-dose rIL-2 therapy ideal for pursuing immune modulation in states of minimal residual disease or as a preventative therapy for malignancy in congenital and acquired immune deficiencies.

In summary, adoptive immunotherapy with mobilized PBMC highly enriched for human NK cells is only now undergoing careful evaluation in the clinical setting. While in vitro laboratory and in vivo animal studies suggest that NK cells are truly capable of mediating an antitumor cytolytic effect, preliminary results from the clinical trials would suggest that by themselves, NK cells are not consistently homing to the tumor bed, thus limiting their cytolytic potential. With the development of both in vitro and in vivo models to expand, activate, and infuse enriched populations of human NK cells, we will need to develop novel techniques to deliver these effector cells to sites of malignant disease. Such approaches may involve the use of tumor-specific Ab, other exogenously administered cytokines, or novel strategies to deliver cytokine genes to malignant tissues in vivo.

REFERENCES

Abrams, J.S., Rayner, A.A., Wiernik, P.H., et al. (1990) High-dose recombinant interleukin-2 alone: a regimen with limited activity in the treatment of advanced renal cell carcinoma. *Journal of the National Cancer Institute*, **82**, 1202–6.

Alderson, M.R., Sassenfeld, H.M., and Widmer, M.B. (1990) Interleukin 7 enhances cytolytic T lymphocyte generation and induces lymphokine-activated killer cells from human peripheral blood. *Journal of Experimental Medicine*, **172**, 577–87.

Bajorin, B.F., Sell, K.W., Richards, J.M., et al. (1990) A randomized trial of interleukin-2 plus lymphokine activated killer cells versus interleukin-2 alone in renal cell carcinoma. *Proceedings of the American Association of Cancer Research*, **31**, A1106.

Bancroft, G.J. (1993) The role of natural killer cells in innate resistance to infection. *Current Opinion in Immunology*, **5**, 503–10.

Bar, M.H., Sznol, M., Atkins, M.B., et al. (1990) Metastatic malignant melanoma treated with combined bolus and continuous infusion interleukin-2 and lymphokine-activated killer cells. *Journal of Clinical Oncology*, **8**, 1138–47.

Basse, P., Herberman, R.B., Nannmark, U., et al. (1991) Accumulation of adoptively transferred adherent lymphokine-activated killer cells in murine metastases. *Journal of Experimental Medicine*, **174**, 479–88.

Bernstein, Z.P., Porter, M., Grimes, P., and Caligiuri, M.A. (1994) Phase I study of daily subcutaneous (SQ) low dose interleukin-2 (IL-2) in HIV-associated malignancies. *Proceedings of the American Association of Clinical Oncology*, **13**, 19.

Bluman, E.M., Lindemann, M.J., Porter, M.M., Pixley, L., Frankel, S.R., and Caligiuri, M.A. (1994) Low dose interleukin-2 (IL-2) expands natural killer (NK) cell populations in vivo by selective prevention of apoptosis. *Blood*, **84**, 1139.

Brown, E., Atkinson, J.P., and Fearon, D.T. (1994) Innate immunity: 50 ways to kill a microbe. *Current Opinion in Immunology*, **6**, 73–4.

Caligiuri, M.A. (1993) Low-dose recombinant interleukin-2 therapy: rationale and potential clinical applications. *Seminars in Oncology*, **20**, 3–10.

Caligiuri, M.A., Murray, C., Robertson, M.J., et al. (1993b) Selective modulation of human natural killer cells in vivo after prolonged infusion of low dose recombinant interleukin-2. *Journal of Clinical Investigation*, **91**, 123–32.

Caligiuri, M.A., Murray, C., Soiffer, R.J., et al. (1991) Extended continuous infusion of low-dose recombinant interleukin-2 in advanced cancer: prolonged immuno-modulation without significant toxicity. *Journal of Clinical Oncology*, **9**, 2110–19.

Caligiuri, M.A., Zmuidinas, A., Manley, T.J., Levine, H., Smith, K., and Ritz, J. (1990) Functional consequences of interleukin 2 receptor expression on resting human lymphocytes. Identification of a novel natural killer cell subset with high affinity receptors. *Journal of Experimental Medicine*, **171**, 1509–26.

Charak, B.S. and Mazumder, A. (1993) Preclinical studies with interleukin-2 in tumor bearing animals. In M.B. Atkins and J.W. Mier (Eds.) *Therapeutic applications of interleukin-2*, pp. 49–71. New York, Marcel Dekker.

Crump, W.L., Owen-Schaub, L.B., and Grimm, E.A. (1989) Synergy of human recombinant interleukin 1 with interleukin 2 in the generation of lymphokine-activated killer cells. *Cancer Research*, **49**, 149–53.

Dianzani, U., Zarcone, D., Pistoia, V., et al. (1989) CD8+ CD11b+ peripheral blood T lymphocytes contain lymphokine-activated killer cell precursors. *European Journal of Immunology*, **19**, 1037–44.

Dillman, R.O., Oldham, R.K., Tauer, K.W., et al. (1991) Continuous interleukin-2 and lymphokine-activated killer cells for advanced cancer: a National Biotherapy Study Group trial. *Journal of Clinical Oncology*, **9**, 1233–40.

Dutcher, J.P., Creekmore, S., Weiss, G.R., et al. (1989) Phase II study of high dose interleukin-2 and lymphokine-activated killer cells in patients with metastatic malignant melanoma. *Journal of Clinical Oncology*, **7**, 477–85.

Dutcher, J.P., Gaynor, E.R., Boldt, D.H., et al. (1991) A phase II study of high dose continuous infusion interleukin-2 with lymphokine-activated killer cells in humans. *Journal of Clinical Oncology*, **9**, 641–8.

Finke, J.H., Rayman, P., Alexander, J., et al. (1990) Characterization of the cytolytic activity of CD4+ and CD8+ tumor-infiltrating lymphocytes in human renal cell carcinoma. *Cancer Research*, **50**, 2363–70.

Fisher, R.I., Coltman, C.A., Doroshow, J.H., et al. (1988) Metastatic renal cancer treated with interleukin-2 and lymphokine-activated killer cells: a phase II clinical trial. *Annals of Internal Medicine*, **108**, 518–23.

Fox, B.A. and Rosenberg, S.A. (1989) Heterogeneous lymphokine-activated killer cell precursor population. Development of a monoclonal antibody that separates two populations of precursors with distinct culture requirements and separate target-recognition repertoires. *Cancer Immunology and Immunotherapy*, **29**, 155–66.

Frankel, S.R., Pixlie, L., Porter, M., Herzig, G.P., and Caligiuri, M.A. (1994) Low dose IL-2 in first remission acute myeloid leukemia. *Proceedings of the American Association of Cancer Research*, **35**, 1344.

Gaynor, E.R., Weiss, G.R., Margolin, K.A., et al. (1990) Phase I study of high-dose continuous-infusion recombinant IL-2 and autologous lymphokine-activated killer cells in patients with metastatic or unresectable malignant melanoma and renal cell carcinoma. *Journal of the National Cancer Institute*, **82**, 1397–402.

Grimm, E.A., Mazumder, A., Zhang, H.Z., and Rosenberg, S.A. (1982) Lymphokine activated killer cell phenomenon. Lysis of natural killer cell-resistant solid tumor cells by interleukin 2 activated autologous human peripheral blood lymphocytes. *Journal of Experimental Medicine*, **155**, 1823–41.

Hawkins, M.J. (1988) IL-2/LAK: current status and possible future directions. In V.T. DeVita, S. Hellman, and S.A. Rosenberg (Eds.) *Principles and practice of oncology updates*, pp. 1–14. Philadelphia, J.B. Lippincott Company.

Herberman, R.B., Hiserodt, J.C., Vujanovic, N.L., et al. (1987) Lymphokine activated killer cell activity: characterization of effector cells and progenitor cells in blood and spleen. *Immunology Today*, **8**, 178–81.

Hercend, T., Farace, F., Baume, D., et al. (1990) Immunotherapy with lymphokine activated natural killer cells and recombinant interleukin-2: a feasibility trial in metastatic renal cell carcinoma. *Journal of Biological Response Modifiers*, **9**, 546–55.

Hiserodt, J.C. (1993) Lymphokine-activated killer cells: biology and relevance to disease. *Cancer Investigation*, **11**, 420–39.

Kawamoto, K., Fujihara, H., Numa, Y., and Matsumara, H. (1991) Antineoplastic effects of natural killer cells sorted with flow cytometry on brain tumors. *Human Cell*, **4**, 157–64.

Kehrl, J.H., Dukovich, M., Whalen, G., et al. (1988) Novel interleukin 2 (IL-2) receptor appears to mediate IL-2-induced activation of natural killer cells. *Journal of Clinical Investigation*, **81**, 200–5.

Kolitz, J.E. and Mertelsmann, R. (1991) The immunotherapy of human cancer with interleukin 2: present status and future directions. *Cancer Investigation*, **9**, 529–42.

Kuppen, P.J., Basse, P.H., Goldfarb, R.H., et al. (1994) The infiltration of experimentally induced lung metastases of colon carcinoma CC531 by adoptively transferred interleukin-2-activated natural killer cells in WAG rats. *International Journal of Cancer*, **56**, 574–9.

Lafreniere, R. and Rosenberg, S.A. (1985) Adoptive immunotherapy of murine hepatic metastases with lymphokine-activated killer (LAK) cells and recombinant interleukin-2 (IL-2) can mediate the regression of both immunogenic and non-immunogenic sarcomas and an adenocarcinoma. *Journal of Immunology*, **134**, 3895–900.

Lanier, L.L., Kipps, T.J., and Phillips, J.H. (1985) Functional properties of a unique subset of cytotoxic CD3+ T lymphocytes that express Fc receptors for IgG (CD16/Leu11 antigen). *Journal of Experimental Medicine*, **163**, 2089–116.

Lotze, M.T., Frana, L.W., Sharrow, S.O., et al. (1985a) In vivo administration of purified human interleukin 2. I. Half-life and immunologic effects of the Jurkat cell line-derived interleukin-2. *Journal of Immunology*, **134**, 157–66.

Lotze, M.T., Line, B.R., Mathiesen, D.J., et al. (1980) The in vivo distribution of autologous human and murine lymphoid cells grown in T cell growth factor (TCGF): implications for the adoptive immunotherapy of tumors. *Journal of Immunology*, **125**, 1487–93.

Lotze, M.T., Matory, Y.L., Ettinghausen, S.E., et al. (1985b) In vivo administration of purified human interleukin 2. II. Half-life and immunologic effects, and expansion of peripheral lymphoid cells in vivo with recombinant IL-2. *Journal of Immunology*, **135**, 2865–75.

Marincola, F.M. (1994) Interleukin-2. In V.T. DeVita, S. Hellman, and S.A. Rosenberg (Eds.) *Biologic therapy of cancer updates*, Vol. 4, no. 3, pp. 1–16. Philadelphia, J.B. Lippincott Company.

McCabe, M.S., Stablein, D., and Hawkins, M.J. (1991) The modified group C experience–phase III randomized trials of IL-2 versus IL-2/LAK in advanced renal cell carcinoma and advanced melanoma. *Proceedings of the American Association of Clinical Oncology*, **10**, A174.

McMannis, J.D., Fischer, R.I., Creekmore, S.P., et al. (1988) In vivo effects of recombinant IL-2; isolation of circulating Leu-19+ lymphokine activated killer effector cells from cancer patients receiving recombinant IL-2. *Journal of Immunology*, **140**, 1335–40.

Melder, R.J., Rosenfeld, C.S., Herberman, R.B., and Whiteside, T.L. (1989) Large-scale preparation of adherent lymphokine-activated killer (A-LAK) cells for adoptive immunotherapy in man. *Cancer Immunology and Immunotherapy*, **29**, 67–73.

Melder, R.J., Whiteside, T.L., Vujanovic, N.L., et al. (1988) A new approach to generating antitumor effectors for adoptive immunotherapy using human adherent lymphokine-activated killer cells. *Cancer Research*, **48**, 3461–9.

Meropol, N.J., Porter, M., Perez, R.P., et al. (1994) Low dose interleukin-2 (IL-2): daily subcutaneous injection results in selective in vivo expansion of natural killer (NK) cells with minimal toxicity. *Proceedings of the American Association of Clinical Oncology*, **13**, 965.

Mule, J.J., Ettinghausen, S.E., Speiss, P.J., et al. (1986) Anti-tumor efficacy of lymphokine-activated killer cells and recombinant interleukin-2 in vivo: survival benefit and mechanisms of tumor escape in mice undergoing immunotherapy. *Cancer Research*, **46**, 676–83.

Munari, L., Silvani, A., Passerini, C.G., et al. (1990) Adoptive immunotherapy with adherent lymphokine-activated killer (A-LAK) cells in glioblastoma multiforme. *Journal of Neurosurgical Sciences*, **34**, 283–8.

Nagler, A., Lanier, L.L., and Phillips, J.H. (1990) Constitutive expression of the high affinity interleukin 2 receptors on human CD16⁻ natural killer cells. *Journal of Experimental Medicine*, **171**, 1527–33.

Ortaldo, J.R., Mason, A., and Overton, R. (1986) Lymphokine activated killer cells. Analysis of progenitors and effectors. *Journal of Experimental Medicine*, **165**, 1193–1205.

Owen-Schaub, L.B., Gutterman, J.U., and Grimm, E.A. (1988) Effect of tumor necrosis factor alpha and IL-2 in the generation of human lymphokine activated killer cell toxicity. *Cancer Research*, **48**, 788–92.

Palmer, P.A., Vinke, J., Evers, P., et al. (1992) A review of patients treated by continuous infusion of recombinant interleukin-2 (rIL-2) with or without autologous lymphokine activated killer cells for the treatment of advanced renal cell carcinoma. *European Journal of Cancer*, **28**, 1038–43.

Papa, M.Z., Mule, J.J., and Rosenberg, S.A. (1986) Anti-tumor efficacy of lymphokine-activated killer cells and recombinant interleukin-2 in vivo: successful immunotherapy of established pulmonary metastases from weakly immunogenic and non-immunogenic murine tumors of different histological types. *Cancer Research*, **46**, 4973–8.

Parkinson, D.R., Abrams, J.S., Wiernik, P.H., et al. (1990a) Interleukin-2 therapy in patients with metastatic malignant melanoma: a phase II study. *Journal of Clinical Oncology*, **8**, 1650–6.

Parkinson, D.R., Fisher, R.I., Rayner, A.A., et al. (1990b) Therapy of renal cell carcinoma with interleukin-2 and lymphokine-activated killer cells: phase II experience with a hybrid bolus and continuous infusion interleukin-2 regimen. *Journal of Clinical Oncology*, **8**, 1630–6.

Phillips, J.H., Gemlo, B.T., Myers, W.W., et al. (1987) In vivo and in vitro activation of natural killer cells in advanced cancer patients undergoing combined recombinant interleukin-2 and LAK-cell therapy. *Journal of Clinical Oncology*, **5**, 1933–41.

Phillips, J.H. and Lanier, L.L. (1986) Dissection of the lymphokine activated killer phenomenon. Relative contribution of peripheral blood natural killer cells and T lymphocytes to cytolysis. *Journal of Experimental Medicine*, **164**, 814–25.

Rabinowich, H., Sedimayr, P., Herberman, R.B., and Whiteside, T.L. (1991) Increased proliferation, lytic activity, and purity of human natural killer cells cocultured with mitogen-activated feeder cells. *Cellular Immunology*, **135**, 454–70.

Rabinowich, H., Vitolo, D., Alarac, S., et al. (1992) Role of cytokines in the adoptive immunotherapy of an experimental model of human head and neck cancer by human IL-2-activated natural killer cells. *Journal of Immunology*, **149**, 340–49.

Richards, J.M., Bajorin, D.F., Vogelzang, N.J., et al. (1990) Treatment of metastatic melanoma with continuous intravenous IL-2 ± LAK cells: a randomized trial. *Proceedings of the American Society of Clinical Oncology*, **9**, 279.

Robertson, M.J. and Ritz, J. (1990) Biology and clinical relevance of human natural killer cells. *Blood*, **76**, 2421–38.

Rosenberg, S.A. and Lotze, M.T. (1986) Cancer immunotherapy using interleukin-2 activated lymphocytes. In W.E. Paul, C.G. Fatham, and H. Metzger (Eds.) *Annual review of immunology*, Vol. 4, pp. 681–709. Palo Alto, CA, Annual Reviews.

Rosenberg, S.A., Lotze, M.T., Muul, L.M., et al. (1985) Observations on the systemic administration of autologous lymphokine-activated killer cells and recombinant interleukin-2 to patients with metastatic cancer. *New England Journal of Medicine*, **313**, 1485–92.

Rosenberg, S.A., Lotze, M.T., Muul, L.M., et al. (1987) A progress report on the treatment of 157 patients with advanced cancer using lymphokine-activated killer cells and interleukin-2 or high dose interleukin-2 alone. *New England Journal of Medicine*, **316**, 889–97.

Rosenberg, S.A., Lotze, M.T., Yang, J., et al. (1989) Experience with the use of high-dose interleukin-2 in the treatment of 652 cancer patients. *Annals of Surgery*, **210**, 474–85.

Rosenberg, S.A., Lotze, M.T., Yang, J.C., et al. (1993) Prospective randomized trial of high-dose interleukin-2 alone or in conjunction with lymphokine-activated killer cells for the treatment of patients with advanced cancer. *Journal of the National Cancer Institute*, **85**, 622–32.

Ruffini, P.A., Rivoltini, L., Boiardi, A., and Parmiani, G. (1993) Factors, including transforming growth factor beta, released in the glioblastoma residual cavity, impair activity of adherent lymphokine-activated killer cells. *Cancer Immunology and Immunotherapy*, **36**, 409–16.

Sacchi, M., Snyderman, C.H., Heo, D.S., et al. (1990) Local adoptive immunotherapy of human head and neck cancer xenografts in nude mice with lymphokine-activated killer cells and interleukin 2. *Cancer Research*, **50**, 3113–18.

Schmidt, R.E., Murray, C., Daley, J.F., et al. (1986) A subset of natural killer cells in peripheral blood displays a mature T cell phenotype. *Journal of Experimental Medicine*, **164**, 351–7.

Schwarz, R.E., Iwatsuki, S., Herberman, R.B., and Whiteside, T.L. (1989a) Unimpaired ability to generate adherent lymphokine-activated killer (A-LAK) cells in patients with primary or metastatic liver tumors. *Cancer Immunology and Immunotherapy*, **30**, 312–16.

Schwarz, R.E., Vujanovic, N.L., and Hiserodt, J.C. (1989b) Enhanced antimetastatic activity of lymphokine-activated killer cells purified and expanded by their adherence to plastic. *Cancer Research*, **49**, 1441–6.

Siegel, J.P., Sharon, M., Smith, P.L., and Leonard, W.J. (1987) The IL-2 receptor b chain (p70): role in mediating signals for LAK, NK, and proliferative activities. *Science*, **238**, 75–8.

Smith, K.A. (1993) Lowest dose interleukin-2 therapy. *Blood*, **81**, 1414–23.

Sondel, P.M., Kohler, P.C., Hank, J.A., et al. (1988) Clinical and immunological effects of recombinant interleukin-2 given by repetitive weekly cycles of patients with cancer. *Cancer Research*, **48**, 2561–7.

Sparano, J.A. and Dutcher, J.P. (1993) High dose IL-2 treatment of melanoma. In M.B. Atkins and J.W. Mier (Eds.) *Therapeutic applications of interleukin-2*, pp. 99–117. New York, Marcel Dekker.

Taniguchi, T. and Minami, Y. (1993) The IL-2/IL-2 receptor system: a current overview. *Cell*, **73**, 5–8.

Trinchieri, G. (1989) Biology of natural killer cells. *Advances in Immunology*, **47**, 187–337.

Trinchieri, G., O'Brien, T., Shade, M., et al. (1984) Phorbol esters enhance spontaneous cytotoxicity of human lymphocytes, abrogate F_c receptor expression, and inhibit antibody-dependent lymphocyte-mediated cytotoxicity. *Journal of Immunology*, **133**, 1869–77.

Tsudo, M., Goldman, C.K., Bongiovanni, K.F., et al. (1987) The p75 peptide is the receptor for interleukin 2 expressed on large granular lymphocytes and is responsible for the interleukin 2 activation of these cells. *Proceedings of the National Academy of Sciences of the United States of America*, **84**, 5394–8.

Verfaille, C., Kay, N., Miller, W., and McGlave, P. (1990) Diminished A-LAK cells cytotoxicity and proliferation accompany disease progression in chronic myelogenous leukemia. *Blood*, **76**, 401–8.

Voss, S.D., Sondel, P.M., and Robb, R.J. (1992) Characterization of the interleukin 2 receptors (IL-2R) expressed on human natural killer cells activated in vivo by IL-2: association of the p64 γ chain with the IL-2R β chain in functional intermediate-affinity IL-2R. *Journal of Experimental Medicine*, **176**, 531–41.

Vujanovic, N.L., Rabinowich, H., Lee, Y.J., et al. (1993) Distinct phenotypes and functional characteristics of human natural killer cells obtained by rapid interleukin-induced adherence to plastic. *Cellular Immunology*, **151**, 133–57.

Waleski, J., Paietta, E., Dutcher, J., and Wiernik, P.H. (1989) Evaluation of natural killer and lymphokine-activated killer (LAK) cell activity in vivo in patients treated with high-dose interleukin-2 and adoptive transfer of autologous (LAK) cells. *Journal of Cancer Research and Clinical Oncology*, **115**, 170–9.

Weiss, G.R., Margolin, K.A., Aronson, F.R., et al. (1992) A randomized phase II trial of continuous infusion interleukin-2 or bolus injection interleukin-2 plus lymphokine-activated killer cells for advanced renal cell carcinoma. *Journal of Clinical Oncology*, **10**, 275–81.

West, W.H. (1989) Continuous infusion recombinant interluekin-2 (IL-2) in adoptive cellular therapy of renal carcinoma and other malignancies. *Cancer Treatment Review*, **16**, 83–9.

West, W.H., Tauer, K.W., Yanelli, J.R., et al. (1987) Constant-infusion recombinant interleukin-2 in adoptive immunotherapy of advanced cancer. *New England Journal of Medicine*, **316**, 898–905.

Whitehead, R.P., Kopecky, K.J., Samson, M.K., et al. (1989) A phase II study of IV bolus recombinant interleukin 2 in metastatic malignant melanoma: a Southwest Oncology Group study. *Proceedings of the American Society of Clinical Oncology*, **8**, 284.

Yasumura, S., Lin, W., and Hirabayashi, H., et al. (1994) Immunotherapy of liver metastases of human gastric carcinoma with interleukin 2-activated natural killer cells. *Cancer Research*, **54**, 3808–16.

26

Autologous Tumor Cell Vaccines

LORI MINASIAN

Immunization against cancer has been a provocative but elusive goal in tumor immunology. Vaccines against certain infectious diseases have been successful because well-defined antigens (Ag) were found on the specific viral or bacterial organisms that were not found on normal human cells. This results in humoral and cellular responses, and evaluation for the efficacy of these vaccines can easily be determined serologically, by measuring antibody (Ab) titers against the specific Ag.

The goal of antitumor immunization, however, is to induce a cellular or T-lymphocyte response rather than a serological response. A cellular-cytotoxic response results in lysis of existing cancer cells as well as the development of immunological memory. The generation of a cytotoxic T-cell response requires two independent steps: one to activate $CD4^+$ cells and another to activate $CD8^+$ cells. Ag-presenting cells, such as macrophages or dendritic cells, must endocytose the Ag and present it via a major histocompatibility complex (HC) class II molecule to $CD4^+$ T cells. The Ag-presenting cell also has a co-stimulatory molecule that must bind a receptor on the $CD4^+$ T cell simultaneously in order to activate the $CD4^+$ T cell (Linsley et al. 1991). If the co-stimulatory molecule is not present, T-cell anergy will occur (Jenkins et al. 1991). Once the $CD4^+$ cells are activated, they release specific cytokines. Independently, $CD8^+$ T cells must recognize the Ag that is presented by a major HC class I molecule. The cytokines released by the $CD4^+$ cells impact upon those $CD8^+$ cells that have recognized Ag.

For such immunization to be successful against cancer, unique Ag (tumor-associated Ag [TAA]) must exist on the tumor cells, but not on the normal host cells (Oettgen and Old 1991). Since malignant transformation occurs in normal cells, it is difficult to define Ag specific to the tumor. In some cases, malignant transformation results in increased expression of normally occurring Ag (Albino et al. 1986). Unique Ag have been found on melanoma cells (Van der Bruggen, Knuth, and Boon 1991), although for the vast majority of human malignancies TAA have not been identified.

■ IMMUNIZATION WITH AUTOLOGOUS TUMOR CELLS

One means of investigating antitumor vaccines without identifying TAA is to immunize with autologous tumor cells. The patient's own cancer cells act as the source for the Ag. Merely presenting the TAA is insufficient, as vaccines utilizing autologous tumor cells alone rarely induce an antitumor response (Krementz et al. 1971; McCarthy et al. 1973). This suggests that despite the presence of unique Ag, the malignant cells survive by escaping host-defense mechanisms, preventing the development of a T-cell response.

In an attempt to improve the host immune response to autologous tumor-cell vaccines, highly immunogenic adjuvants, such as bacille Calmette-Guérin (BCG), *Corynebacterium parvum*, or viral oncolysates have been added to vaccine preparations. These adjuvants were added to create a local, nonspecific inflammatory reaction that recruits lymphocytes to the vaccine site. Ag processing can occur in the transformation from acute to chronic inflammation, and Ag-specific cytotoxic T cells can be generated (Hanna, Peters, and Hoover 1991). Many clinical trials using autologous tumor cells for vaccinating cancer patients have been done, with few showing conclusively either the development of a specific immunological response or a survival advantage (Livingston 1991). Although one small pilot study of colorectal cancer patients given an autologous tumor-cell vaccine and BCG showed an improvement in survival (Hoover et al. 1985), a large, randomized trial of colorectal cancer patients failed to confirm any survival benefit for the immunizations (Harris et al. 1994). Two other randomized trials (Morton et al. 1978; Morton 1986) failed to show a benefit for use of the adjuvant plus tumor cells as compared with tumor cells alone.

Despite the inability to prove efficacy, isolated patients have had significant tumor regression after multiple vaccinations. One patient with metastatic melanoma received irradiated autologous tumor cells along with BCG for 2 years before developing high titers of $CD8^+$ T cells that efficiently lysed his tumor cells both in vitro and in vivo (Livingston et al. 1979). This patient remains alive without disease for more than 10 years (Gansbacher et al. 1992a). This case and others suggest the possibility of developing a successful antitumor vaccine.

A more recent design strategy for antitumor vaccines is to circumvent the need for $CD4^+$ cytokine production by having the tumor cell secrete the cytokine as well as provide the TAA. By introducing the gene for the cytokine directly into the tumor cell, an increased amount of cytokine can be produced at the site of cytotoxic T-cell engagement with little or no systemic toxicity.

This strategy has been shown to increase the immunogenicity of tumor cells in animal models. In one model (Gansbacher et al. 1990), a retroviral vector containing the gene for interleukin-2 (IL-2) was introduced into a CMS-5 sarcoma cell line. Balb/c mice were injected with either the transfected cells or control cells (CMS-5 cell with no vector or CMS-5 cells with an empty vector). Those mice given the control cells died of progressive tumor. Those given the transfected cells rejected the tumor cells and lived. These immune mice were then rechallenged with parental, unmodified CMS-5 cells and were able to reject the parental cells. Hence, tumorigenicity was abrogated by the constitutive secretion of the cytokine by the tumor cells. Lymphocytes removed from the spleens of the immune mice were able to lyse tumor cells in vitro. While a weak and short-lived cytolytic response was seen in mice receiving only the unmodified tumor cells, the cytolytic response from the immune mice lasted for more than 75 days. Thus, immunologic memory was induced as well.

Similar studies using different murine tumor models have shown that transduction of various cytokine genes induces rejection of the gene-modified tumor cells in syngeneic hosts. In these studies, the mice did not have established cancer, and were injected with lethal numbers of either unmodified tumor cells or cytokine-secreting tumor cells. The following cytokines have increased immunogenicity of tumor cells in specific tumor models: IL-2 (Fearon et al. 1990; Gansbacher et al. 1990; Porgador et al. 1993); IL-4 (Tepper et al. 1989; Golumbek, Lazenby, and Levitsky 1991); IL-6 (Mullen et al. 1992; Porgador et al. 1992); IL-7 (Hock et al. 1991; Jicha, Mulé, and Rosenberg 1991; Aoki et al. 1992); interferon-γ (IFN-γ) (Watanabe et al. 1989; Gansbacher et al. 1992b); tumor necrosis factor-α (TNF-α) (Asher, Mulé, and Kasid 1991; Blankenstein et al. 1991); granuclocyte colony-stimulating factor (G-CSF) (Colombo et al. 1991; Stoppacciaro et al. 1993); and granulocyte-macrophage colony-stimulating factor (GM-CSF) (Dranoff et al. 1993). Some cytokines, such as IL-5, are not capable of inducing rejection of lethal numbers of tumor cells (Kruegar-Krasagakes et al. 1993). Other cytokines do not have the same effect in all tumor models. Transduction of J558L tumor cells with the gene for TNF-α led to tumor cell rejection, but not when the gene for IL-6 was used (Blankenstein et al. 1991).

The mechanism by which the gene-modified cells are rejected depends upon the cytokine. Each cytokine has specific and different effects upon the various cells in the immune system. Secretion of IL-2 induced tumor-specific cytotoxic T cells, which when depleted, abrogated the antitumor response (Fearon et al. 1990; Gansbacher et al. 1990). IFN-γ led to up-regulation of major HC class I Ag and other adhesion molecules, increasing the tumor cells' immunogenicity (Watanabe et al. 1989; Gansbacher et al. 1992b). By stimulating both $CD4^+$ and $CD8^+$ lymphocytes, specific immunity is augmented by IL-6 (Mullen et al. 1992; Porgador et al. 1992), GM-CSF (Dranoff et al. 1993), and TNF-α (Asher et al. 1991; Blankenstein et al. 1991). A localized inflammatory reaction at the site of tumor can be induced by IL-4 with an infiltration of eosinophils and macrophages (Tepper et al. 1989; Golumbek et al. 1991) and by G-CSF with an infiltration of neutrophils (Colombo et al. 1991; Stoppacciaro et al. 1993). With both IL-4 or G-CSF, no T-cell response was generated and no immunologic memory induced.

While secretion of cytokines can result in the rejection of gene-modified tumor cells, the regression of previously established tumor has more clinical relevance. In some tumor models, vaccination with cytokine-secreting tumor cells leads to tumor regression. Secretion of IL-2 by MBT-2 bladder carcinoma cells resulted in the regression of established bladder cancer in 60% of the mice injected (Connor et al. 1993). Additionally, when these mice were rechallenged with unmodified tumor cells, they were able to reject those cells. Secretion of IL-2 in murine mammary tumors (Cavallo et al. 1993), IL-6 in Lewis lung carcinoma cells (Porgador et al. 1992), and GM-CSF in B16 melanoma cells (Dranoff et al. 1993) also resulted in the regression of established murine cancer. These cytokines, IL-2, IL-6, and GM-CSF, are capable of augmenting a T-cell–dependent mediated response, necessary for the development of immunologic memory and a long-lasting antitumor response. In a different study (Tepper, Coffman, and Leder 1992), local inflammation consisting primarily of eosinophils was generated by the secretion of IL-4 and led to tumor regression both locally and at distant sites. Despite the regression of distant metastases, no T-cell–mediated response was induced. For an antitumor vaccine to be successful, a long-lasting immunological response must be generated, otherwise the cancer will regrow after the initial regression.

Modification of tumor cells by transduction of genes other than cytokines also has biological effects. Major HC genes have been introduced into tumor cells, in order to have the tumor cell act as an Ag-presenting cell. Abnormalities in major HC class I (Alexander, Bennicelli, and Guerry 1989; Momburg et al. 1989; Nouri et al. 1990) and class II (Alexander et al. 1989; Clements et al. 1992) Ag have been found in human malignancies, and may be an important factor in allowing the tumor cells to escape immune surveillance (Nouri and Oliver 1994). Transduction of major HC class I Ag genes can decrease tumorigenicity in some murine models (Hui, Grosveld, and Festenstein 1984; Wallich et al. 1985). One major difficulty with introducing major HC class II into tumor cells is that the tumor cells do not express a co-stimulatory molecule, and enhanced major HC expression without the simultaneous recognition of the co-stimulatory molecule allows the tumor cells to escape immune recognition (Jenkins et al. 1991). When both the major HC class II molecule and the co-stimulatory molecule were introduced into the tumor cell, enhanced immunogenicity was seen (Baskar et al. 1993).

Thus, the immunogenicity of murine tumor cells can be increased by genetically engineering constitutive expression of either cytokine or major HC genes. To examine this strategy in patients with cancer, several clinical trials have been initiated and are actively accruing patients. The intention is to enhance the immunogenicity of the patients' own tumor cells and, it is hoped, lead to the rejection of the patients' existing cancer. The primary objective of these early trials is to determine safety and feasibility of cytokine gene transfer.

■ PERSPECTIVES ON THE DEVELOPMENT OF CYTOKINE-SECRETING AUTOLOGOUS TUMOR CELL VACCINES

Several technical problems in the development of autologous tumor-cell vaccines exist. These include the ability to grow the tumor cells in culture, the ability to incorporate the gene into the tumor cells, the safety issues regarding gene transfer into the cells, the ability to determine the vaccine's efficacy, and the immune status of the patients to be vaccinated.

The initial step is growing the autologous tumor cells in culture. All autologous tumor cells are obtained by surgical excision of existing cancer. For many human tumor explants, stable, long-term tumor-cell cultures cannot be established, and in some cases, tumor cells grown in long-term cultures may lose some antigenicity (Degiovanni et al. 1988; Knuth et al. 1989). Currently, several of the clinical trials using autologous tumor cell vaccines are being conducted in patients with melanoma, as these cells are readily grown in culture.

One alternative cell source for cytokine secretion is skin fibroblasts. The fibroblasts can be quickly expanded in vitro, easily transduced with the retroviral vector, and used to deliver the cytokine (Lotze et al. 1994). These cytokine gene-modified fibroblasts would be admixed with the autologous tumor cells which would provide the TAA. This mixture would obviate the need to grow the autologous cells in culture for prolonged periods; however, it is unclear if this approach would be as stimulatory as cytokine-secreting tumor cells. One study (Tsai et al. 1993) showed inferior results with cytokine-secreting fibroblasts. Tumorigenicity was abrogated by IL-2–secreting murine mammary tumor cells, 4TO7, and not altered by IL-2–secreting fibroblasts mixed with unmodified 4TO7 cells. Further study is needed to determine if this is a viable alternative.

The second step is to incorporate the gene into the tumor cells. Viral vectors are the most common means of gene transfer currently being used because a virus can rapidly and efficiently infect cells. Retroviral vectors are the "gold standard" for high-efficiency gene transfer.

In well-established human tumor cell lines, transduction with cytokine-containing retroviral vectors can result in stable and continued secretion of the cytokine (Gansbacher et al. 1992b; Gastl et al. 1992). Recent data have suggested that short-term cultures of tumor cells can be generated and efficiently transduced with retroviral vectors (Jaffee et al. 1993; Yanelli et al. 1993; Patel et al. 1994). Currently, no information exists regarding the optimal number of tumor cells per vaccination nor the number of immunizations needed to induce an antitumor response in cancer patients, and thus it is unclear if short-term cultures will be sufficient to generate adequate numbers of tumor cells for immunization.

Third, the safety issues regarding gene transfer include the toxicity secondary to the exogenous gene, the possibility of introducing new Ag to the immune system, the potential for in vivo recombination of viral particles, and the generation of replication-competent retrovirus. The cytokines currently being used in cytokine gene-transfer clinical trials (IL-2, IL-4, TNF-α, IFN-γ, and GM-CSF) have all been investigated pharmacologically, and little toxicity is associated with the low doses secreted by the tumor cells.

The introduction of exogenous proteins into patients can result in the development of an immune response against that protein. The potential exists to either develop Ab against the protein encoded by the cytokine DNA, and thereby inactivate the immunization, or to develop an autoimmune response against normal tissues that express similar Ag. In the preliminary clinical trials, no autoimmune reactions have yet been reported. One advantage for the retroviral vector is that no foreign proteins are expressed. The parental murine virus itself does not infect the target cells, which limits the patient's exposure to foreign Ag that may precipitate an autoimmune reaction.

The major concern associated with using retroviral vectors for human gene therapy is its potential for recombination with other virally derived sequences and generation of a replication-competent retrovirus. In one primate study (Donahue et al. 1992), rhesus monkeys received autologous bone-marrow transplant (ABMT) with CD34$^+$ hemopoietic cells transduced with a retroviral vector. A replication-competent retrovirus had contaminated the retroviral-producer cell line. Three of the primates developed productive infections with the replication-competent retrovirus, and 6 months later these monkeys had a progressive lymphoma. It is not the retroviral vector itself but its potential to recombine and form a replication-competent retrovirus that is the concern (Anderson 1994). To date, more than 200 patients have participated in gene therapy trials using a retroviral vector, and none have developed a malignancy as a consequence of the retroviral vector (Anderson 1994). Nonetheless, other vectors, such as adenovirus (Brody et al. 1994), vaccinia virus, and nonviral vectors are being examined for use in gene transfer. The drawback of these other vectors is that they are DNA viruses that are not permanently incorporated into the host genome, so that the gene expression is transient.

Fourth, beyond the technical issues of creating the vaccine itself, there is the issue of determining the vaccine's efficacy. As the TAA have not been identified, serologic titers cannot be used to determine efficacy. The standard means to assess a cytotoxic T-cell response is a cumbersome and labor-intensive cytotoxicity assay. In some cases, the immune response measured in these assays were nonspecific (Livingston et al. 1979, 1982). Rapid and objective methods for assessing effectiveness are essential to guide the development of an antitumor vaccine. This would enable issues regarding dose and schedule of vaccination to be determined prior to initiating the effort and expense of large randomized clinical trials.

The fifth problem in developing an autologous vaccine is the patient's immune status. The current clinical trials using cytokine gene transfer in antitumor vaccines have safety and toxicity as their primary end point. Eligible patients must have end-stage cancer that has failed conventional therapy; however, patients with metastatic cancer have impaired immune function as manifested by decreased cell-mediated cytotoxicity (Takasugi, Ramseyer, and Takasugi 1977) and decreased lymphocyte proliferation. These patients may not have the immunological capacity to respond to an effective vaccine. Thus, a lack of efficacy in these early trials may not truly indicate an ineffective vaccine strategy. Initially, cytokine gene transfer must be proven safe and tolerable in patients who have a limited life expectancy before trials in patients with much earlier stage cancer can be conducted. Ultimately, the best use of any autologous tumor vaccine will be in the adjuvant setting. Patients who have had all their macroscopic cancer surgically resected, but who are at high risk for recurrence, would be most likely to respond immunologically and benefit from this approach.

In summary, numerous investigators have utilized autologous tumor-cell vaccines against malignancies. While few clinical trials have shown significant benefit for immunization with autologous tumor-cell vaccines, a few patients have demonstrated impressive clinical remission, suggesting that with the correct design strategy, effective antitumor immunization is possible. Cytokine gene transfer in autologous tumor cells has the potential to provide an innovative vaccine strategy. With an increased understanding of tumor immunology, the effects of cytokines, and methods to overcome the associated technical difficulties, the goal of production of an effective anticancer vaccine may be attained.

REFERENCES

Albino, A.P., Houghton, A.N., Eisinger, M., et al. (1986) Class II major histocompatibility antigen expression in human melanocytes transformed by Harvey murine sarcoma virus (Ha-MSV) and Kirsten MSV (Ki-MSV) retroviruses. *Journal of Experimental Medicine*, **164**, 1710–22.

Alexander, M.A., Bennicelli, J., and Guerry, D.I.V. (1989) Defective antigen presentation by human melanoma cell lines cultured from advanced but not biologically early disease. *Journal of Immunology*, **142**, 4070–8.

Anderson, W.F. (1994) Editorial: Was it just stupid or are we poor educators? *Human Gene Therapy*, **5**, 791–92.

Aoki, T., Tashiro, K., Miyatake, S., et al. (1992) Expression of murine interleukin-7 in a murine glioma cell line results in reduced tumorigenicity in vivo. *Proceedings of the National Academy of Sciences of the United States of America*, **89**, 3850–4.

Asher, A.L., Mulé, J.J., and Kasid, A. (1991) Murine tumor cells transduced with the gene for tumor necrosis factora. *Journal of Immunology*, **146**, 3227–34.

Baskar, S., Ostrand-Rosenberg, S., Nabavi, N., et al. (1993) Constitutive expression of B7 restores immunogenicity of tumor cells expressing truncated major histocompatibility complex class II molecules. *Proceedings of the National Academy of Sciences of the United States of America*, **90**, 5687–90.

Blankenstein, T., Qin, Z., Uberla, K., et al. (1991) Tumor suppression after tumor cell-targeted tumor necrosis a gene transfer. *Journal of Experimental Medicine*, **173**, 1047–52.

Brody, S.L., Jaffe, H.A., Han, S.K., et al. (1994) Direct in vivo gene transfer and expression in malignant cells using adenovirus vectors. *Human Gene Therapy*, **5**, 437–47.

Cavallo, F., Di Pierro, F., Giovanelli, M., et al. (1993) Protective and curative potential of vaccination with interleukin-2 gene transfected cells from a spontaneous mouse mammary adenocarcinoma. *Cancer Research*, **53**, 5067–70.

Clements, V.K., Baskar, S., Armstrong, T.D., et al. (1992) Invariant chain alters the malignant phenotype of MHc class II tumour cells. *Journal of Immunology*, **149**, 2391–6.

Colombo, M.P., Ferrari, G., Stoppacciaro, A., et al. (1991) Granulocyte colony stimulating factor gene transfer suppresses tumorigenicity of a murine adenocarcinoma in vivo. *Journal of Experimental Medicine*, **173**, 889–97.

Connor, J., Bannerji, R., Saito, S., et al. (1993) Regression of bladder tumors in mice treated with interleukin-2 gene-modified tumor cells. *Journal of Experimental Medicine*, **177**, 1127–34.

Degiovanni, G., Lahaye, T., Herin, M., et al. (1988) Antigenic heterogeneity of a human melanoma tumor detected by autologous CTL clones. *European Journal of Immunology*, **18**, 671–6.

Donahue, R.E., Kessler, S.W., Bodine, D., et al. (1992) Helper virus induced T cell lymphoma in non human primates after retroviral mediated gene transfer. *Journal of Experimental Medicine*, **176**, 1125–35.

Dranoff, G., Jaffee, E., Lazenby, A., et al. (1993) Vaccination with irradiated tumor cells engineered to secrete murine granulocyte-macrophage colony-stimulating factor stimulates potent, specific, and long-lasting antitumor immunity. *Proceedings of the National Academy of Sciences of the United States of America*, **90**, 3539–43.

Fearon, E.R., Pardoll, D.M., Itaya, T., et al. (1990) Interleukin-2 production by tumor cells bypass T helper function in generation of an antitumor response. *Cell*, **60**, 397–403.

Gansbacher, B., Houghton, A.N., Livingston, P., et al. (1992a) Clinical protocol: a pilot study of immunization with HLA-A2 matched allogeneic melanoma cells that secrete interleukin-2 in patients with metastatic melanoma. *Human Gene Therapy*, **3**, 677–90.

Gansbacher, B., Zier, K., Cronin, K., et al. (1992b) Retroviral gene transfer induced constitutive expression of interleukin-2 or interferon-γ in irradiated human melanoma cells. *Blood*, **80**, 2817–25.

Gansbacher, B., Zier, K., Daniels, B., et al. (1990) Interleukin-2 gene transfer abrogates tumorigenicity and induces protective immunity. *Journal of Experimental Medicine*, **172**, 1217–24.

Gastl, G., Finstad, C.L., Guarini, A., et al. (1992) Retroviral vector-mediated lymphokine gene transfer into human renal cancer cells. *Cancer Research*, **52**, 6229–36.

Golumbek, P.T., Lazenby, A.J., and Levitsky, H.I. (1991) Treatment of established renal cancer by tumor cells engineered to secrete interleukin-4. *Science*, **254**, 713–16.

Hanna, M.G., Peters, L.C., and Hoover, H.C. (1991) Immunotherapy by active specific immunization: basic principles and preclinical studies. In V.T. DeVita, S. Helman, and S.A. Rosenberg (Eds.) *Biologic therapy of cancer*, pp. 651–69. Philadelphia, J.B. Lippincott Company.

Harris, J., Ryan, L., Adams, G., et al. (1994) Survival and relapse in adjuvant autologous tumor vaccine therapy for Duke's B and C colon cancer- EST 5283. *Proceedings of the American Society of Clinical Oncology*, **13**, 955a.

Hock, H., Dorsch, M., Diamantstein, T., et al. (1991): Interleukin-7 induces CD4$^+$ T cell-dependent tumor rejection. *Journal of Experimental Medicine*, **174**, 1291–8.

Hoover, H.C., Surdyke, M.G., Dangel, R.B., et al. (1985) Prospectively randomized trial of adjuvant active-specific immunotherapy for human colorectal cancer. *Cancer*, **55**, 1236–43.

Hui, K., Grosveld, F., and Festenstein, H. (1984) Rejection of transplantable AKR leukaemia cells following MHc DNA-mediated cell transformation. *Nature*, **311**, 750–2.

Jaffee, E.M., Dranoff, G., Cohen, L.K., et al. (1993) High efficiency gene transfer into primary tumor explants without cell selection. *Cancer Research*, **53**, 2221–6.

Jenkins, M.K., Taylor, P.S., Norton, S.D., et al. (1991) CD28 delivers a costimulatory signal involved in antigen-specific IL-2 production by human T cells. *Journal of Immunology*, **147**, 2461–6.

Jicha, D.L., Mule, J.J., and Rosenberg, S.A. (1991) Interleukin 7 generates antitumor cytotoxic T lymphocytes against murine sarcomas with efficacy in cellular adoptive immunotherapy. *Journal of Experimental Medicine*, **174**, 1511–15.

Knuth, A., Wolfel, T., Klegman, E., et al. (1989) Cytolytic T-cell clones against an autologous human melanoma: specificity study and definition of three Ag by immunoselection. *Proceedings of the National Academy of Sciences of the United States of America*, **86**, 2804–8.

Krementz, W.H., Samuels, M.S., Wallace, J.H., et al. (1971) Clinical experiences in immunotherapy of cancer. *Surgery, Gynecology and Obstetrics*, **133**, 209–17.

Kruegar-Krasagakes, S., Li, W., Richter, G., et al. (1993) Eosinophils infiltrating interleukin-5 gene-transfected tumors do not suppress tumor growth. *Europoean Journal of Immunology*, **23**, 992–95.

Linsley, P.S., Brady, W., Grosmaire, L., et al. (1991) Binding of the B cell activation antigen B7 to CD28 costimulates T cell proliferation and interleukin-2 mRNA accumulation. *Journal of Experimental Medicine*, **173**, 721–30.

Livingston, P. (1991) Active specific immunotherapy in the treatment of patients with cancer. *Immunology and Allergy Clinics of North America*, **11**, 401–23.

Livingston, P.O., Shiku, H., Pinsky, C.M., et al. (1979) Cell-mediated cytotoxicity for cultured autologous melanoma cells. *International Journal of Cancer*, **24**, 34–44.

Livingston, P.O., Watanabe, T., Shiku, H., et al. (1982) Serologic response of melanoma patients receiving melanoma cell vaccines. I. Autologous cultured melanoma cells. *International Journal of Cancer*, **30**, 413–22.

Lotze, M.T., Rubin, J.T., Carty, S., et al. (1994) Gene therapy of cancer: a pilot study of IL-4 gene-modified fibroblasts admixed with autologous tumor to elicit an immune response. *Human Gene Therapy*, **5**, 41–55.

McCarthy, W.H., Cotton, G., Carlton, A., et al. (1973) Immunotherapy of malignant melanoma. A clinical trial. *Cancer*, **32**, 97–103.

Momburg, F., Ziegler, A., Harpprecht, J., et al. (1989) Selective loss of HLA-A or HLA-B antigen expression in colon carcinoma. *Journal of Immunology*, **14**, 352–58.

Morton, D.L. (1986) Adjuvant immunotherapy of malignant melanoma: status of clinical trials at UCLA. *International Journal of Immunotherapy*, **2**, 31.

Morton, D.L., Eilber, F.R., Holmes, E.C., et al. (1978) Preliminary results of a randomized trial of adjuvant immunotherapy in patients with malignant melanoma who have lymph node metastases. *Australian and New Zealand Journal of Surgery*, **48**, 49.

Mullen, C.A., Coale, M., Levy, A.T., et al. (1992) Fibrosarcoma cells transduced with the IL-6 gene exhibit reduced tumorigenicity, increased immunogenicity and decreased metastatic potential. *Cancer Research*, **52**, 6020–4.

Nouri, A.M.E. and Oliver, R.T.D. (1994) The frequency of major histocompatibility complex antigen abnormalities in urological tumours and their correction by gene transfection or cytokine stimulation. *Cancer Gene Therapy*, **1**, 119–23.

Nouri, A.M.E., Smith, M.E.F., Crosby, D., et al. (1990) Selective and non-selective loss of immunoregulatory molecules (HLA-A, B, CAg and LFA-3) in transitional cell carcinoma. *British Journal of Cancer*, **62**, 603–6.

Oettgen, H.F., and Old, L.J. (1991) The history of cancer immunotherapy. In V.T. DeVita, S. Helman, and S.A. Rosenberg (Eds.) *Biologic therapy of cancer*, pp. 87–119. Philadelphia, J.B. Lippincott Company.

Patel, P.M., Flemming, C.L., Fisher, C., et al. (1994) Generation of interleukin-2-secreting melanoma cell populations from resected metastatic tumors. *Human Gene Therapy*, **5**, 577–84.

Porgador, A., Gansbacher, B., Bannerji, R., et al. (1993) Anti-metastatic vaccination of tumor-bearing mice with IL-2 gene-inserted tumor cells. *International Journal of Cancer*, **53**, 471–7.

Porgador, A., Tzehoval, E., Katz, A., et al. (1992) Interleukin 6 gene transfection into Lewis lung carcinoma tumor cells suppresses the malignant phenotype and confers immunotherapeutic competence against parental metastatic cells. *Cancer Research*, **52**, 3679–86.

Stoppacciaro, A., Melani, C., Parenza, M., et al. (1993) Regression of an established tumor genetically modified to release granulocyte colony-stimulating factor requires granulocyte-T cell cooperation and T cell produced interferon-γ. *Journal of Experimental Medicine*, **178**, 151–61.

Takasugi, M., Ramseyer, A., and Takasugi, J. (1977) Decline of natural non-selective cell-mediated cytotoxicity in patients with tumor progression. *Cancer Research*, **37**, 413–18.

Tepper, R.I., Coffman, R.L., and Leder, P. (1992) An eosinophil-dependent mechanism for the antitumor effect of interleukin-4. *Science*, **257**, 548–51.

Tepper, R.I., Pattengal, P.K., Leder, P., et al. (1989) Murine interleukin-4 displays potent antitumor activity in vivo. *Cell*, **57**, 503–12.

Tsai, S.C.J., Gansbacher, B., Tait, L., et al. (1993) Induction of antitumor immunity by interleukin-2 mouse mammary tumor cells versus transduced mammary stromal fibroblasts. *Journal of the National Cancer Institute*, **85**, 546–53.

Van der Bruggen, P., Knuth, A., and Boon, T. (1991) A gene encoding an antigen recognized by cytolytic T cells on a human melanoma. *Science*, **254**, 1643–8.

Wallich, R., Bulbuc, N., Hammerling, G.J., et al. (1985) Abrogation of metastatic properties of tumour cells by *de novo* expression of H-2k Ag following H-2 gene transfection. *Nature*, **315**, 301–5.

Watanabe, Y., Kuribayashi, K., Miyatake, S., et al. (1989) Exogenous expression of mouse interferon gamma cDNA in mouse neuroblastoma C1300 cell: results in reduced tumorigenicity by augmented antitumor immunity. *Proceedings of the National Academy of Sciences of the United States of America*, **86**, 9456–60.

Yanelli, J.R., Hyatt, C., Johnson, S., et al. (1993) Characterization of human tumor cell lines transduced with the cDNA encoding either tumor necrosis-α (TNF-α) or interleukin-2 (IL-2). *Journal of Immunological Methods*, **161**, 77–90.

-27

Allogeneic Cellular Vaccines Against Tumors

SUSANNE OSANTO AND PETER SCHRIER

The use of autologous cancer cells as vaccines to augment anti-tumor immunity has been extensively explored throughout the last decades (Hoover et al. 1985; Rao et al. 1988; Berd 1990; Hersey 1990). Although a few patients have appeared to benefit from this approach, the responses observed generally have been only partial and short lived. Recently obtained insights in antigen (Ag) presentation, identification of human tumor rejection Ag, and the demonstration of HLA class I restricted–cytotoxic T lymphocyte (CTL) recognition of tumor Ag-derived peptides, have renewed the interest and enthusiasm for the concept of cancer vaccines and has provided us with the knowledge to design novel immunotherapy strategies.

Immunogenic tumor Ag have long since been sought. In the past, the nature of tumor-rejection Ag has proven difficult to elucidate. Recently, it was demonstrated that cytotoxic T cells, in contrast to antibodies (Ab), recognize short peptides derived from endogenous proteins that are presented at the cell surface in the Ag-presenting groove of major histocompatibility complex (HC) class I molecules (Townsend et al. 1990; Parham 1990; Brodsky and Guagliardi 1991). Since all endogenous cellular proteins can be presented to the immune system in this way, any tumor-specific structure in the cell may function as a potential tumor-specific Ag. The concept of immuno-surveillance thus becomes more likely, since many tumor-specific proteins recognized by T cells are intracellular proteins. It is now generally accepted that T lymphocytes are the most powerful effector arm of the specific immune response that can lead to tumor rejection (Greenberg 1991; Melief 1992), underscoring the importance to aim at specific T-cell–mediated immune responses in new immunotherapy trials.

Tumor-rejection Ag may arise from point mutations in normal genes. This may result in new antigenic peptides, either because these peptides are now able to bind major HC class I molecules or because new epitopes are generated. Strong new rejection Ag that can be recognized by T cells are frequently generated (De Plaen et al. 1988; Boon, van Pel, and de Plaen 1989a, b; Szikora et al. 1990). Such point mutations affecting normal genes may be different for every tumor (and thus highly specific for every individual tumor). Experimental animal tumors caused by chemicals and UV light are indeed strongly immunogenic and mutations have been demonstrated to occur in random cellular genes, thus explaining the diverse tumor-rejection Ag observed in such tumors.

Tumor-rejection Ag may also arise from the activation of a gene that is silent in normal tissues and for which no natural tolerance has been established. In contrast to tumor Ag arising from mutations, such genes may be activated in different tumors but also in histologically identical tumors. Because individuals differ in their HLA haplotype and thus in their Ag-presenting molecules, one and the same Ag may give rise to different CTL epitopes in individuals, depending on their HLA alleles. Since different major HC haplotypes in general bind nonoverlapping sets of peptides, it is likely that, with the exception of common shared major HC haplotypes (such as HLA-A*0201), the specific epitopes recognized by the immune system will differ from individual to individual. In general, the immunogenicity of spontaneous tumors is low compared with that of chemically induced tumors. Most human tumors, perhaps with the exception of melanoma, are only weakly immunogenic or nonimmunogenic. With the recently obtained insights in Ag processing and the oncogenic events leading to deregulation of normal cells, it becomes feasible to manipulate the immune system such that a more efficient immune response against human tumors can be elicited; however, additional immunotherapeutic measures are necessary to fully exploit the power of cellular, and in particular, specific T-cell immunity.

■ TUMOR ANTIGENS AND T-CELL DEFENSE AGAINST CANCER CELLS

Experimental Tumor Antigens Defined by CTL

Assuming that T cells might be able to eradicate the majority of cancer cells as effectively as they lyse virus-infected cells, investigators have long hoped to identify tumor-rejection Ag: structures that T lymphocytes can recognize on tumor cells in the body. Evidence for immunogenicity of tumors and the presence of tumor-rejection Ag on cancer cells came from experiments in the 1950s. Tumors that developed in mice after exposure to large doses of carcinogens or UV irradiation were surgically removed. The primary host was able to reject a subsequent challenge with its own resected tumor, but not a challenge with an independently induced tumor (Prehn and Main 1957; Klein et al. 1960; Kripke 1974). These observations demonstrated the presence of immunogenic tumor Ag that were named tumor-associated transplantation antigens (TATA). Each individual tumor carries unique Ag, capable of inducing recognition of itself but not of other similarly induced tumors (Old et al. 1962; Prehn 1962; Globerson and Feldman 1964; Basombrio 1970). Tumor-specific CTL were shown to be the most important effector cells mediating tumor rejection in these experimental models (Uyttenhove, Maryanski, and Boon 1983). Both chemical carcinogenesis and UV light induce (random) point mutations in cellular genes. This may result in highly immunogenic peptides that differ by only one amino acid and that can be recognized by CTL.

In the case of viral oncogenesis, T cells have also been shown to play a key role in surveillance against viral oncogenes through recognition of peptides encoded by viral genes (Kast et al. 1989; Melief et al. 1989; Melief and Kast 1990; Greenberg 1991). In the 1970s, however, Hewitt et al. (1976) demonstrated in a large series of experiments that in contrast to experimental animal tumors, spontaneous murine tumors in general were not immunogenic. Since the majority of human tumors are to be classified as spontaneous, this would implicate that most human tumors are nonimmunogenic or weakly immunogenic and that immunotherapy would only be beneficial to a selected number of patients with immunogenic tumors.

Human Cancer Antigens Defined by Cytotoxic T Lymphocytes

Recently, evidence has been obtained for the existence of CTL-defined Ag shared by human tumors of different histological origin. CTL recognizing autologous and allogeneic human sarcoma cells sharing HLA-A*0201 as a common HLA class I allele were identified (Slovin et al. 1986). This suggests the presence of a common Ag on human sarcomas recognized by CTL in association with HLA-A*0201. Also in other human tumor types evidence has been obtained for the presence of common tumor Ag. HLA-A*0201–restricted lysis of renal cell carcinoma (RCCA) cells and HLA-B5–restricted lysis of ovarian carcinoma cells by CTL have been reported (Wang et al. 1992; Schendel et al. 1993). Furthermore, HLA class I–restricted T cell lysis of CTL obtained from patients with leukemia and head and neck tumors has also been demonstrated (Faber et al. 1992; Falkenburg et al. 1993; Yasamura et al. 1993).

Melanoma and HLA-A*0201–Cross-Reactive Cytotoxic T Lymphocytes

Melanoma is the most striking example of an immunogenic tumor in humans that is able to elicit T-cell–mediated antitumor immunity in vivo. Spontaneous regressions have been reported in a small fraction of patients, and tumor-infiltrating lymphoctyes (TIL) have been identified in such spontaneously regressing lesions (Gromet, Epstein, and Blois 1978). TIL are also frequently found in non-regressing lesions and, when cultured in vitro with interleukin-2 (IL-2), display antimelanoma cytolytic activity. Adoptive transfer of such TIL has been shown to mediate the regression of metastases in about 40% of patients with metastatic melanoma. Specific T-lymphocyte responses to melanoma have been well documented. Several groups have identified stable cytotoxic T lymphocytes, derived from either peripheral blood (PB), lymph nodes, or TIL, with melanoma-restricted pattern of lytic activity (Degiovanni et al. 1988; Anichini et al. 1989; Topalian, Solomon, and Rosenberg 1989; Wölfel et al. 1989; Mukherji, Chakraborty, and Sivanandham 1990; Notter and Schirrmacher 1990; Platsoucas 1991). These melanoma-related Ag are typically recognized by CD8[+] CTL, in association with HLA class I molecules. HLA-A*0201 is the most commonly expressed class I allele in the white population (about 45% of individuals) and has been identified as a restricting allele for many melanoma-specific CTL generated in vitro following stimulation with autologous melanoma cells (Darrow, Slingluff, and Seigler 1989; Crowley et al. 1991). Also, following transfection with the HLA-A*0201 gene, HLA-A*0201[−] melanomas are recognized and lysed by HLA-A*0201–restricted CTL (Kawakami et al. 1992). The cumulative data suggest that HLA-A*0201 can serve as a dominant class I allele for presentation of melanoma antigens to autologous cytotoxic T cells and that most tumors from HLA-A*0201[+] patients share common melanoma Ag seen by CTL. Studies using immunoselected melanoma cell clones and autologous T-cell clones, as well as studies analyzing high-performance liquid chromatography (HPLC) –fractionated peptides from melanoma cells (Slingluff et al. 1993; Storkus et al. 1993; Cox et al. 1994), all indicate that multiple antigenic peptides can provoke an immune response against melanomas. Recently, several human melanoma rejection Ag recognized by T lymphocytes have been isolated (see below) and it is likely that additional genes will be identified in the near future.

Identification of Human Cancer Antigens

The search for tumor-related Ag in melanoma has led to the identification of an antigenic peptide MZ2-E, which is encoded by the MAGE-1 gene and presented in association with HLA-A*0101 (Van der Bruggen et al. 1991; Traversari et al. 1992). The MAGE-1 gene expressed in melanoma was found to have a sequence identical to the germ-line gene. The gene is expressed by approximately 40% of melanoma cells and also other tumor cells of different histological origin (e.g., breast and lung carcinomas). MAGE-1 is the first example of an embryonic gene product that can be reactivated in tumors. This stresses the point that self-peptides encoded by nonmutated genes can be potential targets for T-cell responses against tumor cells. The MAGE-1 gene belongs to a family of 12 closely related genes that are 60% to 85% identical. Two other genes of this family, MAGE-2 and MAGE-3, are frequently expressed in human tumors. Another CTL clone of patient MZ2 was found to recognize a peptide encoded by gene MAGE-3 and presented by HLA-A*0101 (Gaugler et al. 1994).

More recently, three other Ag, namely tyrosinase, gp100 and MART-1 (melanoma Ag recognized by T cells-1) or Melan-Aa, were found to be expressed in melanoma cells as well as in their normal cellular counterpart (i.e., melanocytes) (Brichard et al. 1993; Bakker et al. 1994; Coulie et al. 1994; Kawakami et al. 1994a). All three Ag have been shown to generate HLA-A*0201–binding CTL epitopes and the HLA-A*0201–restricted CTL lyse not only the neoplastic A*0201$^+$ cells but also A*0201$^+$ melanocytes (Brichard et al. 1993; Bakker et al. 1994; Kawakami et al. 1994b). Tyrosinase is a key enzyme for the melanin pathway in pigmented cells and is expressed in melanoma cells as well as in melanocytes. The function of the melanocyte lineage-specific Ag glycoprotein gp100 and MART-1 protein is unknown at present.

The immunogenicity of these three melanocyte differentiation antigens demonstrates that an immune mechanism against non-mutated autoantigens can be mounted in tumor patients and may lead to destruction of melanomas and melanocytes in vivo. These findings provide evidence that it is indeed possible to alter a state of tolerance to self-antigens. Furthermore, because TIL lines were used to identify the gp100 as well as the MART-1 Ag, this may suggest that conditions at the site of metastases are favorable to induce T-cell responses against self-Ag that otherwise would induce anergy.

Immune Suppression

There are several factors that may contribute to ineffective tumor rejection. Failure to reject the tumor may result from an excess of suppressor T cells (North 1982), or alterations in the T-cell repertoire and in the T-cell receptor (Nossal 1989; Mizoguchi et al. 1992; Finke et al. 1993). Aberrant presentation of tumor Ag by Ag-presenting cells, including the tumor cells, may lead to T-cell anergy due to a failure to provide the co-stimulatory signals necessary to activate Ag-specific T cells (Mueller, Jenkins, and Schwartz 1989; Restifo et al. 1991; Restifo et al. 1993). Also, release of immune suppressive factors by the tumor cells themselves (De Martin et al. 1987; Ranges et al. 1987; Carel et al. 1990; Torre-Amione et al. 1990; Inge et al. 1992) and loss of major HC Ag and consequent loss of tumor peptide presentation (Möller and Hammerling 1992; Schrier and Peltenburg 1993) may contribute to ineffective tumor rejection; however, the suppression of helper T-cell function provides us a rationale for several immuno-therapeutic strategies.

■ STRATEGIES TO ENHANCE TUMOR IMMUNOGENICITY

Several lines of evidence now indicate that although tumors may seem nonimmunogenic or weakly immunogenic, immunological tolerance can be abolished. Lack of antigenicity of spontaneous tumors could be overcome by artificial modification of such cells. This modification has been called the "xenogenization of tumor cells" and can be achieved by various methods. On acquiring a new Ag, the neoantigen somehow provides a co-stimulus and the xenogenized tumors can now engender a response not only to the neoantigen, but also to their TATA. For instance, a deficient T-helper arm may be bypassed by local production of cytokines such as IL-2 by tumor cells. Another explanation for enhanced immunogenicity is that following modification of tumor cells, higher amounts of tumor Ag are expressed and the existing tolerance is overcome due to the higher concentration of T-cell epitopes.

Mutagenization

Following in vitro mutagenization of weakly immunogenic tumor cells, strong immunogenic (tum$^-$) Ag were induced and expressed at the cell surface of the tumor cells. When such mutagenized cells were injected, the presence of these strong immunogenic Ag induced an immune response against the much weaker immunogenic Ag, already present on the original tumor cells (Frost et al. 1983, 1984; Boon et al. 1989a, b). Therefore, the presence of tum$^-$ Ag (the name "tum$^-$ Ag" relates to the fact that these tumor-cell variants, in contrast to the original tumorigenic tum$^+$ cell line, no longer cause tumors in vivo) somehow acts as a co-stimulus to enhance the immune response against the tumor. The acquired immune memory in mice immunized with tum$^-$ variants can be adoptively transferred with T lymphocytes.

Introduction of Viral Antigens

Immunization with an allogeneic virus-induced tumor has been shown to effectively protect against a subsequent challenge with a poorly immunogenic syngeneic tumor induced by the same virus (Azuma, Phillips, and Green 1987). This method requires processing of allogeneic tumor proteins by host Ag-presenting cells to generate memory T cells for the syngeneic tumor. Therefore, common tumor Ag shared between allogeneic and syngeneic tumors are necessary, a requirement met by virus-induced tumors, but in humans also by melanoma, for instance. Infection of nonimmunogenic tumor cells with viruses or transfection of tumor cells with a gene encoding for a viral Ag may induce rejection responses against the original unmodified tumor cells, perhaps as a result of improved helper effects (Lindenmann and Klein 1967; Kobayashi et al. 1969; Boone et al. 1974; Kuzumaki et al. 1978; Yamaguchi et al. 1982; Hosokawa et al. 1983; Shimizu et al. 1984; Fearon et al. 1988; Von Hoegen, Weber, and Schirrmacher 1988). Modification of tumor cells by Newcastle disease virus specifically augmented the tumor-specific CTL response, but did not induce a CTL response against viral Ag or new antigenic determinants (Von Hoegen et al. 1988). Studies in cancer patients immunized with a virus-modified autologous tumor cell vaccine are underway, and a correlation between disease-free interval and an increase in delayed-type hypersensitivity (DTH) skin reaction against autologous tumor cells has been found (Liebrich et al. 1991).

Introduction of Major Histocompatibility Complex Genes

Molecular technology enables us to insert genes into tumor cells as well as in immune effector cells in order to improve their immunogenicity or therapeutic efficacy, respectively. The introduction of foreign genes, (e.g., foreign major HC genes) by gene transfer techniques, and subsequent expression of these genes in weakly immunogenic, chemically, or UV-induced tumors (three distinct possibilities), may somehow act as co-stimulus, rendering the cells highly immunogenic. Such cells failed to grow in the host or lost metastatic ability and, moreover, protected normal animals from a subsequent challenge with otherwise lethal doses of parental nontransfected cells (Hui, Grosveld, and Festenstein 1984; Gelber et al. 1989; Hui et al. 1989; Isobe et al. 1989; Ostrand-Rosenberg et al. 1991). In the case of individually unique tumor Ag of weakly immunogenic, chemically, or UV-induced tumors, the principle of an allogeneic stimulus can be succesfully applied by introduction of allogeneic major HC class I or major HC class II genes into the tumor cells.

Introduction of Cytokine Genes

To circumvent the toxicity of systemic cytokine administration, the effect of tumor cells that secrete cytokines following genetic engineering has been examined. Immunization with genetically modified rodent tumor cells, in which cytokine genes such as IL-2 (Fearon et al. 1990) are inserted, have been shown to result in enhanced immunogenicity, decreased tumorigenicity (Fig. 27.1), and long-lasting immunity against wild-type parental tumor cells. Similar results (i.e., decreased tumorigenicity and rejection of nonmodified parental tumor cells) have been obtained in animal studies following the use of tumor cells producing various cytokines (e.g., IL-4, IL-7, interferon-γ [IFN-γ], tumor necrosis factor-α [TNF-α], granulocyte colony-stimulating factor [G-CSF], and granulocyte-macrophage colony-stimulating factor [GM-CSF]) (Watanabe et al. 1989; Bubenik, Simova, and Jandlova 1990; Gansbacher et al. 1990; Li, Diamantstein, and Blankenstein 1990; Asher et al. 1991; Blankenstein et al. 1991; Colombo et al. 1991; Golumbek et al. 1991; Hock et al. 1991; Maruguchi et al. 1991; Tepper, Pattengale, and Leder 1991; Dranoff et al. 1993). Interestingly, melanoma-bearing mice immunized with IL-2–secreting, melanoma-associated-antigen–positive (MAA[+]) allogeneic mouse fibroblasts survived significantly longer than tumor-bearing mice treated with non–IL-2–secreting MAA[+] allogeneic cells, indicating

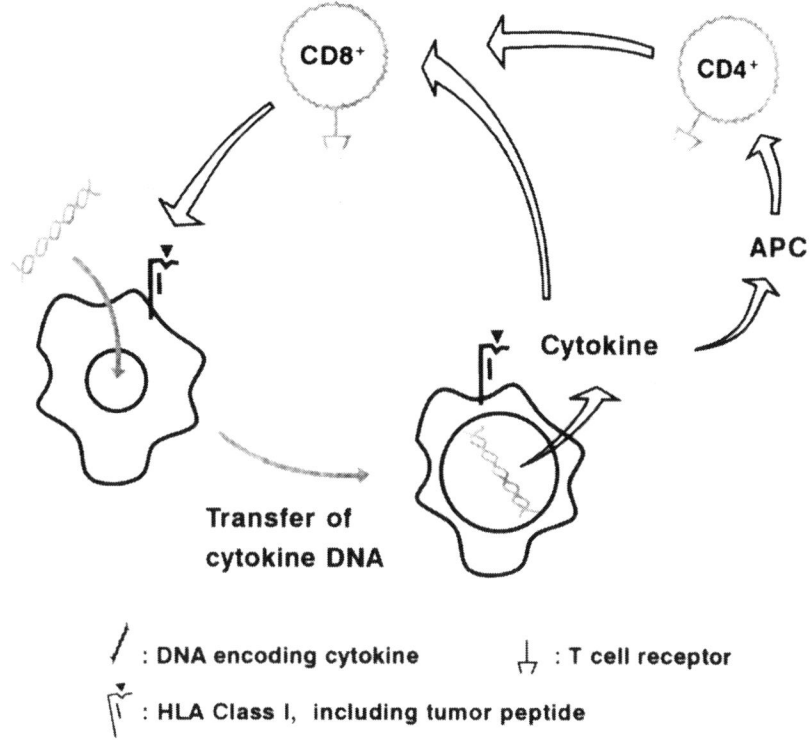

/ : DNA encoding cytokine   ⊥ : T cell receptor

Ⅰ : HLA Class I, including tumor peptide

Figure 27.1 Schematic respresentation of the effect of vaccination with cytokine-modified tumor cells. Two alternative routes are depicted: 1, The cytokine in combination with HLA class I-bound tumor peptide enhances stimulation of CD8+ T cells. 2, The cytokine enhances stimulation of Ag-presenting cells that present tumor peptide derived from degraded tumor protein, to CD4+ T cells.

that optimal therapy required the expression of tumor antigens combined with IL-2 secretion when stimulated with allogeneic cells (Kim et al. 1993).

The effector cells that mediated the observed tumor regression may differ depending on the tumor type as well as on the cytokine used. For instance, in the case of IL-2–transfected cells, the effectiveness of the model probably relies on circumvention of a deficient CD4+ group (see Fig. 27.1), whereas memory for both the genetically modified tumor cells as well as for the parental cells depends on CD8+ cells. Most reports indicate that this approach is highly effective in protecting animals from subsequent tumorigenic doses of nonmodified tumor cells. Until now, there were only a few animal studies indicating that this approach is also effective in eradication of already established tumors (Tepper et al. 1991).

■ INTRODUCTION OF GENES ENCODING CO-STIMULATORY MOLECULES

A number of experiments have indicated that introduction of the accessory molecule B7.1 in weakly immunogenic tumors may not only result in the rejection of the genetically modified tumor cells but also protects the animals from a subsequent challenge with wild-type parental tumor cells and even induces lasting memory for both the genetically modified and unmodified tumor cells (Chen et al. 1992; Townsend and Alisson 1993; Chen et al. 1994).

■ HISTORY OF CLINICAL STUDIES

Tumor Vaccines

For the last decades, whole tumor vaccines have been used to treat cancer patients. These vaccines consisted of either irradiated autologous or allogeneic tumor cells (Hoover et al. 1985; Morton 1986; Rao et al. 1988; Berd et al. 1990; McCune et al. 1990; Mitchell et al. 1990), tumor cell lysates (Cassel, Murray, and Philips 1983), and soluble tumor Ag (Hollinshead et al. 1987; Bystryn et al. 1992). In general, most of these vaccine strategies have involved co-injection of cells with adjuvants such as bacille Calmette-Guérin (BCG). In rare instances, remissions have been reported for melanoma and RCCA. In some reports, the remission rate and disease-free survival were shown to correlate with the return of delayed-type hypersensitivity responses to recall Ag and the development of such a response to autologous tumor cells, suggesting that the patient's immune system is activated by the vaccination.

Cytokine Therapy and Cellular Adoptive Transfer

Based on animal studies (Mazumder and Rosenberg 1984; Mule et al. 1984; Lafreniere and Rosenberg 1985), clinical trials using recombinant IL-2 and adoptive transfer of lymphocytes with lymphocyte-activated killer cell (LAK) activity were initiated in cancer patients in 1984. Overall response rates of about 30% and 20% have been obtained in patients with metastatic RCCA and melanoma, respectively, and some remissions lasted for several years (Rosenberg, Lotze, and

Muul 1985; Rosenberg et al. 1987; West, Tauer, and Yanelli 1987). Although clinical remissions have been obtained with IL-2 and LAK cell treatment, LAK cells could not be demonstrated to specifically home to metastatic sites.

In contrast to LAK cells, administration of cultured T lymphocytes derived from the tumor itself together with IL-2 results in homing of these cells to metastatic sites in the patient and clinical remission in a higher percentage of patients with metastatic melanoma (Rosenberg et al. 1988; Rosenberg, Lotze, and Yang 1989). Generation of activated CTL with reactivity specific for the tumor thus may provide a more effective approach in the treatment of cancer patients.

Despite the encouraging complete and partial responses, toxicity of the treatment is high and cures are relatively rare, which makes the routine use of such expensive, elaborate, and time-consuming therapy difficult to justify.

Genetic Engineering of Tumor Cells to Modify Their Immunogenicity

Molecular biology techniques enable us to explore strategies to transform weakly immunogenic or nonimmunogenic tumors into strongly immunogenic tumors. Most of the tumor-specific Ag to which we might direct the immune system are still not identified. It is therefore more efficient to produce the vaccine by using the patient's own tumor cells as the source of the Ag.

The feasibility and safety of gene therapy with genetically modified human cells has been demonstrated by Rosenberg et al., who reported the first gene-marking study (Rosenberg et al. 1990). For this observation to be exploited in the treatment of human malignant disease, two approaches could be attempted. First, in vivo delivery of genes to established tumors might lead to local cytokine secretion and ultimately tumor rejection. The second approach would be to genetically modifiy tumor cells ex vivo and to use the modified tumor cells as a therapeutic vaccine for eliminating minimal residual disease. This would require the culture of cells from resected tumor material and their in vitro modification followed by injection of the modified cells.

Rationale for Genetically Modified Allogeneic Human Tumor Vaccines

There are several problems to overcome before patients can routinely be immunized with genetically modified autologous tumor cells. Growing autologous tumor cells in vitro is time consuming, and establishment of tumor cell lines is not successful in all cases and requires a considerable amount of time. The recent identification of common tumor Ag presented by HLA-A*0201 and HLA-A*0101 to CTL justifies the use of HLA-A*0201$^+$ and HLA-A*0101$^+$ allogeneic melanoma cells as a vaccine in melanoma patients sharing the same alleles. Approximately 60% to 70% of white patients will be HLA-A*0201 and/or HLA-A*0101. Therefore, such a vaccine is expected to be applicable in a considerable number of melanoma patients. Furthermore, the use of allogeneic tumor cells, that are genetically engineered to secrete cytokines, combines the advantages of "cytokine gene therapy" and "foreign major HC gene therapy."

Both the local secretion of cytokines as well as the allogeneic stimulus may enhance the processes of local influx of cellullar infiltrate including tumor-specific CTL precursors at the site of vaccination, tumor-cell degradation, and release of tumor Ag. In the case of GM-CSF, activity of Ag-presenting cells may be specifically stimulated, resulting in improved Ag presentation (Dranoff et al. 1993). Following immunization of patients with genetically modified allogeneic tumor cells that share an HLA class I allele, such cells may in vivo either directly present shared tumor peptides to already existing class I restricted CTL of the patient (if the shared class I allele indeed presents a shared immunodominant tumor peptide) or may first be degraded and serve as a source of tumor Ag for professional Ag-presenting cells (Fig. 27.2). These cells will then process and select the appropriate epitopes, which will enter the class II route to stimulate CD4$^+$ T cells, or even the class I route (these epitopes are therefore matched to the patient's tumor) to directly stimulate CD8$^+$ T cells (Huang et al. 1994). In the case of a fully allogeneic tumor cell vaccine, stimulation of an efficient immune response can only occur via Ag-presenting cells (Fig. 27.2). Tumor peptides that bind to the patient's HLA alleles will be

Figure 27.2 Induction of a CD8$^+$ T-cell–mediated antitumor response by vaccination with gene-modified tumor cells. Three situations are shown as indicated: vaccination with (*1*) autologous tumor cells; (*2*) allogeneic tumor cells, sharing one or more HLA class I alleles; or (*3*) completely allogeneic tumor cells. All vaccination strategies lead to a CD8$^+$-mediated immune response against the patient's own tumor cells (shown on the right side). The cells used for vaccination are shown on the left side. Autologous tumor cells or autologous HLA molecules are depicted in gray, allogeneic tumor cells or allogeneic HLA-molecules are depicted in black.

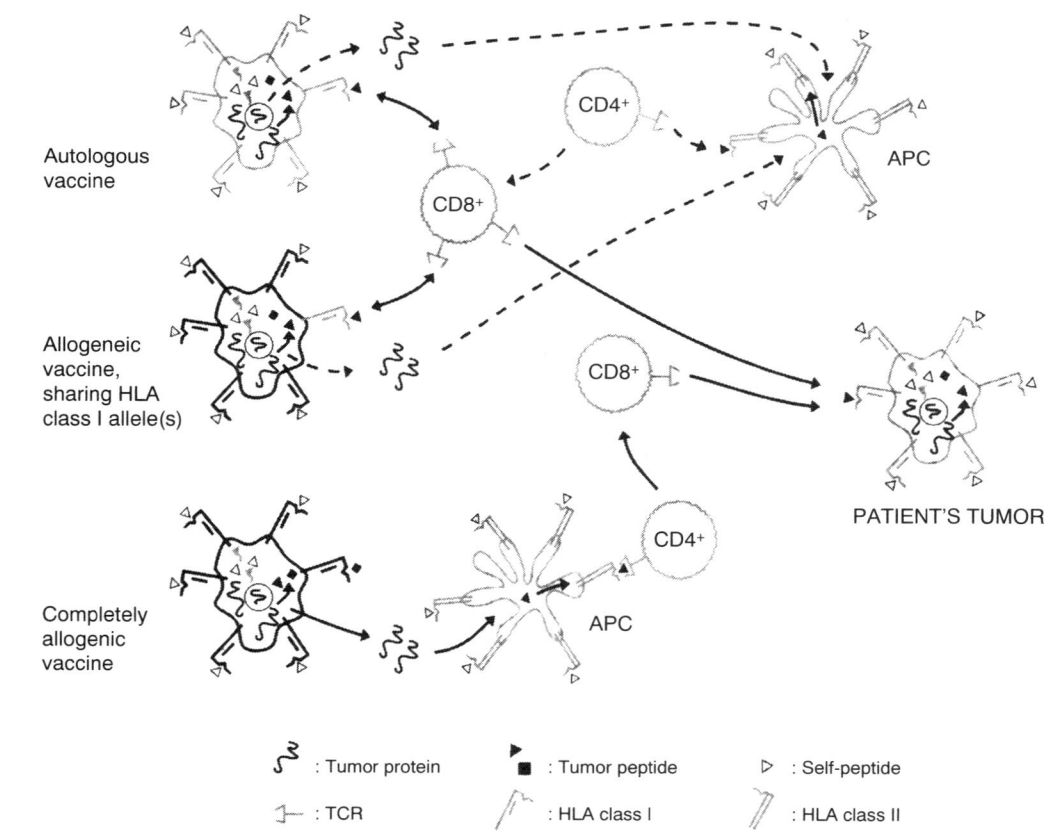

Autologous vaccine

Allogeneic vaccine, sharing HLA class I allele(s)

Completely allogenic vaccine

CD4+

CD8+

CD4+

CD8+

APC

APC

PATIENT'S TUMOR

🗝 : Tumor protein   ◣■ : Tumor peptide   ▷ : Self-peptide

⊥ : TCR   ⎰ : HLA class I   ⎰ : HLA class II

generated and presented to the immune system. Following vaccination with autologous tumors, both direct as well as indirect stimulation of T cells may occur (Fig. 27.2).

In February 1992, we initiated the first clinical study, in which HLA-A*0101[+] or HLA-A*0201[+] melanoma patients were immunized with HLA-A*0101, *0201, B8 allogeneic melanoma cells, that have been genetically modified by transfection to secrete IL-2. These cells have a high expression of HLA-A, -B, and -C alleles and are, therefore, an attractive candidate to use as a vaccine. Moreover, the cell line expresses all MAGE genes, tyrosinase, and gp100. The choice of IL-2 is based on the fact that clinical remissions were obtained in patients with metastatic melanoma following IL-2–based treatment regimens. Furthermore, evidence exists for the presence of CTL precursors in melanoma patients, while animal studies employing genetically engineered tumor cells producing IL-2 have shown that an active CD8[+] effector group can be generated. In addition, there is evidence that IL-2 secretion by tumor cells increases the frequency of tumor-specific CTL and CTL precursors and this correlates with tumor rejection (Ley et al. 1991). The IL-2 gene was transfected with the neo[r] gene into melanoma cell line Mel518A. We cloned the IL-2 cDNA behind the immediate early cytomegalovirus (CMV) promoter. This promoter is well expressed in melanoma cell lines, as determined by reporter assays. G418-resistant clones were selected and tested for IL-2 production by a CTL-L2 bioassay and enzyme-linked immunosorbent assay (ELISA) assay. Clones produce IL-2 in the range of 0.1 μg IL-2/10[6] tumor cells/24 h. At 100 Gy, a dose that completely inhibited proliferation of the cells in vitro, the secretion of biologically active IL-2 on a per-cell basis increased in the first days and decreased in the second week following irradiation.

The purpose of our study is to evaluate the toxicity and antitumor efficacy of weekly subcutaneous (SC) injections of these IL-2–secreting, allogeneic melanoma cells. No toxicities were observed. Thus far we have observed inflammatory reactions and regressions of distant metastases (Osanto et al. 1994). The nature of the cellular infiltrate in metastases and at the site of vaccination and HLA class I and II expression in metastatic cells is being investigated. Other human gene therapy trials have now been started using a similar approach, with either IL-2–, IFN-γ–, and IL-4–secreting tumor cells.

Nabel et al. (1993) reported another approach to enhance the antitumor immune response by in vivo injection of a foreign HLA class I gene directly into tumor deposits (i.e., HLA B7 using DNA liposome complexes). HLA-B7 protein expression was demonstrated in the tumor cells near the site of injection. No systemic toxicity was observed, while a fivefold increase in the frequency of HLA-B7–reactive CTL precursors was demonstrated following immunization. Furthermore, a distant lung metastasis regressed in one of the five reported patients, suggesting that allogeneic effects may indeed enhance the antitumor immune response (Nabel et al. 1993). Altogether, these data look promising and definitely merit further investigation of immunization with gene-modified tumor cells.

■ PERSPECTIVES OF CANCER IMMUNOTHERAPY

The perspective of cancer immunotherapy has changed dramatically since cancer Ag, which are potential targets for attack by the immune system, have been defined at the molecular level. All immunotherapy trials in the past have been hampered by the fact that tumor-rejection Ag expressed on the patient's tumor and on the vaccines used to stimulate the patient's immune system were not properly identified, precluding specific monitoring of immunological effects in vivo. We are now able to identify those patients whose tumor expresses a well-defined Ag and who may therefore benefit from specific immunization.

Though the approach of immunization with well-characterized genetically modified tumor cell vaccines is certainly promising, several factors may counteract the beneficial effects of vaccination (e.g., immune suppression, see above). In addition, local overproduction of cytokines by the modified cell may lead to enhanced growth in some tumors through a paracrine loop.

Further data from clinical studies must be awaited in order to optimize the immunization regimens. Based on animal experiments, the optimum moment to initiate immunotherapy is at the time of a low-tumor burden. It may be necessary to augment the antitumor effects mediated by preexisting in vivo–sensitized T cells either by in vivo administration of cytokines such as IL-2 or by adoptive transfer of in vitro–expanded autologous cytotoxic T cells (obtained by a secondary in vitro stimulation). Crucial to the progress of cancer immunotherapy will be the monitoring of cellular immune responses to the identified cancer Ag. In the case of immunization with HLA class I–matched genetically modified allogeneic tumor cells, this may require in vitro studies with targets loaded with known class I–binding tumor peptides instead of the classical determination of CTL precursor frequencies.

REFERENCES

Anichini, A., Mazzocchi, A., Fossati, G., and Parmiani, G. (1989) Cytotoxic T lymphocyte clones from peripheral blood and from tumor site detect intratumor heterogeneity of melanoma cells. Analysis of specificity and mechanisms of interaction. *Journal of Immunology*, **142**, 3692–701.

Asher, A.L., Mulé, J.J., Kasid, A., et al. (1991) Murine tumor cells transduced with the gene for tumor necrosis factor α. *Journal of Immunology*, **146**, 3227–34.

Azuma, H., Phillips, J.D., and Green, W.R. (1987) Clonal heterogeneity of anti-AKR/Gross leukemia virus cytotoxic T lymphocytes. *Journal of Immunology*, **139**, 2464–73.

Bakker, A.B.H., Schreurs, M.J.W., De Boer, A.J., et al. (1994) Melanocyte lineage-specific antigen gp100 is recognized by melanoma derived tumor infiltrating lymphocytes. *Journal of Experimental Medicine*, **179**, 1005–9.

Basombrio, M. (1970) Search for common antigenicity among twenty-five sarcomas induced by methylcholanthrene. *Cancer Research*, **30**, 2458–62.

Berd, D., Maguire, H.C., McCue, P., and Mastrangelo, M.J. (1990) Treatment of metastatic melanoma with an autologous tumor-cell vaccine: clinical and immunological results in 64 patients. *Journal of Clinical Oncology*, **8**, 1858–67.

Blankenstein, T., Qin, Z., Überla, K., et al. (1991) Tumor suppression after tumor cell-targeted tumor necrosis factor α gene transfer. *Journal of Experimental Medicine*, **173**, 1047–52.

Boon, T., van Pel, A., and De Plaen, E. (1989a) Tum⁻ transplantation antigens, point mutations and antigenic peptides: a model for tumor-specific transplantation antigens. *Cancer Cells*, **1**, 25–8.

Boon, T., van Pel, A., De Plaen, E., et al. (1989b) Genes coding for T-cell-defined tum transplantation antigens: point mutations, antigenic peptides, and subgenic expression. *Cold Spring Harbor Symposia on Quantitative Biology*, **54**, 587–96.

Boone, C.W., Paranjpe, M., Orme, T., and Gillette, R. (1974) Virus-augmented tumor transplantation antigens. Evidence for a helper antigen mechanism. *International Journal of Cancer*, **13**, 543–51.

Brichard, V., Van Pel, A., Wölfel, T., et al. (1993) The tyrosinase gene codes for an antigen recognized by autologous cytolytic T-lymphocytes on HLA-A2 melanomas. *Journal of Experimental Medicine*, **178**, 489–95.

Brodsky, F.M., and Guagliardi, L.E. (1991) The cell biology of antigen processing and presentation. *Annual Review of Immunology*, **9**, 707–44.

Bubenik, J., Simova, J., and Jandlova, T. (1990) Immunotherapy of cancer using local administration of lymphoid cells transformed by IL-2 cDNA and constitutively producing IL-2. *Immunology Letters*, **23**, 287–92.

Bystryn, J.C., Oratz, R., Roses, D., Harris, M., Henn, M., and Lew, R. (1992). Relationship between immune response to melanoma vaccine immunization and clinical outcome in stage-II malignant melanoma. *Cancer*, **69**, 1157–64.

Carel, J.C., Schreiber, R.D., Falqui, L., and Lacy, P.E. (1990) Transforming growth factor-beta decreases the immunogenicity of rat islet xenografts (rat to mouse) and prevents rejection in association with treatment of the recipient with a monoclonal antibody to interferon-gamma. *Proceedings of the National Academy of Sciences of the United States of America*, **87**, 1591–5.

Cassel, W.A., Murray, D.R., and Philips, H.S. (1983) A phase II study on the postsurgical management of stage II malignant melanoma with a Newcastle disease virus oncolysate. *Cancer*, **52**, 856–60.

Chen, L., Ashe, S., Brady, W.A., et al. (1992) Costimulation of antitumor immunity by the B7 counterreceptor for the T lymphocyte molecules CD28 and CTLA-4. *Cell*, **71**, 1093–102.

Chen, L., McGowan, P., Ashe, S., et al. (1994) Tumor immunogenicity determines the effect of B7 costimulation on T cell-mediated tumor immunity. *Journal of Experimental Medicine*, **179**, 523–31.

Colombo, M.P., Ferrara, G., Stoppacciaro, A., et al. (1991) Granulocyte colony-stimulating factor gene transfer suppresses tumorigenicity of a murine adenocarcinoma in vivo. *Journal of Experimental Medicine*, **173**, 889–97.

Coulie, P.G., Brichard, V., Pel, A.V., et al. (1994) A new gene coding for a differentiation antigen recognized by autologous cytolytic T-lymphocytes on HLA-A2 melanomas. *Journal of Experimental Medicine*, **180**, 35–42.

Cox, A.L., Skipper, J., Chen, Y., et al. (1994) Identification of a peptide recognized by five melanoma-specific human cytotoxic T cell lines. *Science*, **264**, 716–19.

Crowley, N.J., Darrow, T.L., Quinn-Allen, M.A., and Seigler, H.F. (1991) Major HC-restricted recognition of autologous melanoma by tumor-specific cytotoxic T-cells – evidence for restriction by a dominant HLA-A allele. *Journal of Immunology*, **146**, 1692–9.

Darrow, T.L., Slingluff, C.L., Jr., and Seigler, H.F. (1989) The role of HLA class I antigens in recognition of melanoma cells by tumor-specific cytotoxic T lymphocytes. Evidence for shared tumor antigens. *Journal of Immunology*, **142**, 3329–35.

de Martin, R., Haendler, B., Hofer-Warbinek, R., et al. (1987) Complementary DNA for human glioblastoma-derived T cell suppressor factor, a novel member of the transforming growth factor-beta gene family. *EMBO Journal*, **6**, 3673–7.

Degiovanni, G., Lahaye, T., Herin, M., Hainaut, P., and Boon, T. (1988) Antigenic heterogeneity of a human melanoma detected by autologous CTL clones. *European Journal of Immunology*, **18**, 671–6.

De Plaen, E., Lurquin, C., Van Pel, A., et al. (1988) Immunogenic (tum⁻) variants of mouse tumor P815: cloning of the gene of tum⁻ antigen P91A and identification of the tum⁻ mutation. *Proceedings of the National Academy of Sciences of the United States of America*, **85**, 2274–8.

Dranoff, G., Jaffee, E., Lazenby, A., et al. (1993) Vaccination with irradiated tumor cells engineered to secrete murine granulocyte-macrophage colony-stimulating factor stimulates potent, specific and long-lasting anti-tumour immunity. *Proceedings of the National Academy of Sciences of the United States of America*, **90**, 3539–43.

Faber, L.M., Luxemburg-Heijs, S.A.P.V., Willemze, R., and Falkenburg, J.H.F. (1992) Generation of leukemia-reactive cytotoxic T lymphocyte clones from the HLA-identical bone marrow donor of a patient with leukemia. *Journal of Experimental Medicine*, **176**, 1283–9.

Falkenburg, J.H.F., Faber, L.M., Elshout, M.V., et al. (1993) Generation of donor-derived anti-leukemic cytotoxic T lymphocyte responses for treatment of relapsed leukemia after allogeneic HLA-identical bone marrow transplant. *Journal of Immunotherapy*, **14**, 305–9.

Fearon, E.R., Itaya, T., Hunt, B., Vogelstein, B., and Frost, P. (1988) Induction in a murine tumor of immunogenic tumor variants by transfection with a foreign gene. *Cancer Research*, **38**, 2975–80.

Fearon, E.R., Pardoll, D.M., Itaya, T., et al. (1990) Interleukin-2 production by tumor cells bypasses T-helper function in the generation of an antitumor response. *Cell*, **60**, 397–403.

Finke, J.H., Zea, A.H., Stanley, J., et al. (1993) Loss of T-cell receptor zeta-chain and p56(lck) in T-cells infiltrating human renal cell carcinoma. *Cancer Research*, **53**, 5613–16.

Frost, P., Kerbel, R.S., Bauer, E., Tartamella-Biondo, R., and Cefalu, W. (1983) Mutagen treatment as a means for selecting immunogenic variants from otherwise poorly immunogenic malignant murine tumors. *Cancer Research*, **43**, 125–32.

Frost, P., Liteplo, R.G., Donaghue, T.P., and Kerbel, R.S. (1984) Selection of strongly immunogenic 'tum⁻' variants from tumors at high frequency using 5-aza cytidine. *Journal of Experimental Medicine*, **159**, 1491–501.

Gansbacher, B., Zier, K., Daniels, B., Cronin, K., Bannerji, R., and Gilboa, E. (1990) Interleukin 2 gene transfer into tumor cells abrogates tumorigenicity and induces protected immunity. *Journal of Experimental Medicine*, **172**, 1217–24.

Gaugler, B., Van den Eynde, B., Van der Bruggen, P., et al. (1994) Human gene MAGE-3 codes for an antigen recognized on a melanoma by autologous cytotolytic T lymphocytes. *Journal of Experimental Medicine*, **179**, 921–30.

Gelber, C., Plaksin, D., Vadai, E., Feldman, M., and Eisenbach, L. (1989) Abolishment of metastasis formation by murine tumor cells transfected with "foreign" H-2K genes. *Cancer Research*, **49**, 2366–73.

Globerson, A., and Feldman, M. (1964) Antigenic specificity of benzo[a]pyrene-induced sarcomas. *Journal of the National Cancer Institute*, **32**, 1229–43.

Golumbek, P.T., Lazenby, A.J., Levitsky, H.I., et al. (1991) Treatment of established renal cancer by tumor cells engineered to secrete interleukin-4. *Science*, **254**, 713–16.

Greenberg, P.D. (1991) Adoptive T-cell therapy of tumors – mechanisms operative in the recognition and elimination of tumor cells. *Advances in Immunology*, **49**, 281–355.

Gromet, M.A., Epstein, W.A., and Blois, M. (1978) The regressing thin malignant melanoma: a distinctive lesion with metastatic potential. *Cancer*, **42**, 2282.

Hersey, P. (1990) Evaluation of the current status of active specific immunotherapy of melanoma. In P. Rümke (Ed.) *Therapy of advanced melanoma*, pp. 183–200. Basel, Karger.

Hewitt, H.B., Blake, E.R., and Walder, A.S. (1976) A critique of the evidence for active host defence against cancer, based on personal studies of 27 murine tumours of spontaneous origin. *British Journal of Cancer*, **33**, 241–59.

Hock, H., Dorsch, M., Diamantstein, T., and Blankenstein, T. (1991) Interleukin-7 induces CD4⁺ T-cell-dependent tumor rejection. *Journal of Experimental Medicine*, **174**, 1291–8.

Hollinshead, A., Stewart, T.H.M., Takita, H., Dalbow, M., and Concannon, J. (1987) Adjuvant specific active lung cancer immunotherapy trials. *Cancer*, **60**, 1249–62.

Hoover, H.C., Surdyke, M., Dangel, R.B., Peters, L.C., and Hanna, M.A. (1985) Prospectively randomized trial of adjuvant active-specific immunotherapy for human colorectal cancer. *Cancer*, **55**, 1236–43.

Hosokawa, M., Okayasu, T., Ikeda, K., Katoh, H., Suzuki, Y., and Kobayashi, H. (1983) Alteration of immunogenicity of xenogenized tumor cells in syngeneic rats by the immune response to virus-associated antigens produced on immunizing cells. *Cancer Research*, **43**, 2301–5.

Huang, A.Y.C., Golumbek, P., Ahmadzadeh, M., Jaffee, E., Pardoll, D., and Levitsky, H. (1994) Role of bone marrow-derived cells in presenting major HC class I-restricted tumor antigens. *Science*, **264**, 961–5.

Hui, K., Grosveld, F., and Festenstein, H. (1984) Rejection of transplantable AKR leukaemia cells following major HC DNA-mediated cell transformation. *Nature*, **311**, 750–2.

Hui, K.M., Sim, T.F., Foo, T.T., and Oei, A.A. (1989) Tumor rejection mediated by transfection with allogeneic class-I histocompatibility gene. *Journal of Immunology*, **143**, 3835–43.

Inge, T.H., Hoover, S.K., Susskind, B.M., Barrett, S.K., and Bear, H.D. (1992) Inhibition of tumor-specific cytotoxic lymphocyte-T responses by transforming growth factor-beta1. *Cancer Research*, **52**, 1386–92.

Isobe, K., Hasegawa, Y., Iwamoto, T., et al. (1989) Induction of antitumor immunity in mice by allo-major histocompatibility complex class-I gene transfectant with strong antigen expression. *Journal of the National Cancer Institute*, **81**, 1823–8.

Kast, W.M., Offringa, R., Peters, P.J., et al. (1989) Eradication of adenovirus E1-induced tumors by E1A-specific cytotoxic T lymphocytes. *Cell*, **59**, 603–14.

Kawakami, Y., Eliyahu, S., Delgado, C.H., et al. (1994a) Cloning of the gene for a shared human melanoma antigen recognized by autologous T cells infiltrating into tumor. *Proceedings of the National Academy of Sciences of the United States of America*, **91**, 3515–19.

Kawakami, Y., Eliyahu, S., Sakaguchi, K., et al. (1994b) Identification of the immunodominant peptides of the MART-1 human melanoma antigen recognized by the majority of HLA-A2-restricted tumor infiltrating lymphocytes. *Journal of Experimental Medicine*, **180**, 347–52.

Kawakami, Y., Zakut, R., Topalian, S.L., Stotter, H., and Rosenberg, S.A. (1992) Shared human melanoma antigens – recognition by tumor-infiltrating lymphocytes in HLA-A2.1-transfected melanomas. *Journal of Immunology*, **148**, 638–43.

Kim, T.S., Russell, S.J., Collins, M.K.L., and Cohen, E.P. (1993) Immunization with interleukin-2-secreting allogeneic mouse fibroblasts expressing melanoma-associated antigens prolongs the survival of mice with melanoma. *International Journal of Cancer*, **55**, 865–72.

Klein, G., Sjögren, H., Klein, E., and Hellström, K.E. (1960) Demonstration of resistance against methylcholanthrene-induced sarcomas in the primary autochthonous host. *Cancer Research*, **20**, 1561–72.

Kobayashi, H., Sendo, F., Shirai, T., Kaji, H., Kodama, T., and Saito, H. (1969) Modification in growth of transplantable rat tumors exposed to Friend virus. *Journal of the National Cancer Institute*, **42**, 413–19.

Kripke, M.L. (1974) Antigenicity of murine skin tumors induced by ultraviolet light. *Journal of the National Cancer Institute*, **53**, 333–6.

Kuzumaki, N., Fenyo, E.M., Giovanella, B., and Klein, G. (1978) Increased immunogenicity of low-antigenic rat tumors after superinfection with endogenous murine C-type virus in nude mice. *International Journal of Cancer*, **21**, 62–6.

Lafreniere, R. and Rosenberg, S.A. (1985) Successful immunotherapy of murine experimental hepatic metastases with lymphokine-activated killer (LAK) cells. *Cancer Research*, **45**, 3735–41.

Ley, V., Langlade-Demoyen, P., Kourilsky, P., and Larsson-Sciard, E.L. (1991) Interleukin 2-dependent activation of tumor-specific cytotoxic T lymphocytes in vivo. *European Journal of Immunology*, **21**, 851–4.

Li, W., Diamantstein, T., and Blankenstein, T. (1990) Lack of tumorigenicity of interleukin 4 autocrine growing cells seems related to the anti-tumor function of interleukin 4. *Molecular Immunology*, **27**, 1331–7.

Liebrich, W., Schlag, P., Manasterski, M., et al. (1991) In vitro and clinical characterisation of a Newcastle disease virus-modified autologous tumour cell vaccine for treatment of colorectal cancer patients. *European Journal of Cancer*, **27**, 703–10.

Lindenmann, J. and Klein, P.A. (1967) Viral oncolysis. Increased immunogenicity of host cell antigen associated with influenza virus. *Journal of Experimental Medicine*, **126**, 93–108.

Maruguchi, Y., Toda, K.I., Fujii, K., Imamura, S., and Watanabe, Y. (1991) Survival period of tumor-bearing mice is prolonged after the interferon-gamma-producing gene transfer. *Cancer Letters*, **60**, 41–9.

Mazumder, A. and Rosenberg, S.A. (1984) Successful immunotherapy of NK-resistent established pulmonary melanoma metastases with LAK cells and recombinant IL-2. *Science*, **225**, 1487–9.

McCune, C.S., O'Donnell, R.W., Marquis, D.M., and Sahasrabudhe, D.M. (1990) Renal cell carcinoma treated by vaccines for active specific immunotherapy: correlation of survival with skin testing by autologous tumor cells. *Cancer Immunology and Immunotherapy*, **32**, 62–6.

Melief, C.J.M. (1992) Tumor eradication by adoptive transfer of cytotoxic T lymphocytes. *Advances in Cancer Research*, **58**, 143–75.

Melief, C.J.M. and Kast, W.M. (1990) Efficacy of cytotoxic T-lymphocytes against virus-induced tumors. *Cancer Cells*, **2**, 116–20.

Melief, C.J.M., Vasmel, W.L., Offringa, R., et al. (1989) Immunosurveillance of virus-induced tumors. *Cold Spring Harbor Symposia on Quantitative Biology*, **54**, 597–603.

Mitchell, M.S., Harel, W., Kempf, R.A., et al. (1990) Active-specific immunotherapy for melanoma. *Journal of Clinical Oncology*, **8**, 856–69.

Mizoguchi, H., O'Shea, J.J., Longo, D.L., Loefller, C.M., McVicar, D.W., and Ochoa, A.C. (1992) Alterations in signal transduction molecules in T-lymphocytes from tumor-bearing mice. *Science*, **258**, 1795–8.

Morton, D.L. (1986) Active immunotherapy against cancer. Present status. *Seminars in Oncology*, **13**, 180–5.

Möller, P. and Hämmerling, G.J. (1992) The role of surface HLA-A,B,C molecules in tumour immunity. *Cancer Surveys*, **13**, 101–27.

Mueller, D.L., Jenkins, M.K., and Schwartz, R.H. (1989) Clonal expansion versus functional clonal inactivation: a co-stimulatory signalling pathway determines the outcome of T cell antigen receptor occupancy. *Annual Review of Immunology*, **7**, 445–80.

Mukherji, B., Chakraborty, N.G., and Sivanandham, M. (1990) T-cell clones that react against autologous human tumors. *Immunology Reviews*, **116**, 33–62.

Mule, J.J., Shu, S., Schwarz, S.L., and Rosenberg, S.A. (1984) Adoptive immunotherapy of established pulmonary metastases with LAK cells and recombinant interleukin-2. *Science,* **225**, 1487–9.

Nabel, G.J., Nabel, E.G., Yang, Z.Y., et al. (1993) Direct gene transfer with DNA-liposome complexes in melanoma: expression, biologic activity, and lack of toxicity in humans. *Proceedings of the National Academy of Sciences of the United States of America,* **90**, 11307–11.

North, R.J. (1982) Cyclophosphamide-facilitated adoptive immunotherapy of an established tumor depends on elimination of tumor-induced suppressor T-cells. *Journal of Experimental Medicine,* **55**, 1063–74.

Nossal, G.J.V. (1989) Immunologic tolerance: collaboration between antigen and lymphokines. *Science,* **245**, 147–53.

Notter, M. and Schirrmacher, V. (1990) Tumor-specific T-cell clones recognize different protein determinants of autologous human malignant melanoma cells. *International Journal of Cancer,* **45**, 834–41.

Old, L.J., Boyse, E.A., Clarke, D.A., and Carswell, E.A. (1962) Antigenic properties of chemically induced tumors. II. Antigens of tumor cells. *Annals of the New York Academy of Sciences,* **101**, 80–106.

Osanto, S., Brouwenstijn, N., Vaessen, N., et al. (1994) Gene therapy of metastatic melanoma patients with IL-2 transfected melanoma cells. *Proceedings of the American Society of Clinical Oncology,* **13**, 950a.

Ostrand-Rosenberg, S., Roby, C., Clements, V.K., and Cole, G.A. (1991) Tumor-specific immunity can be enhanced by transfection of tumor cells with syngeneic major HC-class-II genes or allogeneic major HC-class-I genes. *International Journal of Cancer,* **6**, 61–8.

Parham, P. (1990) Antigen processing. Transporters of delight. *Nature,* **348**, 674–5.

Platsoucas, C.D. (1991) Human autologous tumor-specific T-cells in malignant melanoma. *Cancer Metastasis Reviews,* **10**, 151–76.

Prehn, R.T. (1962) Specific isoantigenicities among chemically-induced tumors. *Annals of the New York Academy of Sciences,* **101**, 107–13.

Prehn, R.T. and Main, J.M. (1957) Immunity to methylcholanthrene-induced sarcomas. *Journal of the National Cancer Institute,* **18**, 769–78.

Ranges, G.E., Figari, I.S., Espevik, T., and Palladino, M.A., Jr. (1987) Inhibition of cytotoxic T cell development by transforming growth factor beta and reversal by recombinant tumor necrosis factor alpha. *Journal of Experimental Medicine,* **166**, 991–8.

Rao, V.S., Wiseman, C., Mazumder, A., et al. (1988) Effect of cholesterylhemisuccinate (CHS) on cell mediated immunity in melanoma patients treated with active intralymphatic immunotherapy. *Proceedings of the American Association of Cancer Research,* **29**, 409.

Restifo, N.P., Esquivel, F., Asher, A.L., et al. (1991) Defective presentation of endogenous antigens by a murine sarcoma – implications for the failure of an anti-tumor immune response. *Journal of Immunology,* **147**, 1453–9.

Restifo, N.P., Esquivel, F., Kawakami, Y., et al. (1993) Identification of human cancers deficient in antigen processing. *Journal of Experimental Medicine,* **177**, 265–72.

Rosenberg, S.A., Aebersold, P., Cornetta, K., et al. (1990) Gene transfer into humans – immunotherapy of patients with advanced melanoma, using tumor-infiltrating lymphocytes modified by retroviral gene transduction. *New England Journal of Medicine,* **323**, 570–8.

Rosenberg, S.A., Lotze, M.T., and Muul, L.M. (1985). Special report: observations on the systemic administration of autologous lymphokine-activated killer cells and recombinant interleukin-2 to patients with metastatic cancer. *New England Journal of Medicine*, **313**, 1485–92.

Rosenberg, S.A., Lotze, M.T., Muul, L.M., et al. (1987) A progress report on the treatment of 157 patients with advanced cancer with lymphokine-activated killer cells and interleukin-2 or high dose interleukin-2 alone. *New England Journal of Medicine*, **316**, 889–97.

Rosenberg, S.A., Lotze, M.T., and Yang, C.J. (1989) Experience with the use of high-dose interleukin-2 in the treatment of 652 cancer patients. *Annals of Surgery*, **210**, 474–85.

Rosenberg, S.A., Packard, B.S., Aebersold, P.M., et al. (1988) Use of tumor-infiltrating lymphocytes and interleukin-2 in the immunotherapy of patients with metastatic melanoma. *New England Journal of Medicine*, **319**, 1676–80.

Schendel, D.J., Gansbacher, B., Oberneder, R., et al. (1993) Tumor-specific lysis of human renal cell carcinomas by tumor-infiltrating lymphocytes. I. HLA-A2-restricted recognition of autologous and allogeneic tumor lines. *Journal of Immunology*, **151**, 4209–20.

Schrier, P.I. and Peltenburg, L.T.C. (1993) Relationship between myc oncogene activation and major HC Class I expression. *Advances in Cancer Research*, **60**, 181–246.

Shimizu, Y., Fujiwara, H., Ueda, S., Wakamiya, N., Kato, S., and Hamaoka, T. (1984) The augmentation of tumor specific immunity by virus help. II. Enhanced induction of cytotoxic T lymphocyte and antibody response to tumor antigens by vaccinia virus reactive helper T cells. *European Journal of Immunology*, **14**, 839–43.

Slingluff, C.L., Cox, A.L., Henderson, R.A., Hunt, D.F., and Engelhard, V.H. (1993) Recognition of human melanoma cells by HLA-A2.1-restricted cytotoxic T-lymphocytes is mediated by at least 6 shared peptide epitopes. *Journal of Immunology*, **150**, 2955–63.

Slovin, S.F., Lackman, R.D., Ferrone, S., Kiely, P.E., and Mastrangelo, M.J. (1986). Cellular immune response to human sarcomas: cytotoxic T cell clones reactive with autologous sarcomas. *Journal of Immunology*, **137**, 3042–8.

Storkus, W.J., Zeh, H.J., III, Salter, R.D., and Lotze, M.T. (1993) Identification of T-cell epitopes: rapid isolation of class I-presented peptides from viable cells by mild acid elution. *Journal of Immunotherapy*, **14**, 94–103.

Szikora, J.P., Van Pel, A., Brichard, V., et al. (1990) Structure of the gene of tum⁻ transplantation antigen P35B: presence of a point mutation in the antigenic allele. *EMBO Journal*, **9**, 1041.

Tepper, R.I., Pattengale, P.K., and Leder, P. (1991) Murine interleukin-4 displays potent anti-tumor activity in vivo. *Cell*, **57**, 503–12.

Topalian, S.L., Solomon, D., and Rosenberg, S.A. (1989) Tumor-specific cytolysis by lymphocytes infiltrating human melanomas. *Journal of Immunology*, **142**, 3714–25.

Torre-Amione, G., Beauchamp, R.D., Koeppen, H., et al. (1990) A highly immunogenic tumor transfected with a murine transforming growth factor type-beta-1 cDNA escapes immune surveillance. *Proceedings of the National Academy of Sciences of the United States of America*, **87**, 1486–90.

Townsend, A., Elliott, T., Cerundolo, V., Foster, L., Barber, B., and Tse, A. (1990) Assembly of major HC class I molecules analyzed in vitro. *Cell*, **62**, 285–95.

Townsend, S.E. and Allison, J.P. (1993) Tumor rejection after direct costimulation of CD8$^+$ T-cells by B7-transfected melanoma cells. *Science,* **259,** 368–70.

Traversari, C., Van der Bruggen, P., Luescher, I.F., et al. (1992) A nonapeptide encoded by human gene MAGE-1 is recognized on HLA-A1 by cytolytic T-lymphocytes directed against tumor antigen-MZ2-E. *Journal of Experimental Medicine,* **176,** 1453–7.

Uyttenhove, C., Maryanski, J., and Boon, T. (1983) Escape of mouse mastocytoma P815 after nearly complete rejection is due to antigen-loss variants rather than immunosuppression. *Journal of Experimental Medicine,* **157,** 1040–52.

Van der Bruggen, P., Traversari, C., Chomez, P., et al. (1991) A gene encoding an antigen recognized by cytolytic lymphocytes-T on a human melanoma. *Science,* **254,** 1643–7.

Von Hoegen, P., Weber, E., and Schirrmacher, V. (1988) Modification of tumor cells by a low dose of Newcastle disease virus. II. Augmented tumor-specific T cell response in the absence of an anti-viral response. *European Journal of Immunology,* **18,** 1159–66.

Wang, P., Vegh, Z., Vanky, F., and Klein, E. (1992) HLA-B5-restricted auto-tumor specific cytotoxic T-cells generated in mixed lymphocyte-tumor-cell culture. *International Journal of Cancer,* **52,** 517–22.

Watanabe, Y., Kuribayashi, K., Miyatake, S., et al. (1989) Exogenous expression of mouse interferon-τ cDNA in mouse C1300 neuroblastoma cells results in reduced tumorigenicity by augmented anti-tumor immunity. *Proceedings of the National Academy of Sciences of the United States of America,* **86,** 9456–60.

West, W.H., Tauer, K.W., and Yannelli, J.R. (1987) Constant-infusion recombinant interleukin-2 in adoptive immunotherapy of advanced cancer. *New England Journal of Medicine,* **316,** 898–905.

Wölfel, T., Klehmann, E., Muller, C.A., Schutt, K.H., Meyer zum Buschenfelde, K.H., and Knuth, A. (1989) Lysis of human melanoma cells by autologous cytolytic T cell clones. Identification of human histocompatibility leukocyte antigen A2 as a restriction element for three different antigens. *Journal of Experimental Medicine,* **170,** 797–810.

Yamaguchi, H., Moriuchi, T., Hosokawa, M., and Kobayashi, H. (1982) Increased or decreased immunogenicity of tumor-associated antigen according to the amount of virus-associated antigen in rat tumor cells infected with Friend virus. *Cancer Immunology and Immunotherapy,* **12,** 119–23.

Yasumura, S., Hirabayashi, H., Schwartz, D.R., et al. (1993) Human cytotoxic T-cell lines with restricted specificity for squamous cell carcinoma of the head and neck. *Cancer Research,* **53,** 1461–8.

–28

Neutrophil Transfusions for Treatment of Infections

KIRSTEN MAAKESTAD, ROSEMARY MAZANET,
W. CONRAD LILES, AND DAVID C. DALE

Background Information

Bacterial and fungal infections are significant causes of treatment-related morbidity and mortality among cancer and bone-marrow transplant (BMT) patients (Strauss 1993). Recently, the expanding use of dose-intensive cancer treatment strategies (chemotherapy and immunosuppressive therapies) has increased the frequency of prolonged neutropenia and, consequently, increased the risk of infection in these patients (Aisner, Schimpff, and Wiernick 1977; Manzullo 1994). Despite improvements in antimicrobial regimens and use of hemopoietic growth factors, severe neutropenia remains the most important risk factor leading to hospitalization of patients during cancer chemotherapy (Pizzo 1993). Therefore, investigators continue to explore methods to treat profound and prolonged neutropenia, including transfusion of neutrophils to replace the endogenous neutrophils these patients lack. This chapter summarizes progress to date in developing neutrophil transfusion therapy and explores the new directions for making this therapy more effective and more widely available.

Physiological Principles Underlying Neutrophil-Transfusion Therapy

Neutrophils are produced extravascularly in the bone marrow (BM); approximately 10 to 14 days are normally required to produce each mature cell that is ready to enter the blood. Once released from the marrow into circulation, neutrophils are found in two compartments of approximately equal size: the freely flowing, circulating pool; and the marginating pool, in which the neutrophils are loosely adherent to the vessel walls throughout the body (Table 28.1). These two pools are in a dynamic equilibrium, with neutrophils moving back and forth between the pools; however, only the circulating population is accessible when collecting cells for therapeutic use.

A normal person (70 kg) produces about 1×10^{11} neutrophils per day (Boggs 1974). With their short blood half-life (about 6 to 8 hours), only about 2.0×10^{10} neutrophils, or 20% of the daily production, are in the circulating population at any time and available for collection (Table 28.1). Neutrophil levels for collection can be increased by stress, excitement, or exercise (all cause cells to shift from the marginal to the circulating pool) and by a variety of agents that release cells from the marrow neutrophil reserves. Because the marrow reserve represents roughly ten times the circulating pool, it is the most important source of cells for the acute response to inflammation and infection of normal persons. Additionally, the marrow reserve is an available supply of neutrophils for collection, if it can be readily mobilized without untoward effects.

■ THE EFFICACY OF NEUTROPHIL TRANSFUSION THERAPY

The first report of a neutrophil transfusion was in 1934 (Strumia 1934). A "leukocyte cream" was injected intramuscularly into neutropenic patients, which increased the neutrophil count in nine of ten patients. In the 1960s, Freireich et al. (1964) bypassed the need for improved collection technology, by using patients with chronic myelogenous leukemia (CML) as donors, which allowed up to 3×10^{11} neutrophils to be collected (Morse et al. 1966). In febrile leukopenic cancer recipients, 54% of the transfused patients became afebrile within 36 hours. The lack of availability of CML donors and the risk of transferring infections and malignant cells to the recipient limited the use of this approach.

By the mid 1960s, investigations turned to the development of adequate collection methods from normal donors, using centrifugation and filter-adherence techniques. Steady progress in cell collection and separation soon led to initiation of several controlled trials (Table 28.2). The first controlled trial in cancer patients with documented or suspected gram-negative sepsis that had not responded to the standard antimicrobial therapy, by Graw et al. (1972), provided important information and encouraged other studies. They reported 100% sur-

Table 28.1. Key Blood Cell Kinetic Measurements Related to Neutrophil Transfusion Therapy[a]

Neutrophil Kinetics

Average life span: 10 hours
$T_{1/2}$: 6.6 hours
Turnover rate (daily production):
180×10^7/kg body weight/day
Released into circulation daily: 1.0×10^{11}

Comparison	Average Life Span	% of Circulating Cells Consumed Daily
Red Blood Cell:	90 days	0.8%
Platelet:	10 days	10%
Neutrophils:	0.4 days	200% to 300%

Approximate Quantities of Neutrophils in Various Pools

Marrow storage pool (mobilizable)	1.3×10^{11}
Circulating pool (available for collection)	2.0×10^{10}
Marginating pool (unavailable for collection)	2.0×10^{10}

[a]Adapted from Athens, J.W. (1961) Leukokinetic studies. IV. The total blood, circulating, and marginal granulocyte pools and the granulocyte turnover rate in normal subjects. *Journal of Clinical Investigation*, **40**, 989–95; and Wright, D. G. (1984) Symposium on infectious complications of neoplastic disease (part II). Leukocyte transfusions: thinking twice. *American Journal of Medicine*, **76**, 637–44.

Table 28.2. Controlled Trials of Neutrophil Transfusions in Adults[a]

First Author	Year	No. of Patients Transfused	% Survival Transfused	Control	Efficacy
Graw	1972	76	46%	30%	Partial
Higby	1975	36	76%	26%	Yes
Fortuny	1975	39	78%	80%	No
Vogler	1977	30	59%	15%	Yes
Alavi	1977	31	80%	62%	Partial
Herzig	1977	27	75%	36%	Yes
Winston	1982	95	63%	72%	No

[a]Adapted from Strauss, R.G. (1993) Therapeutic granulocyte transfusions in 1993. *Blood*, **81**, 1675–8.

vival with four transfusions, 80% survival with three transfusions, and 30% survival in the control group, a group lacking a suitable donor.

This study used two methods of leukapheresis, centrifugation and filtration, and noted many more adverse reactions and fewer circulating neutrophils with filtration leukapheresis (Graw et al. 1972), suggesting that neutrophils were damaged during the collection process (Menitove and Abrams 1987; McCullough et al. 1976). They also noted that ABO- and, probably, HLA-matching resulted in higher posttransfusion counts (Graw et al. 1972).

The six studies that followed (1972 to 1982) were less convincing of the value of neutrophil transfusion therapy, but study design issues and the size of these trials limited their conclusiveness. Higby et al. (1975) limited the therapy to four transfusions instead of clinical improvement, but showed a treatment benefit. Vogler and Winston (1977) demonstrated efficacy, especially for patients with prolonged neutropenia and noted that patients receiving transfusions containing less than 0.3×10^{10} neutrophils did not appear to respond. Fortuny et al. (1975) had a very high survival in the control group with antibiotics alone (80%), suggesting that the study included patients who were not critically ill. Alavi et al. (1977) initiated neutrophil transfusions for patients with febrile neutropenia, including many patients destined to do well with antibiotics alone. This study concluded that neutrophil transfusions were efficacious for patients with documented infections and suggested that neutrophil transfusions prevent fungal infections (Alavi et al. 1977). Herzig et al. (1977) confirmed that the greatest benefit was for patients with prolonged neutropenia.

The study of Winston et al. (1982) was designed well, but showed a lack of efficacy. The patients had documented infections and BM suppression, and the donors' cells were collected by centrifugation leukapheresis; however, the lack of efficacy was not surprising considering the mean number of cells per transfusion was only 0.5×10^{10}. The high survival rate of control patients on standard therapy also suggested either that the antibiotics used were more effective than in the past or that the study included many patients without serious infections.

Strauss (1993) and Wright (1984) summarized these trials (Table 28.1). The positive studies were by Higby, Vogler, and Herzig, and the negative studies were by Winston and Fortuny. The Graw study showed partial efficacy in patients who received adequate transfusions, and the Alavi study showed partial benefits in the subset of neutropenic patients with persistent BM failure. Overall, the results of these controlled trials fail to establish unequivocally whether neutrophil transfusions are beneficial, especially considering the improved combinations of antimicrobial therapies now available; however, they do set out the clinical requirements for the most appropriate use of neutrophil-transfusion therapy. These are documented bacterial or fungal infection, proven neutropenia, decreased BM neutrophil production that is expected to last for more than 7 days, and lack of response to antibiotic therapy after 48 hours (Schiffer and Wade 1987). All four conditions should be present together. Neutrophil-transfusion therapy should not be used in patients who have a neutrophil count greater than 0.5×10^9/L; febrile neutropenia without a likely or proven infection; or a depleted BM storage pool if recovery of blood counts are expected soon.

■ TECHNICAL CONSIDERATIONS

Donor Stimulation to Induce Neutrophilia

Patients with untreated CML often have blood neutrophil counts greater than 50×10^9/L. From these donors, Freireich et al. (1964) and others were able to routinely collect approximately 7×10^{10} neutrophils (Morse et al. 1966; Schiffer et al. 1983; Schiffer and Wade 1987). An advantage of CML cells may be that myelocytes and other incompletely matured neutrophil forms have a prolonged circulating half-life and comprise much of the transfusate. This results in persistence of these cells in the circulation; however, the overall interest in CML donors has waned significantly because of the lack of donors, the possibility of CML cell engraftment, and the risk of transmission of potential pathogens (Strauss 1993; Schiffer et al. 1983; Schiffer and Wade 1987).

In the 1970s, studies focused on pharmacological methods to increase blood neutrophils in normal donors, with a goal of increasing mean collections from 0.5×10^{10} to 3.0×10^{10} cells (Shogi and Vogler 1974). Corticosteroids effectively increased blood neutrophil levels principally by mobilizing the marrow-neutrophil reserves (Dale et al. 1975). For the next 15 years, a variety of doses and types of steroids were tested. Most studies employed dexamethasone or prednisone in doses that increased neutrophil yields to about 2 to 3×10^{10} neutrophils (Mannoni, Rodet, and Vernant 1979; French, Lolomon, and Fratantoni 1982; Strauss 1993). Side effects were minimal. The possibility of steroid-induced functional defects was a concern, but controlled trials using steroids for donor stimulation showed positive results (Higby et al. 1975; Alavi et al. 1977; Vogler and Winton 1977).

As an alternative to steroids, recombinant human granulocyte colony-stimulating factor (rHuG-CSF) recently has been used to increase the circulating pool and stimulate production in donors (Bensinger, Price, and Dale 1993; Caspar et al. 1993). Compared with steroids, rHuG-CSF therapy causes a greater increase in blood counts (Table 28.1) (Chatta et al. 1994a, b). The study by Caspar et al. (1993) investigated the administration of a single dose of rHuG-CSF followed by a single collection of neutrophils. Bensinger et al. (1993) collected cells a mean of 7.6 times over approximately 12 days from individual donors. Both studies used 300-μg doses of rHuG-CSF administered subcutaneously (SC) approximately 12 hours before leukapheresis and both harvested a mean greater than 4.0×10^{10} neutrophils per collection (Bensinger et al. 1993; Caspar et al. 1993). A single dose of rHuG-CSF increased the circulating neutrophil count by mobilization of neutrophils from the BM storage pool. Prolonged administration of rHuG-CSF–stimulated neutrophil production and accelerated BM transit time (Price, Chatta, and Dale 1992). Chemotaxis, phagocytosis, and superoxide anion production appear normal in the neutrophils collected for these studies when tested in vitro (Caspar et al. 1993). It is also noteworthy that neutrophil counts remain elevated longer in recipients of rHuG-CSF–stimulated cells, suggesting the transfusions contain immature cells or neutrophils with a prolonged life span (Bensinger et al. 1993; Caspar et al. 1993; Freireich 1994).

In the donors stimulated with rHuG-CSF, only minimal side effects have been observed, chiefly bone pain and headaches, as in other studies (Bensinger et al. 1993; Caspar et al. 1993; Nagler, Naparstek, and Engelhard 1994). In one instance, daily rHuG-CSF administration was discontinued after a donor's neutrophil count exceeded 50×10^9/L for two consecutive days, but no adverse side effects were associated with these elevated levels (Bensinger et al. 1993).

Neutrophil Collection

Advances in collection techniques were fundamental to the development of neutrophil-transfusion therapy. Since the advent of leukapheresis in 1962, several methods have been tested, including filtration leukapheresis, gravity, intermittent-flow centrifugation, and continuous-flow centrifugation (Menitove and Abrams 1987). Filtration leukapheresis was the method of choice for several years because it is relatively inexpensive and yields 2.5 to 5.0×10^{10} neutrophils/apheresis from steroid-treated donors (McCullough et al. 1976). The process involved the filtration of whole blood through a nylon filter, which traps neutrophils. The neutrophils were removed with chelating agents and by physical means such as shaking and tapping the filters. Function studies, however, revealed that many of the collected neutrophils were defective in both in vitro and in vivo assays (Hammerschmidt et al. 1978; Price and Dale 1979; Menitove and Abrams 1987). Although two- to threefold more cells were collected by filtration than centrifugation, less than 20% of the these cells were circulating after 1 hour compared with 50% of the cells collected by centrifugation. Filtration leukapheresis cells were also found to have a shortened life span and impaired tissue response (McCullough et al. 1976). The filters appeared to activate cells and rupture membranes, allowing granule release and complement activation (McCullough et al. 1976; Hammerschmidt et al. 1978). Various adverse reactions in both donors and recipients were linked to this method, including excessive flushes and chills (Graw et al. 1972; Herzig et al. 1977). Consequently, filtration leukapheresis is no longer used (Strauss 1993).

With intermittent-flow centrifugation, more platelets and fewer granulocytes are collected, so it is sometimes used when a combined transfusion of both platelets and granulocytes is required (Menitove and Abrams 1987). Gravitational leukapheresis may still be used in place of centrifugation methods when a cell separator is not available, but it is very inefficient (Dutcher 1990).

Most apheresis units now use continuous-flow centrifugation leukapheresis, which selectively removes leukocytes, mostly neutrophils, and returns the red cells and platelets to the donor (Dutcher 1990). Side effects for the donor include a slightly decreased hematocrit and, occasionally, shivering and abdominal cramps. Blood from one antecubital vein travels to a pump, where an anticoagulant (usually trisodium citrate) and then hydroxyethyl starch (HES) are added. The HES increases erythrocyte sedimentation by causing roleaux formation. The blood then passes through a specially designed centrifuge. Leukocytes are removed and the remaining blood components are returned to the donor. The efficiency of leukapheresis doubles with HES, while allowing the greatest quantity of erythrocytes to be returned to the donor. Donor fluid retention is the only significant side effect of HES, and no long-term side effects have been reported. Recently, it has been suggested that rHuG-CSF and HES may interact, causing additional weight gain and edema (Caspar et al. 1993; Strauss 1993).

Neutrophil Storage

Neutrophils harvested by any method deteriorate rapidly, with at least a 50% loss of function in less than 24 hours of storage (Price and Dale 1978). Most cells are currently collected and transfused as quickly as possible. Thus far, techniques for extended storage have been largely unsuccessful. The half-life of normal neutrophils in the circulation is approximately 6 to 10 hours in vivo and only slightly greater in vitro.

The optimal storage conditions for neutrophils are not known; when storage is necessary, some centers prefer 22°C and others 4°C (French, Lolomon, and Fratantoni 1982). Glucose is essential for the neutrophils to maintain metabolic function during storage (Glasser, Fiederlein, and Huestis 1985). Investigations on storage by freezing with the cryoprotectant dimethyl sulfoxide (DMSO) in liquid nitrogen indicated that 60% of the cells can maintain some functional capacity after 8 months of storage (Richman 1983), but it is doubtful that these cells would have preserved in vivo functions. Recent studies show that several cytokines and growth factors can extend the neutrophil half-life in vitro by two- to threefold (Begley et al. 1986; Colotta 1993; Liles, Waltersdorph, and Klebanoff 1994). These factors may prove useful to facilitate neutrophil storage.

Neutrophil Dosage

The optimal dose of neutrophils per transfusion is not known. The minimum effective dose has been established at about 1×10^{10} neutrophils, but some believe the recommended dose should be increased to 2 to 3×10^{10} neutrophils, or higher (McCullough 1989; Schiffer 1990).

Graw et al. (1972) established a dose schedule of one transfusion per day for a minimum of 4 days. In studies involving fewer than four transfusions, efficacy dropped significantly (Schiffer 1990). For practical reasons, the schedule has remained at one transfusion per day, but increased efficacy could result from two transfusions per day. The duration of therapy has also not been established.

Associated Risks of Transfusion

Common side effects of neutrophil transfusions are chills and fever (Menitove and Abrams 1987). Alloimmunization is a more serious risk (Schiffer et al. 1979; Herzig 1989). Donors and recipients should be matched by ABO blood type. Some transfusion reactions may be due to HLA incompatibilities, but HLA matching does not necessarily prevent these reactions (Graw et al. 1972; Schiffer et al. 1979; Strauss et al. 1981; Schiffer and Wade 1987). The standard procedure is to check for antibodies (Ab) to ABO antigens and to test for leukoagglutination, but the value of the leukoagglutination tests is uncertain. Until testing methods improve, the best way to minimize risk for alloimmunized patients is to tranfuse cells from HLA-compatible donors whenever possible, but this is not often practical.

A second concern about HLA incompatibility is its possible contribution to transfusion-associated graft-versus-host disease (taGVHD) (Weiden et al. 1981). Most HLA antigens are found on lymphocytes (transfused in small quantities with neutrophil transfusion), but they are also found on neutrophils. To avoid taGVHD, cell products have usually been irradiated with 1,500 to 3,000 rads from a cesium source (Weiden et al. 1981; Menitove and Abrams 1987). Although irradiation effectively reduces the number and function of lymphocytes, neutrophils are relatively insensitive to irradiation. There is still uncertainty, however, about the effects of irradiating the cells.

Pulmonary toxicity also has been attributed to neutrophil-transfusion therapy, especially when cells and amphotericin are given concomitantly (Hammerschmidt et al. 1980). Pulmonary toxicities, however, are often difficult to recognize in severely ill patients. Pulmonary infiltrates have been ascribed to granule release from damaged neutrophils and complement activation (Hammerschmidt et al. 1980), causing localized enzyme release in the pulmonary microvasculature (Strumia 1934). Pulmonary toxicities have probably been reduced by screening of donors for cytomegalovirus (CMV). Avoiding filtration leukapheresis and separation of amphotericin B and neutrophil-transfusion therapy by several hours are generally recommended.

■ APPLICATIONS

Congenital Diseases

Neutrophil-transfusion therapy has been used successfully in patients with congenital diseases, such as chronic granulomatous disease (CGD) and the leukocyte adhesion deficiency syndrome (LAD) (Raubitoschek et al. 1973; Bujak, Kwon-Chung, and Chusid 1974; Haddad, Beatty, and Dowdle 1976; Yomtovian et al. 1980). Although there have been no large clinical trials, neutrophil-transfusion therapy in CGD patients with serious infections not responding to antibiotics has become a common practice. Patients have shown a resolution of bacterial and fungal infections, including invasive aspergillosis and *Staphylococcus aureus* abscesses.

Neonates

Incomplete development of the immune system in the neonatal period is evidenced by deficiencies of both humoral and cellular constituents. Neonates may have reduced BM progenitor cells, smaller BM storage pools, and neutropenia (Cairo 1990). A severe infection in a neonate can cause a depletion of the BM storage pool and release of immature cells to the blood that are less capable of phagocytosis, oxidative metabolism, and chemotaxis (Strauss 1989). The mechanisms of these deficiencies are not fully understood, but the reduced phagocytosis may be due, in part, to decreased expression of C3bi complement receptors on immature cells (Bruce et al. 1986).

These qualitative and quantitative deficiencies predispose neonates to an increased risk of overwhelming infections. The incidence of bacterial sepsis in neonates is from 1 to 10 per 1,000 live births, and the mortality rate is high (Cairo 1990). The first study demonstrating efficacy of neutrophil-transfusion therapy in this population was a nonrandomized retrospective study (Laurenti et al. 1981) that reported a reduction in mortality from 91% in the group receiving standard therapy alone to 10% in the group receiving neutrophil transfusions plus standard therapy. Subsequently, a larger prospective study by Cairo showed a significant increase in survival of transfused septic neonates (97%) compared with nontransfused septic neonates (52%) receiving supportive care (Cairo et al. 1992). This study used an average neutrophil dose of 0.75×10^9. In contrast, the two negative studies collected whole blood and transfused the buffy coat (Strauss 1989; Cairo 1990).

Questions have been raised as to the safety of transfusions in neonates (O'Conner et al. 1988). Cairo (1991) stated that neonates in their study experienced few of the complications typically seen in adult transfusions, such as pulmonary reactions and transfusion-related infectious diseases.

Gram-Negative Sepsis

Several investigators have used neutrophil transfusions to treat neutropenic patients with acute leukemia and gram-negative sepsis using cells from CML or normal donors. Overall, these trials suggest that this therapy can increase the survival of patients who meet all of the following criteria: a culture-proven infection, proven neutropenia, decreased BM storage pool that is expected to last for more than a week, and unresponsiveness to antibiotic therapy after 48 hours (Clift 1984). Whether antibiotic therapy has improved enough since then to invalidate this result is not known.

Fungal Infections

Yeast and fungal infections are a major problem for myelosuppressed patients. Neutrophil-transfusion therapy has been used successfully to overcome fungal infections in patients with neutrophil dysfunction disorders (Raubitoscheck et al. 1973; Bujak et al. 1974; Haddad et al. 1976), but has not been studied systematically in neutropenic cancer patients.

Standard antifungal therapy for most serious mycotic infections remains amphotericin B. Because neutrophils are ultimately required for resolution of fungal infection, the rate of hemopoietic recovery is an important prognostic factor (Hetherington 1993). A retrospective study in BMT patients recently reported a lack of benefit of neutrophil transfusions (Bhatia et al. 1994). Another report of neutrophil transfusion therapy for patients with acute leukemia and established severe fungal infections reported that 15% to 20% of the patients responded to the transfusions. In this study, donors were treated with rHuG-CSF before leukapheresis, which increased the donor neutrophil count by four- to tenfold (Nagler et al. 1994).

Neutrophils stimulated with rHuG-CSF exhibit improved functional activity against fungi. An increase in oxidative burst over unstimulated neutrophils in response to blastoconidia and pseudohyphae of *Candida albicans* and *Aspergillus fumigatus* hyphae was measured by superoxide production (Roilides et al. 1993). The present level of morbidity and mortality from fungal infections among neutropenic cancer patients encourages the continued investigation of this application.

Prophylactic Treatment

Prophylactic neutrophil-transfusion therapy has been tested in multiple clinical trials as a regimen to prevent infections in acute myeloid leukemia (AML) patients undergoing initial induction chemotherapy and in BMT recipients (Clift et al. 1978; Winston et al. 1980; Strauss et al. 1981; Winston et al. 1981). Several studies reported a lower overall incidence of infection, but none of the studies could show that prophylactic neutrophil transfusion increased survival, nor that its efficacy outweighed the associated risks. The extended time needed for prophylactic treatment greatly increases the risk of adverse reactions (e.g., pulmonary toxicities, transmission of CMV, and alloimmunization reactions). Some researchers maintain that there is therapeutic potential for prophylactic treatment and investigations should continue, but most do not currently recommend it as a routine part of therapy.

■ CONCLUSIONS

Clinical trials suggest that neutrophil-transfusion therapy is an effective treatment for patients with severe neutropenia and gram-negative or neonatal sepsis and for severe infections in patients with defective neutrophil function; however, many of the studies had flaws in their basic design or are obsolete because of changes in clinical practice. Interest in neutrophil transfusions has been rekindled through use of the hemopoietic growth factor rHuG-CSF in normal donors to mobilize neutrophils from the marrow to the blood and enhance cell production. Clinical testing of this possibility is just now beginning. Review of the history of the development of this therapy suggests that neutrophils collected from rHuG-CSF–stimulated donors should be carefully studied in randomized trials in gram-negative sepsis and fungal infections, both of which are often unresponsive to current therapies and have a high mortality rate.

REFERENCES

Aisner, J., Schimpff, S.C., and Wiernik, P.H. (1977) Treatment of invasive aspergillosis: relation of early diagnosis and treatment to response. *Annals of Internal Medicine*, **86**, 539–43.

Alavi, J.B., Root, R.K., Djerassi, I., et al. (1977) A randomized clinical trial of granulocyte transfusions for infection in acute leukemia. *New England Journal of Medicine*, **296**, 706–11.

Athens, J.W. (1961) Leukokinetic studies. IV. The total blood, circulating, and marginal granulocyte pools and the granulocyte turnover rate in normal subjects. *Journal of Clinical Investigation*, **40**, 989–95.

Begley, C.G., Lopez, A.F., Nicola, N.A., et al. (1986) Purified colony-stimulating factors enhance the survival of human neutrophils and eosinophils in vitro: a rapid and sensitive microassay for colony-stimulating factors. *Blood*, **68**, 162–6.

Bensinger, W.I., Price, T.H., and Dale, D.C. (1993) The effects of daily recombinant human granulocyte colony-stimulating factor administration on normal granulocyte donors undergoing leukapheresis. *Blood*, **81**, 1883–8.

Bhatia, S., McCullough, J.J., Perry, E.H., et al. (1994) Granulocyte transfusions: efficacy in fungal infections in neutropenic patients following bone marrow transplantation. *Transfusion*, **34**, 226–32.

Boggs, D.R. (1974) Transfusion of neutrophils as prevention or treatment of infection in patients with neutropenia. *New England Journal of Medicine*, **290**, 1055–62.

Bruce, M.C., Baley, J.E., Medvik, K.A., et al. (1986) Impaired surface membrane expression of C3bi but not C3b receptors on neonatal neutrophils. *Pediatric Research*, **21**, 306–11.

Bujak, J.S., Kwon-Chung, K.J., and Chusid, M.J. (1974) Osteomyelitis and pneumonia in a boy with chronic granulomatous disease of childhood caused by a mutant strain of *Aspergillus nidulans*. *American Journal of Clinical Pathology*, **61**, 361–7.

Cairo, M.S. (1990) The use of granulocyte transfusions in neonatal sepsis. *Transfusion Medicine Reviews*, **4**, 14–22.

Cairo, M.S. (1991) The role of granulocyte transfusions as adjuvant therapy in the treatment of neonatal sepsis. *Transfusion Science*, **12**, 247–56.

Cairo, M.S., Worcester, C.C., Rucker, R.W., Hanten, S., et al. (1992) Randomized trial of granulocyte transfusions versus intravenous immune globulin therapy for neonatal neutropenia and sepsis. *Journal of Pediatrics*, **120**, 281–5.

Caspar, C.B., Seger, R.A., Burger, J., et al. (1993) Effective stimulation of donors for granulocyte transfusions with recombinant methionyl granulocyte colony-stimulating factor. *Blood*, **81**, 2866–71.

Chatta, G.S., Price, T.H., Allen, R.C., and Dale, D.C. (1994a) Effects of in vivo recombinant methionyl human granulocyte colony-stimulating factor on the neutrophil response and peripheral blood colony-forming cells in healthy young and elderly adult volunteers. *Blood*, **84**, 2923–9.

Chatta, G.S., Price, T.H., Stratton, J.R., and Dale, D.C. (1994b) Aging and marrow neutrophil reserves. *Journal of the American Geriatrics Society*, **42**, 77–81.

Clift, R.A. (1984) Granulocyte transfusions. *American Journal of Medicine*, **76**, 631–6.

Clift, R.A., Sanders, J.E., Thomas, E.D., et al. (1978) Granulocyte transfusions for the prevention of infection in patients receiving bone-marrow transplants. *New England Journal of Medicine*, **298**, 1052–7.

Colotta, F. (1993) Granulocyte transfusions from granulocyte colony-stimulating factor-treated donors: also a question of cell survival? *Blood*, **82**, 2258.

Dale, D.C., Fauci, A.S., Guerry, D., and Wolff, S.M. (1975) Comparison of agents producing a neutrophilic leukocytosis in man: hydrocortisone, prednisone, endotoxin and etiocholanolone. *Journal of Clinical Investigation*, **56**, 808–13.

Dutcher, J.P. (1990) Granulocyte transfusion therapy in patients with malignancy. In J.P. Dutcher (Ed.) *Modern transfusion therapy*, pp. 135–56. Boca Raton, FL, CRC Press.

Fortuny, I.E., Bloomfield, C.D., Hadlock, D.C., et al. (1975) Granulocyte transfusion: a controlled study in patients with acute non-lymphocytic leukemia. *Transfusion*, **15**, 548.

Freireich, E.J. (1994) White cell transfusions born-again. *Leukemia and Lymphoma*, **11**, 161–5.

Freireich, E.J., Levin, R.H., Whang, J., et al. (1964) The function and fate of transfused leukocytes from donors with chronic myelocytic leukemia in leukopenic recipients. *Annals of the New York Academy of Sciences*, **113**, 1081–9.

French, J.E., Lolomon, J.M., and Fratantoni, J.C. (1982) Survey on the current use of leukapheresis and the collection of granulocyte concentrates. *Transfusion*, **22**, 220–5.

Glasser, L., Fiederlein, R.L., and Huestis, D.W. (1985) Granulocyte concentrates: glucose concentrations and glucose utilization during storage at 22C. *Transfusion*, **25**, 68–9.

Graw, R.G., Herzig, G., Perry, S., et al. (1972) Normal granulocyte transfusion therapy: treatment of septicemia due to gram-negative bacteria. *New England Journal of Medicine*, **287**, 367–71.

Haddad, H.L., Beatty, D.W., and Dowdle, E.B. (1976) Chronic granulomatous disease of childhood. *South African Medical Journal*, **50**, 2068–72.

Hammerschmidt, D.E., Craddock, P.R., McCullough, J., et al. (1978) Complement activation and pulmonary leukostasis during nylon fiber filtration leukapheresis. *Blood*, **51**, 721–30.

Hammerschmidt, D.E., Weaver, L.J., Hudson, L.D., Craddock, P.R., and Jacob, H.S. (1980) Association of complement activation and elevated plasma-C5a with adult respiratory distress syndrome. Pathophysiological relevance and possible prognostic value. *Lancet*, **1**, 947–9.

Herzig, R.H. (1989) The negative aspects of granulocyte transfusions. *Cancer Investigation*, **7**, 589–92.

Herzig, R.H., Henig, G.P., Graw, R.G., et al. (1977) Successful granulocyte transfusion therapy for gram negative septicemia. *New England Journal of Medicine*, **296**, 701–5.

Hetherington, S.V. (1993) Prevention of fungal infections in neutropenic patients. *Infectious Medicine*, **10**, 40–7.

Higby, D.J., Yates, J.W., Henderson, E.S., et al. (1975) Filtration leukapheresis for granulocyte transfusion therapy. *New England Journal of Medicine*, **292**, 761–6.

Laurenti, F., Ferro, R., Isachi, G., et al. (1981) Polymorphonuclear leukocyte transfusion for the treatment of sepsis in the newborn infant. *Journal of Pediatrics*, **98**, 118–22.

Liles, C.W., Waltersdorph, A.M., and Klebanoff, S.J. (1994) Regulation of apoptosis in human neutrophils: effects of proinflammatory mediators, protein kinase inhibitors, and antibodies directed against b2-integrins. *Clinical Research*, **42**, 148a.

Mannoni, P., Rodet, M., and Vernant, J.P. (1979) Efficiency of prophylactic granulocyte transfusions in preventing infections in acute leukaemia. *Blood Transfusion and Immunohaematology*, **22**, 503–18.

Manzullo, E.F. (1994) Sepsis: the role of steroids and monoclonal antibodies in treatment. *Oncology*, **8**, 115–20.

McCullough, J. (1989) Granulocyte transfusion. In L.D. Petz and S.N. Swisher (Eds.) *Transfusion medicine*, pp. 469–84. New York, Churchill Livingstone.

McCullough, J., Weiblen, B.J., Deinard, A.R., et al. (1976) In vitro function and post transfusion survival of granulocytes collected by continuous-flow centrifugation and by filtration leukapheresis. *Blood*, **48**, 315–26.

Menitove, J.E. and Abrams, R.A. (1987) Granulocyte transfusion in neutropenic patients. *Critical Reviews in Oncology/Hematology*, **7**, 89–113.

Morse, E.E., Freireich, I.J., Carbone, P.P., et al. (1966) The transfusion of leukocytes from donors with chronic myelocytic leukemia to patients with leukopenia. *Transfusion*, **6**, 183–92.

Nagler, A., Naparstek, E., and Engelhard, D. (1994) Combined therapy of granulocyte transfusions, intravenous opsonins and antibiotics for gram-negative pneumonia in neutropenic cancer patients. *Acta Haematology*, **91**, 42–5.

O'Conner, J.C., Strauss, R.G., Goeken, N.E., et al. (1988) A near-fatal reaction during granulocyte transfusion of a neonate. *Transfusion*, **28**, 173–6.

Pizzo, P.A. (1993) Management of fever in patients with cancer and treatment induced neutropenia. *New England Journal of Medicine*, **328**, 1323–32.

Price, T.H., Chatta, G.S., and Dale, D.C. (1992) The effect of recombinant granulocyte colony-stimulating factor (G-CSF) on neutrophil kinetics in normal human subjects. *Blood*, **80**, 350a.

Price, T.H. and Dale, D.C. (1978) Neutrophil transfusion: the effect of storage and collection method on neutrophil blood kinetics. *Blood*, **51**, 789–98.

Price, T.H. and Dale, D.C. (1979) Blood kinetics and in vivo chemotaxis of transfused neutrophils: effect of collection method donor corticosteroid treatment and short term storage. *Blood*, **54**, 977–86.

Raubitoschek, A.A., Levin, A.L., Stites, D.P., et al. (1973) Normal granulocyte infusion therapy for aspergillosis in chronic granulomatous disease. *Pediatrics*, **51**, 230–3.

Richman, C.M. (1983) Prolonged cryopreservation of human granulocytes. *Transfusion*, **23**, 508–11.

Roilides, E., Uhlig, K., Venzon, D., et al. (1993) Enhancement of oxidative response and damage caused by human neutrophils to *Aspergillus fumigatus* hyphae by granulocyte colony-stimulating factor and gamma interferon. *Infection and Immunity*, **61**, 1185–93.

Schiffer, C.A. (1990) Granulocyte transfusions: an overlooked therapeutic modality. *Transfusion Medicine Reviews*, **4**, 2–7.

Schiffer, C.A., Aisner, J., Daly, P.A., et al. (1979) Alloimmunization following prophylactic granulocyte transfusion. *Blood*, **54**, 766–74.

Schiffer, C.A., Aisner, J., Dutcher, J.P., et al. (1983) Sustained post-transfusion granulocyte count increments following transfusion of leukocytes obtained from donors with chronic myelogenous leukemia. *American Journal of Hematology*, **15**, 65–74.

Schiffer, C.A. and Wade, J.C. (1987) Supportive care: issues in the use of blood products and treatment of infection. *Seminars in Oncology*, **14**, 454–67.

Shogi, M. and Vogler, W.R. (1974) Effects of hydrocortisone on the yield and bactericidal function of granulocytes collected by continuous-flow centrifugation. *Blood*, **44**, 435–43.

Strauss, R.G. (1989) Current status of granulocyte transfusions to treat neonatal sepsis. *Journal of Clinical Apheresis*, **5**, 25–9.

Strauss, R.G. (1993) Therapeutic granulocyte transfusions in 1993. *Blood*, **81**, 1675–8.

Strauss, R.G., Connett, J.E., Gale, R.P., et al. (1981) A controlled trial of prophylactic granulocyte transfusions during initial induction chemotherapy for acute myelogenous leukemia. *New England Journal of Medicine*, **305**, 597–603.

Strumia, M.M. (1934) The effect of leukocytic cream injections in the treatment of the neutropenias. *American Journal of the Medical Sciences*, **187**, 527–44.

Vogler, W.R. and Winton, E.F. (1977) A controlled study of the efficacy of granulocyte transfusions in patients with neutropenia. *American Journal of Medicine*, **63**, 548–55.

Weiden, P.L., Zuckerman, N., Hansen, J.A., et al. (1981) Fatal GVHD in a patient with lymphoblastic leukemia following normal granulocyte transfusions. *Blood*, **57**, 328–32.

Winston, D.J., Ho, W.G., Gale, R.P., et al. (1981) Prophylactic granulocyte transfusion therapy during chemotherapy of acute nonlymphocytic leukemia. *Annals of Internal Medicine*, **94**, 616–22.

Winston, D.J., Ho, W.G., Gale, R.P., et al. (1982) Therapeutic granulocyte transfusions for documented infections. *Annals of Internal Medicine*, **97**, 509–15.

Winston, D.J., Ho, W.G., Young, L.S., et al. (1980) Prophylactic granulocyte transfusions during human bone marrow transplantation. *American Journal of Medicine*, **68**, 893–7.

Wright, D.G. (1984) Symposium on infectious complications of neoplastic disease (part II). Leukocyte transfusions: thinking twice. *American Journal of Medicine*, **76**, 637–44.

Yomtovian, R., Abramson, J., Quie, P., et al. (1980) Granulocyte transfusion therapy in chronic granulomatous disease. *Transfusion*, **21**, 739–43.

29

Experimental and Clinical Cellular Immunotherapy in Bone-Marrow Transplantation

ARNON NAGLER, SHOSHANA MORECKI,
ALIZA ACKERSTEIN, REUVEN OR,
ELIZABETH NAPARSTEK, AND SHIMON SLAVIN

Bone-marrow transplantation (BMT) is recognized as a conventional, occasionally even front-line, mode of therapy for an increasing number of hemooncological malignancies not curable by other therapeutic modalities (Thomas 1963; O'Reilly 1983; Slavin and Nagler 1991). Relapse of the basic disease after BMT occurs in a substantial percentage of patients depending on the biology of the malignancy, disease status at transplantation, and type of BMT (Working Party on Leukemia 1988), with a higher relapse rate following autologous BMT in comparison to allogeneic BMT (Fefer et al. 1987; Gale, Goldman, and Horowitz 1991; Kersey et al. 1987). Interestingly, the risk of relapse following unrelated BMT is lower (Gajewski et al. 1990). The higher risk of relapse after autologous or syngeneic BMT is due to the lack of graft-versus-tumor effect (Bucker et al. 1989; Horowitz et al. 1990). The existence of graft-versus-leukemia (GVL) effect is well documented and based on several clinical observations that include association of acute and chronic graft-versus-host disease (GVHD) with decreased incidence of leukemic relapse, higher relapse rates of leukemia following T-cell–depleted marrow grafts, and higher relapse rates of leukemia after intensive posttransplant immunosuppression (Weiden et al. 1979, 1981; Apperley et al. 1986; Marmont et al. 1989; Weiss, Reich, and Slavin 1990b; Bacigalupo et al. 1991; Mehta 1993). Recent experimental and clinical evidence demonstrates antitumor effects similar to GVL in mice with solid tumors and graft-versus-lymphoma effect in patients with lymphoma (Moscovitch and Slavin 1984; Phillips et al. 1986; Jones et al. 1991; Chopra et al. 1992). Several effector cells of the immune system including $CD3^+$ T cells (both the $CD4^+$ and $CD8^+$ T-cell subsets) as well as $CD3^-$ $CD56^+$ natural killer (NK) cells may play a role in the graft-versus-tumor effect (Korngold and Sprent 1987; Slavin et al. 1990c; Weiss et al. 1990b; Champlin et al. 1991; Truitt and Atasoylu 1991; Slavin et al. 1992a; Cohen et al. 1993). It is tempting to try to prevent or treat cytogenetic and overt clinical relapse following BMT by adoptive transfer of immunocompetent cells of the immune system. This strategy attempts to induce immune-specific or tumor-associated effector mechanisms against residual tumor cells that have escaped the radiochemotherapy given as pretransplant conditioning. In addition, a variety of recombinant cytokines may potentially be used for preventing or treating relapse following BMT. Some of the cytokines may have antitumor effects by themselves; others may facilitate immunological reconstitution following BMT, thus enhancing the reactivity of cells involved in either the afferent division (antigen [Ag] processing, Ag-presentation, and priming) or efferent division (humoral responses and cell-mediated effector cells) of the immune system. Others may amplify the antitumor effector cells by rendering the malignant cells more antigenic and/or immunogenic, thus more susceptible to the T-cell–dependent and –independent antitumor-effector mechanisms (Fabian, Kletter, and Slavin 1988; Ackerstein, Kedar, and Slavin 1991; Givon et al. 1992; Weiss, Reich, and Slavin 1992; Benyunes et al. 1993; Giralt et al. 1993; Uchiyama et al. 1993). In the last few years, several groups have used both the effector cells of the immune system (allogeneic cell-mediated immunotherapy [allo-CMI]) as well as cytokines (in vivo and in vitro) or a combination of both (allogeneic cell-mediated cytokine-activated immunotherapy [allo-CCI]) to prevent and treat relapse following BMT. This chapter reviews and discusses the recent international experience, focusing on our own post-BMT experimental and clinical cellular immunotherapy studies.

■ ALLOGENEIC CELL-MEDIATED CYTOKINE-ACTIVATED IMMUNOTHERAPY FOLLOWING ALLOGENEIC BONE-MARROW TRANSPLANTATION

Allogeneic cell-mediated immunotherapy consists of infusion of HLA-matched donor cells after BMT for either prevention or treatment of relapse.

Prevention of Relapse by Allo-CMI

A murine model of B-type lymphoid leukemia (BCL1) has shown that GVL effects can be induced by administration of allogeneic lymphocytes following initial transplantation with T-lymphocyte–

depleted marrow allografts. Moreover, GVL effects induced by administration of gradual increments of immunocompetent allogeneic donor lymphocytes after BMT can be significantly potentiated by concomitant administration of a short course of well-tolerated, low-dose recombinant interleukin-2 (rIL-2) in vivo (Slavin et al. 1992a; Weiss et al. 1992).

The possible potentiation of GVL effects by allo-(CMI was investigated using the same murine model under experimental conditions designed for simulating minimal residual disease (MRD) following allogeneic BMT. Lethally irradiated (BALB/c × C57BL/6) F_1 recipients ($H-2^{d/b}$) were reconstituted with $20 × 10^6$ T-lymphocyte–depleted allogeneic BM cells obtained from C57BL/six donors ($H-2^b$) mixed with 10^4, 10^5, or 10^6 BCL1 cells. This was followed by administration of sequential increments of allogeneic donor-type spleen cells: 10^6 cells on day +1, 10^7 cells on day +5, and $5 × 10^7$ on day +9, with or without concomitant administration of rIL-2 ($12 × 10^4$ IU twice daily for 3 days, IP) together with each spleen-cell administration. All control mice receiving 10^4 to 10^6 BCL1 cells developed marked splenomegaly by day +21 and all secondary BALB/c adoptive recipients of 10^5 spleen cells obtained from each of these mice, serving as live test tubes to assess the presence or successful elimination of clonogenic BCL1, developed leukemia within 21 to 36 days, and died. Treatment of mice that received 10^4 BCL1 cells with either three courses of low-dose rIL-2, three increments of allogeneic spleen cells alone, or a combination of both, resulted in normalization of splenomegaly on day +21, but only adoptive recipients of 10^5 spleen cells obtained from mice treated with both allogeneic spleen cells and rIL-2 (100%) or allogeneic spleen cells alone (80%) were disease free. Low-dose rIL-2 alone was insufficient to cure any of the mice inoculated with 10^4 BCL1 (Weiss et al. 1992).

Previously published data suggest that both immunocompetent allogeneic lymphocytes and high-dose rIL-2 alone (Ackerstein et al. 1991) may play an important role in preventing leukemia relapse in mice with MRD; low-dose rIL-2 seems ineffective by itself even against MRD (Ackerstein et al. 1991). The combination of both allogeneic cells and low-dose rIL-2 is synergistic and much more effective than any of the agents used alone, particularly when the tumor load increases (Weiss et al. 1992). Thus, cell-mediated immunotherapy might be applied therapeutically to prevent relapse or treat established MRD after BMT even following initial reconstitution with T-cell–depleted BM cells. This strategy permits the use of allogeneic BMT procedures without posttransplant immunosuppression with cyclosporin A, which suppresses GVL in experimental animals (Weiss et al. 1992) and humans (Bacigalupo et al. 1991).

One additional important observation is the further reduction of the risk of GVHD induced by inoculation of immunocompetent donor T cells for induction of GVL by increasing the time interval between BMT and cell therapy (Slavin et al. 1978; Johnson, Drobyski, and Truitt 1993). The longer the time interval between BMT and cell therapy, the larger the number of donor T cells can be given safely without any appreciable GVHD; however, cell dose and schedules may vary between mouse strains and human individuals.

Based on the above data derived in mice, GVL effects mediated by allogeneic lymphocytes following BMT may be optimized by concomitant administration of low well-tolerated doses of rIL-2, while controlling for GVHD. In humans, rIL-2 doses comparable to the high doses that seem effective in mice cannot be given because of irreversible toxicity. Therefore, it cannot be anticipated that rIL-2 without allogeneic lymphocytes will be curative in humans.

Based on this type of preclinical data, we have recently applied a similar strategy. Eighty-one leukemic patients underwent T-cell depletion at the time of BMT using the Campath 1 antibody (monoclonal rat anti-human CDW52; Waldmann et al. 1984; Slavin et al. 1985). Patients were subsequently given allo-CMI consisting of increments of HLA-matched donor peripheral blood leukocytes (PBL) to a total cell dose corresponding to 10^4, 10^5, 10^6, and 10^7 T cells/kg on days +1, +7, +14, and +21, respectively. If no GVHD developed, patients were scheduled to receive an additional dose of 10^7 T cells/kg (Naparstek et al. 1995). Forty percent of the patients treated with donor cells developed acute GVHD and were unable to complete the scheduled T-cell repletion protocol; however, the above methodology permitted titration of allo-CMI on an individual basis, since no additional allo-CMI may be required once any evidence for GVHD develops. The incidence of chronic GVHD was also greater in patients treated with allo-CMI compared with controls; however, the probability of remaining in remission was also higher among recipients of T-cell–depleted allografts who received donor T lymphocytes (78%) compared with patients not receiving donor T cells (60%) ($p < 0.05$). The efficacy of allo-CMI was demonstrated in different categories of patients with acute leukemia. Leukemic patients in first complete remission (CR) treated with allo-CMI were more likely to remain in remission when compared with untreated controls (90% versus 74% at 2 years, respectively). A similar trend was observed in patients with acute leukemia transplanted in second CR. More impressive were the findings in acute lymphocytic leukemia (ALL) patients. Irrespective of the stage of leukemia, ALL patients who received donor T cells and developed GVHD had only a 14% probability of relapse by 2 years, compared with 61% for patients who received T cells but had no GVHD, and 56% for patients who had neither T cells nor GVHD. Recently, the same strategy has been proposed for chronic myeloid leukemia (CML) patients (van Rhee et al. 1994). The protocol seems feasible and the results are encouraging. Determination of optimal cell doses and timing of administration, and perhaps use of better defined cell subsets, may help to maximize GVL while reducing the incidence or controlling the severity of GVHD.

Treatment of Established Relapse by Allo-CMI, Allo-CCI, and rIL-2

Despite major advances in the field of clinical transplantation, relapse of the original disease remains a major cause of treatment failure, even for those patients transplanted during first complete remission and certainly in more advanced stages of disease. Recently, the procedure of allo-CMI or donor leukocyte transfusions has been confirmed to result in hematological and cytogenetic remissions in CML patients and to a lesser extent other hematological malignancies in patients who relapsed following BMT (Slavin et al. 1988b; Kolb et al. 1990; Slavin et al. 1990a, b, c; Cullis et al. 1992; Drobysky et al. 1992; Slavin et al. 1992a, c, d, e; Bär et al. 1993; Drobyski et al. 1993; Helg et al. 1993; Slavin et al. 1993a, b; Szer et al. 1993; Porter et al. 1994). Pilot studies were performed at Hadassah Hospital in Jerusalem in patients relapsing following allogeneic BMT who would normally be considered incurable, and used allogeneic donor PBL given late following BMT. Our first patient, a 2.5-year-old boy with pre-B ALL was transplanted in second relapse from his sister and had overt hematological and extramedullary relapse 2 months following BMT. The patient was treated with minimal amounts of chemotherapy that did not result in remission, followed by repeated infusions of donor PBL. He is now more than 7 years post BMT without evidence of disease and has a negative polymerase chain reaction (PCR) test for male (Y) sex chromosome in BM and peripheral blood (PB) cells. Subsequently we have given HLA-matched donor cells to 16 additional patients with various hematological malignancies (ALL, five; CML, five; AML, three, Burkitt's lymphoma/leukemia, one; and myelodysplastic syndromes (MDS), one) who had cytogenetic or overt hematological relapse following HLA-matched allogeneic BMT. Ten of the 17 patients responded with disappearance of the malignant clone documented by PCR, cytogenetics, or morphology. In one patient with MDS, the response was only transient. Another patient with CML died of severe chronic GVHD 15 months following BMT in full remission defined by negative *bcr/abl* by reverse transcriptase PCR (RT-PCR). The other eight patients are alive and well with follow-up of greater than 8 months to greater than 7 years following BMT (Slavin et al. 1988b, 1990b, 1992c; Slavin et al. submitted). We recently reported a 17-year-old man who had cytogenetic and hematological relapse 4 months after non–T-cell–depleted allogeneic BMT for CML in accelerated phase. Two sequential transfusions of donor buffy coat cells (4.8 to 8.7 × 10^7/kg) followed by 3 days of subcutaneous (SC) rIL-2 (3 × 10^6 IU/m^2) failed to induce remission. The patient finally responded to 3.7 × 10^7 allogeneic lymphokine-activated killer (LAK) cells per kilogram followed by 3 days of SC rIL-2 with complete elimination of *bcr/abl* transcripts by RT-PCR and reappearance of 100% cells with normal female karyotype. Complete cytogenetic remission was accompanied by GVHD grade II, and has been maintained with follow-up of 8 months (Kapelushnik et al. submitted). This unique case may indicate that LAK cells through allo-CCI may provide a more effective immunotherapy than allo-CMI, and should be kept as an option for reinduction of remission in CML patients who relapse following BMT and are resistant to transfusion of buffy coat cells alone. Allo-CCI provides a most powerful mode of immunotherapy, as the in vitro incubation of the donor effector cells with rIL-2 may cause direct or indirect stimulation of a variety of major histocompatibility complex (HC) –restricted and nonrestricted effector cell subsets, as well as production of secondary cytokines with potent antileukemic effect (Kapelushnik et al. submitted). A larger number of patients and longer observation periods are required to assess the full potential of allo-CMI and allo-CCI; however, the preliminary results from our own center and the cumulative international experience in patients considered incurable until recently are encouraging.

■ ALLOGENEIC CELL THERAPY FOLLOWING ABMT/ASCT

Allo-CMI with rIL-2 Using HLA-Mismatched PBL for Prevention and Treatment of Relapse

In treating a variety of chemoradiosensitive malignancies, ABMT or autologous stem-cell transplant (ASCT) is becoming more popular as an alternative to allogeneic BMT, either because of lack of fully matched donors or because of the lower incidence of procedure-related risks, especially rejection and GVHD. In addition, life-threatening infectious complications are less frequent in recipients of autografts. The only major disadvantage of ASCT/ABMT in comparison with allogeneic BMT is the higher risk of relapse due to lack of graft-versus-tumor or GVL effects. Our goal was to introduce a GVL or graft-versus-tumor equivalent in the setting of MRD following ABMT/ASCT through allo-CMI/CCI plus transient in vivo potentiation of donor cells with rIL-2.

We have recently assessed the feasibility of cell therapy in 27 patients (15 females and 12 males), median age 17 (range 1.5 to 42) years, autografted for AML (19), ALL (6), and CML (2) who received, following transplant, some form of allo-CMI using HLA-mismatched haploidentical allogeneic PBL and rIL-2. Twelve high-risk patients were transplanted in first CR; 15 had advanced disease. Conditioning included busulfan 16 mg/kg and cyclophosphamide 200 mg/kg (BU/CY) or busulfan 16 mg/kg and cyclophosphamide 120 mg/kg supplemented with thiotepa 10 mg/kg (BU/THIO/CY). Bone-marrow cells were purged with mafosfamide. Sixteen patients (group A) were treated with gradual increments of donor PBL (10^4, 10^5, 10^6, and 10^7 T cells/kg on days +1, +7, +14, and +28, respectively) with another dose of 10^7 T cells/kg plus rIL-2 (6×10^6 IU/m^2 for 5 days IV) 1 month later, in the absence of GVHD. Three patients developed grade I GVHD proven by skin biopsy. Engraftment was normal. Using a male (Y) probe, donor cells were detected 12 to 48 hours after PBL administration peaking at 24 hours. Twelve of the 16 patients (seven with advanced disease) relapsed 4.5 months (median) after ABMT. Eleven patients (group B) were treated with a median of 10^7 T cells/kg of donor PBL starting at +1 day after ABMT with rIL-2 6×10^6 IU/m^2 for 1 to 3 days IV administration. Three patients who received greater than 0.5×10^8 PBL/kg with rIL-2 for 3 days developed acute GVHD at days 4 to 7. Three of 11 patients (group B) are alive, median follow-up of 39 months following ABMT (Nagler et al. 1992). Based on these preliminary data, the following conclusions may be reached: (1) It seems feasible to induce GVHD in the setting of ABMT; (2) PBL dose of greater than 0.5×-10^8 T cells/kg with 3 days rIL-2 induced lethal GVHD; and (3) adoptive immunotherapy may not adversely affect engraftment as long as no GVHD develops (Nagler et al. 1992).

Allo-CMI with rIL-2 Using HLA-matched PBL for Prevention and Treatment of Relapse

HLA-matched PBL have a better chance of engrafting and thus inducing more effective GVL with a substantially smaller risk of severe GVHD. As previously indicated, one of the most important goals in

ASCT is to induce potential immune-mediated interactions against autologous residual tumor cells or to introduce potentially alloreactive major HC/minor HC-mismatched donor immune cells in an attempt to replace the missing GVL effects, since host immune cells are unable to recognize or are tolerant of autologous tumor determinants.

A clinical trial of ABMT/ASCT for patients with malignant hematological diseases and a fully matched sibling who decline or are not qualified for allogeneic BMT has been initiated. This study uses matched-sibling PBL following autologous BMT/ASCT in an attempt to induce GVL with smaller risk of GVHD at the stage of MRD. Therapy consisted of administration of 5×10^7 T cells/kg on an outpatient basis 8 weeks after ABMT as soon as hemopoietic reconstitution seemed adequate and stable. For patients showing no evidence of GVHD, a second dose of donor PBL consisting of 5×10^7 T cells/kg was given plus in vivo activation of effector cells with rIL-2 6×10^6 IU/m^2 SC for 3 days to further potentiate GVL. To date, six patients with leukemia have entered the study. Patients were conditioned prior to ABMT with BU/THIO/CY (for AML) or CY and fractionated total-body irradiation (TBI) (for CML). Prompt engraftment was observed in all patients. No anti-GVHD prophylaxis was given. Presently, with a median observation of 4 to 29 (median 14) months, five of six patients are alive and relapse was observed in one. Two elderly patients with CML are doing extremely well (currently receiving interferon-α [IFN-α]) and are in full hematological remission but with positive yet constantly decreasing *bcr/abl* PCR signal (Slavin et al. 1993a).

Our data suggest that allogeneic cell therapy at the stage of MRD may be safely induced by HLA-matched allogeneic PBL obtained from matched siblings following ABMT. More patients and longer observation periods are needed to assess the efficacy and safety of this approach. We are now trying this approach of cell therapy in leukemic patients who relapsed following ABMT. We are also investigating the role of allo-CMI and allo-CCI with in vivo rIL-2 for prevention of relapse in patients at high risk following ASCT for lymphomas and solid tumors (Or et al. submitted).

■ LYMPHOKINE-MEDIATED IMMUNOTHERAPY

This section summarizes attempts to induce "autoimmune" responses against autologous tumor cells for patients with no indication for allogeneic BMT or for patients with no matched donor available for allo-CMI. This avoids the risk of GVHD inducible by mismatched PBL. The use of lymphokine-mediated immunotherapy (LMI) is based on outpatient administration of lymphokines in an attempt to potentiate and stimulate cellular immunity against MRD.

Development of LMI Protocol in a Murine Model of B-Cell Leukemia/Lymphoma (BCL1)

We have demonstrated that administration of high-dose rIL-2 following syngeneic BMT in BALB/c mice resulted in tumor dormancy with eventual elimination of clonogenic BCL1 (Ackerstein et al. 1991; Slavin et al. 1992b). Similarly, the same model documented the efficacy of LMI following syngeneic (corresponding to ABMT) BMT, at the stage of MRD (Ackerstein et al. 1991). BALB/c mice inoculated with BCL1 were treated 1 day later with CY (100 mg/kg) and transplanted with normal syngeneic BM cells on the following day (day 0). High-dose rIL-2 (600,000 IU intraperitoneally (IP) three times daily) for five consecutive days was initiated on day +1, +7, or +21 following BMT. Mice receiving no rIL-2 therapy relapsed and died within 50 days following BMT, whereas mice receiving high-dose rIL-2 showed long-term disease-free survival. The optimal time for rIL-2 initiation was determined to be 3 weeks after BMT, with 90% of the mice surviving with no evidence of disease for more than 1 year. Kinetics of lymphocyte reconstitution following syngeneic BMT indicated a steep increase in the absolute number of PBL on days 17 through 24. It is conceivable that maximal efficacy of rIL-2 therapy was elicited when rIL-2 was administered at the time of peak regeneration of lymphocytes because lymphocytes, rather than tumor cells, appear to be target cells for rIL-2. Similarly, when 10^4 BCL1 cells were given 1 day after syngeneic BMT to simulate quantitative MRD following ABMT, rIL-2 therapy given at 14 days after BMT seemed effective in prolonging disease-free survival, in contrast to the same regimen given 1 day after BMT (Ackerstein et al. 1991).

Our recent data suggest that posttransplant immunotherapy with rIL-2 could be further amplified by coadministration of IFN-α.

LMI Protocol in Lymphoma Patients

Based on animal data, we subsequently investigated the feasibility of induction of a lymphokine-mediated antitumor effect by administration of IL-2 concomitantly with IFN-α in patients with malignant lymphoma, at the stage of MRD following ABMT (Slavin et al. 1992d; Nagler et al. 1993). At 3 months following ABMT, 45 patients (28 non-Hodgkin's lymphoma [NHL] and 17 Hodgkin's disease [HD]) received

LMI consisting of a combination of rIL-2 and IFN-α, while 45 patients (26 NHL and 19 HD) received no immunotherapy. No significant differences in either grade, stage of disease, or status at time of transplant were observed between the two groups of patients. Recombinant IL-2 (provided by EruoCetus) and IFN-α (Roferon A, provided by Hoffmann-La Roche) were self-administered SC on an outpatient basis. All patients were treated with IFN-α given as 3×10^6 U SC daily for 5 days a week for 4 weeks followed by, or in combination with, rIL-2 SC 3 to 6×10^6 IU/m^2 daily for 5 days a week for 4 weeks. After a 4-week interval, a second cycle was given. Toxicity was usually mild and reversible and included fever, anorexia, nausea and vomiting, rash, and flu-like symptoms (Schechter et al. 1992; Klapholz et al. 1993).

Among patients receiving no immunotherapy, 23 of 45 (14 NHL and 9 HD) (51%) relapsed ($p < 0.05$). In contrast, only 2 of the 17 patients with HD and 7 of the 28 patients with NHL who received LMI relapsed a median of 22.5 (14 to 36) months after ABMT. Of those seven, three did not complete the immunotherapy protocol. All of them were very-high-risk patients, transplanted at a very advanced stage of their disease (third CR, three; second PR, three; and refractory disease, one). Overall, 36 of 45 patients (80%) of those receiving LMI, and 22 of 45 (49%) receiving no immunotherapy, are alive with no evidence of disease.

Preliminary data suggest that immunotherapy by a combination of rIL-2 and IFN-α can be reasonably well tolerated on an outpatient basis and may intensify remission, by reducing relapse rate with an overall increased disease-free survival in patients with MRD following ABMT for lymphoma. A controlled, prospectively randomized study in a larger number of lymphoma patients is indicated to confirm these results.

■ ADOPTIVE IMMUNOTHERAPY OF HEPATITIS B FOLLOWING BMT BY ALLO-CMI

Recipients of BMT remain profoundly immunosuppressed for many months. Attempts to immunize patients against a variety of pathogens before and after BMT have usually been unsuccessful, presumably because of chemoradiotherapy-related impairment of T- and B-cell–dependent functions (Binder 1994).

In an attempt to circumvent this impairment, several investigators have previously suggested that adoptive transfer of donor immunity to recipient may be accomplished following BMT by actively immunizing the HLA-identical donor before donation of marrow.

This concept was confirmed in preclinical models in mice successfully potentiated against influenza virus (Mumcuoglu et al. 1987) and *Pseudomonas aeruginosa* infection (Avichezer et al. 1989) and subsequently in patients undergoing BMT (Saxon et al. 1986; Gottlieb et al. 1990; Engelhard et al. 1991, 1993). Immunity to a variety of pathogens including *Pseudomonas aeruginosa*, tetanus, varicella, diphtheria, and influenza virus, as well as to cytomegalovirus and human immunodeficiency virus (HIV), can be transferred to the BMT recipient, presumably through the transfer of functionally activated B cells (Gottlieb et al. 1990; Saxon et al. 1986; Engelhard et al. 1993, 1991; Lane et al. 1990). Ag-driven, donor-type B cells can expand in the new recipient, conferring immunity to the new host. Adoptive transfer of specific immune responses against tumor-specific Ag, as well as viral Ag, were also accomplished by cultured memory T cells and T-cell clones (Cheever et al. 1986; Riddell et al. 1992).

We have previously seen successful adoptive transfer of immunity to tetanus and diphtheria by PBL obtained from donors intentionally immunized prior to BMT, as part of adoptive transfer of donor PBL for cell therapy of leukemia. We were recently able to document successful adoptive transfer of immunity of hepatitis B virus (HBV) following active immunization of BM donors prior to T-cell–depleted allogeneic BMT (Ilan et al. 1993a). In one HBSAg$^+$ patient, immune reconstitution following BMT from the anti-HBc$^+$/anti-HBs$^+$ BM donor resulted in clearance of the circulating HBsAg as well as HBV DNA by PCR (Ilan et al. 1993b). Recently we succeeded in inducing immunity to HBV by adoptive transfer of HBV-immune PBL after autologous as well as allogeneic BMT in three patients (Ilan et al. 1994). The three patients seroconverted to anti-HBs within 18 to 35 (median 29) days following administration of HBV-immune PBL. In one of the patients a booster effect was documented in the BMT recipient who was immunized with a recombinant HBsAg vaccine. The two remaining patients lost their antibodies (Ab) to HBsAg in association with relapse of their leukemia. The Ab levels generated through adoptive transfer of HBV-immune PBL were relatively low; however, the anti-HBs titers obtained were above the conventionally accepted protective concentration of 10 IU/mL.

A similar immunological maneuver may also be applicable to HBsAg carriers in whom persistent HBV infection is believed to be the result of deficient T-cell–dependent B-cell responses. Furthermore, HBV-immune PBL may be evaluated in the future as a better potential substitute to the high-cost, hepatitis B immune globulin currently used to protect recipients of liver transplantation for end-stage HBV-induced liver disease from infection of the allograft by host HBV.

■ IMMUNOLOGICAL EVALUATION OF PATIENTS TREATED BY LMI AND ALLO-CMI FOLLOWING AUTOLOGOUS AND ALLOGENEIC BMT

Reconstitution of a functional immune system after BMT is crucial. Immune deficiency due to ablative chemoradiotherapy given before transplant is usually profound during the first 3 months after BMT, but tends to recover within 1 to 2 years (Friedrich et al. 1982; Witherspoon et al. 1984; Wimperis et al. 1987; Lum 1990). Acceleration of hemopoietic and immune reconstitution has been attempted using biological response modifiers such as recombinant granulocyte-macrophage colony-stimulating factor (rGM-CSF) or rIL-2. These agents shorten the recovery period and activate cellular immune reconstitution in experimental animals (Kedar et al. 1988; Slavin et al. 1989) and in humans (Blaise et al. 1990; Heslop et al. 1991; De Witte et al. 1992; Morecki et al. 1992; Fefer et al. 1993).

Immunological activation after BMT for hematological malignant diseases is designed both to achieve an improved immune defense against infectious agents and to stimulate antitumor effector mechanisms for control of minimal residual tumor cell growth that has escaped the high-dose chemotherapy.

Attempts to activate the host immune system use mainly two immunotherapy modalities: (1) LMI, using low (i.e., safe) doses of rIL-2 and IFN-α given concomitantly or sequentially over 1 or 2 months, with most of the patients undergoing two cycles of cytokine treatment; and (2) allo-CMI and allo-CCI, using gradual graded increments of allogeneic-matched PBL at different time intervals following BMT, with or without concomitant administration of rIL-2 and/or allogeneic LAK cells, respectively, depending on the lack of GVHD. Both modalities are given in an outpatient therapy setting.

Immune Status in Recipients of CMI Following ABMT/ASCT

LMI consisting of rIL-2 and IFN-α can stimulate the host immune system (Morecki et al. 1992). Immunological evaluation was done in 28 patients entering the LMI protocol. Of 26 patients with hematological malignancies (CML, AML, HD, NHL), 24 were treated at remission and 2 with progressive disease. LMI was given to ten patients 2 to 5 months after autologous BMT, and to one patient after allogeneic BMT. Eleven of 26 patients with hematological malignancies and both patients with metastatic melanoma received their LMI treatment following conventional therapy without previous BMT. Non–major HC-restricted cytotoxicity either in fresh PB samples (spontaneous activity) or after in vitro IL-2 activation (LAK) was evaluated before and after LMI. Spontaneous killing activity was low before therapy, but increased upon termination of the course of LMI in 10 of 15 evaluated cycles. LAK cell activity was markedly elevated in 14 of 20 evaluated cycles of sequential treatment as well as in 8 of 14 evaluated cycles of concomitant treatment. The two effector mechanisms of non–major HC-restricted cytotoxicity (spontaneous and LAK-induced activity) were not linearly correlated after LMI. This might indicate that the status of patients' NK activity may not always reflect the potential capacity of LAK precursor cells to be further stimulated in vitro following in vivo cytokine administration. Activation of T-cell–dependent mitogenic response was demonstrated in six of nine patients after concomitant LMI, while no such effect was observed following sequential LMI in ten evaluable patients. The increased T-cell responses observed after concomitant LMI was significantly correlated to the augmentation of LAK activity in these patients; however, in the absence of measurable disease, these immunological variables could not be directly correlated to in vivo antitumor effects.

Significant LAK activity was seen in 22% of patients treated with concomitant rIL-2 and rIFN-β (Krigel et al. 1988). Cytokine administration has shown previously a moderate but encouraging response in patients with advanced solid tumors (Lee et al. 1989; Atzpodien et al. 1990; Hirsh et al. 1990).

Immune Status in Recipients of Cell Therapy Following BMT

Immunological variables were evaluated in three groups of patients with hematological malignancies: (1) patients after ABMT/ASCT who received HLA-matched PBL; (2) patients after ABMT/ASCT who received HLA-mismatched PBL; and (3) patients after allogeneic BMT who received donor HLA-matched PBL. In all three groups, the ability to activate the patient's immune system was evaluated prior to and 3 days following rIL-2 treatment that was given concomitantly with the highest dose of PBL (10^7 to 10^8 T cells/kg). Spontaneous non–major HC-restricted cytotoxic activity was significantly increased in five of seven and four of four patients after ABMT/ASCT who were treated with HLA-matched or -mismatched PBL, respectively. Such a marked increase could not be shown after cell therapy with matched donor PBL following allogeneic BMT.

Nonspecific T-cell–dependent mitogenic responses were mostly decreased after ABMT/ASCT plus allo-CMI, mostly increased after allo-CMI plus allogeneic BMT, and inconsistent after mismatched PBL plus ABMT.

No major changes of T-cell or NK-cell characteristic markers were observed after rIL-2 treatment given concomitantly with HLA-matched PBL following autologous or allogeneic BMT. Analysis of cell-surface markers of PB mononuclear cells (MNC) samples taken 3 months and 1 year after autologous or allogeneic BMT revealed that in both groups of patients, CD4$^+$ cells were always lower, while CD8$^+$ cells were mostly higher than in a group of ten healthy volunteers. There were no marked differences in NK phenotypic markers between the two groups of patients and healthy volunteers.

Three to 4 months following autologous or allogeneic BMT, the absolute numbers and the proportions of CD3$^+$ cells are near normal values, while the CD4$^+$/CD8$^+$ ratio is inverted. Low absolute numbers of CD4$^+$ cells persist up to 6 months after BMT (Friedrich et al. 1982; Gratama et al. 1984; Charmot et al. 1987). Following allo-CMI, this pattern was not altered.

Other reports using rIL-2 therapy after ABMT have emphasized the increase in CD16$^+$ and CD56$^+$ cells (Blaise et al. 1990; Fefer et al. 1993). After cell therapy using the original BM donor-derived lymphocytes to treat relapse after allogeneic T-cell–depleted BMT, CD57$^+$ cells increase (Bär et al. 1993) and the proportion of CD3$^+$ cells is normal (Small et al. 1993).

Most of the cell-therapy programs following BMT in various centers consisted of either autologous MNC or lymphocytes from the original BM donor. A few of these clinical studies have included reports on immune evaluation of treated patients in which activation of non–major HC-restricted cytotoxicity was demonstrated (Fefer et al. 1993; Small et al. 1993; Soiffer et al. 1993). Jiang et al. (1993) have demonstrated an increase in cytotoxic T-lymphocyte precursor frequency directed against the patient's leukemia cells in two relapsed CML patients who were treated with donor buffy coat after allogeneic BMT.

Altogether, posttransplant immunotherapy seems to offer new effective modalities capable of stimulating, replacing, or supplementing host-defense mechanisms in a significant proportion of treated patients and may be helpful in mediating an effective antitumor response in vivo.

■ CONCLUSIONS AND FUTURE GOALS

We have shown both in experimental animals and in pilot clinical studies that it may be possible to decrease relapse rates and even to reinduce remissions in patients who relapse following allogeneic BMT, using a variety of approaches based on administration of donor PB T cells. Moreover, it seems feasible to induce a GVL effect, especially in the setting of MRD, for patients with leukemia and lymphoma, and possibly other cancers, by administration of HLA-matched or partially mismatched PBL following ABMT/ASCT, and allogeneic BMT. This GVL-like effect can be amplified by in vivo or in vitro treatment of effector cells with rIL-2. Furthermore, optimal cytokine combinations (e.g., rIL-2 plus IFN-α) may intensify remission and prolong disease-free survival in patients with lymphoma and leukemia treated at the stage of MRD following ABMT or ASCT; however, allo-CMI–based immunotherapy strategies were associated with both increased risk of GVHD and life-threatening BM aplasia that may respond to early administration of donor stem cells. There is an immediate need to evaluate the role of the different cell subsets present in PBL as well as to establish optimal cell doses and schedules. The risk of serious antihost responses following autologous and allogeneic BMT must also be minimized. The use of well-defined cell subsets and optimal combinations of cytokines in vitro and in vivo may provide safer approaches for improved cell therapy. In addition, various cytokine combinations should be explored in order to facilitate immunohemopoietic reconstitution and amplification of the antitumor effects of autologous or allogeneic immune cells. This approach could be tested following conventional as well as high-dose chemotherapy.

In parallel with continuous research in animal models of human diseases to further characterize optimal effector cells and the most effective in vitro and in vivo activation of anticancer effector cells, prospective randomized clinical trials are needed to formally document the efficacy of allogeneic cell therapy for prevention of relapse in patients with no evidence of disease who are at high risk of relapse. Such patients are probably easier to cure, but it would be much more difficult to prove that posttransplant immunotherapy improves the overall outcome unless a sufficient number of patients and sufficiently long observation periods are available for proper statistical analysis. In addition, it must be documented that the potential advantages of therapy for prevention of relapse are worth the potential risk of procedure-related GVHD, which may cause marrow aplasia or classical systemic acute and chronic GVHD. The feasibility of elimination of antihost responses by eradication of donor T cells by a variety of methods, including introduction of suicide genes before cell therapy, may help in reducing the risks involved in allo-CMI and allo-CCI.

Other attractive therapeutic options include genetic manipulation of tumor cells or donor immunocompetent effector cells prior to adoptive cell therapy, by insertion of specific cytokine genes to amplify immunogenicity and antitumor potential, respectively. Genetically modified tumor cells of the patient can be used as vaccines to increase the chance of specific immunization of host T cells against weak immunogeneic or nonimmunogeneic tumor cells, in order to establish a "custom-made" vaccine while reducing the risk of nonspecific sensitization against non–tumor-associated determinants. In vitro generation of tumor-specific cytotoxic cells, although technically difficult and perhaps not feasible for every tumor, is an elegant and safe approach for adoptive transfer of tumor-specific immunity. At present, such an approach still remains speculative. Recombinant cytokines and possibly other biological response modifiers will undoubtedly play a major role in up-regulating some of these effects either alone or in conjunction with cellular immunotherapy.

ACKNOWLEDGMENTS

This work was supported by a research grant from Baxter Healthcare Corporation and the German Israel Foundation (GIF) (to SS).

REFERENCES

Ackerstein, A., Kedar, E., and Slavin, S. (1991) Use of recombinant human interleukin-2 in conjunction with syngeneic bone marrow transplantation as a model for control of minimal residual disease in malignant hematological disorders. *Blood*, **78**, 1212–5.

Apperley, J.F., Jones, L., Hale, G., et al. (1986) Bone marrow transplantation for patients with chronic myeloid leukemia: T-cell depletion with Campath-1 reduces the incidence of graft-versus-host disease but may increase the risk of leukemic relapse. *Bone Marrow Transplantation*, **1**, 53–66.

Atzpodien, J., Korfer, A., Franks, C.R., Poliwoda, H., and Kirchner, H. (1990) Home therapy with recombinant interleukin-2 and interferon-a2b in advanced human malignancies. *Lancet*, **335**, 1509–12.

Avichezer, D., Gilboa-Garber, N., Mumcuoglu, M., and Slavin, S. (1989) Adoptive transfer of resistance to *Pseudomonas aeruginosa* infection by splenocytes and bone marrow cells from BALB/c mice immunized by *Pseudomonas aeruginosa* lectin preparations. *Infection*, **17**, 407–10.

Bacigalupo, A., Van Lint, M.T., Occhini, D., et al. (1991) Increased risk of leukemia relapse with high-dose cyclosporine A after allogeneic marrow transplantation for acute leukemia. *Blood*, **77**, 1423–8.

Bär, B.M., Schattenberg, A., Mensink, E.J., et al. (1993) Donor leukocyte infusions for chronic myeloid leukemia relapsed after allogeneic bone marrow transplantation. *Journal of Clinical Oncology*, **11**, 513–9.

Benyunes, M.C., Massumoto, C., York, A., et al. (1993) Interleukin-2 with or without lymphokine-activated killer cells as consolidative immunotherapy after autologous bone marrow transplantation for acute myelogenous leukemia. *Bone Marrow Transplantation*, **12**, 159–63.

Binder, H.J. (1994) Immunity to hepatitis B virus: passing the torch. *Gastroenterology*, **106**, 1388–94.

Blaise, D., Olive, D., Stoppa, A.M., et al. (1990) Hematologic and immunologic effects of the systemic administration of recombinant interleukin-2 after autologous bone marrow transplantation. *Blood*, **76**, 1092–7.

Bucker, C.D., Sander, J.E., Hill, R., et al. (1989) Allogeneic versus autologous marrow transplantation for patients with acute lymphoblastic leukemia in first or second marrow remission. In K.E. Dicke, G. Spitzer, S. Jagannath, and M.J. Evinger-Hodges (Eds.) *Autologous bone marrow transplantation*, pp. 145–50. University of Texas, M.D. Anderson Cancer Center.

Champlin, R., Jansen, J., Ho, W., et al. (1991) Retention of graft-versus-leukemia using selective depletion of CD8-positive T lymphocytes for prevention of graft-versus-host disease following bone marrow transplantation for chronic myelogenous leukemia. *Transplantation Proceedings*, **23**, 1695–6.

Charmot, D., Ragueneau, M., Olive, D., et al. (1987) Generation of CD8 cytolytic T cells early after autologous or allogeneic bone marrow transplantation. *Bone Marrow Transplantation*, **2**, 183–94.

Cheever, M.A., Thompson, D.B., Klarnet, J.P., and Greenberg, P.D. (1986) Antigen-driven long term-cultured T cells proliferate in vivo, distribute widely, mediate specific tumor therapy, and persist long-term as functional memory T cells. *Journal of Experimental Medicine*, **163**, 1100–12.

Chopra, R., Goldstone, A.H., Pearce, R., et al. (1992) Autologous vs allogeneic bone marrow transplantation for non-Hodgkin's lymphoma: a case controlled analysis of the European Bone Marrow Transplant Group Registry data. *Journal of Clinical Oncology*, **10**, 1690–5.

Cohen, P., Vourka-Karussis, U., Weiss, L., and Slavin, S. (1993) Spontaneous and IL-2-induced anti-leukemic and anti-host effects against tumor and host specific alloantigens. *Journal of Immunology*, **151**, 4803–10.

Cullis, J.O., Jiang, Y.Z., Schwarer, A.P., Hughes, T.P., Barrett, A.J., and Goldman, J.M. (1992) Donor leukocyte infusions for chronic myeloid leukemia in relapse after allogeneic bone marrow transplantation. *Blood*, **79**, 1379–81.

De Witte, T., Gratwohl, A., Van Der Lely, N., et al. (1992) Recombinant human granulocyte-macrophage colony-stimulating factor accelerates neutrophil and monocyte recovery after allogeneic T-cell-depleted bone marrow transplantation. *Blood*, **79**, 1359–65.

Drobyski, W.R., Keever, C.A., Roth, M.S., et al. (1993) Salvage immunotherapy using donor leukocyte infusions as treatment for relapsed chronic myelogenous leukemia after allogeneic bone marrow transplantation: efficacy and toxicity of a defined T-cell dose. *Blood*, **82**, 2310–18.

Drobyski, W.R., Roth, M.S., Thibodeau, S.N., and Gottschall, J.L. (1992) Molecular remission occurring after donor leukocyte infusions for the treatment of relapsed chronic myelogenous leukemia after allogeneic bone marrow transplantation. *Bone Marrow Transplantation*, **10**, 301–4.

Engelhard, D., Handsher, R., Naparstek, E., et al. (1991) Immune response to polio vaccination in bone marrow transplant recipients. *Bone Marrow Transplantation*, **8**, 295–300.

Engelhard, D., Nagler, A., Hardan, I., et al. (1993) Antibody response to a two-dose regimen of influenza vaccine in allogeneic T cell-depleted and autologous BMT recipients. *Bone Marrow Transplantation*, **11**, 1–5.

Fabian, I., Kletter, Y., and Slavin, S. (1988) The therapeutic potential of recombinant colony-stimulating factor and interleukin-3 in murine B cell leukemia. *Blood*, **72**, 913–18.

Fefer, A., Benyunes, M.C., Massumoto, C., et al. (1993) Interleukin-2 therapy after autologous bone marrow transplantation for hematologic malignancies. *Seminars in Oncology*, **20**, 41–5.

Fefer, A., Sullivan, K.M., Weiden, P., et al. (1987) Graft versus leukemia effect in man: the relapse rate of acute leukemia is lower after allogeneic than after syngeneic marrow transplantation. *Progress in Clinical and Biological Research*, **244**, 401–8.

Friedrich, W., O'Reilly, R.J., Koziner, B., et al. (1982) T-lymphocyte reconstitution in recipients of bone marrow transplants with and without GVHD: imbalance of T-cell subpopulations having unique regulatory and cognitive functions. *Blood*, **59**, 696–701.

Gajewski, J.L., Ho, W.G., Feig, S.A., Hunt, L., Kaufman, N., and Champlin, R.E. (1990) Bone marrow transplantation using unrelated donors for patients with advanced leukemia or bone marrow failure. *Transplantation*, **40**, 244–9.

Gale, R.P., Goldman, J.M., and Horowitz, M.M. (1991) Bone marrow transplants in twins with chronic myelogenous leukemia. *Blood*, **78**, 244a.

Giralt, S., Escudier, S., Kantarjian, H., et al. (1993) Preliminary results of treatment with filgrastim for relapse of leukemia and myelodysplasia after allogeneic bone marrow transplantation. *New England Journal of Medicine*, **329**, 757–61.

Givon, T., Slavin, S., Haran-Ghera, N., Michalevicz, R., and Revel, M. (1992) Antitumor effects of human recombinant interleukin-6 on acute myeloid leukemia in mice and in cell cultures. *Blood*, **79**, 2392–8.

Gottlieb, D.J., Furer, C.E., Que, J.U., Prentice, H.G., Duncombe, A.S., and Brenner, M.K. (1990) Immunity against *Pseudomonas aeruginosa* adoptively transferred to bone marrow transplant recipients. *Blood*, **76**, 2470–5.

Gratama, J.W., Maipal, A., Olijans, R., et al. (1984) T lymphocyte repopulation and differentiation after bone marrow transplantation. Early shifts in the ratio between $T4^+$ and $T8^+$ T lymphocytes correlate with the occurrence of acute graft-versus-host disease. *Blood*, **63**, 1416–23.

Helg, C., Roux, E., Beris, P., et al. (1993) Adoptive immunotherapy for recurrent CML after BMT. *Bone Marrow Transplantation*, **12**, 125–9.

Heslop, H.E., Duncombe, A.S., Reittie, J.E., et al. (1991) Interleukin 2 infusion after autologous bone marrow transplantation enhances hemopoietic regeneration. *Transplantation Proceedings*, **23**, 1704–5.

Hirsh, M., Lipton, A., Harvey, H., et al. (1990) Phase I study of interleukin-2 and interferon alfa-2a as outpatient therapy for patients with advanced malignancy. *Journal of Clinical Oncology*, **8**, 1657–63.

Horowitz, M.M., Gale, R.P., Sondel, P.M., et al. (1990) Graft-versus-leukemia reactions after bone marrow transplantation. *Blood*, **75**, 555–62.

Ilan, Y., Nagler, A., Ackerstein, A., et al. (1994) Development of antibodies to hepatitis B virus surface antigen in bone marrow transplant recipient following treatment with peripheral blood lymphocytes from immunized donors. *Journal of Clinical and Experimental Immunology*, **97**, 299–302.

Ilan, Y., Nagler, A., Adler, R., et al. (1993a) Adoptive transfer of immunity to hepatitis B virus after T cell-depleted allogeneic bone marrow transplantation. *Hepatology*, **18**, 246–52.

Ilan, Y., Nagler, A., Adler, R., Tur-Kaspa, R., Slavin, S., and Shouval, D. (1993b) Ablation of persistent hepatitis B by bone marrow transplantation from a hepatitis B-immune donor. *Gastroenterology*, **104**, 1818–21.

Jiang, Y.Z., Cullis, J.O., Kanfer, E.J., Goldman, J.M., and Barrett, A.J. (1993) T cell and NK cell mediated graft-versus-leukemia reactivity following donor buffy coat transfusion to treat relapse after marrow transplantation for chronic myeloid leukemia. *Bone Marrow Transplantation*, **11**, 133–8.

Johnson, B.D., Drobyski, W.R., and Truitt, R.L. (1993) Delayed infusion of normal donor cells after MHc-matched bone marrow transplantation provides an antileukemia reaction without graft-versus-host disease. *Bone Marrow Transplantation*, **11**, 329–36.

Jones, R.J., Ambinder, R.F., Pintadosi, S., and Santos, G.W. (1991) Evidence of graft-versus-lymphoma effect associated with allogeneic bone marrow transplantation. *Blood*, **77**, 649–53.

Kapelushnik, J., Nagler, A., Or, R., et al. (submitted) Donor leukocyte activated killer (LAK) cell transfusions for treatment of relapsed chronic myelogenous leukemia (CML) not responding to donor buffy coat post allogeneic bone marrow transplantation (BMT).

Kedar, E., Tsuberi, B., Landesberg, A., et al. (1988) In vitro and in vivo cytokine-induced facilitation of immunohemopoietic reconstitution in mice undergoing BMT. *Bone Marrow Transplantation*, **33**, 297–314.

Kersey, J.H., Weisdorf, D., Nesbit, M.E., LeBien, T.W., Goldman, A.I., and Bostrom, B. (1987) Comparison of autologous and allogeneic bone marrow transplantation for treatment of high-risk refractory acute lymphoblastic leukemia. *New England Journal of Medicine*, **317**, 461–7.

Klapholz, L., Ackerstein, A., Goldenhersh, M.A., Vardy, D., and Nagler, A. (1993) Local cutaneous reaction induced by subcutaneous interleukin-2 and interferon alpha-2a immunotherapy following ABMT. *Bone Marrow Transplantation*, **11**, 443–6.

Kolb, H.J., Mittermüller, J., Clemm, C., et al. (1990) Donor leukocyte transfusions for treatment of recurrent chronic myelogenous leukemia in marrow transplant patients. *Blood*, **76**, 2462–5.

Korngold, R. and Sprent, J. (1987) T cell subsets and graft-versus-host disease. *Transplantation*, **44**, 335–9.

Krigel, R.L., Padavic-Shaller, K.A., Rudolph, A.R., et al. (1988) A phase I study of recombinant interleukin 2 plus recombinant β-interferon. *Cancer Research*, **48**, 3875–81.

Lane, H.C., Zunich, K.M., Wilson, W., et al. (1990) Syngeneic bone marrow transplantation and adoptive transfer of peripheral blood lymphocytes combined with zidovudine in human immunodeficiency virus (HIV) infection. *Annals of Internal Medicine*, **113**, 512–9.

Lee, K.H., Talpaz, M., Rothberg, J.M., et al. (1989) Concomitant administration of recombinant human interleukin-2 and recombinant interferon alpha-2A in cancer patients: a phase I study. *Journal of Clinical Oncology*, **7**, 1726–32.

Lum, L.G. (1990) Immune recovery after bone marrow transplantation. *Hematology/Oncology Clinics of North America*, **4**, 659–75.

Marmont, A.M., Gale, R.P., Butturini, A., et al. (1989) T-cell depletion in allogeneic bone marrow transplantation: progress and problems. *Haematologica*, **74**, 235–48.

Mehta, J. (1993) Graft-versus-leukemia reactions in clinical bone marrow transplantation. *Leukemia and Lymphoma*, **10**, 427–32.

Morecki, S., Revel-Vilk, S., Nabet, C., et al. (1992) Immunological evaluation of patients with hematological malignancies receiving ambulatory cytokine-mediated immunotherapy with recombinant human interferon-alpha 2a and interleukin-2. *Cancer Immunology and Immunotherapy*, **35**, 401–11.

Moscovitch, M. and Slavin, S. (1984) Anti-tumor effects of allogeneic bone marrow transplantation in (NZB × NZW) F1 hybrids with spontaneous lymphosarcoma. *Journal of Immunology*, **132**, 997–1000.

Mumcuoglu, M., Zakay-Rones, Z., Parag, G., Weiss, L., and Slavin, S. (1987) The effect of T lymphocyte depletion on susceptibility to influenza virus infection and development of anti-viral immunity in lethally irradiated mice reconstituted with syngeneic bone marrow grafts. *Bone Marrow Transplantation*, **2**, 403–12.

Nagler, A., Ackerstein, A., Or, R., et al. (1992) Adoptive immunotherapy with mismatched allogeneic peripheral blood lymphocytes (PBL) following autologous bone marrow transplantation (ABMT). *Experimental Haematology*, **20**, 705.

Nagler, A., Drakos, P., Ackerstein, A., et al. (1993) Autologous bone marrow transplantation for non-Hodgkin's lymphoma and Hodgkin's disease: the role of immunotherapy. *European Journal of Cancer*, **29A**, S173.

Naparstek, E., Or, R., Nagler, A., et al. (1995) depleted allogeneic bone marrow transplantation for acute leukemia using Campath-1 antibodies and post transplant administration of donor's peripheral blood lymphocytes for prevention of relapse. *Blood*, **89**, 506.

Or, R., Nagler, A., Ackerstein, A., et al. (submitted) Allogeneic cell-mediated immunotherapy at the minimal residual disease stage following autologous stem cell transplantation for malignant lymphoma.

O'Reilly, R.J. (1983) Allogeneic bone marrow transplantation: current status and future directions. *Blood*, **62**, 941–64.

Phillips, G.L., Herzig, R.H., Lazarus, H.M., Fay, J.W., Griffith, R., and Herzig, G.P. (1986) High-dose chemotherapy, fractionated total-body irradiation, and allogeneic marrow transplantation for malignant lymphoma. *Journal of Clinical Oncology*, **4**, 480–8.

Porter, D.L., Roth, M.S., McGarigle, C., Ferrara, J.L., and Antin, J.H. (1994) Induction of graft-versus-host disease as immunotherapy for relapsed chronic myeloid leukemia. *New England Journal of Medicine*, **330**, 100–6.

Riddell, S.R., Watanabe, K.S., Goodrich, J.M., Li, C.R., Agha, M.E., and Greenberg, P.D. (1992) Restoration of viral immunity in immunodeficient humans by the adoptive transfer of T cell clones. *Science*, **257**, 238–41.

Saxon, A., Mitsuyasu, R., Stevens, R., Champlin, R.E., Kimata, H., and Gale, R.P. (1986) Designed transfer of specific immune responses with bone marrow transplantation. *Journal of Clinical Investigation*, **78**, 959–67.

Schechter, D., Nagler, A., Ackerstein, A., et al. (1992) Recombinant interleukin-2 and interferon alpha immunotherapy following autologous bone marrow transplantation. A case report of cardiovascular toxicity with serial echocardiographic evaluation. *Cardiology*, **80**, 168–71.

Slavin, S., Ackerstein, A., Kedar, E., et al. (1991a) Induction of cell-mediated IL2-activated antitumor responses in conjunction with autologous and allogeneic bone marrow transplantation. *Transplantation Proceedings*, **23**, 802–3.

Slavin, S., Ackerstein, A., Kedar, E., and Weiss, L. (1990a) IL-2 activated cell-mediated immunotherapy: control of minimal residual disease in malignant disorders by allogeneic lymphocytes and IL-2. *Bone Marrow Transplantation*, **6**, 86–90.

Slavin, S., Ackerstein, A., Nagler, A., Naparstek, E., and Weiss, L. (1990b) Cell mediated cytokine activated immunotherapy (CCI) of malignant hematological disorders for eradication of minimal residual disease (MRD) in conjunction with conventional chemotherapy or bone marrow transplantation (BMT). *Blood*, **76**(Suppl. 1), 566a.

Slavin, S., Ackerstein, A., Naparstek, E., Or, R., and Weiss, L. (1990c). The graft-versus-leukemia (GVL) phenomenon: is GVL separable from GVHD. *Bone Marrow Transplantation*, **6**, 155–61.

Slavin, S., Ackerstein, A., Weiss, L., Nagler, A., Or, R., and Naparstek, E. (1992a) Immunotherapy of minimal residual disease by immunocompetent lymphocytes and their activation by cytokines. *Cancer Investigation*, **10**, 221–7.

Slavin, S., Ackerstein, A., Weiss, L., Nagler, A., Or, R., and Naparstek, E. (1992b) Induction of tumor dormancy in BALB/c mice against nonimmunogenic B cell leukemia. In T.H. Stewart and E.F. Wheelock (Eds.) *Cellular immune mechanisms and tumor dormancy*, pp. 99–110. Boca Raton, FL, CRC Press.

Slavin, S., Fuks, Z., Kaplan, H.S., and Strober, S. (1978) Transplantation of allogeneic bone marrow without graft-versus-host disease using total lymphoid irradiation. *Journal of Experimental Medicine*, **147**, 963–72.

Slavin, S., Mumcuoglu, M., Landesberg-Weisz, A., and Kedar, E. (1989) The use of recombinant cytokines for enhancing immuno-hemopoietic reconstitution following bone marrow transplantation. I. Effects of in vitro culturing with IL-3 and GM-CSF on human and mouse bone marrow cells purged with mafosfamide (ASTA-Z). *Bone Marrow Transplantation*, **4**, 459–64.

Slavin, S. and Nagler, A. (1991) New developments in bone marrow transplantation. *Current Opinion in Oncology*, **3**, 254–71.

Slavin, S., Naparstek, E., Nagler, A., et al. (1993a) Cell mediated immunotherapy (CMI) for the treatment of malignant hematological diseases in conjunction with autologous bone marrow transplantation (ABMT). *Blood*, **82**, 292a.

Slavin, S., Naparstek, E., Nagler, A., Amar, A., and Or, R. (1995) Allogeneic cell mediated immunotherapy following allogeneic bone marrow transplantation: a modality for prevention and treatment of relapse in malignant hematologic disorders in conjunction with bone marrow transplantation. *Experimental Hematology*, (in press).

Slavin, S., Or, R., Kapelushnik, Y., et al. (1992c) Immunotherapy of minimal residual disease in conjunction with autologous and allogeneic bone marrow transplantation (BMT). *Leukemia*, **6**, 164–6.

Slavin, S., Or, R., Naparstek, E., et al. (1992d) Eradication of minimal residual disease (MRD) following autologous (ABMT) and allogeneic bone marrow transplantation (BMT) by cytokine-mediated immunotherapy (CMI) and cell-mediated cytokine-activated immunotherapy (CCI) in experimental animals and man. *Blood*, **80**, 535a.

Slavin, S., Or, R., Naparstek, E., et al. (1992e) Eradication of minimal residual disease (MRD) following autologous (ABMT) and allogeneic bone marrow transplantation (BMT) by cytokine mediated immunotherapy (CMI) and cell mediated cytokine activated immunotherapy (CCI) in experimental animals and man. *Blood*, **80**, 535a.

Slavin, S., Or, R., Naparstek, E., et al. (1993b) Amplified graft vs leukemia effects (CVL) to prevent and treat relapse post-BMT with donor's peripheral blood lymphocytes and in recombinant cytokines. *9th Annual Meeting EBMT Proceedings*, p. 981.

Slavin, S., Or, R., Naparstek, E., Ackerstein, A., and Weiss, L. (1988b) Cellular mediated immunotherapy of leukemia in conjunction with autologous and allogeneic bone marrow transplantation in experimental animals and man. *Blood*, **72**, 407a.

Slavin, S., Waldmann, H., Or, R., et al. (1985) Prevention of graft vs host disease in allogeneic bone marrow transplantation for leukemia by T cell depletion in vitro prior to transplantation. *Transplantation Proceedings*, **17**, 465.

Small, T.N., Papadopoulos, E., Kernan, N.A., and O'Reilly, R.J. (1993) Effects on immune reconstitution of unirradiated donor leukocyte infusions for the treatment or prophylaxis of EBV. Lymphoproliferative disorders following unrelated bone marrow transplantation (BMT). *Blood*, **82**, 214a.

Soiffer, R.J., Canning, C., Gonin, R., and Ritz, J. (1993) Influence of low dose interleukin-2 on relapse rate after T-cell depleted allogeneic BMT. *Blood*, **82**, 215a.

Szer, J., Grigg, A.P., Phillipos, G.L., and Sheridan, W.P. (1993) Donor leucocyte infusions after chemotherapy for patients relapsing with acute leukaemia following allogeneic BMT. *Bone Marrow Transplantation*, **11**, 109–11.

Thomas, E.D. (1963) The role of marrow transplantation in the eradication of malignant disease. *Cancer*, **49**, 1963.

Truitt, R.L. and Atasoylu, A.A. (1991) Impact of pretransplant conditioning and donor T cells on chimerism, graft-versus-host disease, graft-versus-leukemia reactivity, and tolerance after bone marrow transplantation. *Blood*, **77**, 2515–23.

Uchiyama, A., Hoon, D.S., Morisaki, T., Kaneda, Y., Yuzuki, D.H., and Morton, D.L. (1993) Transfection of interleukin 2 gene into human melanoma cells augments cellular immune response. *Cancer Research*, **53**, 949–52.

van Rhee, F., Feng, L., Cullis, J.O., et al. (1994) Relapse of chronic myeloid leukemia after allogeneic bone marrow transplant: the case for giving donor leukocyte transfusions before the onset of hematological relapse. *Blood*, **83**, 3377.

Waldmann, H., Polliack, A., Hale, G., et al. (1984) Elimination of graft-versus-host disease by in-vitro depletion of alloreactive lymphocytes with a monoclonal rat anti-human lymphocyte antibody (Campath-l). *Lancet*, **2**, 483–6.

Weiden, P.L., Flournoy, N., Thomas, E.D., et al. (1979) Antileukemic effect of graft-versus-host disease in human recipients of allogeneic-marrow grafts. *New England Journal of Medicine*, **300**, 1068–73.

Weiden, P.L., Sullivan, K.M., Flournoy, N., Storb, R., and Thomas, E.D. (1981) Antileukemic effect of chronic graft-versus-host disease: contribution to improved survival after allogeneic marrow transplantation. *New England Journal of Medicine*, **304**, 1529–33.

Weiss, L., Reich, S., and Slavin, S. (1992) Use of recombinant human interleukin-2 in conjunction with bone marrow transplantation as a model for control of minimal residual disease in malignant hematological disorders: I. Treatment of murine leukemia in conjunction with allogeneic bone marrow transplantation and IL-2-activated cell mediated immunotherapy. *Cancer Investigation*, **10**, 19–26.

Weiss, L., Weigensberg, M., Morecki, S., et al. (1990b) Characterization of effector cells of graft vs. leukemia following allogeneic bone marrow transplantation in mice inoculated with murine B-cell leukemia. *Cancer Immunology and Immunotherapy*, **31**, 236–42.

Wimperis, J.Z., Brenner, M.K., Prentice, H.G., et al. (1987) B cell development and regulation after T cell-depleted marrow transplantation. *Journal of Immunology*, **138**, 2445–50.

Witherspoon, R.P., Matthew, D., Storb, R., et al. (1984) Recovery of in vivo cellular immunity after human marrow grafting. Influence of time postgrafting and acute graft-versus-host disease. *Transplantation*, **37**, 145–50.

Working Party on Leukaemia, European Group for Bone Marrow Transplantation. (1988) Allogeneic bone marrow transplantation for leukaemia in Europe. *Lancet*, **1**, 1379–82.

30

Donor Lymphocyte Therapy in Bone-Marrow Transplantation

FRITS VAN RHEE AND JOHN GOLDMAN

Bone-marrow transplantation (BMT) aims to eradicate leukemia cells with use of lethal myeloablative therapy composed of high-dose chemotherapy and total-body irradiation (TBI). Transplantation of normal stem cells from a suitable allogeneic donor will result in the repopulation of BM with donor blood cells and allows for rescue of the patient. Immune reconstitution of the host by donor lymphoid cells provides protection against both exogenous infection and reactivation of latent pathogens. Before the era of clinical BMT, Barnes and Loutit (1957) suggested that lymphoid cells present in the infused donor marrow might also play an important role in the elimination of leukemic hemopoiesis after transplant by mediating a direct antitumor effect. Their early observations, made in murine transplant models, are now widely accepted; the graft-versus-leukemia (GVL) effect also contributes significantly to cure after BMT for leukemia in humans.

The Seattle group first reported that the relapse rate after transplant for acute leukemia was greater with use of syngeneic than with HLA-identical sibling donors. This supported the idea of a clinical antitumor effect mediated by allogeneic donor cells. The exclusion of graft-versus-host disease (GVHD) as an independent variable eliminated the difference in relapse between the two groups, suggesting that GVHD accounted for most of the observed antileukemic effect (Weiden et al. 1979). The contribution of GVHD to the GVL effect was further demonstrated by the same group in a study of 163 patients treated for acute leukemia; fewer relapses were observed if acute and/or chronic GVHD occurred following BMT (Weiden et al. 1981). Data from the International Bone Marrow Transplant Registry (IBMTR) and other studies implied that donor T lymphocytes play a crucial role in the mediation of the GVL effect, and that removal of

550

T lymphocytes from the marrow inoculum greatly increased the risk of relapse after transplant (Goldman et al. 1988; Horowitz et al. 1990). This effect of T-cell depletion is particularly evident after transplant for chronic myeloid leukemia (CML), where the actuarial incidence of relapse may be as great as 70%.

Allogeneic BMT establishes partial or complete donor chimerism of the lymphoid system and results in tolerance to donor cells. This allows the opportunity to infuse immunocompetent donor cells after BMT to induce immunological effects in the recipient. The GVL effect can be exploited for therapeutic advantage in patients who relapse after BMT. Thus, transfusions of buffy coat cells from the original marrow donor to patients with leukemic relapse can restore complete remission and provide convincing evidence for the existence of the GVL effect. This novel form of adoptive immunotherapy, also referred to as donor leukocyte or lymphocyte therapy, shows particular promise in the treatment of relapsed CML. Immune modulation of the recipient by donor lymphocyte therapy is also an important new approach for the management of posttransplant Epstein-Barr virus (EBV)–induced lymphoproliferative disorders that may occur especially after T-cell–depleted BMT.

■ DONOR LYMPHOCYTE THERAPY FOR RELAPSE OF LEUKEMIA

Relapse after allogeneic BMT occurs in 10% to 30% of patients transplanted with unmanipulated donor cells for CML in chronic phase (CP) or acute leukemia in first remission (Goldman et al. 1986; Thomas et al. 1986). Relapse rates are considerably greater in patients transplanted in a more advanced phase of their disease, indicating that biologically aggressive leukemia cells are more difficult to eradicate. It is now well established that residual disease can be demonstrated by molecular techniques in many patients in apparent complete remission after BMT for CML, which suggests that some leukemia cells commonly survive the myeloablative regimen (Hughes et al. 1991). In CML, residual cells have been detected by reverse transcriptase polymerase chain reaction (RT-PCR) in some long-term survivors more than 10 years after BMT (van Rhee et al. 1994a). These findings and the experience with T-cell depletion must mean that the immunological competence of donor cells is of paramount importance for the control and elimination of the residual leukemic clone after transplant.

Sullivan et al. (1989) were the first to attempt to modulate the immune system after transplant to reduce the incidence of relapse in a group of patients with advanced hematological malignancies. GVL was induced in vivo either by transfusion of donor buffy coat cells in the immediate posttransplant period or by deliberate reduction of immunosuppressive therapy. No clinical benefit was observed, as the patients who received donor cells experienced more acute GVHD and infections with no reduction in leukemic relapse. This study was confined to patients with advanced disease and did not include patients with CML in CP, which may account for the failure to observe a reduction in the relapse rate. It seems reasonable to speculate that transfusions of donor buffy coat cells in the acute transplant setting are more likely to cause significant GVHD. Tissue injury after BMT due to the conditioning regimen and infection results in the induction of cytokines and in the up-regulation of adhesion molecules, and major histocompatibility complex (HC) antigens (Ag), all of which may enhance GVHD. In contrast, animal studies suggest that delayed infusion of donor lymphocytes after transplantation results in less GVHD due to the development of donor-host tolerance (Weiden et al. 1976; Johnson, Drobyski, and Truitt 1993).

Kolb et al. (1990) first reported that therapeutic use of donor buffy coat cells in combination with interferon-α (IFN-α) in three patients with frank relapse of CML and observed complete hematological and cytogenetic remissions. These exciting initial observations have now been confirmed by several other groups, and donor lymphocyte therapy has become an accepted treatment option for relapse after transplant (Cullis et al. 1992; Bar et al. 1993; Drobyski et al. 1993; Hertenstein et al. 1993; Porter et al. 1994; van Rhee et al. 1994a).

■ DONOR LYMPHOCYTE THERAPY FOR CHRONIC MYELOID LEUKEMIA IN RELAPSE AFTER ALLOGENEIC MARROW TRANSPLANT

The management of relapse of CML after allogeneic transplant is a major therapeutic challenge, as palliative therapy with oral cytotoxic drugs will merely alleviate symptoms by controlling blood cell counts and the size of the spleen, but does not have the capacity for cure. Data from the European Group for Blood and Marrow Transplantation (EBMT) suggest that IFN-α can suppress the leukemic clone and prolong life (Arcese et al. 1993). Posttransplant immunosuppressive therapy with cyclosporin A can suppress the donor lymphocyte subsets that mediate GVL, and complete remissions following cessation of cyclosporin A have been documented in a few instances (Collins et al. 1992). A second transplant may be an option in selected cases, but has a high morbidity and mortality and a long-term survival of approximately 30% to 50% (Barrett et al. 1991; Cullis et al. 1992; Mrsic et al. 1992).

Leukocyte transfusion from the original BM donor induces both hematological and cytogenetic responses in approximately 70% to 80% of patients (Fig. 30.1). A number of variables have been identified that correlate with response (Kolb et al. 1995). Patients with CML are more likely to obtain a complete remission (CR) than those with other hematological malignancies, although transformation of CML to accelerated or blast phase is associated with a poor response to therapy. Interestingly, more responses have been observed in patients who experienced little or no GVHD (grade 0 to 1) after the original transplant procedure (Kolb et al. 1995). This suggests that in some instances the GVL effect was abrogated after BMT by unidentified factors, whereas later a powerful antileukemic effect could be established by infusion of more donor cells at the time of relapse. The occurrence of GVHD after donor lymphocyte therapy also correlates with response of the leukemia, and this provides further evidence that GVHD and GVL are to some extent linked.

A complete cytogenetic response is usually obtained between 1 and 4 months after donor lymphocyte therapy. This time interval presumably reflects the period required for the activation and amplification of immune-effector mechanisms responsible for the GVL ef-

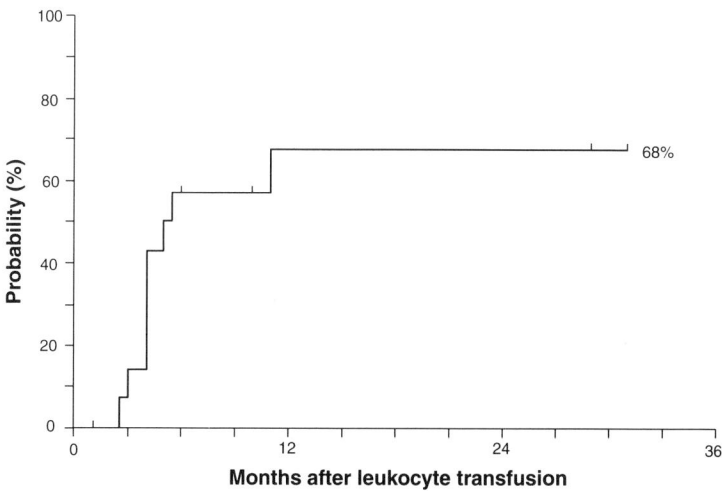

Figure 30.1 Probability of obtaining a complete cytogenetic or molecular response after donor lymphocyte transfusion for CML in 14 patients treated as the Hammersmith Hospital.

fect. Approximately 80% of responders will achieve RT-PCR negativity, but the elimination of residual disease at the molecular level is gradual and may take several months or longer (Antin 1993; Drobyski et al. 1993). In one study, the mean time to PCR negativity was 6 months and progressive reduction in size of the leukemic clone could be documented by competitive PCR (van Rhee et al. 1994b). Second relapses after donor lymphocyte therapy for CML in CP have not been reported, and the remissions appear to be durable. This is in stark contrast to results obtained with IFN-α or second BMT, where second relapses are not infrequent.

The cell dose infused has been highly variable in different studies and does not correlate with response (Bar et al. 1993; Kolb et al. 1995; van Rhee et al. 1994b). Most investigators have transfused 1 to 2 x 10^8 mononuclear cells per kilogram (MNC) collected in one to three leukaphereses. In one study, a target T-cell dose of 2.5 to 5×10^8 cells/kg was transfused (Drobyski et al. 1993), but responses have been seen with as few as 0.34×10^8 MNC kg. It seems likely that both features of the disease phase such as leukemic cell expression of minor HC Ag and donor immune-effector mechanisms are more important in determining response than the number of cells infused. The minimum number of cells required to induce GVL is not known and may vary with different donor-recipient pairs. The idea of transfusing fewer cells is attractive, since there is some evidence to suggest that the severity of GVHD after BMT depends on the number of T cells infused with the donor marrow (Kernan et al. 1986; Lowenberg et al. 1986). It is possible, but not certain, that a similar correlation between cell dose and GVHD applies in the setting of donor lymphocyte therapy.

In most studies, IFN-α has been administered in conjunction with donor lymphocyte therapy for CML. Several studies now suggest that IFN-α alone can improve survival in patients with CML both before BMT and after BMT in the case of relapse (Talpaz et al. 1991; Arcese et al. 1993); however, in both situations cure is not obtained and residual leukemia cells can usually be identified by cytogenetic or molecular methods (Higano, Raskind, and Singer 1992; Lee et al. 1992; Opalka et al. 1991). The exact mechanism of action of IFN-α is not known, but is thought to exert an antiproliferative effect on the leukemic clone or to alter the adhesive properties of CML progenitors to stroma (Dowding et al. 1991). The effect is not selective for CML, but is also seen in other malignancies such as hairy cell leukemia. Analysis of European data indicates that treatment with IFN-α does not improve the response rate to donor lymphocyte therapy (Kolb et al. 1995) and responses to donor lymphocyte therapy have been reported without concomitant IFN-α (Cullis et al. 1992; Drobyski et al. 1993;

van Rhee et al. 1994b). It is possible that IFN-α might increase the toxicity of donor lymphocyte therapy by enhancing GVHD. IFN-α can both increase minor HC Ag presentation by up-regulating HLA-Ag expression and induce expression of co-stimulatory molecules such as LFA-3 and CD58 (Herberman et al. 1981; Balkwill 1989; Upadhyaya et al. 1991). It has been suggested that the combination of IFN-α and donor lymphocyte therapy should be used for those who do not respond to donor lymphocyte therapy alone (van Rhee et al. 1994b).

The optimal timing of donor lymphocyte therapy has not been determined, but it is generally agreed that results are poorer when the disease is in advanced or blastic phase. The tempo of relapse of CML is slow and regular cytogenetic monitoring of BM may allow for the early identification of disease recurrence. The presence of Philadelphia chromosome-positive (Ph[+]) metaphases in the marrow, while hematological values are still normal, is commonly referred to as cytogenetic relapse. Residual disease can also be studied at the molecular level by RT-PCR for *bcr/abl* mRNA. In the first year after transplant, leukemia cells can be detected by PCR in many patients, but such findings are not associated with relapse (Hughes et al. 1991). In contrast, PCR positivity more than 12 months after BMT does carry an increased risk of relapse, but qualitative PCR data do not yield sufficient information to predict relapse in any particular individual (Cross et al. 1993a). In contrast, serial quantitative PCR assays can identify individual patients with increasing numbers of leukemia-specific transcripts who have proliferating leukemic cells, and these patients are likely to progress to hematological relapse (Cross et al. 1993b; Lion et al. 1993; Lion 1994). Criteria for the definition of molecular relapse have not been firmly established, although suggestions have included an increase in transcript numbers of at least 1 log on three consecutive PCR assays or the detection of more than 1,000 transcripts/μg RNA by competitive PCR (Lion et al. 1993; van Rhee et al. 1994b).

Cytogenetic and molecular diagnosis of early relapse makes it possible to consider instituting donor lymphocyte therapy before progression to hematological relapse, as illustrated in Figure 30.2. It has not been established whether early therapy results in an increased response rate, although in one series all seven patients who received donor lymphocyte transfusions for cytogenetic or molecular relapse responded, compared with three of seven patients in hematological relapse (van Rhee et al. 1994b). It is important to note that cytogenetic relapse may be transient in approximately 20% of patients, particularly if the percentage of Ph[+] metaphases in BM remains less than

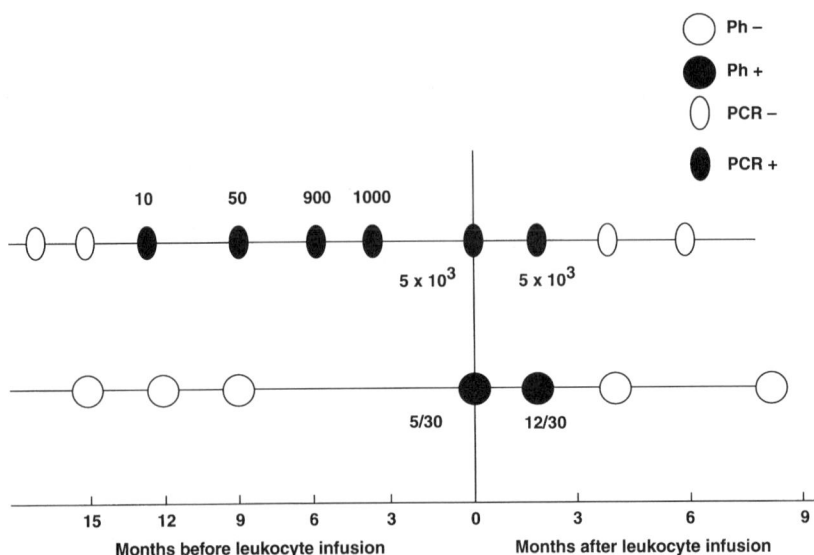

Figure 30.2 Use of competitive PCR for *bcr/abl* mRNA to initiate early therapy for a patient with relapse of CML after allogeneic BMT. PCR results (*solid line*) are shown as: open ellipse = PCR-negative, black ellipse = PCR-positive. Quantitative PCR results are shown above positive results and expressed as the number of *bcr/abl* molecules detected per microgram of RNA. Cytogenetic results are shown as: open circle if all metaphases examined were Ph^- or filled circle if Ph^+ metaphases were detected. The number of Ph^+ metaphases detected and the total number of metaphases examined are shown in italics.

40% (Apperley et al. 1986; Arthur et al. 1988; Zaccaria et al. 1988). Analogous instances of transient molecular relapse have also been observed in our laboratory (Feng et al. 1994). Early treatment has the disadvantage that it may unnecessarily expose some patients with transient relapse to adverse effects of GVHD.

Routine treatment of molecular relapse with donor lymphocyte infusions is at present not advisable and is, perhaps, best restricted to research protocols. IFN-α is less toxic than donor lymphocyte therapy, but the role of IFN-α in the management of molecular relapse has not been explored. Hemopoietic growth factors (e.g., granulocyte colony-stimulating factor [G-CSF]) could also be employed (Giralt et al. 1993), particularly in cases where there is poor or sluggish engraftment. Preferential stimulation of normal hemopoiesis with competition of leukemic and normal hemopoiesis for BM niches could account for the mechanism of action of G-CSF.

We have designed an algorithm that outlines our current management of CML in cytogenetic relapse (Fig. 30.3). Regular cytogenetic analysis of the marrow and PCR monitoring of the peripheral blood (PB) at 3-month intervals in the first year after transplant and 6-month intervals thereafter, will assist in the early identification of disease recurrence. Patients with less than 40% Ph$^+$ metaphases in BM should be observed in the first instance and BM should be reexamined in 6 weeks. Cessation of immunosuppressive therapy is relatively innocuous and may induce disease regression. Patients with progressive cytogenetic relapse should receive donor leukocyte transfusion before the BM is completely replaced by Ph$^+$ metaphases. Nonresponders who have progressed to hematological relapse could be subsequently

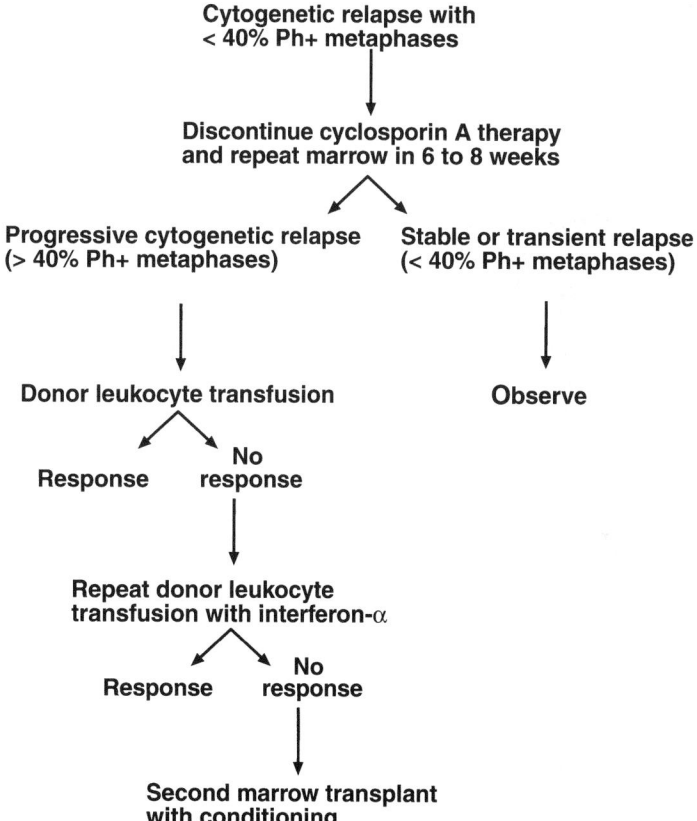

Figure 30.3 Algorithm for the management of cytogenetic relapse of CML after allogeneic BMT.

treated by the combination of IFN-α and donor leukocyte transfusion. The last option as salvage therapy is a second BMT.

■ DONOR LYMPHOCYTE THERAPY FOR OTHER HEMATOLOGICAL MALIGNANCIES

A comparison of the relapse rates after T-cell–depleted and unmanipulated BMT in patients reported to the IBMTR indicates that the GVL effect is operational not only after transplant for CML, but also after transplant for acute leukemias (Horowitz et al. 1990); however, efforts to exploit a GVL effect in other hematological malignancies by donor lymphocyte therapy have been much less successful than in CML. Donor lymphocyte therapy CR have been reported in a small number of patients with acute myeloid leukemia (AML), but the remissions may not be as durable as those obtained after donor lymphocyte transfusion for CML (Kolb et al. 1995). The possible benefit of combining intensive chemotherapy and donor lymphocyte therapy remains undefined.

The IBMTR data regarding relapse rates after transplant and the experience with donor lymphocyte therapy suggest that the GVL effect in the acute leukemias is considerably less potent than in CML. This may be because the bulk of acute leukemia stem cells are intrinsically more aggressive and more difficult to eradicate, but it is also possible that acute leukemia cells are less amenable to immunological control by donor cells due to reduction or lack of relevant Ag presentation or inability to provide co-stimulatory signals.

■ DONOR LYMPHOCYTE THERAPY FOR EBV-INDUCED LYMPHOPROLIFERATIVE DISORDERS

Transplantation with BM from an EBV-seropositive donor can produce a rapidly fatal lymphoproliferative disorder, also referred to as EBV-associated lymphoma, in the immunosuppressed recipient. EBV lymphoma has also been described in individuals receiving immunosuppressive therapy after renal, hepatic, and cardiac transplantation. After BMT, EBV lymphoma originates in the B-lymphocyte population from the donor, and EBV DNA has been shown by PCR in the malignant cells. The lymphoma is usually of diffuse large-cell type and the syndrome typically develops within the first 6 months after transplant when the host is still immunosuppressed. Methods of lymphoid-cell depletion that selectively remove T cells from the marrow graft predispose to the development of EBV lymphomas, and reported incidences vary from 0.6% to 12% (Zutter et al. 1988; Antin et al. 1991). In contrast, EBV lymphoproliferative disorders are rare after T-replete BMT or with BM depleted of lymphocytes with the panlymphoid antibody (Ab) Campath-1, which removes both B and T cells (Hale and Waldmann 1994). These findings suggest that donor T cells play a central role in the suppression of EBV-immortalized B cells transferred to the recipient at the time of transplant and that T-cell depletion may abrogate this specific anti-EBV response.

Treatment of EBV lymphoma has proven difficult, although oligo- or polyclonal tumors may respond to treatment with acyclovir or B-cell monoclonal antibodies (mAB) (Fisher et al. 1991). The outlook for patients with monoclonal proliferations has been generally dismal. Cytotoxic T-cell precursors specific to EBV are readily demonstrable in the PB of normal EBV-seropositive individuals at high frequencies (Bourgault et al. 1991), and a recent report suggests that unmodified lymphocyte transfusions from the original BM donor can transfer specific cytotoxic T-cell activity to the recipient. Papadopoulos et al. (1994) described five patients with EBV-lymphoproliferative disorders after T-cell–depleted BMT who received one to three lymphocyte transfusions from their original EBV$^+$ BM donor. Rapid regression of EBV lymphomas were observed in all cases and complete remissions have lasted for 16 months. Two patients died of a pulmonary syndrome that has not been reported after lymphocyte therapy for hematological malignancies. Although pulmonary infiltration by EBV lymphoma was suspected, no evidence for this was found at autopsy.

It is of interest to note that in contrast to lymphocyte transfusion for CML, responses were observed within 1 month of transfusions. In addition, the total number of T cells transfused was relatively low in this study and varied from 0.8 to 2.0×10^6 cells/kg. These findings suggest that EBV-specific T-cell precursors were present at relatively high frequencies in the lymphocyte collection.

Recent retrovirally marked EBV-specific cytotoxic T-cell lines have been generated in vitro, and these cell lines have been used to treat reactivation of EBV or EBV-lymphoproliferative disorder after BMT. The genetically marked lymphocyte population persisted in vivo for up to 4 months after infusion and exerted clinically significant antiviral activity with return of EBV DNA levels to baseline values. A single patient was treated for immunoblastic lymphoma and a complete response (Rooney et al. 1995).

■ ADVERSE EFFECTS OF DONOR LYMPHOCYTE THERAPY

GVHD is the single most frequent complication of donor lymphocyte therapy (reviewed by Antin 1993). Both acute and chronic GVHD syndromes have been reported and can be classified clinically according to conventional criteria. The infusion of further immunocompetent cells from the donor precipitates GVHD in 80% of patients and this is clinically significant (grade 2 to 4) in 51%. The incidence of GVHD after donor lymphocyte therapy may be greater than after BMT. Donor lymphocyte therapy usually involves the infusion of large numbers of T cells whose immunocompetence is not usually modulated by cyclosporin A and methotrexate, as happens after BMT. Both these factors could account for the observed difference in GVHD incidence. In individual patients, the occurrence and severity of GVHD after the original transplant procedure does not appear to correlate closely with GVHD after donor lymphocyte therapy (Kolb et al. 1995). Attempts have been made to reduce GVHD after donor lymphocyte infusion by cyclosporin A in four patients who received cells from volunteer donors, but an antileukemic effect was not seen until cyclosporin A had been stopped (van Rhee et al. 1994a). This limited experience suggests that suppression of donor lymphocytes is not selective, but that suppression of GVH and GVL effects occurs pari passu.

Recent studies using escalating doses of T lymphocytes suggest that it may be possible to separate GVL responses from GVHD by infusing low numbers (1.0 to 1.5×10^7 cells/kg) of T cells. Mackinnon et al. (1995) treated eight patients with a T-cell dose of only 1.0×10^7 cells/kg and observed complete remissions without GVHD in seven patients.

Marrow aplasia is a further important complication of donor lymphocyte therapy and develops in approximately half of the patients treated in hematological relapse. A variable period of pancytopenia may follow donor lymphocyte therapy in these patients and usually indicates a response to therapy with suppression or eradication of the leukemic clone. Hemopoietic reconstitution may originate from residual donor stem cells in the marrow, although it is possible that transfused stem cells in the lymphocyte collection also contribute. The pancytopenia is fatal in 10% of patients, with death due to infection or bleeding.

The initial management of aplasia can be expectant with transfusion support and growth factors, but a second stem-cell infusion from the original marrow donor may be required if hematological recovery does not occur. A second stem-cell transfusion does not require further preparatory treatment to prevent rejection of the donor hemopoietic stem cells, since the majority of the recipient's T cells are still of donor origin at the time of relapse (Drobyski et al. 1993; van Rhee et al. 1994b). This second stem-cell infusion usually results in hemopoietic reconstitution with donor cells, indicating that a deficiency of stem cells rather than stromal factors was the cause of the aplasia.

Small quantities of residual donor hemopoiesis can be demonstrated in most patients with hematological relapse by using molecular methods such as restriction fragment length polymorphism (RFLP) analysis and in situ hybridization with X and Y chromosome probes in sex-mismatched transplants (Drobyski et al. 1993; Hertenstein et al. 1993). In one instance, detection of donor cells in the myeloid compartment during pancytopenia appeared to predict for recovery from aplasia (Garicochea et al. 1994), but other studies have not yielded such consistent results (Hertenstein et al. 1993). The cytogenetic detection of donor cells in the BM appears to correlate better with the potential for spontaneous recovery from aplasia (Bar et al. 1993; van Rhee et al. 1994b).

There is some preliminary evidence that aplasia can be prevented by introducing therapy with leukocyte transfusions at the stage of molecular or cytogenetic relapse when significant residual donor hemopoiesis is still present in BM (Bar et al. 1993; van Rhee et al. 1994b). This may be of considerable importance and obviate the need for a second stem-cell infusion.

It is of interest to note that only half of the patients treated in hematological relapse develop aplasia and a period of pancytopenia is not a sine qua non for the repopulation of the marrow by donor-type hemopoiesis. Infusion of hemopoietic stem cells with the lymphocyte collection could in principle prevent or reduce the period of pancytopenia, although stem-cell engraftment might not occur in all instances due to competition with leukemia stem cells for BM niches. Pretreatment of the donor with G-CSF (see Chapter 12) would allow for the simultaneous collection of both lymphocytes and adequate numbers of stem cells at the time of leukapheresis.

■ FUTURE PROSPECTS

The experience with donor lymphocyte therapy for relapsed CML and EBV-lymphoproliferative disorder illustrates the enormous potential for the use of adoptive immunotherapy after BMT. The availability of effective treatment for relapse of CML will renew the interest in T-cell depletion for the initial transplant procedure. This offers the prospect of infusing specific numbers of T cells after the transplant either at predetermined intervals or guided by leukemia-specific transcript levels measured by competitive PCR.

The antileukemic effect mediated by allogeneic cells is very powerful, but immunotherapy is not selective and still carries significant risk to the patient. Neither the target antigens nor the effector cells involved in GVL are well defined. The important challenge is to elucidate the immunological mechanisms responsible for GVHD and GVL that could result in novel treatment strategies. Selection and/or amplification of leukemia-selective or -specific GVL responses could allow for the separation of GVHD and GVL. Cytotoxic donor T cells specific to CMV have been generated and expanded in vitro (Riddell et al. 1992). Infusion of these cells produces detectable levels of anti-CMV activity, but it is not certain if this translates into clinical benefit. The Ph chromosome carries the *bcr/abl* oncogene that encodes a p210 *bcr/abl* protein with tyrosine kinase activity. The fusion region of this peptide is unique to leukemia cells and could potentially serve as a leukemia-specific Ag. It has been suggested that the *bcr/abl* peptide, after presentation by HLA class I or II at the cell surface, could elicit a leukemia-specific T-cell response. There is some evidence for the existence of specific T-cell responses directed at *bcr/abl* synthetic peptides (Chen et al. 1992; ten Bosch et al. 1993), but it is not certain if such T cells also recognize CML cells. Cytotoxic T cells selectively reacting with leukemia cells have been generated (Falkenberg et al. 1992), but these cells might not retain their specificity in vivo (Sondel et al. 1994). In addition, there is no augmentation of CTL frequencies directed against *bcr/abl* peptides after BMT for CML (Barrett et al. 1993).

Differences in minor HC Ag are the target for the powerful GVH alloimmune response. Such Ag, if presented by leukemic cells, could also form the basis of the GVL. T-cell clones specific to minor HC Ag on CML progenitors have been raised from HLA-identical donor and recipient pairs (Falkenberg et al. 1991). Minor HC Ag can be restricted to hemopoietic cells (de Buerger et al. 1992), which could explain why some responders do not develop GVHD after donor lymphocyte transfusion.

Deletion of unwanted alloresponses rather than amplification of leukemia-specific T-cell responses may be an alternative approach to separating GVHD and GVL. In the case of CML, non–leukemic-host, PHA-stimulated lymphoblasts, presenting host-specific minor HC Ag, can be used to stimulate donor lymphocytes. Activated donor lymphocyte populations can be deleted by use of a ricin-conjugated anti-

CD25 mAB. After depletion, proliferative responses to CML cells were preserved, while responses to the patient's lymphocytes were abrogated (Datta et al. 1994). The transduction of a thymidine kinase suicide gene into lymphocytes prior to immunotherapy may also prove useful in the control of GVHD (Tiberghien et al. 1994) and has already been reported in a patient treated for EBV lymphoma (Servida et al. 1993).

REFERENCES

Antin, J.H. (1993) Graft-versus-leukemia: no longer an epiphenomenon. *Blood*, **82**, 2273–7.

Antin, J.H., Bierer, B.E., Smith, B.R., et al. (1991) Selective depletion of bone marrow T lymphocytes with anti-CD5 monoclonal antibodies: effective prophylaxis for graft-versus-host disease in patients with hematological malignancies. *Blood*, **78**, 2139–49.

Apperley, J.F., Rassool, F., Parreira, A., et al. (1986) Philadelphia-positive metaphases in the marrow after bone marrow transplantation for chronic granulocytic leukemia. *American Journal of Hematology*, **22**, 199–204.

Arcese, W., Goldman, J.M., D'Arcangelo, E., et al. (1993) Outcome for patients who relapse after allogeneic bone marrow transplantation for chronic myeloid leukemia. *Blood*, **82**, 3211–9.

Arthur, C.K., Apperley, J.F., Guo, A.P., Rassool, F., Gao, L.M., and Goldman, J.M. (1988) Cytogenetic events after bone marrow transplantation for chronic myeloid leukemia in chronic phase. *Blood*, **71**, 1179–86.

Balkwill, F.R. (1989) Interferons. *Lancet*, **1**, 1060–3.

Bar, B.M., Schattenberg, A., Mensink, E.J., et al. (1993) Donor leukocyte infusions for chronic myeloid leukemia relapsed after allogeneic bone marrow transplantation. *Journal of Clinical Oncology*, **11**, 513–9.

Barnes, D.W. and Loutit, J.F. (1957) Treatment of murine leukemia with X-rays and homologous bone marrow. *British Medical Journal*, **3**, 241–52.

Barrett, A.J., Guimaraes, A., Cullis, J.O., and Goldman, J.M. (1993) Immunological characterization of the tumor specific bcr/abl junction of Philadelphia chromosome positive chronic myeloid leukemia. *Stem Cells*, **11**, 104–8.

Barrett, A.J., Locatelli, F., Treleaven, J.G., Gratwohl, A., Szydlo, R.M., and Zwaan, F.E. (1991) Second transplants for leukemic relapse after bone marrow transplantation: high early mortality but favourable effect of chronic GVHD on continued remission. *British Journal of Haematology*, **79**, 567–74.

Bourgault, I., Gomez, A., Gomard, E., and Levy, J.P. (1991) Limiting-dilution analysis of the HLA restriction of anti-Epstein-Barr virus specific cytolytic T lymphocytes. *Clinical and Experimental Immunology*, **84**, 501–7.

Chen, W., Peace, B.J., Rovira, D.K., You, S.G., and Cheever, M.A. (1992) T-cell immunity to the joining region of the p210 BCR-ABL protein. *Proceedings of the National Academy of Sciences of the United States of America*, **89**, 1468–71.

Collins, R.H., Jr., Rogers, Z.R., Bennett, M., Kumar, V., Nikein, A., and Fay, J.W. (1992) Hematological relapse of chronic myelogenous leukemia following allogeneic bone marrow transplantation: apparent graft-versus-leukemia effect following abrupt discontinuation of immunosuppression. *Bone Marrow Transplantation*, **10**, 391–5.

Cross, N.C., Feng, L., Chase, A., Bungey, J., Hughes, T.P., and Goldman, J.M. (1993b) Competitive polymerase chain reaction to estimate the number of BCR-ABL transcripts in chronic myeloid leukemia after bone marrow transplantation. *Blood*, **82**, 1929–36.

Cross, N.C., Hughes, T.P., Feng, L., et al. (1993a) Minimal residual disease after allogeneic bone marrow transplantation for chronic myeloid leukemia in first chronic phase: correlations with acute graft-versus-host disease and relapse. *British Journal of Haematology*, **84**, 67–74.

Cullis, J.O., Jiang, Y.Z., Schwarer, A.P., Hughes, T.P., Barrett, A.J., and Goldman, J.M. (1992) Donor leukocyte infusions for chronic myeloid leukemia in relapse after allogeneic bone marrow transplantation. *Blood*, **79**, 1379–81.

Datta, A.R., Jiang, Y.Z., Gordon, A.A., et al. (1994) Distinct donor T-cell populations distinguish between lymphocytes and myeloid cells in marrow recipients with chronic myeloid leukemia. *Bone Marrow Transplantation*, **14**, 517–24.

de Buerger, M., Bakker, A., van Rood, J.J., van der Woude, F., and Goulmy, E. (1992) Tissue distribution of minor histocompatibility antigens. Ubiquitous versus restricted tissue distribution indicates heterogeneity amongst human cytotoxic T lymphocyte-defined non-MHC antigens. *Journal of Immunology*, **149**, 1788–94.

Dowding, C., Guo, A.P., Osterholz, J., Siczkowski, M., Goldman, J., and Gordon, M. (1991) Interferon-alpha overrides the deficient adhesion of chronic myeloid leukemia primitive progenitor cells to bone marrow stromal cells. *Blood*, **78**, 499–505.

Drobyski, W.R., Keever, C.A., Roth, M.S., et al. (1993) Salvage immunotherapy using donor leukocyte infusions as treatment for relapsed chronic myelogenous leukemia after allogeneic bone marrow transplantation: efficacy and toxicity of a defined T-cell dose. *Blood*, **82**, 2310–18.

Faber, L.M., van Luxemburg-Heijs, S.A., Willemze, R., and Falkenburg, J.H. (1992) Generation of leukemia-reactive cytotoxic T lymphocyte clones from the HLA-identical bone marrow donor of a patient with leukemia. *Journal of Experimental Medicine*, **176**, 1283–9.

Falkenburg, J.H., Goselink, H.M., van der Harst, D., et al. (1991) Growth inhibition of clonogenic leukemic precursor cells by minor histocompatibility antigen-specific cytotoxic T lymphocytes. *Journal of Experimental Medicine*, **174**, 27–33.

Feng, L., Cross, N.C., van Rhee, F., Chase, A., Bungey, J., and Goldman, J.M. (1994) Molecular monitoring of transient relapse after allogeneic BMT for CML. *20th Annual Meeting of EBMT*, Harrogate, UK, March 1994, abstr. 522.

Fischer, A., Blanche, S., Le Bidois, J., et al. (1991) Anti-B-cell monoclonal antibodies in the treatment of severe B-cell lymphoproliferative syndrome following bone marrow and organ transplantation. *New England Journal of Medicine*, **324**, 1451–6.

Garicochea, B., van Rhee, F., Spencer, A., et al. (1994) Aplasia after donor lymphocyte infusion (DLI) in relapse after sex-mismatched BMT: recovery of donor-type haematopoiesis predicted for by non-isotopic in situ hybridisation. *British Journal of Haematology*, **88**, 400–2.

Giralt, S., Escudier, S., Kantarjian, H., et al. (1993) Preliminary results of treatment with filgrastim for relapse of leukemia and myelodysplasia after allogeneic bone marrow transplantation. *New England Journal of Medicine*, **329**, 757–61.

Goldman, J.M., Apperley, J.F., Jones, L., et al. (1986) Bone marrow transplantation for patients with chronic myeloid leukemia. *New England Journal of Medicine*, **314**, 202–7.

Goldman, J.M., Gale, R.P., Horowitz, M.M., et al. (1988) Bone marrow transplantation for chronic myelogenous leukemia in chronic phase. Increased risk for relapse associated with T-cell depletion. *Annals of Internal Medicine*, **108**, 806–14.

Hale, G.H. and Waldmann, H. (1994) Campath-1 antibodies in bone marrow transplantation. *Journal of Hematotherapy*, **3**, 5–31.

Herberman, R.B., Ortaldo, J.R., Rubinstein, M., and Pestka, S. (1981) Augmentation of natural and antibody-dependent cell-mediated cytotoxicity by pure human leukocyte interferon after allogeneic bone marrow transplantation. *Journal of Clinical Immunology*, **1**, 149–53.

Hertenstein, B., Wiesneth, M., Novotny, J., et al. (1993) Interferon-alpha and donor buffy coat transfusions for treatment of relapsed chronic myeloid leukemia after allogeneic bone marrow transplantation. *Transplantation*, **56**, 1114–18.

Higano, C.S., Raskind, W.H., and Singer, J.W. (1992) Use of alpha interferon for the treatment of relapse of chronic myelogenous leukemia in chronic phase after allogenic bone marrow transplantation. *Blood*, **80**, 1437–42.

Horowitz, M.M., Gale, R.P., Sondel, P.M., et al. (1990) Graft-versus-leukemia reactions after bone marrow transplantation. *Blood*, **75**, 555–62.

Hughes, T.P., Morgan, G.J., Martiat, P., and Goldman, J.M. (1991) Detection of residual leukemia after bone marrow transplant for chronic myeloid leukemia: role of polymerase chain reaction in predicting relapse. *Blood*, **77**, 874–8.

Johnson, B.D., Drobyski, W.R., and Truitt, R.L. (1993) Delayed infusion of normal donor cells after MHC-matched bone marrow transplantation provides an antileukemia reaction without graft-versus-host disease. *Bone Marrow Transplantation*, **11**, 329–36.

Kernan, N.A., Collins, N.H., Juliano, L., Cartagena, T., Dupont, B., and O'Reilly, R.J. (1986) Clonable T lymphocytes in T cell-depleted bone marrow transplants correlate with development of graft-v-host disease. *Blood*, **68**, 770–3.

Kolb, H.J., Mittermuller, J., Clemm, C., et al. (1990) Donor leukocyte transfusions for treatment of recurrent chronic myelogenous leukemia in marrow transplant patients. *Blood*, **76**, 2462–5.

Kolb, H.J., Schattenberg, A., Goldman, J.M., et al. (1995) Graft-versus-leukemia effect of donor lymphocyte transfusion in marrow grafted patients. *Blood*, **86**, 2041–50.

Lee, M.S., Kantarjian, H., Talpaz, M., et al. (1992) Detection of minimal residual disease by polymerase chain reaction in Philadelphia chromosome-positive chronic myelogenous leukemia following interferon therapy. *Blood*, **79**, 1920–3.

Lion, T. on behalf of the European Investigators on Chronic Myeloid Leukemia Group. (1994) Clinical implications of qualitative and quantitative polymerase chain reaction analysis in the monitoring of patients with chronic myelogenous leukemia. *Bone Marrow Transplantation*, **14**, 505–9.

Lion, T., Henn, T., Gaiger, A., Kahls, P., and Gadner, H. (1993) Early detection of relapse after bone marrow transplantation in patients with chronic myelogenous leukemia. *Lancet*, **341**, 275–6.

Lowenberg, B., Wagemaker, G., van Bekkum, D.W., et al. (1986) Graft-versus-host disease following transplantation of 'one log' versus 'two log' T-lymphocyte-depleted bone marrow from HLA-identical donors. *Bone Marrow Transplantation*, **1**, 133–40.

MacKinnon, S., Papadopoulos, E.B., and Carabasi, M.H., et al. (1995) Adoptive immunotherapy evaluating escalating doses of donor leukocytes for relapse of chronic myeloid leukemia after bone marrow transplantation: separation of graft-versus-leukemia responses from graft-versus-host disease. *Blood*, **86**, 1261–8.

Mrsic, M., Horowitz, M.M., Atkinson, K., et al. (1992) Second HLA-identical sibling transplants for leukemia recurrence. *Bone Marrow Transplantation*, **9**, 269–75.

Opalka, B., Wandl, U.B., Becher, R., et al. (1991) Minimal residual disease in patients with chronic myelogenous leukemia undergoing long-term treatment with recombinant interferon alpha-2b alone or in combination with interferon-gamma. *Blood*, **78**, 2188–93.

Papadopoulos, E.B., Lananyi, M., Emanuel, D., et al. (1994) Infusions of donor leukocytes to treat Epstein-Barr virus-associated lymphoproliferative disorders after allogeneic bone marrow transplantation. *New England Journal of Medicine*, **330**, 1185–91.

Porter, D.L., Roth, M.S., McGarigle, C., Ferrara, J.L., and Antin, J.H. (1993) Induction of graft-versus-host disease as immunotherapy for relapsed chronic myeloid leukemia. *New England Journal of Medicine*, **33**, 100–6.

Riddell, S.R., Watanabe, K.S., Goodrich, J.M., Li, C.R., Agha, M.E., and Greenberg, P.D. (1992) Restoration of viral immunity in immunodeficient humans by the adoptive transfer of T cell clones. *Science*, **257**, 238–41.

Rooney, C.M., Smith, C.A., Ng, C.Y.C., et al. (1995) Use of gene-modified virus-specific T lymphocytes to control Epstein-Barr-virus-related lymphoproliferation. *Lancet*, **345**, 9–13.

Servida, P., Rossini, S., Traversari, C., et al. (1993) Gene transfer into peripheral blood lymphocytes for in vivo modulation of donor antitumor immunity in a patient affected by EBV lymphoma. *35th Annual meeting of the American Society of Hematology*, St Louis, MO, 1993, abstr. 843.

Sullivan, K.M., Storb, R., Buckner, D., et al. (1989) Graft-versus-host disease as adoptive immunotherapy in patients with advanced hematological neoplasms. *New England Journal of Medicine*, **320**, 828–34.

Talpaz, M., Kantarjian, H., Kurzrock, R., Trujillo, J.M., and Gutterman, J.U. (1991) Interferon-alpha produces sustained cytogenetic responses in Philadelphia chromosome-positive chronic myelogenous leukemia patients. *Annals of Internal Medicine*, **114**, 532–8.

ten Bosch, G.J., Toomvliet, A.C., Melief, C.J., and Leeksma, O.C. (1993) Specific recognition of peptides corresponding to the joining region of p210 BCR-ABL by human T-cells. *Blood*, **82**, 521a.

Thomas, E.D., Clift, R.A., Fefer, A., et al. (1986) Marrow transplantation for the treatment of chronic myelogenous leukemia. *Annals of Internal Medicine*, **104**, 155–63.

Tiberghien, P., Reynolds, C.W., Keller, J., et al. (1994) Ganciclovir treatment of herpes simplex thymidine kinase-transduced primary T lymphocytes:

an approach for specific in vivo donor T-cell depletion after bone marrow transplantation. *Blood*, **84**, 1333–41.

Uphadhyaya, G., Gupta, S.C., Sih, S.A., et al. (1991) Interferon-alpha reduces the deficient expression of the cytoadhesion molecule lymphocyte antigen-3 by chronic myelogenous leukemia cells. *Journal of Clinical Investigation*, **88**, 2131–6.

van Rhee, F., Lin, F., Cross, N.C., et al. (1994a) Detection of residual leukaemia more than 10 years after allogeneic bone marrow transplantation for chronic myelogenous leukaemia. *Bone Marrow Transplantation*, **14**, 609–13.

van Rhee, F., Lin, F., Cullis, J.O., et al. (1994b) Relapse of chronic myeloid leukemia after allogeneic bone marrow transplant: the case for giving donor lymphocyte transfusions before the onset of hematological relapse. *Blood*, **83**, 3377–83.

Weiden, P.L., Flournoy, N., Thomas, E.D., et al. (1979) Antileukemic effect of graft-versus-host disease in human recipients of allogeneic marrow grafts. *New England Journal of Medicine*, **300**, 1068–73.

Weiden, P.L., Storb, R., Tsoi, M.S., Graham, T.C., Lerner, K.G., and Thomas, E.D. (1976) Infusion of donor lymphocytes into stable canine radiation chimeras: implications for mechanism of transplantation tolerance. *Journal of Immunology*, **116**, 1212–9.

Weiden, P.L., Sullivan, K.M., Flournoy, N., Storb, R., and Thomas, E.D. (1981) Antileukemic effect of graft-versus-host disease: contribution to improved survival after allogeneic marrow transplantation. *New England Journal of Medicine*, **304**, 1529–33.

Zaccaria, A., Rosti, G., Sessarego, M., et al. (1988) Relapse after allogeneic bone marrow transplantation for Philadelphia chromosome positive chronic myeloid leukemia: cytogenetic analysis of 24 patients. *Bone Marrow Transplantation*, **3**, 413–23.

Zutter, M.M., Martin, P.J., Sale, G.E., et al. (1988) Epstein-Barr virus lymphoproliferation after bone marrow transplantation. *Blood*, **72**, 520–9.

Graft-Versus-Leukemia Effect in Bone-Marrow Transplantation

DAVID L. PORTER AND JOSEPH H. ANTIN

The treatment of hematological malignancies with allogeneic bone-marrow transplantation (BMT) involves the administration of myeloablative doses of chemotherapy and radiation to patients, followed by the infusion of normal donor bone marrow (BM) to allow hemopoietic reconstitution; however, despite the very intensive conditioning therapy, small numbers of residual leukemia cells often survive that ultimately can lead to clinical relapse. Residual malignant cells would be expected to survive, since chemotherapy and radiation kill cells by first-order kinetics; fortunately, fewer relapses are seen than might be anticipated. Seemingly, other factors are involved in eradicating residual disease. It is now clear that the donor BM can result in an antitumor reaction independent of the conditioning regimen. This graft-versus-leukemia (GVL) effect appears to be mediated by the adoptive transfer of immunocompetent donor cells present in the marrow graft, and is an important component of successful allogeneic BMT. The rationale for some of the earliest clinical trials of BMT were based on the use of allogeneic BM as adoptive immunotherapy, and not just as a convenient source for hemopoietic rescue after myeloablative therapy (Mathe et al. 1965).

Over the past four decades, the GVL reaction has been studied and defined in detail in animal models of transplantation. It has been more difficult to unequivocally demonstrate a GVL reaction in humans, and for many years the evidence for significant GVL in clinical BMT has been largely circumstantial. Recently, the successful use of donor mononuclear cell (MNC) infusions to reestablish remission in patients with relapsed leukemia after BMT has provided a direct demonstration of the clinical potency of the GVL reaction. The target antigens (Ag) and the effector cells and/or molecules responsible for

GVL still remain largely undefined. It is also unclear whether the GVL effects are separable from the generalized graft-versus-host reaction; attempts to prevent graft-versus-host disease (GVHD) often result in a loss of the GVL effect, and attempts to enhance GVL often result in greater toxicity from GVHD. Ultimately, the ability to harness the GVL effects of donor cells for clinical benefit independent of the toxic GVHD reaction may allow allogeneic BMT to be performed for greater numbers of patients in a safer, more effective manner.

■ DEFINING THE GRAFT-VERSUS-LEUKEMIA REACTION IN ANIMAL MODELS

It has been suspected since the earliest experiments in BMT that adoptive transfer of the donor immune system could contribute to the cure of leukemia. Barnes and colleagues first demonstrated that leukemic mice treated with a subtherapeutic dose of radiation were more likely to be cured if they received an allogeneic rather than a syngeneic donor BM graft (Barnes et al. 1956; Barnes and Loutit 1957). These experiments also demonstrated that mice receiving allogeneic grafts, though less likely to relapse, developed a lethal wasting syndrome now recognized as GVHD. These observations revealed for the first time the importance of the GVL effect for eradicating residual leukemia and highlighted the intimate relationship between GVL and GVHD. After 40 years of investigation, the ability to control GVHD without sacrificing the critical GVL effects remains a difficult and central challenge for successful BMT.

Murine models of BMT have been useful to dissect out the critical components responsible for GVHD and GVL. It is now generally accepted that donor T cells mediate acute GVHD (Korngold and Sprent 1987). In some models, the same subset of T cells are responsible for GVL, and the beneficial antileukemic properties of the donor cells are inseparable from the toxic GVHD effects (Truitt, LeFever, and Shih 1987). In other systems, it has been possible to separate GVL from GVHD (Slavin et al. 1981; Truitt et al. 1983; Sykes, Romick, and Sachs 1990; Truitt et al. 1990). For instance, Sykes and colleagues (1990) have developed a model of fully mismatched BMT (A/J into B10 across major histocompatibility complex [HC] barriers) where GVHD and GVL are induced by different lymphocyte populations. They have shown that the CD4$^+$ subset of donor T cells primarily mediates GVHD, while the CD8$^+$ T cells are necessary for GVL effects (Sykes et al. 1993); however, in the strain combination A/J into *balb/c*, both CD4$^+$ and CD8$^+$ appear to contribute to GVL (Sykes et al. 1994). Furthermore, the administration of a brief course of interleukin-2 (IL-2) early in the transplant to these mice minimized GVHD while preserving GVL, largely through selective inhibition of the $CD4^+$ T cells (Sykes et al. 1993, 1990).

In another extensively studied murine model, Truitt et al. (1983) have also shown that donor T cells mediate the GVL reaction after allogeneic BMT; however, these cells were only effective if obtained from donor mice that had been preimmunized against host Ag (Truitt et al. 1983, 1990). Interestingly, alloimmunization before adoptive transfer does not necessarily result in an increase in GVHD, implying that GVHD and GVL may also be separable in this model. In this system, a distinct population of activated killer cells were also identified with GVL reactivity. These investigators have isolated cell clones that will cause a lethal GVHD reaction, and others that will mediate GVL effects, further supporting the conclusion that, at least in mice, GVL and GVHD reactivity may be separable.

These examples highlight that while murine models are extremely useful for modeling GVL, the conclusions regarding the effector cells causing GVHD and GVL must be evaluated with caution. It seems clear that experimental results may vary depending on the leukemia model, the mouse strain combinations under study, and on the degree of HC variation between the donor and host. Effectors likely to be important for GVL reactivity might include cytotoxic T cells, natural killer (NK) cells that function in a major HC-unrestricted manner, and cytokines elaborated by activated lymphocytes (Slavin, Eckerstein, and Weiss 1988). It is most likely that more than one cell population or effector mechanism is responsible for the GVL reaction, and different effectors may be of varying importance depending on the model system under investigation. Another caveat is that many of these studies were done using virally induced leukemia, and the role of a specific antiviral effect is difficult to exclude. While these models will continue to serve as a useful guide, they may not be directly applicable for clinical use.

■ EVIDENCE FOR A GRAFT-VERSUS-LEUKEMIA REACTION IN CLINICAL MARROW TRANSPLANTATION

Despite the demonstration of a GVL reaction in murine models, it has been difficult to identify a direct GVL effect in clinical BMT. Although retrospective data are very suggestive that the GVL effect may be crucial for successful BMT for some patients, until recently the evidence has been largely circumstantial, and primarily has con-

Table 31.1. Indirect Evidence for a Graft-Versus-Leukemia Reaction in Clinical Bone-Marrow Transplantation

- Abrupt withdrawal of immunosuppression, or a flare of graft-versus-host disease, may reestablish remission in patients with relapsed leukemia after BMT (anecdotal).
- Syngeneic marrow grafts are associated with a higher risk of relapse than allogeneic marrow grafts.
- Graft-versus-host disease after BMT is associated with a lower risk of relapse.

sisted of three indirect but important clinical observations (Table 31.1). The first line of evidence comes from several anecdotal reports of patients who relapsed with leukemia after allogeneic BMT but reentered remission associated with either a flare of GVHD (Odom et al. 1978), or after rapid withdrawal of immunosuppression (Sullivan and Shulman 1989; Higano et al. 1990; Collins et al. 1992). Although intriguing, only a very small number of such cases have been reported, and many patients with relapse undoubtedly do not respond to withdrawal of immunosuppression, even when a flare of GVHD can be induced.

The second clinical observation implicating an important GVL component of allogeneic BMT is that recipients of syngeneic BM grafts have a significantly higher risk of leukemic relapse compared with patients receiving allogeneic BM grafts. This effect was first suggested by the Seattle group (Weiden et al. 1979). An update of these data compared 785 recipients of HLA-matched allogeneic BM grafts with 53 recipients of syngeneic BM, and confirmed the higher probability of relapse after syngeneic BMT (Fefer et al. 1987). For patients with acute myeloid leukemia (AML), Gale and Champlin (1984) reported that transplantation with syngeneic marrow was associated with an almost threefold higher risk of relapse compared with allogeneic marrow grafting. This finding has also been confirmed in large retrospective analyses from the International Bone Marrow Transplant Registry (IBMTR) (Horowitz et al. 1990; Gale et al. 1994) (Fig. 31.1).

The IBMTR data have further suggested that recipients of syngeneic BM have a higher risk of relapse independent of GVHD, implying that an allogeneic graft is associated with a significant GVL effect that may be separable from GVHD (Horowitz et al. 1990; Gale et al. 1994) This is seen in Figure 31.1, where the probability of relapse for 70

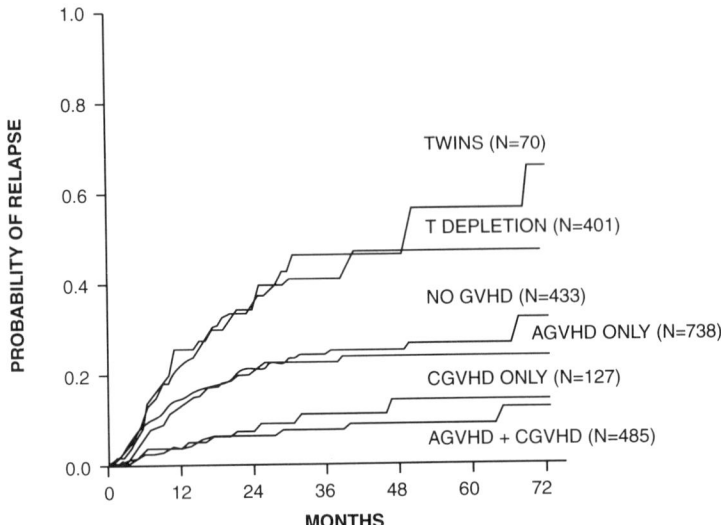

Figure 31.1 Probability of relapse after BMT depending on the type of graft and the extent of GVHD. (Reprinted with permission from Horowitz et al. 1990.)

recipients of syngeneic grafts was higher than for 433 recipients of allogeneic grafts who did not experience clinical GVHD. These findings have been noted both in standard-risk patients transplanted with AML in first remission or chronic myeloid leukemia (CML) in chronic phase (Gale and Champlin 1984; Horowitz et al. 1990) and for patients at high risk for relapse (BMT performed for AML or acute lymphocytic leukemia [ALL] in second or greater remission, or at relapse) (Fefer et al. 1987). It is noteworthy that while some analyses demonstrate similar findings for patients with ALL transplanted in first remission, a recent update from the IBMTR found no significant increase in the relapse rate following syngeneic BMT for these patients (Gale et al. 1994).

The higher risk of relapse after syngeneic BM grafting suggests that HC Ag may be important and necessary for a GVL reaction. Many authors caution against overinterpretation of these findings, however. Although the conditioning regimens tend to be similar, recipients of non–T-cell–depleted allogeneic BM grafts typically receive methotrexate, with or without cyclosporine, as GVHD prophylaxis; recipients of syngeneic grafts receive no such therapy. Although the total dose of methotrexate is relatively low, it is difficult to exclude the unlikely possibility that antileukemic effects of either GVHD prophylaxis or GVHD therapy contribute to the GVL effects of allogeneic BMT. Another improbable explanation for a higher rate of relapse after syngeneic BMT is that leukemia could arise from donor cells; these cells might be impossible to distinguish from the recipients' original leukemia in syngeneic twins.

Finally, there are considerable data demonstrating that GVHD is protective against relapse after BMT, suggesting that GVL and GVHD are similar or overlapping processes. Data from the Seattle group show that patients transplanted with advanced leukemia (AML or ALL in relapse or CML in accelerated phase or blast crisis) who develop acute and/or chronic GVHD have a lower risk of relapse compared with patients who have no GVHD (Weiden et al. 1979; Sullivan et al. 1989c). Similar results have been demonstrated for both high-risk and standard-risk patients (Goldman et al. 1988). The IBMTR summarized the risk of relapse after BMT for more than 2,200 patients transplanted with early leukemia (AML or ALL in first remission or CML in chronic phase) (Horowitz et al. 1990) (Table 31.2). The development of acute and chronic GVHD was associated with a lower risk of relapse compared with patients who developed no GVHD. The magnitude of the protective effects of GVHD against relapse appear to be disease dependent. For instance, the IBMTR data showed that for patients receiving unmanipulated donor BM grafts, acute GVHD was protective against relapse for patients with ALL, while the combination of acute and chronic GVHD was protective against relapse for patients with ALL, AML, and CML (Table 31.2). Taken together, these clinical observations provide important but indirect evidence to suggest that allogeneic bone marrow supplies a significant immune-mediated antileukemic effect.

■ WHAT ARE THE EFFECTOR CELLS FOR THE GRAFT-VERSUS-LEUKEMIA REACTION IN HUMANS?

The identity of the effector cells for GVL remains unknown, but it is likely that more than one cell type participates in the antileukemic reaction. Current data support the conclusion that at least a subset of donor T cells are involved in generating the GVL effect. Because donor T cells are critical effectors of GVHD, T-cell depletion of the donor BM graft has been used as one of the most successful means of limiting the occurrence and severity of GVHD (Maraninchi

Table 31.2. Relative Risk of Relapse After Allogeneic Bone-Marrow Transplantation[a]

Patient Group	ALL (p)	AML (p)	CML (p)	All Patients (p)
Allogeneic, non–T-depleted				
No GVHD	1.00	1.00	1.00	1.00
Acute GVHD only	0.36 (0.004)	0.78 (0.26)	1.15 (0.75)	0.68 (0.03)
Chronic GVHD only	0.44 (0.16)	0.48 (0.12)	0.28 (0.16)	0.43 (0.01)
Acute and chronic GVHD	0.38 (0.02)	0.34 (0.0003)	0.24 (0.03)	0.33 (0.0001)
Allogeneic, T-depleted				
All patients	1.20 (0.61)	1.30 (0.33)	5.14 (0.0001)	1.76 (0.002)
No GVHD	1.48 (0.33)	1.57 (0.12)	6.91 (0.0001)	2.14 (0.0001)
Acute and/or chronic GVHD	0.98 (0.97)	0.80 (0.60)	4.45 (0.003)	1.32 (0.25)

[a]Adapted from Horowitz et al. 1990, with permission.

et al. 1987; Apperley et al. 1988; Antin et al. 1991; Marmont et al. 1991; Soiffer et al. 1992). Although pan–T-cell depletion of the donor BM improves peritransplant-related mortality rates as initially anticipated, there is a significant increase in subsequent relapse rates (Maraninchi et al. 1987; Apperley et al. 1988; Horowitz et al. 1990; Marmont et al. 1991), and overall long-term survival remains unchanged. This suggests that there are similar or overlapping effector mechanisms for the GVHD and GVL reactions, and that loss of GVHD after T-cell depletion is accompanied by a loss of vital GVL mechanisms. For unclear reasons, this GVL effect of donor T cells is most significant in patients transplanted for CML (Table 31.2). There is a 6.9-fold increase in relative risk of relapse for recipients of T-cell–depleted allografts who have no GVHD compared with patients who receive unmanipulated grafts and develop no GVHD (Horowitz et al. 1990). To further support the role of T cells in the GVL reaction, it has been noted that the presence of greater numbers of circulating cytotoxic T-cell precursors directed against the patients' leukemia cells after BMT may correlate with leukemia-free survival (Jiang et al. 1991). Furthermore, T-cell–depletion strategies that leave NK cells behind (e.g., CD5 or CD6 purging) still have high relapse rates (Antin et al. 1991; Soiffer et al. 1992). Taken together, these observations implicate donor T cells as effective mediators of both GVL and GVHD.

It is likely that $CD4^+$ cells are at least one subset of T cells that are important for the GVL reaction. For instance, some patients will have $CD4^+$ T cells that will specifically lyse leukemic cells in vitro (Sosman et al. 1990; Jiang et al. 1991). Nimer et al. (1994) have reported that allografts selectively depleted of $CD8^+$ T cells result in a low incidence of GVHD, yet preserve a GVL effect similar to allogeneic donor BM. While these findings do not directly implicate $CD4^+$ cells in the GVL reaction, they suggest that $CD8^+$ cells may not be necessary.

Another likely candidate effector-cell population participating in the GVL reaction is NK cells. NK cells can lyse cells of the CML-derived cell line K562 in vitro, and NK cell numbers and activity are increased in the peripheral blood (PB) after BMT (Reittie et al. 1989; Hauch et al. 1990). The NK cells isolated from some patients after BMT are capable of lysing cryopreserved host leukemic cells (Hauch et al. 1990; Jiang et al. 1993) and inhibiting leukemic progenitor colony growth (Mackinnon, Hows, and Goldman 1990). In recipients of T-cell–depleted allografts for CML, the ability of IL-2–stimulated peripheral blood MNC to lyse leukemic targets may correlate with subsequent risk of relapse (Hauch et al. 1990).

▪ ADOPTIVE IMMUNOTHERAPY WITH DONOR MONONUCLEAR CELL INFUSIONS: A DIRECT DEMONSTRATION OF A GRAFT-VERSUS-LEUKEMIA REACTION

The evidence discussed above for a clinically significant GVL reaction has been indirect. Recently, several groups have provided direct evidence for a GVL reaction by administering donor MNC to patients with relapsed leukemia without additional chemoradiotherapy. Kolb et al. (1990) first reported that three patients with CML in relapse after allogeneic BMT achieved complete cytogenetic remissions following the administration of IFN-α and infusions of buffy coat cells obtained from the original BM donor. These results have since been confirmed and expanded at several transplant centers, and donor MNC infusions have now been used to treat more than 100 patients with relapsed leukemia worldwide (Kolb et al. 1990; Frassoni et al. 1992; Bar et al. 1993; Drobyski et al. 1993; Helg et al. 1993; Hertenstein et al. 1993; Kolb et al. 1993a; Szer et al. 1993; van Rhee et al. 1993; Porter et al. 1994b, c). Donor MNC infusions have typically been given with a short course of IFN-α, although the contribution of IFN-α to the antileukemic effect remains unclear (Kolb et al. 1993b; Porter and Antin 1994). The donor MNC, with or without IFN-α, provide a direct and very potent GVL effect. Complete remissions have been obtained in 60% to 80% of patients with relapse of CML treated in the CP of the disease (Table 31.3, and reviewed by Kolb et al. 1993b; Porter and Antin 1994). The dramatic antileukemic effect of donor MNC is further highlighted by the fact that the majority of patients who achieve complete cytogenetic remissions have no cells with detectable *bcr/abl* mRNA transcripts when assayed by reverse transcriptase polymerase chain reaction (RT-PCR) (Bar et al. 1993; Drobyski et al. 1993; Helg et al. 1993; Hertenstein et al. 1993; van Rhee et al. 1993; Porter et al. 1994b). This assay is capable of detecting one leukemic cell in 10^6 normal cells (Roth et al. 1992). For patients with CML, this likely represents at least a 6-log reduction in leukemic cells (Antin 1993).

Donor MNC are given without GVHD prophylaxis, and the majority of patients who respond also develop acute and chronic GVHD; however, acute GVHD tends to be generally mild to moderate (grade 0 to 2), and the severity appears to be less than might be anticipated considering the dose of T cells administered may be up to ten times more than that typically contained in an unmodified marrow graft. It is intriguing that several patients have achieved complete remissions (CR) without developing clinical GVHD, further suggesting that

Table 31.3. Response to Immunotherapy[a]

Disease	N	Complete Cytogenetic Response	Complete Molecular Response
CML CP	48[b]	33 (69%)	26/44 (59%)
CML AP/BC	9	1/9 (11%)	0/11 (0%)
Acute leukemia, myelodysplasia	11[c]	2/11 (14%)[d]	NA

[a]This table is modified from Porter and Antin (1994) with permission. Data are compiled from published articles and abstracts that provide data on response for patients who received donor mononuclear cell infusions for relapsed leukemia (Kolb et al. 1990; Bar et al. 1993; Drobyski et al. 1993; Helg et al. 1993; Hertenstein et al. 1993; Szer et al. 1993; van Rhee et al. 1993; Porter et al. 1994c). Kolb et al. (1993b) have summarized responses for 81 patients treated at various European centers, and some, but not all of these patients, are included in this table.
[b]The majority of the patients were treated at the time of hematological relapse. Several patients are included who were treated at the time of cytogenetic relapse (Bar et al. 1993; Helg et al. 1993; van Rhee et al. 1993) and one patient was treated at the time of molecular relapse (van Rhee et al. 1993).
[c]Ten patients have been previously reported (Szer et al. 1993; Porter et al. 1994c) and one patient, who was a complete responder, is from unpublished data.
[d]Represents a complete remission. Cytogenetic abnormalities were not reported for most patients.

CML = chronic myelogenous leukemia, CP = chronic phase, AP = accelerated phase, BC = blast crisis, NA = not applicable.

GVHD and GVL may be dissociated (Hertenstein et al. 1993; Kolb et al. 1990; van Rhee et al. 1993). Transient pancytopenia because of BM hypoplasia is a frequent complication and occasionally BM aplasia has occurred (Frassoni et al. 1992; Drobyski et al. 1993; Porter et al. 1994b). It is also notable that donor MNC infusions appear to be most effective when given in earlier stages of relapse, as very few patients with clinically advanced CML (accelerated phase or blast crisis) have achieved CR.

Adoptive immunotherapy with donor MNC infusions appears to be less effective for patients who relapse with diseases other than CML for unclear reasons; however, this finding is in keeping with data from the IBMTR suggesting the GVL reaction is most significant in patients with CML (Horowitz et al. 1990). Only a small number of patients have been treated with donor MNC infusions for relapse of acute leukemia or myelodysplastic syndromes (MDS). Szer et al. (1993) reported only one response in four patients treated with relapsed AML; Kolb et al. (1993a) summarized European experiences and reported complete responses in four of nine patients with AML and in 4 of 11 patients with ALL. A remission was also induced in a patient with relapse of non-Hodgkin's lymphoma (NHL). At Brigham and Women's Hospital, one patient with recurrent refractory anemia entered complete remission, while no responses were noted in six other patients with relapsed acute leukemia or MDS (unpublished results).

Adoptive immunotherapy with donor MNC infusions has also been useful in situations other than relapsed leukemia. Donor MNC have been successfully administered to patients with Epstein-Barr virus (EBV) –related B-cell–lymphoproliferative disease (BLPD) after BMT. These very aggressive lymphomas occur at higher frequency in recipients of T-cell–depleted BM grafts; they are typically donor in origin, and because they are usually unresponsive to standard therapy, they are most often fatal (Shapiro et al. 1988). Donor MNC given to a small number of patients with this disorder have resulted in complete regression of disease and unmaintained remissions in several patients (Papadopoulos et al. 1994; Porter et al. 1994a) In addition, donor MNC infusions have been effective in reversing life-threatening adenovirus infection occurring after BMT (Hromas, Cornetta, and Srour 1994). It should be noted, however, that these situations are not necessarily analogous to the GVL response. The reaction against BLPD is in essence an autologous response (donor cells reactive against donor tumor). Additionally, in each case, prior exposure of the donor to viral antigens likely resulted in generation of precursor cytotoxic T cells at frequencies much higher than those expected against potential leukemic antigens. Therefore, one might predict that lower doses of donor cells would be effective for these complications than are necessary to induce GVL.

■ MANIPULATION OF THE GRAFT-VERSUS-LEUKEMIA REACTION IN CLINICAL MARROW TRANSPLANTATION

Relapse after BMT remains a significant cause of treatment failure, and patients who do relapse have a very poor prognosis (Mrsic et al. 1992; Arcese et al. 1993; Radich et al. 1993). This has prompted several trials investigating methods to enhance the GVL effects at the time of initial transplantation. The Seattle group found that deletion of prophylactic immunosuppression for GVHD resulted in a higher incidence of significant acute GVHD but had no influence on relapse in patients transplanted with advanced leukemia (Sullivan et al. 1986, 1989b); however, preliminary data from another trial have suggested that withholding prophylactic immunosuppression may enhance the GVL effect, resulting in lower relapse rates and a higher probability of survival (Elfenbein et al. 1987). Another approach to enhance the GVL effects at the time of BMT was taken by the Seattle group by either abbreviating the course of prophylactic immunosuppression (methotrexate) or administering donor buffy coat cells at the time of transplantation (Sullivan et al. 1989a). The incidence and severity of acute GVHD was increased in patients receiving abbreviated methotrexate and donor buffy coat, but no effect on relapse or survival could be detected; however, an abbreviated course of methotrexate or donor buffy coat cells resulted in a higher incidence of non–transplant-related mortality. The reasons that a significant GVL effect could not be demonstrated in these studies is not clear, but all patients were transplanted for advanced leukemia and were at very high risk for relapse. It is possible that similar manipulations would yield different results in more standard-risk patients. Additionally, these maneuvers had no influence on the incidence of chronic GVHD, and it is possible that chronic GVHD is more closely associated with the GVL effect than acute GVHD (Weiden et al. 1981).

Several investigators have attempted to enhance the GVL potential associated with NK-cell activity by administering IL-2 after allogeneic or autologous BMT (Verdonck et al. 1991; Slavin et al. 1992; Benyunes et al. 1993; Soiffer et al. 1994). IL-2 administration can result in a tenfold increase in circulating NK cells after BMT (Soiffer et al. 1994), and initial studies suggest that this approach may enhance GVL and protect against relapse in patients receiving T-cell–depleted transplants for hematologic malignancies (Slavin et al. 1992; Soiffer et al. 1994). Randomized controlled trials will be needed to define GVL effects of post-BMT cytokine administration, although these early studies are promising.

■ SUMMARY

It is now clear that the success of allogeneic BMT is related not only to the intensive conditioning regimen, but also to the immune-mediated GVL reaction. Donor T cells appear to be important effector cells for the GVL reaction, as well as for GVHD, but it is also likely that other effector cells (such as NK cells) and/or cytokines are important for the GVL effects. Unfortunately, efforts to enhance GVL often result in additional toxicity from GVHD, and efforts to limit GVHD often result in a loss of important GVL effect. The use of donor MNC for relapsed patients not only provides a direct demonstration of GVL but may also provide a strategy to harness a potent GVL reaction while minimizing GVHD. Ultimately, a better understanding of the target antigens for the GVL response, and a precise definition of the effector cells, may allow the manipulation of GVL for even greater therapeutic benefit.

ACKNOWLEDGMENTS

This work was supported in part by NIH grants CA58661 and CA39542 (Joseph H. Antin). David L. Porter is a Fellow of the Leukemia Society of America.

REFERENCES

Antin, J.H., Bierer, B.E., Smith, B.R., et al. (1991) Selective depletion of bone marrow T lymphocytes with anti-CD5 monoclonal antibodies: effective prophylaxis for graft-versus-host disease in patients with hematologic malignancies. *Blood*, **78**, 2139–49.

Antin, J.H. (1993) Graft-versus-leukemia: no longer an epiphenomenon. *Blood*, **82**, 2273–7.

Apperley, J.F., Mauro, F.R., Goldman, J.M., et al. (1988) Bone marrow transplantation for chronic myeloid leukaemia in first chronic phase: importance of a graft-versus-leukaemia effect. *British Journal of Haematology*, **69**, 239–45.

Arcese, W., Goldman, J.M., D'Arcangelo, E., et al. (1993) Outcome for patients who relapse after allogeneic bone marrow transplantation for chronic myeloid leukemia. *Blood*, **82**, 3211–9.

Bar, B., Schattenberg, A., Mensink, E., et al. (1993) Donor leukocyte infusions for chronic myeloid leukemia relapsed after allogeneic bone marrow transplantation. *Journal of Clinical Oncology*, **11**, 513–9.

Barnes, D., Corp, M., Loutit, J., and Neal, F. (1956) Treatment of murine leukaemia with X rays and homologous bone marrow. Preliminary communication. *British Medical Journal*, **2**, 626–30.

Barnes, D. and Loutit, J. (1957) Treatment of murine leukaemia with X-rays and homologous bone marrow. *British Journal of Haematology*, **3**, 241–52.

Benyunes, M., Massumoto, C., York, A., et al. (1993) Interleukin-2 with or without lymphokine-activated killer cells as consolidative immunotherapy after autologous bone marrow transplantation for acute myelogenous leukemia. *Bone Marrow Transplantation*, **12**, 159–63.

Collins, R.H., Jr., Rogers, Z.R., Bennett, M., Kumar, V., Nikein, A., and Fay, J.W. (1992) Hematologic relapse of chronic myelogenous leukemia following allogeneic bone marrow transplantation: apparent graft-versus-leukemia effect following abrupt discontinuation of immunosuppression. *Bone Marrow Transplantation*, **10**, 391–5.

Cullis, J., Jiang, Y., Schwarer, A., Hughers, T., Barrett, A., and Goldman, J. (1992) Donor leukocyte infusions for chronic myeloid leukemia in relapse after allogeneic bone marrow transplantation. *Blood*, **79**, 1379–80.

Drobyski, W., Keever, C., Roth, M., et al. (1993) Salvage immunotherapy using donor leukocyte infusions as treatment for relapsed chronic myelogenous leukemia after allogeneic bone marrow transplantation: efficacy and toxicity of a defined T-cell dose. *Blood*, **82**, 2310–8.

Elfenbein, G., Graham-Pole, J., Weiner, R., Goedert, T., and Gross, S. (1987) Consequences of no prophylaxis for acute graft-versus-host disease after HLA-identical bone marrow transplantation. *Blood*, **70**, 305a.

Fefer, A., Sullivan, K., Weiden, P., et al. (1987) Graft versus leukemia effect in man: the relapse rate of acute leukemia is lower after allogeneic than after syngeneic marrow transplantation. In R.L. Truitt, R.P. Gale, and M.M. Bortin (Eds.) *Cellular immunotherapy of cancer*, pp. 401–8. New York, Alan R. Liss.

Frassoni, F., Fagioli, F., Sessarego, M., et al. (1992) The effect of donor leucocyte infusion in patients with leukemia following allogeneic bone marrow transplantation. *Experimental Hematology*, **20**, 712a.

Gale, R.P. and Champlin, R.E. (1984) How does bone-marrow transplantation cure leukaemia? *Lancet*, **2**, 28–30.

Gale, R.P., Horowitz, M.M., Ash, R.C., et al. (1994) Identical-twin bone marrow transplants for leukemia. *Annals of Internal Medicine*, **120**, 646–52.

Goldman, J.M., Gale, R.P., Horowitz, M.M., et al. (1988) Bone marrow tranplantation for chronic myelogenous leukemia in chronic phase. Increased risk for relapse associated with T-cell depletion. *Annals of Internal Medicine*, **108**, 806–14.

Hauch, M., Gazzola, M.V., Small, T., et al. (1990) Anti-leukemia potential of interleukin-2 activated natural killer cells after bone marrow tranplantation for chronic myelogenous leukemia. *Blood*, **75**, 2250–62.

Helg, C., Roux, E., Beris, P., et al. (1993) Adoptive immunotherapy for recurrent CML after BMT. *Bone Marrow Transplantation*, **12**, 125–9.

Hertenstein, B., Wiesneth, M., Novotny, J., et al. (1993) Interferon-alpha and donor buffy coat transfusions for treatment of relapsed chronic myeloid leukemia after allogeneic bone marrow transplantation. *Transplantation*, **56**, 1114–18.

Higano, C.S., Brixey, M., Bryant, E.M., et al. (1990) Durable complete remission of acute nonlymphocytic leukemia associated with discontinuation of immunosuppression following relapse after allogeneic bone marrow transplantation. A case report of a probable graft-versus-leukemia effect. *Transplantation*, **50**, 175–7.

Horowitz, M.M., Gale, R.P., Sondel, P.M., et al. (1990) Graft-versus-leukemia reactions after bone marrow transplantation. *Blood*, **75**, 555–62.

Hromas, R., Cornetta, K., and Srour, E. (1994) Donor leukocyte infusion as therapy of life-threatening adenoviral infections after T-cell-depleted bone marrow transplantation. *Blood*, **84**, 1689–90.

Jiang, Y.Z., Kanfer, E.J., MacDonald, D., Cullis, J.O., Goldman, J.M., and Barrett, A.J. (1991) Graft-versus-leukaemia following allogeneic bone marrow transplantation: emergence of cytotoxic T lymphocytes reacting to host leukaemia cells. *Bone Marrow Transplantation*, **8**, 253–8.

Jiang, Y.Z., Cullis, J.O., Kanfer, E.J., Goldman, J.M., and Barrett, A.J. (1993) T cell and NK cell mediated graft-versus-leukaemia reactivity following donor buffy coat transfusion to treat relapse after marrow transplantation for chronic myeloid leukaemia. *Bone Marrow Transplantation*, **11**, 133–8.

Kolb, H.J., Mittermuller, J., Clemm, C., et al. (1990) Donor leukocyte transfusions for treatment of recurrent chronic myelogenous leukemia in marrow transplant patients. *Blood*, **76**, 2462–5.

Kolb, H.J., deWitte, T., Mittermuller, J., et al. (1993a) Graft-versus-leukemia effect of donor buffy coat transfusions on recurrent leukemia after marrow transplantation. *Blood*, **82**, 840a.

Kolb, H.J., Mittermuller, J., Hertenstein, H., et al. (1993b) Adoptive immunotherapy in human and canine chimeras – the role of interferon alfa. *Seminars in Hematology*, **30**, 37–9.

Korngold, R. and Sprent, J. (1987) T cell subsets and graft-versus-host disease. *Transplantation*, **44**, 335–9.

Mackinnon, S., Hows, J.M., and Goldman, J.M. (1990) Induction of in vitro graft-versus-leukemia activity following bone marrow transplantation for chronic myeloid leukemia. *Blood*, **76**, 2037–45.

Maraninchi, D., Gluckman, E., Blaise, D., et al. (1987) Impact of T-cell depletion on outcome of allogeneic bone-marrow transplantation for standard-risk leukaemias. *Lancet*, **2**, 175–8.

Marmont, A.M., Horowitz, M.M., Gale, R.P., et al. (1991) T-cell depletion of HLA-identical transplants in leukemia. *Blood*, **78**, 2120–30.

Mathe, G., Amiel, J., Schwarzenberg, L., Cattan, A., and Schneider, M. (1965) Adoptive immunotherapy of acute leukemia: experimental and clinical results. *Cancer Research*, **25**, 1525–31.

Mrsic, M., Horowitz, M.M., Atkinson, K., et al. (1992) Second HLA-identical sibling transplants for leukemia recurrence. *Bone Marrow Transplantation*, **9**, 269–75.

Nimer, S.D., Giorgi, J., Gajewski, J.L., et al. (1994) Selective depletion of CD8[+] cells for prevention of graft-versus-host disease after bone marrow transplantation. A randomized controlled trial. *Transplantation*, **57**, 82–7.

Odom, L.F., August, C.S., Githens, J.H., et al. (1978) Remission of relapsed leukaemia during a graft-versus-host reaction. A "graft-versus-leukaemia reaction" in man? *Lancet*, **2**, 537–40.

Papadopoulos, E.B., Ladanyi, M., Emanuel, D., et al. (1994) Infusions of donor leukocytes to treat Epstein-Barr virus-associated lymphoproliferative disorders after allogeneic bone marrow transplantation. *New England Journal of Medicine*, **330**, 1185–91.

Porter, D. and Antin, J. (1995) Adoptive immunotherapy for relapsed leukemia following allogeneic bone marrow transplantation. *Leukemia and Lymphoma*, **17**, 191–7.

Porter, D., Orloff, G., and Antin, J. (1994a) Donor mononuclear cell infusions as therapy for B-cell lymphoproliferative disorder following allogeneic bone marrow transplant. *Transplant Science*, **4**, 11–5.

Porter, D.L., Roth, M.S., McGarigle, C., Ferrara, J.L., and Antin, J.H. (1994b) Induction of graft-versus-host disease as immunotherapy for relapsed chronic myeloid leukemia. *New England Journal of Medicine*, **330**, 100–6.

Porter, D.L., Roth, M.S., McGarigle, C., Ferrara, J.L., and Antin, J.H. (1994c) Induction of graft-vs-leukemia (GVL) reaction as therapy for relapsed leukemia after allogeneic bone marrow transplantation (BMT). *Journal of Cellular Biochemistry*, **18B**, 94a.

Radich, J.P., Sanders, J.E., Buckner, C.D., et al. (1993) Second allogeneic marrow transplantation for patients with recurrent leukemia after initial transplant with total-body irradiation-containing regimens. *Journal of Clinical Oncology*, **11**, 304–13.

Reittie, J.E., Gottlieb, D., Heslop, H.E., et al. (1989) Endogenously generated activated killer cells circulate after autologous and allogeneic marrow transplantation but not after chemotherapy. *Blood*, **73**, 1351–8.

Roth, M.S., Antin, J.H., Ash, R., et al. (1992) Prognostic significance of Philadelphia chromosome-positive cells detected by the polymerase chain reaction after allogeneic bone marrow transplant for chronic myelogenous leukemia. *Blood*, **79**, 276–82.

Shapiro, R.S., McClain, K., Frizzera, G., et al. (1988) Epstein-Barr virus associated B cell lymphoproliferative disorders following bone marrow transplantation. *Blood*, **71**, 1234–43.

Slavin, S., Weiss, L., Morecki, S., and Weigenberg, M. (1981) Eradication of murine leukemia with histoincompatible marrow grafts in mice conditioned with total lymphoid irradiation (TLI). *Cancer Immunology and Immunotherapy*, **11**, 155–9.

Slavin, S., Eckerstein, A., and Weiss, L. (1988) Adoptive immunotherapy in conjunction with bone marrow transplantation – amplification of natural host defence mechanisms against cancer by recombinant IL-2. *Natural Immunity Cell Growth Regulation*, **7**, 180–4.

Slavin, S., Ackerstein, A., Weiss, L., Nagler, A., Or, R., and Naparstek, E. (1992) Immunotherapy of minimal residual disease by immunocompetent lymphocytes and their activation by cytokines. *Cancer Investigation*, **10**, 221–7.

Soiffer, R.J., Murray, C., Mauch, P., et al. (1992) Prevention of graft-versus-host disease by selective depletion of CD6-positive T lymphocytes from donor bone marrow. *Journal of Clinical Oncology*, **10**, 1191–200.

Soiffer, R.J., Murray, C., Gonin, R., and Ritz, J. (1994) Effect of low-dose interleukin-2 on disease relapse after T-cell-depleted allogeneic bone marrow transplantation. *Blood*, **84**, 964–71.

Sosman, J.A., Oettel, K.R., Smith, S.D., Hank, J.A., Fisch, P., and Sondel, P.M. (1990) Specific recognition of human leukemic cells by allogeneic T cells: II. Evidence for HLA-D restricted determinants on leukemic cells that are crossreactive with determinants present on unrelated nonleukemic cells. *Blood*, **75**, 2005–16.

Sullivan, K.M., Deeg, H.J., Sanders, J., et al. (1986) Hyperacute graft-v-host disease in patients not given immunosuppression after allogeneic marrow transplantation. *Blood*, **67**, 1172–5.

Sullivan, K.M. and Shulman, H.M. (1989) Chronic graft-versus-host disease, obliterative bronchiolitis, and graft-versus-leukemia effect: case histories. *Transplantation Proceedings*, **21**, 51–62.

Sullivan, K.M., Storb, R., Buckner, C.D., et al. (1989a) Graft-versus-host disease as adoptive immunotherapy in patients with advanced hematologic neoplasms. *New England Journal of Medicine*, **320**, 828–34.

Sullivan, K.M., Storb, R., Witherspoon, R., et al. (1989b) Deletion of immunosuppressive prophylaxis after marrow transplantation increased hyperacute graft-versus-host disease but does influence chronic graft-versus-host disease or relapse in patients with advanced leukemia. *Clinical Transplants*, **3**, 5–11.

Sullivan, K.M., Weiden, P.L., Storb, R., et al. (1989c) Influence of acute and chronic graft-versus-host disease on relapse and survival after bone marrow transplantation from HLA-identical siblings as treatment of acute and chronic leukemia. *Blood*, **73**, 1720–8.

Sykes, M., Romick, M.L., and Sachs, D.H. (1990) Interleukin 2 prevents graft-versus-host disease while preserving the graft-versus-leukemia effect of allogeneic T cells. *Proceedings of the National Academy of Sciences of the United States of America*, **87**, 5633–7.

Sykes, M., Abraham, V.S., Harty, M.W., and Pearson, D.A. (1993) IL-2 reduces graft-versus-host disease and preserves a graft-versus-leukemia effect by selectively inhibiting CD4$^+$ T cell activity. *Journal of Immunology*, **150**, 197–205.

Sykes, M., Harty, M.W., Szot, G.L., and Pearson, D.A. (1994) Interleukin-2 inhibits graft-versus-host disease-promoting activity of CD4$^+$ cells while preserving CD4- and CD8-mediated graft-versus-leukemia effects. *Blood*, **83**, 2560–9.

Szer, J., Grigg, A.P., Phillips, G.L., and Sheridan, W.P. (1993) Donor leucocyte infusions after chemotherapy for patients relapsing with acute leukaemia following allogeneic BMT. *Bone Marrow Transplantation*, **11**, 109–11.

Truitt, R.L., Shih, C.Y., Lefever, A.V., Tempelis, L.D., Andreani, M., and Bortin, M.M. (1983) Characterization of alloimmunization-induced T lymphocytes reactive against AKR leukemia in vitro and correlation with graft-vs-leukemia activity in vivo. *Journal of Immunology*, **131**, 2050–8.

Truitt, R., LeFever, A., and Shih, C.-Y. (1987) Graft-versus-leukemia reactions: experimental models and clinical trials. In R.P. Gale and R. Champlin (Eds.) *Progress in bone marrow transplantation*. New York, Alan R. Liss.

Truitt, R., LeFever, A., Shih, C.Y., Jeske, J.M., and Martin, T.M. (1990) Graft-vs-leukemia effect. Graft-versus-host disease. In S.J. Burakoff, H.J. Deeg, J. Ferrarra, and K. Atkinson (Eds.) *Immunology, pathophysiology, and treatment*, pp. 177–204. New York, Marcel Dekker.

van Rhee, F., Cullis, J., Feng, L., Cross, N., and Goldman, J. (1993) Donor leukocyte transfusions (DLT) for relapse of chronic myeloid leukemia after allogeneic bone marrow transplant. *Blood*, **82**, 416a.

Verdonck, L.F., van Heugten, H.G., Giltay, J., and Franks, C.R. (1991) Amplification of the graft-versus-leukemia effect in man by interleukin-2. *Transplantation*, **51**, 1120–4.

Weiden, P.L., Flournoy, N., Thomas, E.D., et al. (1979) Antileukemic effect of graft-versus-host disease in human recipients of allogeneic-marrow grafts. *New England Journal of Medicine*, **300**, 1068–73.

Weiden, P.L., Sullivan, K.M., Flournoy, N., Storb, R., and Thomas, E.D. (1981) Antileukemic effect of chronic graft-versus-host disese: contribution to improved survival after allogeneic marrow transplantation. *New England Journal of Medicine*, **304**, 1529–33.

—Index—

Note: Page numbers in italics refer to tables and illustrations

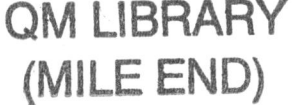